Neuromuscular Essentials

Applying the Preferred Physical Therapist Practice Patterns℠

Neuromuscular Essentials

Applying the Preferred Physical Therapist Practice Patterns ℠

Editor
Marilyn Moffat, PT, DPT, PhD, FAPTA, CSCS
Professor, Physical Therapy Department
New York University
New York, New York

Associate Editors

Joanell A. Bohmert, PT, MS
Itinerant Physical Therapist
Anoka-Hennepin Independent
School District No. 11
Anoka, Minnesota

Janice B. Hulme, PT, MS, DHSc
Clinical Assistant Professor
Doctor of Physical Therapy Program
University of Rhode Island
Kingston, Rhode Island

Assistant Editors

Elaine Rosen, PT, DHSc, OCS, FAAOMPT
Associate Professor
Hunter College Schools of the Health Professions
New York, New York
Partner
Queens Physical Therapy Associates
Forest Hills, New York

Sandra Rusnak-Smith, PT, DHSc, OCS
Partner
Queens Physical Therapy Associates
Forest Hills, New York

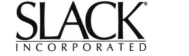

SLACK
INCORPORATED
Delivering the best in health care information and education worldwide

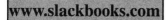

ISBN: 978-1-55642-669-8

The procedures and practices described in this book should be implemented in a manner consistent with the professional standards set for the circumstances that apply in each specific situation. Every effort has been made to confirm the accuracy of the information presented and to correctly relate generally accepted practices. The authors, editor, and publisher cannot accept responsibility for errors or exclusions or for the outcome of the material presented herein. There is no expressed or implied warranty of this book or information imparted by it. Care has been taken to ensure that drug selection and dosages are in accordance with currently accepted/recommended practice. Due to continuing research, changes in government policy and regulations, and various effects of drug reactions and interactions, it is recommended that the reader carefully review all materials and literature provided for each drug, especially those that are new or not frequently used. Any review or mention of specific companies or products is not intended as an endorsement by the author or publisher.

SLACK Incorporated uses a review process to evaluate submitted material. Prior to publication, educators or clinicians provide important feedback on the content that we publish. We welcome feedback on this work.

Published by: SLACK Incorporated
                 6900 Grove Road
                 Thorofare, NJ 08086 USA
                 Telephone: 856-848-1000
                 Fax: 856-848-6091
                 www.slackbooks.com

Some material contained in this book is reprinted with permission from the American Physical Therapy Association. *Guide to Physical Therapist Practice*. 2nd ed. Alexandria, VA: APTA; 2001 and appears courtesy of the APTA. For more information, please contact the APTA directly at www.apta.org.

Contact SLACK Incorporated for more information about other books in this field or about the availability of our books from distributors outside the United States.

Library of Congress Cataloging-in-Publication Data

Neuromuscular essentials : applying the preferred physical therapist practice patterns / editor, Marilyn Moffat ; associate editors, Joanell A. Bohmert ... [et al.].
       p. ; cm. -- (Essentials in physical therapy)
    Includes bibliographical references and index.
    ISBN-13: 978-1-55642-669-8 (alk. paper)
    ISBN-10: 1-55642-669-0 (alk. paper)
    1. Neuromuscular diseases--Physical therapy. 2. Neuromuscular diseases--Patients--Rehabilitation. I. Moffat, Marilyn. II. Bohmert, Joanell A., 1956- III. Series.
    [DNLM: 1. Neuromuscular Diseases--rehabilitation. 2. Physical Therapy Modalities--standards. 3. Case Reports. 4. Central Nervous System Diseases--rehabilitation. 5. Musculoskeletal Manipulations--methods. 6. Patient Care Planning. WE 550 N49445 2008]
    RC925.N445 2008
    616.7'44--dc22
                                          2008015204

Printed in the United States of America.

Last digit is print number: 10   9   8   7   6   5   4   3   2   1

Dedication

Undertaking a task of this magnitude is never possible without the utmost support of many individuals to whom I am deeply indebted. Thus this book is dedicated to: all of my Moffat and Salant families; physical therapy colleagues; APTA staff; faculty, support staff, and students at New York University; and all of my patients and clients who made this endeavor possible.

—*MM*

To Marilyn Woods, PT, a true generalist and servant leader.
Thank you for always seeking the right path for your patients and the profession.
Your memory and spirit will live on in all those you have inspired.

—*JAB*

This is dedicated to all of my patients past and current
who have pushed me to learn and develop my skills throughout the years.
Thank you for allowing me to share your experiences and wisdom.

—*JBH*

Contents

Acknowledgments

This edited book is one of a series of four books that would not have been possible without the dedication, incredibly hard work, and generosity of so many individuals. I am eternally indebted to each of the following outstanding physical therapists for their willingness to share their expertise, their enthusiasm, and their unbelievable patience in seeing this work come to fruition:

- ◆ Associate Editors:
  - Joanell A. Bohmert, PT, MS
  - Janice B. Hulme, PT, MS, DHSc
- ◆ Assistant Editors:
  - Elaine Rosen, PT, DHSc, OCS, FAAOMPT
  - Sandra Rusnak-Smith, PT, DHSc, OCS
- ◆ Contributing Authors:
  - Joanell A. Bohmert, PT, MS
  - Barbara H. Connolly, PT, DPT, EdD, FAPTA
  - Anne-Marie Dupre, PT, DPT, MS, NCS
  - Anne Gallentine, PT
  - Barbara Garrett, PT
  - Laura Gilchrist, PT, PhD
  - Janice B. Hulme, PT, MS, DHSc
  - Gary Krasilovsky, PT, PhD
  - Lisa Kuehn, PT
  - Tsega Andemicael Mehreteab, PT, MS, DPT
  - Patricia C. Montgomery, PT, PhD, FAPTA
  - Kirsten K. Ness, PT, PhD, GCS
  - Sue Sandvik, PT
  - Rose Wichmann, PT
  - Marilyn Woods, PT

The putting together of a book requires the astute skills of both editorial and publishing staff. Working with colleagues and associates at SLACK Incorporated has indeed been a pleasure, and I am indebted to them for their perceptive reviews and their continued encouragement provided along the way. To the following individuals I owe my thanks:

- ◆ Carrie Kotlar, who first approached me with the idea of doing this book and stood by throughout the process with unwavering support
- ◆ John Bond, who jumped in whenever we needed support from the top
- ◆ Jennifer Cahill and Kimberly Shigo, who had the editorial tasks of making our manuscripts into a published book

And last, but not least, are so many who have influenced my life, have challenged me to strive to do the best that I am able, and have supported and encouraged me along the way. My heartfelt thanks are extended to:

- ◆ My mother, for her unconditional support
- ◆ My father and my husband, who were always there for me, were both the epitome of role models, and were both taken from me too early in life
- ◆ My sister and brother-in-law, my stepdaughter, and my grandchildren for always reminding me of what is important in life

- All of my physical therapy colleagues, who have been such an integral part of my life
- The staff at the American Physical Therapy Association, who continually supported me throughout the years and who sometimes met unbelievable demands to see the *Guide* project reach the format it is today
- The faculty and support staff at New York University, my students, and my patients who have taught me so much and made me realize what insight and passion mean in realizing one's goals

Setting an example is not the main means of influencing others; it is the only means—Albert Einstein

—MM

I would like to thank all my many mentors that encouraged me to take risks and explore opportunities. I especially want to thank all the authors, many of whom stretched themselves to put in print their clinical expertise. Two individuals were always there for me, Marilyn Woods, PT, my longtime mentor and friend, and Laura Gilchrist, PT, PhD, my mentee who has become my colleague and friend. I would also like to thank my family, especially my son, Lucas, and my husband, Dave, for their support, encouragement, and faith.

—JAB

I have been and the readers will be the beneficiaries of the wisdom and generosity of all the contributors to this book. I would like to thank all of my colleagues at URI and RICLAS for their unending support and confidence in me. Susan Finn, OTR/L, MA, has been a tremendous source of encouragement, as well as editing and spellchecking assistance. I would also like to thank my children, Clare and Emma, for hanging in there through this "Is it ever going to be done?" project, and my husband, Rich, for supporting this endeavor and for making all those oodles of noodles.

—JBH

About the Editors

Marilyn Moffat, PT, DPT, PhD, FAPTA, CSCS, a recognized leader in the United States and internationally, is a practitioner, a teacher, a consultant, a leader, and an author. She received her baccalaureate degree from Queens College and her physical therapy certificate and PhD degrees from New York University. She is a Full Professor of Physical Therapy at New York University, where she directs both the professional doctoral program (DPT) and the post-professional graduate master's degree program in pathokinesiology. She has been in private practice for more than 40 years and currently practices in the New York area.

Dr. Moffat was one of the first individuals to speak and write about the need for a doctoral entry-level degree in physical therapy. Her first presentation on this topic was given to the Section for Education in 1977.

Dr. Moffat completed a 6-year term as the President of the American Physical Therapy Association (APTA) in 1997. Prior to that she had served on the APTA Board of Directors for 6 years and also as President of the New York Physical Therapy Association for 4 years. During her term as President of the APTA, she played a major role in the development of the Association's *Guide to Physical Therapist Practice* and was project editor of the Second Edition of the *Guide*. Among her many publications is the *American Physical Therapy Association's Book of Body Maintenance and Repair and Age-Defying Fitness*. As part of her commitment to research, Dr. Moffat is currently a member of the Board of Trustees of the Foundation for Physical Therapy, was a previous member of the Financial Advisory Committee, and has done major fundraising for them over the years.

She is currently President of the World Confederation for Physical Therapy (WCPT), and she was a member of the WCPT Task Force to develop an international definition of physical therapy. She coordinated the efforts to develop international guidelines for physical therapist educational programs around the world. She has given more than 800 professional presentations throughout her practice lifetime, and she has taught and provided consultation services in Taiwan, Thailand, Burma, Vietnam, Panama City, Hong Kong, Puerto Rico, Brazil, and Trinidad and Tobago.

Her diversified background is exemplified by the vast number of APTA and New York Physical Therapy Association committees and task forces on which she has served or chaired. She has served as Editor of *Physical Therapy*, the official publication of the Association. She was also instrumental in the early development of the TriAlliance of Rehabilitation Professionals, composed of the APTA, the American Occupational Therapy Association, and the American Speech-Language-Hearing Association. She has been an Associate of the Council of Public Representatives of the National Institutes of Health.

Dr. Moffat is a Catherine Worthingham Fellow of the APTA. She has been the recipient of APTA's Marilyn Moffat Leadership Award; the WCPT's Mildred Elson Award for International Leadership; the APTA's Lucy Blair Service Award; the Robert G. Dicus Private Practice Section APTA Award for contributions to private practice; Outstanding Service Awards from the New York Physical Therapy Association and from the APTA; the Ambassador Award from the National Strength and Conditioning Association; the Howard A. Rusk Humanitarian Award from the World Rehabilitation Fund; the United Cerebral Palsy Citation for Service; the Sawadi Skulkai Lecture Award from Mahidol University in Bangkok, Thailand; New York University's Founders Day Award; the University of Florida's Barbara C. White Lecture Award; the Massachusetts General's Ionta Lecture Award; the Chartered Society of Physiotherapist's Alan Walker Memorial Lecture Award; the APTA Minority Affairs Diversity 2000 Award; and the Section of Health Policy's R. Charles Harker Policy Maker Award. In addition, the New York Physical Therapy Association also named its leadership award after her. She was the APTA's 2004 Mary McMillan Lecturer, the Association's highest award. Dr. Moffat has been listed in *Who's Who in the East, Who's Who in American Women, Who's Who in America, Who's Who in Education, Who's Who in the World*, and *Who's Who in Medicine and Healthcare*.

She is also currently on the Board of Directors of the World Rehabilitation Fund and is a member of the Executive Committee. In addition to her professional associations, she was elected to be a member of Kappa Delta Pi and Pi Lambda Theta.

Dr. Moffat has served on a Citizen's Advisory Council of the New York State Assembly Task Force on the Disabled, has been a member of the State Board for Physical Therapy in New York, has served as a consultant to the New York City Police Department, and has been a member of the Boards of Trustees of Children's Village and the Four Oaks Foundation. The Nassau County Fine Arts Museum, the Howard A. Rusk Rehabilitation Medicine Campaign Committee, Saint John's Church of Lattingtown, and the Nassau County American Red Cross have been the recipients of her volunteer services.

Joanell A. Bohmert, PT, MS, received her BS degree and advanced MS degree from the University of Minnesota. She is a full-time clinician with Anoka-Hennepin School District in Anoka, Minnesota, with a focus of practice on pediatrics and neurology. She has practiced with pediatric and young adult patients and clients for 30 years incorporating the concepts of patient-centered evidence-based practice into patient management, clinical instruction, and clinical research.

Ms. Bohmert completed 7 years on the APTA's Board of Directors, serving 1 year as Vice-President. During her term on the Board she was also a member of the Board of Directors of the American Board of Physical Therapy Specialists (ABPTS) and the Foundation for Physical Therapy. She served as Chair of the Branding Task Force and the Task Force on the Future Role of the Physical Therapist Assistant. Prior to serving on the APTA Board of Directors, Ms. Bohmert served two terms as President of the Minnesota Chapter of the APTA. She was and continues to be actively involved in state legislative affairs, serving as issue expert for direct access.

Ms. Bohmert participated in the development and revision of the APTA's *Guide to Physical Therapist Practice*, Part One, Part Two, and Part Three (Catalog of Tests and Measures) and was a project editor for the Second Edition of the *Guide*. She has lectured extensively on the *Guide*, was a primary faculty for the APTA Guide to Physical Therapist Regional workshops, and was an APTA Trainer for the *Guide*. She participated in the development of the Hooked on Evidence Neuromuscular Clinical Scenarios for individuals with cerebral palsy. Ms. Bohmert has authored two chapters on Applying the Guide to Physical Therapist Practice and one chapter on Physical Therapy in the Educational Environment.

Ms. Bohmert is adjunct faculty for the University of Minnesota, Doctor of Physical Therapy Program, Minneapolis, Minnesota. She is a certified clinical instructor and center coordinator of clinical education for the four Minnesota DPT programs. She is faculty for the development and instruction for the Advanced Credentialed Clinical Instructor Program. She is a member of the Steering Committee and Bottom Line Committee for *Physical Therapy*, the official publication of the Association. Ms. Bohmert is a member of the Steering Committee for the Physical Therapy and Society Summit.

Ms. Bohmert was the recipient of APTA's State Legislative Leadership Award in 1999 and was recognized by the Minnesota Chapter of the APTA in 1999 with the chapter's highest award, the Corinne Ellingham Outstanding Service Award.

Janice B. Hulme, PT, MS, DHSc, received her physical therapy degree from the University of Connecticut in 1976 and an advanced master's degree with a clinical specialization in adult and pediatric neurology from Northeastern University in 1985. She went on to pursue a doctorate from the Institute of Physical Therapy in St. Augustine, Florida, where she studied the clinical application of motor control and motor learning research, graduating in 1999.

Dr. Hulme has specialized in the treatment of adults with neurological dysfunction for most of her career and has been certified by the NDT Association as a coordinator instructor in the treatment of adults with hemiplegia for 15 years. She has been an invited speaker at conferences and workshops throughout the United States and Hong Kong. Currently employed by the University of Rhode Island as a clinical assistant professor, she directs a collaborative program between the State of Rhode Island Department of Developmental Disabilities and the University of Rhode Island Program in Physical Therapy. She shares time teaching in the URI Program and, as the director of physical therapy, overseeing the provision of physical therapy services in 44 group homes.

A clinician at heart, Dr. Hulme has participated in a vast number of continuing education programs to develop expertise in the treatment of adults and children with neurological problems, the integration of motor learning and motor control in clinical practice, as well as the treatment of lymphedema and other women's health issues. She has assisted in research projects, received grant funding, and developed exercise, dancercise, aquatics, and injury prevention programs for people with developmental disabilities.

For more than 30 years, Dr. Hulme has been active in many professional and community service areas. Nationally, she has served on APTA Education Task Forces for curriculum and stroke practice. She has served the Rhode Island Chapter APTA as Treasurer, Finance Committee Chair, and as a member of the legislative, educational programs and professional practice committees. She served on the Rhode Island Board of Examiners in Physical Therapy for 6 years and has had long-term service on the American Heart Association Rehabilitation Committee of Operation Stroke and the Rhode Island Brain Injury Association. Community service activities have included physical therapy presentations in elementary schools; participation in Girl Scouts, Cultural Arts, and Academic Enrichment; and multiple PTA Executive Board positions. More recently, Dr. Hulme has spent time volunteering her professional services in Guatemala.

Dr. Hulme has received awards from the American Stroke Association, the Rhode Island Chapter of the APTA, Vocational Resources Inc, and the Rhode Island Rehabilitation Association for contributions to people with disabilities.

Contributing Authors

Joanell A. Bohmert, PT, MS
Itinerant Physical Therapist
Anoka-Hennepin Independent School District No. 11
Anoka, Minnesota

Barbara H. Connolly, PT, DPT, EdD, FAPTA
Professor and Chairman
Department of Physical Therapy
University of Tennessee Health Services Center
Memphis, Tennessee

Anne-Marie Dupre, PT, DPT, MS, NCS
Clinical Assistant Professor
Doctor of Physical Therapy Program
University of Rhode Island
Kingston, Rhode Island

Anne Gallentine, PT
Physical Therapy Supervisor
Park Nicollet Methodist Hospital
St. Louis Park, Minnesota

Barbara Garrett, PT
Senior Physical Therapist
Kessler Institute for Rehabilitation—
A Select Medical Company
West Orange, New Jersey

Laura Gilchrist, PT, PhD
Associate Professor
Doctor of Physical Therapy Program
College of St. Catherine
Clinical Research Scientist
Children's Hospitals and Clinics of Minnesota
Minneapolis, Minnesota

Janice B. Hulme, PT, MS, DHSc
Clinical Assistant Professor
Doctor of Physical Therapy Program
University of Rhode Island
Kingston, Rhode Island

Gary Krasilovsky, PT, PhD
Associate Professor and Director
Physical Therapy Program, Hunter College of CUNY
Co-Director, DPT Program, Graduate Center of CUNY
New York, New York

Lisa Kuehn, PT
Physical Therapist
Park Nicollet Methodist Hospital
St. Louis Park, Minnesota

Tsega Andemicael Mehreteab, PT, MS, DPT
Clinical Professor
Department of Physical Therapy
New York University
New York, New York

Patricia C. Montgomery, PT, PhD, FAPTA
President
Therapeutic Intervention Programs Inc
Hopkins, Minnesota

Kirsten K. Ness, PT, PhD, GCS
Assistant Member
Department of Epidemiology and Cancer Control
St. Jude Children's Research Hospital
Memphis, Tennessee

Sue Sandvik, PT
Senior Physical Therapist
Park Nicollet Methodist Hospital
St. Louis Park, Minnesota

Rose Wichmann, PT
Program Manager
Struthers Parkinson's Center
Minneapolis, Minnesota

Marilyn Woods, PT
Deceased
Rehabilitation Services—Outcome Management
Park Nicollet Methodist Hospital
St. Louis Park, Minnesota
Senior Physical Therapist
Struthers Parkinson's Center
Minneapolis, Minnesota

Preface

Neuromuscular Essentials: Applying the Preferred Physical Therapist Practice Patterns^{SM} is part of a series of four books (*Musculosketelal Essentials, Neuromuscular Essentials, Cardiovascular/Pulmonary Essentials,* and *Integumentary Essentials*) aimed at promoting an understanding of physical therapist practice and challenging the clinical thinking and decision making of our practitioners. In this book, 15 distinguished contributors have written chapters to take the *Guide to Physical Therapist Practice* to the next level of practice. Each chapter provides the relevant information for the pattern described by the *Guide* and emphasizes the process through which a physical therapist goes to take the patient from the examination to discharge. The Introduction to this book describes what each chapter contains.

It has been a goal of this entire series, and certainly is a strong hope of each of us involved in editing this series, that these *Essentials* will provide students and practitioners with a valuable reference for physical therapist practice.

As a way of introduction to the *Guide to Physical Therapist Practice*, the information below provides a brief overview of its development. Since I was involved in each step of the entire process, I know the unbelievable amount of work done by so many to see that landmark work reach fruition.

DEVELOPMENT OF THE *GUIDE*

The *Guide to Physical Therapist Practice* was developed based on the needs of membership by the American Physical Therapy Association (APTA) under my leadership as President of the Association. As an integral part of all of the groups responsible for writing the *Guide* and as one of three Project Editors for the latest edition of the *Guide*, I was delighted when SLACK Incorporated approached me to take the *Guide* to the next step for students and clinicians.

HISTORY

In the way of history, the development of the *Guide* began in 1992 with a Board of Directors-appointed task force upon which I served and which culminated in the publication of *A Guide to Physical Therapist Practice, Volume I: A Description of Patient Management* in the August 1995 issue of *Physical Therapy*. The APTA House of Delegates approved the development of Volume II, which was designed to describe the preferred patterns of practice for patient/client groupings commonly referred for physical therapy.

In 1997, Volume I and Volume II became Part One and Part Two of the *Guide*, and the first edition of the *Guide* was published in the November 1997 issue of *Physical Therapy*. In 1998, APTA initiated Parts Three and Four of the *Guide* to catalog the specific tests and measures used by physical therapists in the four system areas and the areas of outcomes, health-related quality of life, and patient/client satisfaction. Additional inclusions in the *Guide* were standardized documentation forms and templates that incorporated the patient/client management process and a patient/client satisfaction instrument.

A CD-ROM version of the *Guide* was developed that included not only Part One and Part Two, but also the varied tests and measures used in practice along with their reliability and validity.

FIVE ELEMENTS OF PATIENT/CLIENT MANAGEMENT

The patient/client management model includes the five essential elements of examination, evaluation, diagnosis, prognosis, and intervention that result in optimal outcomes. The patient/client management process is dynamic and allows the physical therapist to progress the patient/client in the process, return to an earlier element for further analysis, or exit the patient/client from the process when the needs of the patient/client cannot be addressed by the physical therapist. The patient/client management process incorporates the disablement model (pathology/pathophysiology, impairments, functional limitations) throughout the five elements and outcomes, but also includes all aspects of risk reduction/prevention; health, wellness, and fitness; societal resources; and patient/client satisfaction. This is the physical therapist's clinical decision-making model.

APPLICATION OF THE *GUIDE* TO CLINICAL PRACTICE

The *Guide* has its practice patterns grouped according to each of the four systems—musculoskeletal, neuromuscular, cardiovascular/pulmonary, and integumentary. Thus, this *Essentials* series continues where the *Guide* leaves off and brings the *Guide* to meaningful, clinically based examples of each of the patterns. In each chapter in each system area, an overview of the pertinent anatomy, physiology, pathophysiology, imaging, and pharmacology is presented; then one to seven cases are presented for each pattern. Each case initially details the physical therapist examination, including the history, systems review, and tests and measures selected for that case. Then the evaluation, diagnosis, and prognosis and plan of care for the case are presented. Prior to the specific interventions for the case is the rationale for the interventions based on the available literature, thus ensuring that, when possible, the interventions are evidence-based. The anticipated goals and expected outcomes for the interventions are put forth as possible in functional and measurable terms. Finally, any special considerations for reexamination, discharge, and psychological aspects are delineated.

Foreword
to the *Essentials in*
Physical Therapy Series

There are many leaders, many educators, and some visionaries, but only a very special few individuals have all three characteristics. The Editor of this series of books, Dr. Marilyn Moffat, certainly has demonstrated these traits and is again helping to guide the profession of physical therapy, as well as all therapists, to a new level of cognitive analysis when implementing and effectively using the *Guide to Physical Therapist Practice*.

Dr. Moffat's dream was for the American Physical Therapy Association to develop the original *Guide*. She nurtured its birth, as well as its development. In 2001, the second edition and evolution of additional practice patterns was introduced to the profession. Although the *Guide* lays the foundation for the entire diagnostic process used by a physical therapist as a movement specialist, many colleagues have difficulty bridging the gap between this model for the entire patient management process and its application to an individual consumer of physical therapy services. Through Dr. Moffat's vision, she recognized this gap and has again tried to link the highest standard of professional process to the patient/client and his or her specific needs.

When you take the leadership of the Editor and combine that with the expertise and clinical mastery of the various chapter authors, the quality of these texts already sets the highest standard of literary reference for an experienced, novel, or student physical therapist.

There are few individuals who could or would take on this dedicated process that will widen the therapist's comprehension of a very difficult and complex process. Dr. Moffat has again contributed, in her typical scholarly fashion, to the world of physical therapy literature and to each practitioner's role as a service provider of health care around the world.

—*Darcy Umphred, PT, PhD, FAPTA*
University of the Pacific
Stockton, California

Introduction

The chapters in *Neuromuscular Essentials* take the *Guide to Physical Therapist Practice*[1] to the next level and parallel the patterns in the *Guide*.

INTRODUCTORY INFORMATION

In each case, where appropriate, a review of the pertinent anatomy, physiology, pathophysiology, imaging, and pharmacology is provided as a means of background material.

PHYSICAL THERAPIST EXAMINATION

Each pattern details one to seven case studies appropriate to that pattern in *Guide* format. Thus, the case begins with the physical therapist examination, which is divided into the three parts of the examination—the history, the systems review, and the specific tests and measures selected for that particular case.

HISTORY

The history provides the first information that will be obtained from the patient/client. The history is a crucial first step in the clinical decision-making process as it enables the physical therapist to form an early hypothesis that helps guide the remainder of the clinical examination. The interview with the patient/client and a review of other available information provide the initial facts upon which further testing will be done to determine the concerns, goals, and eventual plan of care.

SYSTEMS REVIEW

After the history has been completed, the next aspect of the examination is the systems review, which is comprised of a quick screen of the four systems areas and a screen of the communication, affect, cognition, language, and learning style. The cardiovascular/pulmonary review includes assessment of blood pressure, edema, heart rate, and respiratory rate. The integumentary review includes assessing for the presence of any scar formation, the skin color, and the skin integrity. The musculoskeletal review includes assessment of gross range of motion, gross strength, gross symmetry, height, and weight. The neuromuscular review consists of an assessment of gross coordinated movements (eg, balance, locomotion, transfers, and transitions). The screen for communication, affect, cognition, language, and learning style includes an assessment of the patient's/client's ability to make needs known, consciousness, expected emotional/behavioral responses, learning preferences, and orientation.

TESTS AND MEASURES

The specific tests and measures to be selected for the patient/client are based upon the results found during the history taking and during the systems review. These latter two portions of the examination identify the clinical indicators for pathology/pathophysiology, impairments, functional limitations, disabilities, risk factors, prevention, and health, wellness, and fitness needs that will enable one to select the most appropriate tests and measures for the patient/client.

EVALUATION, DIAGNOSIS, AND PROGNOSIS AND PLAN OF CARE

The next step in the patient/client management model is evaluation. All of the data obtained from the examination (history, systems review, and tests and measures) are analyzed and synthesized to determine the diagnosis, prognosis, and plan of care for the patient/client. Then, once the evaluation has been completed and all data have been analyzed, the diagnosis for the patient/client and the pattern(s) into which the patient/client fits are determined.

After a review of the prognosis statement, of the expected range of number of visits per episode, and of the factors that may modify the frequency of visits for the pattern in the *Guide*, the prognosis is determined. Mutually established outcomes and the interventions for the patient/client are determined.

In each case the *Guide* has set the expected course of visits for the patient/client (see Expected Range of Number of Visits Per Episode of Care in each pattern in the *Guide*). This range should be appropriate for 80% of the population. Any additional impairment(s) found during the examination may or may not increase the number of expected visits. There are many factors that may modify the frequency or duration of visits. These may include: the patient's/client's adherence to the program set by the physical therapist, the type and amount of social support and caregiver expertise, the patient's/client's level of impairment, the patient's/client's health insurance plan, and the patient's/client's overall health status. Each patient/client must be looked at individually when determining the frequency and duration of visits.

INTERVENTIONS

Through all the information gathered in the examination and evaluation and with the diagnosis, prognosis, and plan of care in place, the specific interventions for this patient are selected. Whenever possible, interventions that have been shown to be effective through high-quality scientific research are utilized. At the end of all of the interventions is a composite section on anticipated goals and expected outcomes.

REEXAMINATION AND DISCHARGE

Reexamination will be performed throughout the episode of care, particularly as the setting of care changes. Discharge will occur when anticipated goals and expected outcomes have been attained.

PSYCHOLOGICAL ASPECTS

For each case, psychological aspects are important to consider when attempting to motivate patients/clients to comply with a long-range intervention program of exercise and functional training. Among these considerations for all patterns are:

♦ Behavior is governed by expectancies and incentives
♦ The likelihood that people adopt a health behavior depends on three perceptions:
  ● The perception that health is threatened
  ● The expectancy that their behavioral change will reduce the threat
  ● The expectancy that they are competent to change the behavior

It is necessary for physical therapists to understand reasons for noncompliance and formulate intervention plans accordingly. The number one indicator of future noncompliance is past poor compliance. Any psychological considerations beyond these in a particular case will be further detailed in that case.

PATIENT/CLIENT SATISFACTION

And finally for each case, the patient/client satisfaction with the physical therapy management would be determined by using the standard Patient/Client Satisfaction Questionnaire found in the back of the *Guide*.

REFERENCES

1. American Physical Therapy Association. Guide to physical therapist practice. 2nd ed. *Phys Ther.* 2001;81:9-744.

CHAPTER ONE

Primary Prevention/Risk Reduction for Loss of Balance and Falling (Pattern A)

Kirsten K. Ness, PT, PhD, GCS

INTRODUCTION

FALLING

A fall can be defined as the experience of unintentionally coming to rest on the ground, floor, or other lower level. Falls are the leading cause of death in persons older than age 70 years, and 5% to 10% of falls result in fractures and 15% in soft tissue injuries. Thirty percent of elderly who live in the community and 40% of nursing home residents fall each year.[1-25] Falls, or loss of balance control, are not isolated in one system but are the result of the integration of multiple systems of the person within a specific environment.

ANATOMY[26]

MUSCULOSKELETAL SYSTEM

The musculoskeletal requirements of balance control include normal bony alignment, adequate joint range of motion (ROM), and adequate strength.

Bone

The structural integrity of bone is important for posture and balance. Detailed macro- and microscopic anatomy on bone is covered in Musculoskeletal Pattern A: Primary Prevention/Risk Reduction for Skeletal Demineralization.

Joints

A joint is an articulation between two or more bones or parts of bones. Joints come in three types, defined by the type of material that unites the articulating bones. The three major joints of the lower extremity ([LE] hip, knee, and ankle) are synovial joints where the bones are joined by an articular capsule. This capsule encloses the joint cavity and provides a container for synovial fluid. Synovial joints also have articulating surfaces with bone ends that are covered with a protective articular cartilage. The hip, knee, and ankle joints are of particular interest for this practice pattern.

The hip is a freely moving ball-and-socket joint that forms the connection between the lower limb and the pelvic girdle. It is designed for both stability and movement. The round head of the femur articulates with the cup-like acetabulum, which is surrounded by the acetabular labrum to create stability. The head of the femur is covered with cartilage, except at the center, where the femoral ligament arises to provide a pathway for the artery that provides blood supply to the head of the femur. The fibrous joint capsule is comprised of strong ligaments that form a spiral connection between the pelvis and the femur.

The knee is a hinge joint that allows gliding, rolling, and rotation about a vertical access. It connects the distal femur to the proximal tibia and consists of lateral and medial articulations between the femoral condyles and the tibial plateau and an articulation between the femur and patella.

The stability of the knee joint is dependent on the strength of the surrounding muscles and their tendons and the ligaments that connect the femur and tibia.

The ankle joint is also a hinge-type joint formed by an articulation between the distal ends of the tibia and fibula and the pulley-shaped top of the talus (trochlea) and the medial surface of the talus. The tibia and fibula are joined posteriorly by the tibiofibular ligament to form a mortise to grip the talus of the ankle, thereby providing stability for weightbearing. The fibrous capsule of the ankle has strong medial and lateral collateral ligaments to add to the stability of the joint and is lined by loose synovial tissue that may extend superiorly as far as the interosseous ligament of the distal tibiofibular joint. The anatomy and physiology of joints are further detailed in Musculoskeletal Pattern F: Impaired Joint Mobility, Motor Function, Muscle Performance, Range of Motion, and Reflex Integrity Associated With Spinal Disorders and Musculoskeletal Pattern H: Impaired Joint Mobility, Motor Function, Muscle Performance, and Range of Motion Associated With Joint Arthroplasty.

Muscle

Skeletal muscles are called striated or voluntary muscles and are often named for their location in the body or their shapes. Muscles are attached to the skeleton and fascia of limbs, body wall, head, and neck. They are composed of large, long, unbranched, cylindrical fibers with transverse striation arranged in parallel bundles. They contain multiple peripherally located nuclei. The skeletal muscles of the neck, trunk, and LEs are particularly important for the control of balance. The anatomy and physiology of muscle are detailed in Musculoskeletal Pattern C: Impaired Muscle Performance.

NEUROMUSCULAR SYSTEM

Sensory Receptors

In order to utilize the appropriate musculoskeletal response to achieve balance, individuals must have an awareness of the location of their center of gravity in space. They must be able to sense and select the most appropriate motor response. The sensory receptors that provide information for balance control are located in the visual, somatosensory, and vestibular systems.

Visual System

Balance-related visual information is detected in the retina and delivered to two specialized locations in the brain, one specialized for object identification (focal system) and the other specialized for movement control (ambient system).[27] The focal system is related to central vision, and the eye processes this vision primarily through the macula of the retina. Central vision is responsible for the clarity of vision and at what one is looking. The ambient visual system provides

information via nerve fibers from the peripheral portion of the retina to the midbrain about where the body is located in space and where the individual is looking. Therefore, this system contributes to balance and coordination.

Somatosensory System

Information about the body's position is also provided by the somatosensory system. This system is comprised of multiple types of sensation from the body to ascending pathways to the postcentral gyrus in the cerebral cortex. The system is divided into three pathways that are for:

1. Pain and temperature (including sensations of warm or cold)

2. Discriminative touch (including sensations of touch, pressure, vibration, tickling, and itch)

3. Proprioception (including sensations of joint position, muscle movement, and posture)

Cutaneous touch-pressure receptors are located in the skin and subcutaneous tissue of the sole of the foot and provide important sensory input. These touch receptors include Meissner endings and Merkels discs, which are located near the surface of the skin, and Ruffini endings and Pacinian corpuscles, which are located deeper in the skin. Proprioceptive receptors are found in muscles, tendons, and joints, and they detect information about the position of the limbs and body and about muscle length and tension. Proprioceptors include muscle spindles, types I and II; Golgi tendon organs; and joint receptors.[28,29]

Vestibular System

Vestibular inputs also relay important information to the central nervous system (CNS) about the body's position, both at rest and during movement. The receptors of the vestibular system are located in the inner ear and include the semicircular canals that sense velocity changes of movement and the otoliths that provide information about linear acceleration. Vestibular inputs are received primarily by the vestibular nuclei, located in the brainstem.[30-33] The vestibular system is further detailed in Pattern F: Impaired Peripheral Nerve Integrity and Muscle Performance Associated With Peripheral Nerve Injury.

Central Nervous System

Information from the sensory systems is transferred to the CNS (ie, the spinal cord and brain) via afferent pathways, where it is relayed and coordinated to produce appropriate efferent motor outputs to maintain or restore balance. The spinal cord, basal ganglia, cerebellum, thalamus, and multiple areas of the cortex all receive and relay information to produce appropriate motor output.[34] The anatomy and physiology of the CNS is further detailed in Pattern C: Impaired Motor Function and Sensory Integrity Associated With Nonprogressive Disorders of the Central Nervous System—Congenital Origin or Acquired in Infancy or

Childhood and Pattern D: Impaired Motor Function and Sensory Integrity Associated With Nonprogressive Disorders of the Central Nervous System—Acquired in Adolescence or Adult.

PHYSIOLOGY

Sensory receptors convert energy of various forms, such as light, pressure, temperature, and sound, into neuronal signals that travel to the spinal cord and brain where they are processed to determine a response. These processes occur in milliseconds since maintaining an upright position requires rapid processes to select accurate inputs and ignore inaccurate inputs. Persons frequently rely on visual and somatosensory inputs, however, visual and somatosensory inputs are frequently wrong.[35]

Vision influences balance by recording and transmitting information related to an image shift on the retina, resulting in a trigger that stimulates muscle action for postural correction. Visual perception is dependent on visual acuity, visual contrast, object distances, and room illumination. Visual distances less than 2 meters are optimal for balance control.[27]

Receptors in the joint capsules give information about movements and the positions of body parts relative to each other. The receptors in the ankle joints are particularly important, because they sense the torque created about the ankle joint as the body's center of gravity shifts. Muscle spindles provide dynamic afferent signals to the CNS about muscle length and tension or can be activated by a passive stretch of the muscle. Muscle spindles also receive efferent information to their intrafusal component via the alpha motor neuron to maintain tension or set. Neck muscles provide input about the position of the head, and eye muscles provide information about the position of the eyes relative to the head. Pressoreceptors detect body sway. Mechanoreceptors detect the site and depth of skin indentations, accelerations, and pressure changes.[28,29]

The semicircular canals are active at the beginning and the end of movement and are sensitive to velocity changes in the range of 0.2 to 10 Hertz. The otoliths operate at lower frequencies of less than 5 Hertz and provide information about linear acceleration, including gravity. Information from these sensors in the inner ear is transmitted to the vestibular nuclei located in the brainstem, which also receives information from other sensory sources. Coordinated outputs from the vestibular nuclei stabilize vision by stimulating eye movements in the opposite direction of head movements (vestibulo-ocular reflex) and regulate the position of the head on the body (vestibulo-spinal reflex).[30-33]

Input signals about the body's position in space from the sensory systems are relayed to the cortex mostly through the thalamic nuclei, where peripheral input from the spinal cord, basal ganglia, cerebellum, and frontal and parietal lobes are gathered and integrated. The first and fastest responses to a balance challenge occur at the level of the spinal cord and are involuntary. Excitatory afferent synapses between neurons and inhibitory synapses via interneurons mediate nervous system responses. Voluntary responses to postural perturbation are planned within the brain and sent to the muscles via the pyramidal and extrapyramidal systems.[34]

POSTURAL CONTROL[36,37]

Balance is a complex motor control task, requiring the integration of sensory information, neural processing, and biomechanical factors. The control of balance requires an individual to, usually unconsciously, call on postural strategies to keep or restore the body's center of gravity to within the limits of stability, which is the maximum angle from vertical that can be tolerated without either a step, stumble, or fall. A person maintaining equilibrium while standing still will cycle forward and backward approximately 12 degrees and from side to side approximately 16 degrees within a sway envelope. This natural sway functions to align the center of gravity over the base of support and prevent movement outside of the limits of stability. During upright standing, the center of gravity is located in the area of the lower abdomen, with the exact position dependent on the configuration of the body joints at a given time. There are three joints between the center of gravity and the support base during standing: the hip, the knee, and the ankle. Theoretically, the body can assume a variety of positions to keep or return the center of gravity to a position within the limits of stability. Corrective movements are needed to keep the center of gravity within the base of support. To achieve this goal, coordination of the sensory, skeletal muscle, and nervous systems is needed.

Postural strategies are forms or shapes of the body, determined by joint angles that keep or restore the center of gravity to a position within the limits of stability. Postural strategies are both voluntary and automatic. Voluntary postural strategies are diverse and vary between persons as they move to adjust their center of gravity. For example, the knees might bend, the trunk flex, and the arms extend outward as a person searches for postural security. In contrast, automatic postural strategies to control anterior-posterior sway are usually limited to three strategies:

1. The ankle strategy

2. The hip strategy

3. The stepping strategy

The ankle strategy works when the center of gravity is aligned or centered within the limits of stability or when body sway movements are relatively slow (0.3 Hertz). During forward sway, ordered muscular contractions of the gastrocsoleus, hamstrings, and paraspinal muscles gently pull the center of gravity back into the sway envelope. During backward sway, coordinated muscular contractions of the tibialis anterior, quadriceps, and abdominals pull the center of gravity forward into the sway envelope.

The hip strategy is called upon during high frequency sway conditions or when the dimensions of the sway envelope are reduced. The hip strategy produces corrections within the reduced sway envelope during a forward sway with strong contractions of the abdominal and quadriceps muscles. Correction during backward sway requires the coordinated efforts of the paraspinal and hamstring muscles.

The stepping strategy occurs when the center of mass is moved outside of the limits of stability, and a step is required to maintain balance.

These processes occur in the physiological and structural environment of the human body and are controlled by the autonomic nervous system. The ability to maintain the upright position and to superimpose movement for ambulation and daily tasks is dependent on intact sensory, nervous, and musculoskeletal systems and is influenced by disorders in the cardiovascular/pulmonary, gastrointestinal, endocrine, or genitourinary systems.

PATHOPHYSIOLOGY[38,39]

Both aging and disease have effects on the many body systems that regulate or are involved with balance. Reductions in muscle mass and a corresponding loss of muscle strength can impact the effectiveness of the muscle response to balance perturbations. Muscle mass decreases with aging by 25% to 43%, particularly in the LEs. Atrophy of both type 1 (slow twitch) and type 2 (fast twitch) muscle fibers has been reported. Joint contractures, osteoarthritis, osteoporosis, and foot deformity may also interfere with effective balance responses. Bones and joints that are not aligned normally may interfere with appropriate muscular responses.

Inaccurate or reduced sensory inputs may also interfere with normal balance responses. Visual acuity declines with age and/or disease. Older adults have more difficulty with color perception, light/dark adaptation, near/far adaptation, and glare. In addition, the amount of light entering their eyes is diminished, peripheral vision is less sensitive, and limitations in neck ROM may decrease ability to see cues above the level of the head. Disease states that may affect vision include cataracts that cloud the lens, glaucoma that limits peripheral vision, and macular degeneration that results in the gradual decay of the portion of the retina that focuses on an image. Visual perception is also decreased or altered in disease states that cause nerve cell damage within the brain like stroke or traumatic brain injury (TBI). Injury to the vestibular system may also interfere with balance. Normal proprioception allows detection of movement of less than 5 mm at the great toe. Conditions like diabetes, peripheral vascular disease, lumbar myelopathy, and neurodegenerative disorders may all result in a loss of peripheral sensation and interfere with afferent input into the CNS.

Autonomic regulation, CNS disorders, and systemic problems may also impact balance responses. Rapid changes in blood pressure (BP) or reduced sensitivity of the baroreceptors to pressure changes when moving from one position to another may result in a decrease in blood supply to the brain and lightheadedness upon standing. Sedation related to medication use, acute confusion, seizures, cerebral hypoprofusion, dementia, or disorders like Parkinson's disease may all impact the ability of the CNS to accurately process and effectively respond to postural disturbances. Infection, anemia, dehydration, and incontinence may redirect the resource of the body to other tasks and prevent effective responses of the CNS to maintaining the upright position.

Postural instability is reflected as increased body sway, decreased responsiveness of sensory receptors that alert the muscles to contract when movement is away from the center of gravity, slowed reaction time, and increased reliance on visual and proprioceptive input.[40,41] Gait changes are also evident. Step height is decreased and the base of support either widens or narrows. The person with postural instability may shuffle his or her feet and walk very slowly.

IMAGING

Imaging techniques relevant to this practice pattern are dependent on the underlying pathology or organ system impairments that lead to the physical therapy referral. For imaging techniques related to:

- Bone structure, please refer to Musculoskeletal Pattern A: Primary Prevention/Risk Reduction for Skeletal Demineralization and Musculoskeletal Pattern G: Impaired Joint Mobility, Muscle Performance, and Range of Motion Associated With Fracture

- Joint and soft tissue structure, please refer to Musculoskeletal Pattern I: Impaired Joint Mobility, Motor Function, Muscle Performance, and Range of Motion Associated With Bony or Soft Tissue Surgery

- CNS structure, please refer to Pattern C: Impaired Motor Function and Sensory Integrity Associated With Nonprogressive Disorders of the Central Nervous System—Congenital Origin or Acquired in Infancy or Childhood and Pattern D: Impaired Motor Function and Sensory Integrity Associated With Nonprogressive Disorders of the Central Nervous System—Acquired in Adolescence or Adulthood

PHARMACOLOGY

Although no specific medications are designed to prevent falls, physical therapists who treat clients in this practice pattern should consider the side effects and interactions of each medication that is likely being used for another medical problem. Frequent side effects of many medications are dizziness and sedation; both can have a profound impact on maintaining the upright position. Among those drugs that may be used for sedation or that may result in dizziness, the biggest culprits are:

♦ Analgesics (eg, Ultracet, Darvocet, Percocet, morphine sulfate [Astramorph, Duramorph, Infumorph], oxycodone [Darvon, Dilaudid, Hydrostat IR, OxyContin, Roxanol])

♦ Beta-blockers (eg, atenolol [Tenormin], metoprolol [Lopressor, Toprol XL])

♦ Diuretics (eg, Furosemide [Lasix])

♦ Dopamine replacement (eg, levodopa/carbidopa [Sinemet or Atamet], dopamine agonists including bromocriptine [Parlodel], pergolide [Permax], pramipexole [Mirapex], ropinirole [Requip], apomorphine [Apokyn])

♦ Psychotropic medications (eg, Valium [diazepam], Ativan [lorazepam])

♦ Sedatives (eg, amitriptyline)

Case Study #1: Fear of Falls

Ms. Jackson is an 81-year-old female with a recent history of a fall and hypertension and a bladder infection. She continues to have fears of falling.

PHYSICAL THERAPIST EXAMINATION

HISTORY

♦ General demographics: Ms. Jackson is an 81-year-old black female whose primary language is English. She is right-hand dominant. She is a high school graduate.

♦ Social history: Ms. Jackson is a widow. Her husband died 10 years ago. She is a mother of three sons and two daughters, aged 55 to 61 years, and has multiple grandchildren and great-grandchildren.

♦ Employment/work: Ms. Jackson is a retired university secretary. She worked for a famous transplant surgeon for 47 years. She has been retired for 16 years, but provides frequent babysitting support for two of her 11 great-grandchildren. She is afraid she is "getting too old." She reports tripping over a toy and falling last year while taking care of her great-grandchildren.

♦ Living environment: Ms. Jackson lives in a two-story home. There are three steps to enter with a rail on either side. Her bedroom is on the second floor of the house. The stairs have a hand rail on the right side. There is a small bathroom with only a sink and toilet on the main level. The bathroom with the bathtub is on the second floor. The bathtub currently is equipped with a dual level tub rail.

♦ General health status
  • General health perception: Ms. Jackson reports her health status to have deteriorated some over the past year. She occasionally feels dizzy and is very tired at the end of prolonged outings.
  • Physical function: Ms. Jackson has started to use a cane when she leaves the house because she feels unsteady on her feet.
  • Psychological function: Ms. Jackson reports being afraid of falling and wants to do something about it.
  • Role function: Mother, grandmother, great-grandmother, friend to neighbor who is also a widow.
  • Social function: Ms. Jackson is involved in after-school care of two of her great-grandchildren and in a senior group at her church. She enjoys listening to music, spending time with friends and family, and helping "the kids" with homework.

♦ Social/health habits: Ms. Jackson does not smoke or consume alcohol. She limits the salt in her diet.

♦ Family history: Her father died from complications of diabetes, and her mother died soon after having a stroke.

♦ Medical/surgical history: Ms. Jackson has hypertension (HTN) that has been managed with medication for 30 years. She has had one fall in the past year that resulted in a gash on her forehead requiring 12 stitches. She has had occasional low back pain over the years, relieved by nonsteroidal anti-inflammatory drugs (NSAIDs). She had a hysterectomy and bladder repair at age 72 with excellent recovery. Her last menstrual period was at age 52. She has also had a history of elevated cholesterol that is now controlled with medication.

♦ Prior hospitalizations: Ms. Jackson was hospitalized for the birth of her last three children, a hysterectomy and bladder repair, overnight for a fall 8 months ago, and for 2 days 3 months ago with a high fever and urinary tract infection.

♦ Preexisting medical and other health-related conditions: Ms. Jackson has a history of HTN, has had one fall in the past year, and had a recent bladder infection.

♦ Current condition(s)/chief complaint(s): Ms. Jackson is afraid she might fall again. She participated in a screening event at her church that reported her score to be 30 out of 56 on the Berg Balance Test (scores below 45 indicate at risk for falls).[42] The physical therapist from the health fair suggested that she consult with a physical therapist to prevent further falls.

♦ Functional status and activity level: She is independent in her activities of daily living (ADL) but reports having increasing difficulty getting in and out of the bathtub. She prepares her own meals and does her own laundry. She is still able to climb the flight of stairs to the second floor with the aid of the hand rail. Her children assist her with yard work, heavy housework, and grocery shopping. She does not drive.

♦ Medications: Ms. Jackson takes Diuril 0.5 g and Cardizem CD 120 mg for HTN, Mevacor 10 mg for her cholesterol, and 500 mg of calcium, 80 mg aspirin, and a multivitamin each once per day in the morning.

♦ Other clinical tests: Ms. Jackson had a DEXA scan during her hospitalization for the fall. Her t score was -0.8 SD at the femoral neck and -1.0 SD at the lumbar spine, indicating mild low bone mass that is not unexpected for her age.

SYSTEMS REVIEW

♦ Cardiovascular/pulmonary
  ● BP: 120/72 mmHg in supine, initial drop to 100/62 mmHg sitting, 130/84 mmHg after 5 minutes in sitting
  ● Edema: Observation and palpation revealed edema in both LEs
  ● Heart rate (HR): 71 bpm
  ● Respiratory rate (RR): 19 bpm

♦ Integumentary
  ● Presence of scar formation: 2-inch scar, which is well healed, on the left side of her forehead from her fall
  ● Skin color: Darker appearing skin on gaiter areas of legs (the lower half above and around the ankles)
  ● Skin integrity: Intact but shiny, thin, and hairless on lower legs

♦ Musculoskeletal
  ● Gross range of motion: Able to lift arms through 60% of overhead ROM and fully extend knees; can only dorsiflex ankles to neutral bilaterally and does not fully extend hips in standing
  ● Gross strength: Decreased overall
  ● Gross symmetry: Symmetrical movement
  ● Height: 5'4" (1.63 m)
  ● Weight: 155 lbs (70.31 kg)

♦ Neuromuscular
  ● Balance: Unsteady, requires cane or object to support standing
  ● Locomotion, transfers, and transitions: Uses a cane to walk in open spaces, walls or furniture if available; uses hands to pull or push when moving from sit to stand

♦ Communication, affect, cognition, language, and learning style
  ● Communication, affect, cognition: Within normal limits (WNL)
  ● Learning style: Prefers pictures with written directions

TESTS AND MEASURES

♦ Aerobic capacity/endurance
  ● 6-minute corridor walk test revealed a walking distance of 150 meters using a single-end cane and stand-by assist of one
  ● Ms. Jackson stopped frequently to survey surroundings
  ● Her HR was 138 bpm at the end of the walk
  ● Walking distance was shorter than expected for her age and gender[43]

♦ Anthropometric characteristics
  ● Edema: 1+ in both LEs
  ● Body mass index: 26.6 indicates that she is overweight

♦ Arousal, attention, and cognition
  ● Alert and oriented x3
  ● Score 27 on Mini Mental Status Exam (MMSE), which is slightly above normal for her age[44-47]

♦ Assistive and adaptive devices
  ● Uses a single-end cane correctly during ambulation in open spaces, however, uses furniture or walls rather than her cane to maintain balance in closer environments

♦ Cranial and peripheral nerve integrity
  ● No complaints of numbness or tingling
  ● LE sensation intact to light touch
  ● Protective sensation intact at five points on plantar surface of foot to 10 g Semmes-Weinstein monofilament[48]

♦ Environmental, home, and work barriers
  ● Has no working lighting above stairway, no night light in bedroom or bathroom, and multiple throw rugs in kitchen, bathrooms, and entryway[49]
  ● Has dual level grab bar over edge of bathtub
  ● Has lift recliner given to her by children for Christmas 1 year ago[50]

♦ Ergonomics and body mechanics
  ● Uses the end of her cane to pull objects to her
  ● Reports difficulty picking items up off of the floor

♦ Gait, locomotion, and balance
  ● Ambulates with her single-end cane in the left hand using a three-point gait (cane, right foot, left foot) in open spaces with her trunk flexed forward and her

gaze concentrated on her feet

- Stops frequently while walking to look up and survey the environment
- Is unable to look up or to the side when walking without stopping
- Carries on a constant conversation while walking[51]
- Although stops frequently to be sure of balance, no shortness of breath noted
- When in a close environment, uses furniture or the wall for support
- Required 13 seconds to perform the Timed Up and Go,[43] normal for females her age is 11 seconds
- The combined findings on the sensory organization testing (see previous under Cranial and Peripheral Nerve Integrity), a score of 30/56 on the Berg Balance Test[42] at a health fair (see History, Current Condition[s]/Chief Complaint[s]), and a fear of falling[52] all indicate high risk for falls

♦ Motor function
- Has difficulty coordinating observation of environment with movement when upright
- Dexterity and coordination when stability supported (in sitting) WNL

♦ Muscle performance
- Manual muscle testing/dynamometry[53]
  - Gross shoulder motions: 3-/5 R, 3-/5 L
  - Elbow flexion and extension: 3+/5 R, 3+/5 L
  - Hand grip: 22 kg R, 20 kg L
  - Hip flexion (supine): 3-/5 R, 3/5 L
  - Hip extension (side lying): 2/5 R, 2/5 L
  - Hip abduction (side lying): 3/5 R, 3/5 L
  - Hip adduction (side lying): 3-/5 R, 3-/5 L
  - Knee extension (sitting): 3+/5 R, 3+/5 L
  - Knee flexion (standing): 3+/5 R, 3+/5 L
  - Plantarflexion (standing): 3/5 bilaterally (clears heel from floor)
  - Dorsiflexion (sitting): 2/5 bilaterally (cannot move through full ROM)
  - Trunk flexion (supine): 2/5 (flexes cervical spine off of table)
  - Trunk extension (standing): 2-/5 (stands with trunk flexed forward, cannot fully extend)
- Power during activities
  - 22 seconds required for Five Times Sit to Stand[54]: Uses arms to push up for each stand; time above 15 seconds or use of arms is considered at risk for falls

♦ Orthotic, protective, and supportive devices
- Uses a cane for ambulation

♦ Posture
- Observational and grid photographs with client

standing revealed:
- Neck in 30 degrees of cervical flexion
- Trunk flexed forward 20 degrees at the hips
- Scapulae slightly abducted
- Knees locked in extension

♦ Range of motion[55]
- Functional ROM
  - Cervical ROM: WNL except for extension only available to neutral
  - Upper extremity (UE) active range of motion (AROM)
    ▶ Not available through full range, but is functional
    ▶ Can brush hair, put a plate in the cupboard, and fasten her bra
  - UE passive range of motion (PROM)
    ▶ 90% of normal
    ▶ Limitations only in shoulder flexion (160 degrees R, 158 degrees L), abduction (155 degrees R, 150 degrees L), and external rotation (75 degrees bilaterally)
- LE AROM and PROM are presented in Table 1-1

♦ Reflex integrity: WNL

♦ Self-care and home management
- Reported increased difficulty with bathing due to difficulty getting in and out of tub
- Still independent with self-care, cooking, and laundry
- Children assist with housework and yard work
- Functional Status Index (FSI) provides a continuous measure of self-reported need for assistance, pain, and difficulty and consists of the performance of 10 items in the three areas of gross mobility, hand activities, and personal care rated on four-point scale from 1=no pain to 4=severe pain (minimum score is 10 and maximum score is 40)[56,57]
  - Scores were 33 for assistance, 18 for pain, and 34 for difficulty

♦ Sensory integrity
- Vision: Wears "cheaters" for presbyopia, no history of cataracts or glaucoma
- Hearing: Intact to normal conversation with background noise in room
- Demonstrates significantly increased postural sway on firm surface, eyes closed condition, and requires postural support in all conditions while standing on foam on Clinical Test of Sensory Interaction on Balance (CTSIB)[48]
- Incorrect visual information (dome) did not significantly alter sway, although client requested contact guard during test yielding inconclusive test results

	Table 1-1			
	LOWER EXTREMITY ACTIVE AND PASSIVE RANGE OF MOTION			
Motion	**Active**		**Passive**	
	Right	**Left**	**Right**	**Left**
Hip flexion	97 degrees	95 degrees	112 degrees	110 degrees
Hip extension	-10 degrees	-15 degrees	-8 degrees	-10 degrees
Hip abduction	25 degrees	20 degrees	30 degrees	25 degrees
Hip adduction	10 degrees	8 degrees	17 degrees	15 degrees
Hip external rotation (sitting: hip and knee flexed)	22 degrees	20 degrees	30 degrees	28 degrees
Hip internal rotation (sitting: hip and knee flexed)	24 degrees	20 degrees	28 degrees	25 degrees
Knee flexion	95 degrees	98 degrees	110 degrees	114 degrees
Knee extension	0 degrees	0 degrees	0 degrees	0 degrees
Plantarflexion	15 degrees	12 degrees	25 degrees	23 degrees
Dorsiflexion	-3 degrees	-5 degrees	2 degrees	0 degrees
Inversion	5 degrees	5 degrees	5 degrees	5 degrees
Eversion	0 degrees	0 degrees	5 degrees	5 degrees

◆ Work, community, and leisure integration or reintegration
  • Reports fear of falling when out in the community and increased difficulty with providing care for great-grandchildren[58]
  • Reports that she doesn't drive and doesn't walk well enough to take the bus anymore

EVALUATION

Ms. Jackson is an 81-year-old female with a medical diagnosis of HTN and a recent history of a fall and a bladder infection. Her interview revealed increased fear of falling and a pattern of progressive functional limitations in locomotion, ADL, and instrumental activities of daily living (IADL). The client is concerned about her inability to fully participate in her desired life roles. Her physical therapy examination revealed mild LE edema, symptoms of orthostatic hypotension (OH) evidenced by difficulty maintaining BP when moving from supine to sitting, and limitations in AROM and PROM with the biggest deficits in ankle dorsiflexion. Ms. Jackson has significant muscle weakness in the trunk

and LEs. She has adopted a single-end cane and uses it outside and uses furniture or walls inside to help her maintain upright. Her sensation and vestibular function remain intact; however, she relies on visual information for balance control. Her ROM losses, strength impairments, fear of falling, and several environmental barriers in her home (lack of lighting, multiple throw rugs) reduce her ability to transfer or ambulate safely in her home or the community. Ms. Jackson is a client at risk for falls.

DIAGNOSIS

Ms. Jackson is a client who is at risk for loss of balance and falls, has HTN, has symptoms of OH, had a recent history of a fall, and had a bladder infection. She has impaired: aerobic capacity/endurance; anthropometric characteristics; ergonomics and body mechanics; gait, locomotion, and balance; motor function; muscle performance; posture; range of motion; and sensory integrity. She has functional limitations in self-care and home management and in work, community, and leisure actions, tasks, and activities. She has home barriers. These findings are consistent with placement in Pattern A: Primary Prevention/Risk Reduction for Loss of

Balance and Falling. The identified impairments, functional limitations, and barriers will be addressed in determining the prognosis and the plan of care.

PROGNOSIS AND PLAN OF CARE

Over the course of the visits, the following mutually established outcomes have been determined:

♦ Ability to perform physical activities related to self-care, home management, work, community, and leisure is improved with improved body mechanics

♦ Aerobic capacity and endurance are improved

♦ Balance is improved

♦ Fitness is improved

♦ Knowledge of behaviors that foster healthy habits, wellness, and prevention is increased

♦ Muscle performance is increased

♦ Physical capacity is improved

♦ Postural control is improved

♦ Risk factors (decreased physical activity, balance, ROM, muscle performance) are reduced

♦ ROM is increased

♦ Sensory integrity is improved

To achieve these outcomes, the appropriate interventions for this client are determined. These will include: coordination, communication, and documentation; patient/client-related instruction; therapeutic exercise; functional training in self-care and home management; functional training in work, community, and leisure integration or reintegration; and prescription, application, and, as appropriate, fabrication of devices and equipment.

Because of her age, fall history, and extreme deconditioning, it is anticipated that Ms. Jackson will have nine visits over the first 3 weeks. Visit frequency will taper off as she becomes accustomed to exercise and as her strength and mobility increase. Weekly phone calls to encourage exercise will begin when the clinic visit is decreased to one time.

INTERVENTIONS

RATIONALE FOR SELECTED INTERVENTIONS

In 2003, the Centers for Medicare and Medicaid Services (CMS) sponsored a Rand Report[59] to evaluate the effectiveness of fall prevention strategies for older adults. Conclusions of this systematic review of the literature included several recommendations with implications that make them applicable to interventions provided for primary prevention/risk reduction for loss of balance and falls. Successful use of an evidence-based falls prevention and exercise program will improve health and reduce fall-related injuries in older adults. Evidence indicates that in addition to the actual exercise, this program should include a baseline risk assessment so that the intervention can be tailored to modify individual risk factors other than strength, balance, and endurance that contribute to falls among older adults. The program and exercises should be tailored to the individual.

Therapeutic Exercise

Risk Reduction Program for Falls

For Ms. Jackson, an individualized exercise program supervised by a physical therapist based on the work of Campbell and associates,[60] which was cited as an exercise-based fall prevention intervention in the Rand Report,[59] is selected. The original intervention was reviewed and a baseline program determined based on the original program description outlined in their 1997 publication in the *British Medical Journal*.[61] Briefly, this intervention included:

♦ Screening for participation by a health care provider: Ms. Jackson was screened at a church-based health fair by a physical therapist

♦ Baseline assessment of impairments and functional limitations by a physical therapist: Ms. Jackson has completed her examination

♦ Exercise prescription by a physical therapist involves selection of strengthening, balance, and mobility exercises from the program at appropriate and increasing levels of difficulty and a walking program: Ms. Jackson to receive prescription

♦ Exercise instruction includes frequency and provision of an illustrated instruction book: Ms. Jackson to receive exercise program that includes these elements

♦ Regular telephone contact by the physical therapist to encourage exercise: Ms. Jackson to receive regular phone contact as part of her home program

Benefits of Exercise[62]

Persons of any age can generally learn to do and gain benefits from both endurance and strength training. Aerobic training maintains and improves heart and lung function while resistance training helps offset losses in muscle mass and improves strength. Exercise also improves bone health, reduces the risk of osteoporosis, improves postural stability, and increases ROM. All these factors lead to a reduced risk of falls. In addition to these physiological benefits, exercise also has psychological benefits, including the preservation of cognition and the amelioration of depression. Exercising helps individuals take control of their health and improves quality of life. Further information on the benefits of exercise can be found in Musculoskeletal Pattern A: Primary Prevention/Risk Reduction for Skeletal Demineralization and Musculoskeletal Pattern C: Impaired Muscle Performance.

COORDINATION, COMMUNICATION, AND DOCUMENTATION

Communication will occur with Ms. Jackson and her family members to engender support for the home modifications, safety equipment, precautions during movement transitions, and exercise program. All elements of the client's management will be documented. A referral to her primary care physician will be made to ensure that her medication regimen is adequate.

PATIENT/CLIENT-RELATED INSTRUCTION

The client will be instructed in the environmental risk factors for falls, the importance of moving slowly during transitions to allow her BP to normalize, the need for the use of LE compression garments, and the benefits of exercise. Particular emphasis will be placed on the associations between the selected interventions and their association with reducing the risk of another fall. Specific instructions for Ms. Jackson include:

◆ Environmental risk factors for falls[63]
  ● Poor lighting at night and in stairwells
  ● Scatter rugs
  ● Floor clutter
  ● Non-skid mats in tub
◆ Information about OH[64]
  ● Changes in BP and blood flow to brain when moving up from a supine position
  ● Allow time for the body to respond to the change in position
  ● Use of compression garments to reduce this phenomenon

THERAPEUTIC EXERCISE

◆ Aerobic conditioning/endurance conditioning
  ● Progress to walking greater distances using cane for safety and pedometer to count steps
  ● Recumbent bicycle to increase endurance of large muscles in safe position using warm-up, progressively increasing intensity, and cool-down building up to a duration of 20 to 30 minutes each session at least four to five times per week
  ● If possible, progress to treadmill or elliptical machines for aerobic conditioning
◆ Balance, coordination, and agility training
  ● Balance, coordination, and agility exercises
    ■ Balance both feet, one foot, eyes open, eyes closed

    ■ Foam pads for standing to decrease stability of base of support
    ■ Tandem stance and tandem walk
    ■ Toe walking, heel walking
    ■ Side stepping
    ■ Carioca
    ■ Dance
    ■ Figure 8's
    ■ Reaching exercises—forward, backward, sideward
    ■ Tai Chi
    ■ Add obstacles to path as ability increases
◆ Body mechanics and postural stabilization
  ● Postural control training
    ■ Proper alignment of head, cervical and thoracic spines, and shoulders
    ■ Axial extension
    ■ Scapula retraction and depression
    ■ Chicken wing position (hands behind head, horizontal abduction of shoulders)
    ■ Corner stretch
    ■ Transition of position from supine to sitting, standing, and walking
    ■ Transition of position to functional activities
  ● Postural stabilization activities
    ■ Maintenance of axial extension position with bilateral arm raises
    ■ Glut sets
    ■ Core stabilization while sitting on ball
    ■ Arm and leg raises unilateral and then contralateral in quadruped as possible
    ■ Incorporate the use of unstable surfaces like foam rubber cushion in sitting and standing with bilateral and unilateral stance
  ● Postural awareness training
    ■ Postural corrections in standing to achieve upright trunk standing with side to a mirror with grid lines
    ■ Reaching activities in upright posture
◆ Flexibility exercises
  ● Stretching exercises should be done after warming up, using a slow and steady stretch accompanied by deep breathing, and building hold up to 30 to 60 seconds
  ● Heel cord stretching standing one foot forward and one foot back with heel on floor, hands on wall, body well aligned, gently bend forward knee
    ■ Begin with 5-second hold, five repetitions twice per day, progress to 30-second hold, two repetitions twice per day
  ● Active standing trunk movements (eg, gentle rotation, side bends) as tolerated with hands for support on countertop or back of sturdy chair

- Begin with 5-second hold, five repetitions twice per day first trunk, then each leg, progress to 30-second hold, two repetitions twice per day
- ◆ Gait and locomotion training
  - Progress from walking in parallel bars to walking in open spaces with cane and eventually without cane
  - Motor retraining to stand upright, to look ahead, and to move head to survey environment while walking
- ◆ Strength, power, and endurance training[65-68]
  - Hip extensors, abductors, and flexors, knee extensors, ankle dorsiflexors and plantarflexors, shoulder depressors, and elbow extensors using cuff weights and hand-held weights
    - 80% of one repetition maximum
    - 8 to 12 repetitions each group
    - Expect momentary muscular fatigue
    - Progress resistance as strength increases
  - In order to tell if Ms. Jackson is working hard enough, the physical therapist must check for a look of concentration, slight tremor, increased respirations, and perceived exertion as somewhat hard or hard
  - Palpation should reveal a strong contraction
  - Sit to stand exercise
  - Weighted vest to increase strength of trunk musculature while walking

FUNCTIONAL TRAINING IN SELF-CARE AND HOME MANAGEMENT

- ◆ Self-care and home management
  - Injury prevention or reduction
    - Instruction in slow movement from supine to sit and then allowing time for BP to normalize following initial movement
    - Instruction in environmental risk factors for falls
      - ▶ Add lighting to stairwell and use of night lights
      - ▶ Remove or better secure scatter rugs throughout house
      - ▶ Make it part of play routine for great-grandchildren to regularly pick up their toys and place in safe place
    - Develop strategies for safely getting in and out of bathtub
      - ▶ Add non-skid surface to bottom of tub
      - ▶ Purchase an over-the-edge bath seat with back for placement in the tub
      - ▶ Purchase and ask son to install hand-held shower spray
      - ▶ Complete strengthening activities to improve balance and LE strength for transfers

FUNCTIONAL TRAINING IN WORK, COMMUNITY, AND LEISURE INTEGRATION OR REINTEGRATION

- ◆ Community and leisure
  - Progress from walking in church keeping trunk upright, head up, eyes scanning environment first with cane then without cane
  - Progress from walking short distances in community with family and using cane for longer distances as endurance improves

PRESCRIPTION, APPLICATION, AND, AS APPROPRIATE, FABRICATION OF DEVICES AND EQUIPMENT

- ◆ Compression garments
  - Fit and order compression garments for LEs
  - Instruction in use of sock aid for application of low-pressure LE compression garments
  - Instruction in care of LE compression garments

ANTICIPATED GOALS AND EXPECTED OUTCOMES

- ◆ Impact on pathology/pathophysiology
  - Edema is controlled through Ms. Jackson's ability to independently apply low-pressure LE compression garments using sock aid to assist with application.
- ◆ Impact on impairments
  - Aerobic capacity/endurance is increased, and Ms. Jackson can walk 350 feet in 6 minutes while looking forward and without stopping.
  - Muscle strength is improved to WNL in the LEs and trunk so that rising from multiple level surfaces without use of the hands is achieved.
  - Muscle strength is increased, and Ms. Jackson will demonstrate full active hip extension in standing to allow a more upright posture, stabilized center of gravity, and ability to react to external perturbations by using a hip strategy.
  - Posture and postural security in standing is improved, and Mrs. Jackson is able to stand on one foot on foam pad for 10 seconds.
  - ROM is increased to within functional limits (WFL), and 5 degrees of dorsiflexion bilaterally is attained to allow for use of the ankle strategy to maintain upright during quiet standing.

♦ Impact on functional limitations

- Ability to get in and out of her bathtub safely is achieved.
- Ability to move from supine to sit by rolling slowly to her side, pushing into a sitting position without holding her breath, and waiting several minutes in sitting before attempting to rise to a standing position is achieved.
- Ability to perform physical actions, tasks, and activities related to self-care, home management, community, and leisure is improved.
- Increased confidence in ability to travel to her community activities is achieved.
- Increased confidence in mobility is achieved within her home.
- Independent ambulation around her home without gripping furniture or relying on wall support is achieved.

♦ Risk reduction/prevention

- Ability to communicate environmental risk for falls to her family is achieved.
- Ability to identify three benefits of exercise is attained.
- Behaviors that foster healthy habits, wellness, and prevention are acquired; client knowledge of personal and environmental factors associated with the condition is increased.
- Knowledge of need for assistance with lighting, regular toy pick up from preadolescent grandchildren, and either removal or better securing of throw rugs is achieved.[63]
- Risk of recurrence of condition is reduced.
- Safety of client, family, significant others, and caregivers is improved.
- Understanding of and being able to explain the association between dim lighting, throw rugs, alterations in BP, muscle weakness and fall risk is achieved.

♦ Impact on societal resources

- Documentation occurs throughout client management and follows the American Physical Therapy Association's (APTA's) *Guidelines for Physical Therapy Documentation.*[69]
- Risk factors are reduced and safety is improved.

♦ Patient/client satisfaction

- Client and family understanding of anticipated goals and expected outcomes is increased.
- Referrals are made to other professionals or resources whenever necessary or appropriate.

REEXAMINATION

Reexamination is performed throughout the episode of care. It is anticipated that persons placed in this pattern may require additional brief episodes of care to modify their exercise interventions as their abilities change. Periodic reexamination will allow the client to remain safe as she ages and her abilities change.

DISCHARGE

Ms. Jackson is discharged from this physical therapy episode after 16 visits over 3 months. These sessions have covered her entire episode of service. She is discharged because she has achieved goals and expected outcomes. As Ms. Jackson is an older adult with multiple risk factors for falls, she and her family received education regarding factors that may trigger a call to her physical therapist for reexamination and a new episode of physical therapy care.

REFERENCES

1. Commodore DI. Falls in the elderly population: a look at incidence, risks, healthcare costs, and preventive strategies. *Rehabilitation Nursing: The Official Journal of the Association of Rehabilitation Nurses.* 1995;20:84-89.
2. Control NCfIPa. The costs of fall injuries among older adults. Available at: http://www.cdc.gov/ncipc/factsheets/fallcost.htm.
3. DeVito CA, Lambert DA, Sattin RW, Bacchelli S, Ros A, Rodriguez JG. Fall injuries among the elderly. Community-based surveillance. *J Am Geriatr Soc.* 1988;36:1029-1035.
4. Fife D, Barancik JI. Northeastern Ohio Trauma Study III: incidence of fractures. *Ann Emerg Med.* 1985;14:244-248.
5. Finstad M, Pratt L, Rajki S, Wheeler N, Wixon R. Preventing falls among older adults in Hennipin County. April 2000. Available at: http://www.co.hennepin.mn.us/commhlth/reports/SeniorHealth.htm.
6. Fuller GF. Falls in the elderly. *Am Fam Physician.* 2000;61(7):2159-2168, 2173-2174. Review.
7. Luukinen H, Koski K, Laippala P, Kivela SL. Predictors for recurrent falls among the home-dwelling elderly. *Scand J Prim Health Care.* 1995;13:294-299.
8. Nevitt MC, Cummings SR, Hudes ES. Risk factors for injurious falls: a prospective study. *J Gerontol.* 1991;46:M164-M170.
9. O'Loughlin JL, Robitaille Y, Boivin JF, Suissa S. Incidence of and risk factors for falls and injurious falls among the community-dwelling elderly. *Am J Epidemiol.* 1993;137:342-354.
10. Fuller GF. What causes falls in the elderly? How can I prevent a fall? *Am Fam Physician.* 2000;61:2173.
11. Rawsky E. Review of the literature on falls among the elderly. *Image: The Journal of Nursing Scholarship.* 1998;30:47-52.
12. Rizzo JA, Friedkin R, Williams CS, Nabors J, Acampora D, Tinetti ME. Health care utilization and costs in a Medicare population by fall status. *Med Care.* 1998;36:1174-1188.

CHAPTER TWO

Impaired Neuromotor Development (Pattern B)

Barbara H. Connolly, PT, DPT, EdD, FAPTA
Patricia C. Montgomery, PT, PhD, FAPTA
Joanell A. Bohmert, PT, MS

ANATOMY

The nervous system is a highly complex network of inter-connecting neurons and interneurons that form structures that comprise the central (CNS) and peripheral nervous systems (PNS). The nervous system plays a direct or indirect role in the function of all other body systems. It is where information is received, analyzed, synthesized, processed, integrated, conceived, interpreted, felt, labeled, stored, recalled, and distributed. It is considered the control center for movement, emotion, thought, communication, planning, intelligence, and the soul. Much is unknown about why the nervous system develops or works the way it does. Models of neuromotor development and brain function are changing based on new technologies to study and analyze brain function.[1-5]

The nervous system is divided into two parts: the CNS and the PNS. The CNS is comprised of the brain (cortex, cerebellum, brainstem) and spinal cord. The PNS includes the 12 cranial nerves and 31 paired spinal nerves that are grouped to form the somatic and autonomic systems. While the anatomical structures of the brain are the same in all humans there is great individual variation in the function and interaction of the various areas of the brain based on how that individual uses his or her brain.[6,7] The anatomy

and physiology of the CNS are detailed in Pattern C: Impaired Motor Function and Sensory Integrity Associated With Nonprogressive Disorders of the Central Nervous System—Congenital Origin or Acquired in Infancy or Childhood; Pattern D: Impaired Motor Function and Sensory Integrity Associated With Nonprogressive Disorders of the Central Nervous System—Acquired in Adolescence or Adulthood; and Pattern H: Impaired Motor Function, Peripheral Nerve Integrity, and Sensory Integrity Associated With Nonprogressive Disorders of the Spinal Cord. The anatomy and physiology of the PNS are further detailed in Pattern F: Impaired Peripheral Nerve Integrity and Muscle Performance Associated With Peripheral Nerve Injury.

Leonard[7] reports that the human brain is less than 2.5% of body mass; weighs approximately 1500 g; and is composed of 78% water, 10% fat, 8% protein, and 4% other inert materials but receives over 15% of the total blood supply and consumes 25% of the body's total oxygen. The cells that comprise the nervous system are neurons and glial cells. There are over 100 billion neurons in the human body and at least 10x100 billion glial cells.

NEURONS

The basic unit of the nervous system is the neuron. A neuron includes a cell body with multiple projections that receive information, dentrites, and a single projection that sends information to the next neuron, an axon. Neurons are generally tree-like structures with dendrites forming the multiple branches, axons the trunk and roots, and cell bodies the intersection between the trunk and branches. The function of the neuron is to receive, integrate, and respond to information. Information is in the form of an electrochemical signal.

The cell body, or soma, contains a nucleus, cytoplasm, mitochondria, golgi apparatus, and nissl substance. It, along with the dendrites, is responsible for receiving and interpreting information from the body and environment. It is where information is processed and determined if that information will be sent on. It is also responsible for synthesizing macromolecules to produce certain neurotransmitters.

Dendrites are the projectiles that branch off the cell body and receive stimuli through their receptor sites. Generally, dendrites are shorter than axons and may have fine spines as receptors. There is no limit to the number of dendrites per neuron or receptor sites per dendrite. Dendrites will continue to branch or "sprout" to search for information.

The axon is a single projectile from the cell body that conducts the message from the cell body to the nerve terminal presynaptic sites. Generally, axons are covered with myelin that acts as an insulator that increases the speed of conduction and assists in getting the signal to the end of the axon. At the end of the axon are nerve terminals with synaptic vesicles that contain the chemicals that are released as a result of the neuron being stimulated. Neurotransmitters may also be produced in the axon. Axon length varies and can be over 3 feet (1 meter) long as it travels to its target cells.

Neurons have three basic structures:

1. Unipolar

2. Bipolar

3. Multipolar[6]

The structure is based on the number of processes coming out of the cell body, however, in all structures there is only one axon per neuron. Unipolar neurons have just one process from which the dendrite and axon form. These neurons are found in the autonomic nervous system. Bipolar neurons have two processes, a dendrite and axon. While there is only one dendrite arising from the cell body, there is multiple branching of that dendrite to receive information. Bipolar neurons are generally sensory neurons. Multipolar neurons are the most common neuron with multiple processes arising from the cell body. These neurons are found throughout the CNS and PNS.

There are three types of neurons:

1. Sensory

2. Motor

3. Interneurons

Sensory neurons receive internal and external information and send it directly to motor neurons in the spinal cord or to interneurons in the spinal cord or brain. Motor neurons receive information from interneurons in the brain or spinal cord or from sensory neurons in the spinal cord and send information directly to muscle or glands. See Musculoskeletal Pattern C: Impaired Muscle Performance for detailed information on motor neurons and interaction with muscle. Interneurons provide the connection between sensory and motor neurons in the spinal cord or brain. Of the 100 billion neurons in the nervous system, 99.9% are interneurons.[7]

GLIAL CELLS

Glial or glia cells are the support cells for neurons. They produce myelin, guide neural cell migration, respond to injury, and provide support to the internal environment of the brain.

Types of Glial Cells

Astrocytes are located in the brain and spinal cord in both gray and white matter and provide the primary support for neurons. Functions include production and secretion of neurotrophic factors (proteins), metabolism of proteins or chemicals, and response to injury.[6]

Oligodendrocytes are the cells that produce myelin to sheath axons in the CNS and are located in the white matter. Several axons may be wrapped by one oligodendrocyte.

Microglia provide clean up of the white and gray matter in the CNS. They will migrate to the injury site to remove dead and dying cells. They produce cytokines that trigger immune system cells to assist.

Schwann cells are the equivalent to oligodendrocytes in the PNS, but they will only wrap around one axon. Schwann cells are the only glial cells in the PNS and therefore have additional responsibilities including providing nutrients and support, metabolic processing, and facilitating axon regrowth.[6]

DOWN SYNDROME

Children with Down syndrome (DS) have specific neuroanatomical differences that result from the disorder. The overall brain weight of individuals with DS averages 76% of the brain weight of individuals without DS.[8] The combined weight of the cerebellum and brainstem is proportionately even smaller, being an average of 66% of the weight of the cerebellum and brainstem in individuals without DS. Individuals with DS also have been shown to have a decrease in the number of pyramidal neurons in the hippocampus as compared to the hippocampi of individuals of comparable ages who did not have DS.[9]

Of special interest to physical therapists are the orthopedic problems that occur in children with DS. Diamond and associates evaluated the prevalence of orthopedic problems in a large sample of persons with DS.[10] Orthopedic problems included hip subluxations or dislocation, patella instability with resulting subluxation or dislocation, metatarsus varus, pes planus, thoracolumbar scoliosis, and atlantoaxial instability. Atlantoaxial instability, a term used to describe increased mobility of the cervical spine at the level of the first and second vertebrae, has been found to occur in approximately 14% of individuals with DS.[11,12] Radiographs are recommended at 2 years of age and periodically throughout childhood and adolescence. Children with asymptomatic instability typically do not require surgery, but should not engage in contact sports, gymnastics, diving, or other activities that might result in injury to the cervical spine.

Cardiac defects are very common in individuals with DS. Anomalies are present in about 50% of children with ventricular septal defects and complete atrioventricular septal defects among the most prevalent.[11] Survival at 1 year of age is 85% for those without heart defects and 60% for those with congenital heart malformations.

Other congenital anomalies present in children with DS include diastasis recti, duodenal atresia, umbilical hernia, and midface hypoplasia. Most children with DS have very small ear canals that may lead to fluid accumulation, otitis media, and hearing losses.

DEVELOPMENTAL COORDINATION DISORDER

Developmental coordination disorder (DCD) is defined as a developmental disorder in children characterized by motor impairment that interferes with ADL and academic achievements.[13] Since 1994, DCD has been the preferred term to describe the condition of children with motor incoordination, although the terms "clumsy," "gross motor impaired," and "developmental dyspraxia" have been used in the past.[14,15] In DCD, the motor impairment must not be caused by or have the symptoms of an identifiable neurological deficit, such as cerebral palsy or muscular dystrophy.[13] Most investigators agree that children with DCD display deficits in motor coordination that are not due to any identifiable neurological deficit.[16] Therefore, most children with DCD may not have neuroanatomical abnormalities that are obvious.

PHYSIOLOGY

From Neurons to Neighborhoods: The Science of Early Childhood Development[17] describes six phases of brain development. These phases are not discrete but overlap with some continuing into adulthood. The phases are:

1. Neurulation and neurogenesis
2. Neuron proliferation and migration
3. Neuronal differentiation and pathfinding
4. Synaptogenesis
5. Maturation and pruning
6. Gliagenesis or myelination

NEURULATION AND NEUROGENESIS

The nervous system begins to form during the third week of development. It begins as a mass of cells in the ectoderm forming the neural plate that continues to lengthen forming a neural groove in the middle and neural folds on each side. By the end of the third week the neural folds fold inward, meet in the center, and begin to fuse to form the neural tube. The initial fusing of the neural tube occurs approximately in the area that will be the cervical spinal cord. The fusion of the neural tube continues both rostrally and caudally. The rostral end will eventually enlarge into several areas that become the brain. These areas include the forebrain (prosencepalon), midbrain (mesencepalon), and hindbrain (rhombencephalon) with the cavity of the neural tube forming the ventricles. The spinal cord is formed from the rest of the neural tube. Cells that move away from the neural crest (ie, neural crest cells) develop into sensory neurons, Schwann cells, and postganglionic cells of the autonomic nervous system.[6,7,18]

Neural tube defects are a result of failure or incomplete closure of the neural tube and result in permanent damage to the nervous system and development of the fetus. Anaencephalopy occurs when the rostral end of the neural tube fails to close. This results in a lack of the cerebral hemisphere and is always fatal. Spina bifida occurs when the caudal end of the neural tube fails to close. The fetus will continue to develop, however, the amount of defect will depend on how little or much of the neural tube fails to close. See Pattern C: Impaired Motor Function and Sensory Integrity Associated With Nonprogressive Disorders of the Central Nervous System—Congenital Origin or Acquired in Infancy or Childhood for a case study on myelomeningocele.

NEURON PROLIFERATION AND MIGRATION

During prenatal development there is great proliferation and migration of neural cells. The specificity of a neural cell is determined by a number of factors during development including the environmental factors around the cell.[18] In a mature brain all neurons are located in the outermost layer of the cortex. In the developing brain, neurons are produced in the innermost area and must migrate out. Neurons migrate following glial fibers to their specific target area. Neurons are supported in their migration by other glial cells. Once in their designated area, neurons mass together to form the structures of the nervous system. Neural migration is completed before birth in the cerebral cortex but continues after birth in the cerebellum leaving it more susceptible to influences from the environment.[7]

Genetic coding plays an important role in neuron pro-liferation and migration. Defects in the coding can result in a malformation of the nervous and other systems that may result in genetic abnormalities or death of the fetus. The abnormalities may be abnormalities in the brain structures, such as agenesis of the corpus callosum, or may just be abnormal gyral patterns. They may also present as syndromes, such as DS. Environmental factors during development can also impact neural structures and functions. Toxins, such as alcohol or cocaine, can interfere with neural migration resulting in neurons not reaching the appropriate target cells.[18] Fetal alcohol syndrome is the result of alcohol use by the birth mother during pregnancy and presents with abnormalities in neuroanatomy and brain function.[19,20]

NEURAL DIFFERENTIATION AND PATHFINDING

Neural differentiation occurs through prolific growth of dendrites and axons as they lengthen to reach other neurons to establish synaptic connections. Axon growth is facilitated by growth cones that are located on the ends of the axons and assist in the axon's search for its target cell.[6,18] When the axon reaches its target cell a connection is formed and a synapse occurs, thereby establishing a pathway. The specificity of the presynaptic and postsynaptic sites is determined during this development by molecules present in the brain. The developing brain provides an overabundance of neural connections that results in redundancy and lack of precision. The infant has at least twice as many connections as an adult, however, these connections are not necessarily effective or efficient.

As the structures of the brain continue to expand, the cortex, which begins as a smooth surface, quickly develops extensive folds to allow for the massive number of neural and glial cells to be contained within the skull. Areas of the brain are formed by grouping of neurons with like functions or responses to stimulation.

SYNAPTOGENESIS

Synaptogenesis is the development of communication links between neurons. Neurons are separated from each other by a small space called the synaptic cleft. Information received by the neuron through the dendrites is processed in the dendrites and cell body and then conducted down the axon where it is transmitted through release of a chemical from the axon terminals. Signal transmission is an electrochemical process involving neurotransmitters.

Process of Signal Transmission

Neurons are not direct conduits of signals but are rather collectors and assimilators of information. The cell body receives the information and determines if it is worthy to be transmitted through the axon. The process involves the transfer of ions and changes in electrical potentials that result in an action potential and release of chemicals.

Neurons receive information through the transfer of ions across its membrane. The resting membrane potential for neurons is −65 mv. Sensory input to the neuron can have the effect of making the neuron more negatively charged (hyperpolarization) or more positively charged (depolarization). The neuron requires a change in polarization building to a threshold level, the action potential threshold, before a signal is sent down the axon. Neurons modulate the resting membrane potential with each signal it receives. Signals that hyperpolarize the membrane are inhibitory, making it harder for the neuron to reach its threshold. Signals that depolarize are excitatory making it easier to reach the action potential threshold. Therefore, the action potential threshold is the result of the combined inhibitory (hyperpolarization) and excitatory (depolarization) input to the cell.[6,7]

As neurons can receive tens to hundreds of thousands of signals at one time the intensity and duration of the signals have an impact on how quickly the neuron reaches the action potential threshold and how long it continues to transmit the action potential. Sensory receptors respond to stimuli by changing the receptor potential, but not all stimuli will result in reaching the action potential threshold. The sensory signal must be of sufficient amplitude to reach the spike threshold that will result in reaching the action potential. Increasing the amplitude of the signal does not increase the amplitude of the action potential as it operates under the "all or none" phenomenon. Instead the increased amplitude of the sensory input increases the rate of action potentials. Increases in duration of the sensory signal results in increased number of action potentials.[7]

The result of the firing of the action potential is the release of neurotransmitters from synaptic vesicles in the presynaptic terminals. The rate and number of action potentials per unit time determines the amount of transmitter released.[7] The neurotransmitters that are released move across the synaptic cleft looking for receptor sites on the target neuron. If it is the correct receptor, the neurotransmitter binds with the receptor site and causes a synaptic potential in the postsynaptic neuron. Inhibitory postsynaptic potential (IPSP) is the result of hyperpolarization of the receptor site, and excitatory postsynaptic potential (EPSP) is the result of depolarization. The receptor sites, not the neurotransmitter, determine if the action is inhibitory or excitatory.

Again, a single IPSP or EPSP is not likely to significantly change the polarization of the neuron. To have a greater impact, neurons receive input from multiple sources. Neurons use a variety of strategies to elicit an IPSP or EPSP. Temporal summation and spatial summation are two strategies to provide intense input to either hyperpolarize or depolarize the neuron. Convergence is another strategy in which multiple neurons converge on a single receptor neuron. Divergence occurs from axonal branching onto several receptor neurons.

Neurotransmitters

Neurotransmitters are chemicals released from the synaptic vesicles in the presynaptic terminals of axons that cross the synaptic cleft and bind with the receptor site to excite or inhibit the target neuron. Most neurotransmitters belong to one of two categories: small amino molecules (also called amino acids) or neuropeptides.[6] The difference in the two categories is where they are produced. Small amino molecules or amino acids are produced in the individual synaptic endings by cytoplasmic enzymes. This makes them readily available for release and to be recycled back into the presynaptic ending following release.[6] Neuropeptides are produced from larger precursor proteins in the neuron's cell body and must be transported down the axon for storage in the synaptic vesicle. This requires them to be recycled back through the cell body that makes them less available.[6]

Neurotransmitters play a critical role in the development of synaptic connections. Chemicals influence the development of dendrites and axons and the specificity of the receptor sites. The same neurotransmitter may be excitatory or inhibitory, but it must find the specific receptor site to which to bind, as receptor sites are specific to one kind of molecule.

Damage to the receptor sites or in the production areas of the neurotransmitters can result in a depression in transmission that impacts learning and function. Introduction of drugs or toxins to the brain, especially when in rapid development, can interfere with the development and use of synaptic vesicles and postsynaptic receptor sites.[21]

MATURATION AND PRUNING

As the brain develops it goes through periods of excessive proliferation of synapses followed by periods of pruning or eliminating of synapses. These periods are frequently referred to as blossoming and pruning. The result is an increase in the amount of gray matter in the brain through childhood. As the child nears puberty, a significant decrease or thinning of gray matter occurs that continues at least through young adulthood.[22] This process occurs in different areas of the brain at different times but appears to follow a sequential pattern.[22,23]

Critical or sensitive periods appear to exist for certain brain development, such as vision, during which that area of the brain needs input, expects experience, or it will not develop fully or at all.[18,24,25] During these periods there appears to be a peak in the proliferation of connections, and if those connections are not used, they are eliminated. Neurons and pathways also are especially sensitive to damage during these sensitive periods. Other brain areas do not appear to have sensitive periods but rather appear to wait for stimulation, meaning they are dependent on the experiences of the individual to develop.[25,26] This is the process involved in learning to play golf or a musical instrument.[27] This is also the process that makes each brain very individual, allows for reorganization following injury, and provides for the adapt-

ability and plasticity of the brain.[6,17,22,23]

Decisions on which connections to keep and which to eliminate are based on the amount of activity of the connection, making experience essential to proper development. This is referred to as the "use it or lose it" phenomenon. The use it or lose it phenomenon occurs throughout the life span of humans.[7,18,19,21] Experience, good or bad, is used to strengthen synapses in a specific area of the brain.[26]

GLIAGENESIS OR MYELINATION

Glial cells produce myelin, a fatty substance that wraps around the axon insulating it and thereby increasing its speed of conduction. Oligodendrocytes produce myelin in the CNS, while Schwann cells produce myelin in the PNS. Not all axons in the CNS or PNS are myelinated. In the CNS myelination is limited at birth but proceeds rapidly during childhood. Mapping studies of brain development and maturation demonstrate a significant thinning of gray matter and an increase in white matter as the brain matures.[22,23] The motor and sensory areas are the first areas of the cortex to myelinate followed by sensory association areas, then cognitive processes. The areas of the prefrontal brain for executive function are the last to myelinate, occurring in early adulthood.[6,17,22,23,28,29]

POSTNATAL NEUROGENESIS

Until recently it was believed that humans were born with all their neurons, that new neurons were not developed.[30] Loss of neurons over the life span or through injury was considered significant as, unlike other cells in the human body, new neurons were never created. Animal, and now human research, has identified neurogenesis occurring in adults.[31] It has been demonstrated that the hippocampal dentate gyrus and the subventricular zone and its projection through the rostral migratory stream to the olfactory bulb are the only two areas in the adult human brain that develop new neurons.[32,33] While it is still unknown what becomes of these new neurons, researchers are studying the possibilities on brain plasticity and neuroadaptation, nervous system diseases and conditions, and neural cell replacement.[34-38]

DOWN SYNDROME

Trisomy 21, the presence of an extra 21 chromosome that occurs in all types of DS, is the primary cause of the altered pattern of physical and mental development in the child with DS. Trisomy 21, in most incidences, affects all cells of the body and produces a particular blending of physical and mental characteristics.

DEVELOPMENTAL COORDINATION DISORDER

The pertinent physiology for DCD relates to functioning of neurotransmitters or receptor systems within various areas of the CNS. Several theories focus on the etiology of DCD being related to prenatal, perinatal, or neonatal insults since there appears to be a higher incidence of DCD among children with a history of prenatal or perinatal difficulties.[39,40] Hadders-Algra stated that DCD may be the result of damage at the cellular level that occurred prenatally but which cannot be identified through currently available diagnostic techniques.[41]

PATHOPHYSIOLOGY

The pathophysiologies listed under Pattern B: Impaired Neuromotor Development in the *Guide to Physical Therapist Practice*[42] are quite diverse. In addition, this pattern applies to all ages. The *Guide* defines neuromotor development as "the acquisition and evolution of motor skills across the life span."[42] Motor skills continue to develop and be revised across the life span.[43] While this chapter provides a case example of a child with DS, a genetic disorder, and a case of a child with DCD, a condition with unknown etiology, it would also be appropriate to place adults with difficulty acquiring or refining motor skills in this pattern.

DOWN SYNDROME

DS has been recognized as one of the most common causes of developmental delays in children. DS is caused by the presence of an extra, small chromosome on the 21st pair of chromosomes. The incidence of DS becomes greater with increasing maternal age. The likelihood that a woman under 30 who becomes pregnant will have a baby with DS is less than 1 in 1000, but the chance of having a baby with DS increases to 1 in 400 for women who become pregnant at age 35. By age 42, the chance is 1 in 60 that a pregnant woman will have a baby with DS, and by age 49, the chance is 1 in 12.[44]

Three different types of trisomy 21 have been identified. The first type that represents the majority of cases of DS is due to the nondisjunction of two homologous chromosomes during either the first or second meiotic division.[45] A second type is due to a hereditary translocation that is not associated with maternal age and occurs when there is breakage of two nonhomologous chromosomes with subsequent reattachment of the broken chromosomes to other chromosomes. A third type represents a mosaic disorder in which some cells in the individual have a normal complement of the 21st chromosome, while other cells have a trisomy 21.

The pertinent pathophysiology for DS relates to the neurophysiological differences that have been reported. Benda noted a lack of myelinization of the nerve fibers in precentral areas and frontal lobes of the cerebral cortex and in the cerebellum of infants with DS.[46] His findings suggested a lack of CNS maturity in these infants. Other researchers have found that, although prenatal defects of neuro- and synaptogen-

esis are present in infants with DS, neurocytologic changes also occur in individuals with DS as they age.[47] Evidence from post-mortem studies suggests that the neurocytologic changes in DS closely resemble the changes associated with Alzheimer's disease.[47] All adults with DS are thought to have developed the neuropathological changes of Alzheimer's disease by the age of 40 years, but only a small percentage are found to be clinically demented at that time.[48-51]

Seizure disorders are present in approximately 8% of children with DS.[52] It is unknown why there is an increased incidence of seizure disorders in DS, although it has been hypothesized that structural abnormalities and biochemical aberrations of the CNS may be in part responsible.

Immune dysfunction associated with a susceptibility to viral and bacterial infection and acute leukemia have been reported in individuals with DS.[53,54] However, although there is a high incidence of infectious diseases in individuals with DS, the existence of an immunodeficiency has not been firmly established.[55]

One of the most frequently occurring endocrine problems in persons of all ages with DS is thyroid disease.[56] The signs of hypothyroidism, such as lethargy, confusion, constipation, dry skin, dry hair, and fatigue, may be subtle and may be attributed to the DS itself. Therefore, screening is recommended on an annual basis by monitoring thyroid-stimulating hormone and T_4 levels.[11]

DEVELOPMENTAL COORDINATION DISORDER

Children with DCD are thought to have difficulties resulting from problems in neurotransmitters or receptor systems rather than from damage to specific areas of the brain. Ayres described a sensory systems model that defined the "clumsiness" seen in children as a reflection of children's inability to plan and execute a nonhabitual motor task. She attributed these problems to disturbances in the CNS that prevented the normal processing and utilization of sensory information for body scheme development and motor planning.[57] In particular, the tactile, proprioceptive, and vestibular systems were identified as being inadequately utilized. Other researchers have suggested that problems with motor coordination are due to visual perceptual deficits[58-60] or to kinesthetic deficits.[61-63] Smyth and Mason found that children with DCD demonstrated poor proprioceptive function and relied more on visual cues.[64] Smyth and Glencross[65] focused on the speed of processing kinesthetic input as being a dysfunctional system, and Wann and associates[66] reported that children with DCD relied more on vision to maintain their posture, rather than integrating visual and proprioceptive input.

Children with DCD seem to be a heterogeneous group, and questions have arisen about the presence of subtypes. McNab and coworkers[67] using the Bruininks-Oseretsky Test of Motor Proficiency (BOTMP) identified five different subtype profiles of DCD. The first group had better gross motor than fine motor skills; the second group had better speed and dexterity, visuomotor integration, and visual-perceptual skills than kinesthetic abilities; the third group had overall motor problems and difficulties with kinesthetic and visual skills; the fourth group performed well on kinesthetic tasks but poorly on visual and dexterity tasks; and the fifth group had poor performance on running speed and agility but performed well with visual-perceptual skills.

Children with attention deficit/hyperactivity disorders (ADD/ADHD) may fall, bump into things, or knock things over, but this usually is due to distractibility and impulsivity. However, in the *Diagnostic and Statistical Manual of Mental Disorders* (DSM-IV) coding for DCD, ADD/ADHD is identified as a problem associated with DCD and, if criteria for both disorders are met, then both diagnoses can be given.[13] Kaplan and colleagues[68] found that 41% of the children with DCD also had ADHD, while Silver[69] reported that 20% of the children with learning disabilities in his study had coordination problems and almost 75% had attention deficits. These studies seem to indicate that DCD, learning disabilities, and attention deficits may be seen in the same children.

IMAGING

DOWN SYNDROME

Radiographs are recommended at 2 years of age and periodically administered in childhood and adolescence to determine atlantoaxial instability.

♦ Radiographs
  ● Allow for accurate analysis of cervical spine

PHARMACOLOGY

DOWN SYNDROME

Pharmacologic intervention may be indicated to manage a seizure disorder or thyroid disease.

♦ Anticonvulsants
  ● Examples: Carbamazepine (Tegretol), clonazepam (Klonopin), ethosuximide (Zarontin), phenobarbital, phenytoin (Dilantin), primidone (Mysoline), valproic acid (Depakene)[70]
  ● Actions: Inhibit spread of seizure activity; inhibit spike and wave formation; decrease amplitude, frequency, duration, and spread of discharge in seizures
  ● Side effects: Headaches and dizziness; ataxia; skin conditions (dermatitis or rash); very high doses may result in lethargy or drowsiness, interfering with abil-

ity to participate in requested activities; physicians monitor drug level in the bloodstream to determine/adjust dosage

♦ Thyroid drugs
  ● Examples: Levothyroxine (Synthroid, Levoxyl, Levothroid, L-thyroxine, Levotec, Eltroxin, Levo-T), liothyrone (Cytomel)[71]
  ● Actions: Increase metabolism
  ● Side effects: Caution should be used when individuals begin taking medication as there is a risk of angina until the dosage is stabilized[71]

DEVELOPMENTAL COORDINATION DISORDER

Currently no medications are used in the treatment of DCD. However, psychostimulant medications, such as amphetamine (Dexedrine or Adderall) or methylphenidate (Ritalin, Concerta, or Metadate CD), are the most commonly used medications for treatment of the main symptoms of ADHD that often are a comorbidity.[72] These medications have been shown to improve symptoms in about 70% of people who have ADHD.[73-75] Psychostimulants are considered for children with moderate to severe ADHD who have difficulty in at least two different settings, such as school and home.[74] Psychostimulant medications are approved by the US Food and Drug Administration (FDA) to treat people with ADHD age 6 years through adulthood, although occasionally these drugs may be used in younger children. Methylphenidate (such as Ritalin or Concerta) often is the preferred choice for treating ADHD, because it has fewer side effects than other medications and generally works well to control behavior. Dextroamphetamine or the combination dextroamphetamine and amphetamine (Adderall) are usually the second choice when the young child does not improve with methylphenidate. However, either may be the preferred medication in older children. The long-acting form of dextroamphetamine controls behavior for a longer period of time, so fewer doses are required during the day. A typical schedule for giving the medication is after breakfast and lunch and in the afternoon.

Recently, atomoxetine (Strattera) was approved by the FDA for use with individuals with ADHD age 6 years and older. Atomoxetine is not a stimulant but a selective norepinephrine reuptake inhibitor. It has not been shown to have addictive properties. A typical schedule for giving medication is one dose in the morning or dosage divided into two doses with one in the morning and one late afternoon or early evening. Medication is taken daily, and there are not breaks for weekends or vacations as is common with psychostimulant drugs. Common side effects include dizziness, lightheadedness, depressed growth rate, loss of appetite or weight loss, upset stomach, vomiting, constipation, or trouble sleeping.

♦ Psychostimulant drugs

- Examples: Amphetamine (Dexedrine or Adderall) or methylphenidate (Ritalin, Concerta, or Metadate CD)
- Actions: Increase release of dopamine
- Side effects
  - Decreased appetite in about 80% of people who take psychostimulants
    - The appetite is usually least during the daytime, increasing in the evening
    - About 10% to 15% of children have noticeable weight loss[75]
    - However, if the medication is given after meals and if snacks are added to the diet, the child's appetite does not appear to be as affected and weight loss may be prevented
  - Difficulty in going to asleep
    - Many children who report this problem take about an hour to fall asleep[75]
  - Headache and stomachache, but these symptoms usually are only temporary and decrease as the child continues to take the medication

---

Case Study #1: Down Syndrome

Kelsey is a 15-month-old female born at full term with a medical diagnosis of Down syndrome.

PHYSICAL THERAPIST EXAMINATION

HISTORY

- General demographics: Kelsey is a 15-month-old white female. English is the family's primary language.

- Social history: Kelsey lives with her mother and father who are the primary caregivers. Kelsey's grandparents live nearby and provide care for Kelsey on a regular basis.

- Employment/work: Kelsey's play is seldom goal directed. She enjoys listening to musical toys and watching moveable toys. Kelsey enjoys observing other children but does not interact with them.

- Growth and development: Kelsey is small for her stated age of 15 months. However, according to growth charts for children with DS, she is at the 50th percentile for height and weight.[76]

- Living environment: Kelsey lives in a two-level home with her bedroom on the second level.

- General health status
  - General health perception: Kelsey has had numerous ear infections since birth. She has had pressure-equalizing tubes inserted bilaterally.
  - Physical function: Kelsey tires easily during play. She takes frequent naps during the day and is able to sleep well during the night.
  - Psychological function: Kelsey generally is a happy baby. However, she becomes irritable when she is tired.
  - Role function: Daughter, grandchild, playmate.
  - Social function: Kelsey attends a mother–infant early intervention program twice weekly.

- Social/health habits: Kelsey has received routine well baby checkups. Her mother has consulted a nutritionist about Kelsey's dietary habits and is following suggestions made by the nutritionist for supplying Kelsey with a balanced diet.

- Family history: Noncontributory.

- Medical/surgical history: Past medical history includes an esophageal atresia that was not repaired until Kelsey was 6 months old. A gastrostomy was present for the first 6 months of age. She also had a ventricular-septal defect that was surgically repaired at 8 months. A history of chronic otitis media has been documented, and Kelsey now has a mild conductive hearing loss. Pressure-equalizing tubes were placed at 12 months.

- Current condition(s)/chief complaint(s): Kelsey's parents are concerned about her overall development at this time. Her parents are interested in having Kelsey learn to walk, to talk, and to play more appropriately with toys. Although her parents were encouraged to contact local early intervention programs when Kelsey was discharged from the hospital, they did not seek services until she was 10 months old. Kelsey and her mother attend a parent/caregiver-infant early intervention program twice weekly with consultative physical therapy, occupational therapy, and speech therapy services available at each session. The family has declined home-based services.

- Functional status and activity level: Kelsey has a variety of movement patterns but moves slowly, and postural reactions are delayed. She has poor oral motor skills and does not assist in dressing. She observes other children but does not interact with them.

- Medications: None.

- Other clinical tests
  - The Bayley Test of Infant Development II (BSID-II)[77] revealed that Kelsey had a Mental Developmental Index of 85 (1 SD below the mean).
  - The Alberta Infant Motor Scale[78] was administered as a screening instrument when Kelsey was 10 months of age. She scored at the 10th percentile for

her stated age.

- Further testing was done using the Peabody Developmental Motor Scales (PDMS)[79] to determine the degree of gross motor delays. She was found to be functioning at the 11-month level in her stationary skills, at the 9-month level in her locomotion skills, and at the 12-month level in her object manipulation skills. Her gross motor quotient was 76 (>1 SD below the mean).
- The Test of Sensory Function in Infants (TSIF)[80] was used to determine if Kelsey had sensory processing problems, particularly related to tactile processing since she dislikes being placed on her stomach and placing weight on her feet during standing. She scored deficient in her reactivity to tactile deep pressure and in her visual tactile integration. In her adaptive motor function, ocular-motor control and total score, she scored at risk for sensory processing problems.

SYSTEMS REVIEW

- ◆ Cardiovascular/pulmonary
  - BP: WNL
  - Edema: None observed
  - HR: WNL
  - RR: WNL
- ◆ Integumentary
  - Presence of scar formation: Scars are present on the chest and abdomen from the repairs of her esophageal atresia, gastrostomy, and ventricular-septal defect
  - Skin color: Good
  - Skin integrity: Good
- ◆ Musculoskeletal
  - Gross range of motion: Hypermobility is noted in both proximal and distal extremities
  - Gross strength: Decreased in trunk and all extremities
  - Gross symmetry: Symmetrical positioning and postures noted
  - Height: 27" (0.686 m)—at the 50th percentile for children with DS[76]
  - Weight: 15.5 lbs (7.03 kg)—at the 50th percentile for children with DS[76]
- ◆ Neuromuscular
  - Gross coordinated movements
    - Kelsey has good head control in all positions
    - She rolls independently and transitions in and out of sitting and in and out of a hands and knees position
    - She also pulls to stand at furniture
    - She uses increased base of support in both UEs and LEs during transitional movements

- Her postural control decreases when her center of gravity is raised
- ◆ Communication, affect, cognition, language, and learning style
  - Kelsey has been assessed using the BSID-II,[77] and mild mental delays have been documented
  - Kelsey observes other children but does not interact with them
  - Beginning verbal communication
  - Parent requests written home program with diagrams

TESTS AND MEASURES

- ◆ Aerobic capacity/endurance
  - Kelsey tires easily when moving on all-fours and when walking with two hands held
  - While she pulls to stand, standing endurance is limited
- ◆ Anthropometric characteristics
  - Kelsey's height and weight are within the normal range for children her age with DS
  - Facial features are characteristic of children with DS
    - She has epicanthal folds of her eyes, brushfield spots in her iris, low set and posteriorly rotated ears, a flat nasal bridge of her nose, fissured lips, and a small mandible
- ◆ Arousal, attention, and cognition
  - Formal IQ testing has not been completed on Kelsey
  - However, the BSID-II revealed that her mental developmental quotient is 85 (1 SD below the mean of 100 for the test)
  - Cognitive impairment is associated with her medical diagnosis
  - She is a passive child, needing encouragement and stimulation to attend to motor and cognitive tasks
  - She has several words that she uses singly rather than in combination (eg, "more," "mama," "dada")
- ◆ Assistive and adaptive devices: None
- ◆ Cranial and peripheral nerve integrity: WNL
- ◆ Gait, locomotion, and balance
  - Kelsey pulls to stand but is not yet attempting to cruise at furniture
  - She walks with maximal assistance with two hands held
  - She has slow and usually ineffective protective and equilibrium reactions in sitting, all-fours, and standing
- ◆ Integumentary integrity: Normal
- ◆ Joint integrity and mobility: Hypermobility is noted in all UE and LE proximal and distal joints

- Motor function
  - Although Kelsey appears to have a typical variety of movement patterns, her movements are very slow
  - Postural reactions are delayed
  - Kelsey needs multiple repetitions of cognitive and motor tasks for skill achievement and retention
- Muscle performance
  - Kelsey has poor muscle definition throughout her body, particularly noticeable in the shoulders and hips
  - She tends to lock her elbows into extension and externally rotate her arms when making movement transitions
  - She has poor stability in weightbearing positions (eg, all-fours, kneeling)
- Neuromotor development and sensory integration
  - Kelsey has good head control in all positions
  - She rolls independently, transitions in and out of sitting, and in and out of a hands and knees position
  - She also pulls to kneeling and pulls to stand at furniture
  - She tends to use straight plane movements without using trunk rotation
  - She generally is apprehensive about movement activities
  - She grasps objects but cannot release them with control
  - She cannot pick up pellet-sized objects
- Orthotic, protective, and supportive devices: None
- Posture
  - In standing, Kelsey has a wide base of support with lumbar lordosis, knee hyperextension, and foot pronation
  - Her trunk posture is kyphotic in sitting, but lordotic in quadruped
- Range of motion
  - Hypermobility is noted in both proximal and distal joints of the extremities
  - She tends to keep her shoulders elevated with shortened capital extensor muscles
- Reflex integrity
  - Decreased tendon reflexes (hypotonia) are present throughout UEs and LEs
  - Low muscle tone also is noted throughout the face and trunk
- Self-care and home management
  - Kelsey has poor oral motor skills
  - She uses a suckle pattern in feeding
  - Her tongue is thick in contour and protrudes from her mouth
  - She drinks from a cup only at snack time

- Solids are sometimes given to Kelsey by the parents, however, she tends to lose food, both liquids and solids, from her mouth
  - She does not assist in any other self-care
- Sensory integrity
  - Vision is normal
  - Mild conductive hearing loss has been noted
  - Kelsey tends to avoid movement-based activities
  - She also does not like to stand barefooted nor be touched on her face or abdomen (as noted in the test results from the TSIF)
- Ventilation and respiration/gas exchange
  - Kelsey has decreased respiratory-phonatory functioning
  - Her decreased control of the ribcage contributes to a decreased vital capacity
  - She has small nasal passages and is a mouth breather
  - She holds her breath during difficult movement transitions
  - Although the cardiologist reports that Kelsey's heart function is WNL, she occasionally turns blue with breath holding
  - She uses this behavior effectively to avoid activities in which she does not want to participate
- Work, community, and leisure integration or reintegration
  - Kelsey observes other children but does not interact with them
  - She tends to fling objects or toys to dispose of them
  - Play is seldom goal directed

EVALUATION

Kelsey is a 15-month-old child with a medical diagnosis of DS. The physical therapy examination revealed that Kelsey has poor muscle definition throughout her body, with poor stability in weightbearing positions. She has hypermobility in both proximal and distal extremities and has low muscle tone. She is able to pull to standing at furniture but does not cruise. She has slow protective and equilibrium reactions in sitting, all-fours, and standing. She grasps objects but cannot release them with control. She does not assist with any self-care activities. She is a mouth breather and occasionally drools. She has a mild hearing loss.

DIAGNOSIS

Kelsey has a medical diagnosis of DS. She has impaired: arousal, attention, and cognition; gait, locomotion, and balance; joint integrity and mobility; motor function; muscle performance; neuromotor development and sensory integration; posture; reflex integrity; sensory integrity; and ventilation and respiration/gas exchange. She is functionally limited in self-care and in play actions, tasks, and activities. Kelsey's diagnosis for this episode of care is impaired neuromotor development. These findings are consistent with placement in Pattern B: Impaired Neuromotor Development. The identified impairments and functional limitations will be addressed in determining the prognosis and the plan of care.

Prognosis and Plan of Care

Over the course of the visits, the following mutually established goals have been determined:

◆ Kelsey assists with dressing and undressing

◆ Kelsey explores her environment by climbing over objects, on and off the sofa, and into a small rocking chair without assistance

◆ Kelsey maintains a stable trunk during sitting while she plays with a toy with two hands

◆ Kelsey quickly catches herself with her hands when her center of gravity is displaced during sitting

◆ Kelsey takes independent steps between objects (eg, furniture) and adults

◆ Kelsey tolerates touch to her face without crying

◆ Kelsey loses less food and liquids from her mouth during meals

◆ Muscle performance is increased

To achieve these outcomes, the appropriate interventions for Kelsey are determined. These will include: coordination, communication, and documentation; patient/client-related instruction; therapeutic exercise; functional training in self-care and home management; and functional training in work, community, and leisure integration or reintegration.

Based on the diagnosis and prognosis, it is anticipated that over the course of 2 years with 40 to 50 visits, Kelsey will demonstrate optimal neuromotor development and the highest level of functioning in the home and community within the context of her impairments, functional limitations, and disabilities. At this time, the family declined home-based services but agreed that Kelsey and her mother would attend an early intervention program provided two times per week with consultative services from physical therapy, occupational therapy, and speech therapy provided as a part of this program.

Interventions

RATIONALE FOR SELECTED INTERVENTIONS

The emphasis of Kelsey's physical therapy program will be on facilitating ambulation, improving her perceptual motor abilities, improving her balance reactions and postural control, and performing functional activities. Her endurance for gross motor activities and recreational activities also will be addressed. When Kelsey is of preschool age, she will be eligible to attend a school-based early childhood program, half a day, 5 days per week. The primary modes of interventions will be through direct services, training of staff to carry out activities throughout her day at school, plus a home program of activities. When Kelsey enters elementary school, physical therapy intervention will be provided through consultative services.

Therapeutic Exercise

Facilitating Ambulation

Children with DS have a good prognosis for developing motor skills and the average age for achieving independent ambulation is around 2 years of age.[81-83] Exercises to increase trunk stabilization, postural alignment, and LE strength and endurance will enhance ambulation skill acquisition. Ulrich and associates[84] demonstrated that children with DS who participated in treadmill training learned to stand and walk earlier than the control group. In addition, they found that, following initial training and regular support, this training could be done in the home using a small treadmill with the parent providing the practice.

Facilitating Perceptual Motor Skills, Balance, and Postural Control

Through a longitudinal study of children with DS, Connolly and associates documented that specific perceptual motor skills are delayed.[85] Using the BOTMP, these researchers identified that running speed, agility, balance, and coordination were consistently areas of deficits over time with children with DS. They hypothesized that the problems noted in balance and running speed (as related to motor planning) and in coordination (as measured by reaction times) may be related to the neuropathological changes noted with DS.

Shea studied a group of 11- to 14-year-old children with DS using the Peabody Gross Motor Developmental Scales.[86] In this study, best performances were on the receipt and propulsion (ball handling) subscales, with balance (particularly static balance) being the area of greatest difficulty. In an earlier study, Shumway-Cook and Woollacott examined the development of neural control processes underlying stance balance in typically developing children and children with DS.[87] Their study revealed that responses in children with DS showed no adaptive attenuation to changing task conditions and that the onset latencies of responses were slower than in typically developing children. These researchers hypothesized that the balance problems in children with DS do not result from hypotonia, but from deficits within higher level postural mechanisms.

Additionally, Spano and coworkers[88] studied perceptual motor competence in school-age children with DS between 4.5 and 14 years of age. Some aspects of gross motor function showed delayed development, but regular acquisition. All aspects of fine motor skills assessed were more severely impaired and did not show similar development with age. In this sample of children, accuracy and timing of tasks requiring bimanual coordination were most impaired as compared to balance and ball skills that showed more variability.

Improving Fitness and Endurance

Physical inactivity and obesity in persons with mental retardation, including those with DS, is a growing concern. Dichter in a study of 18 children with DS (ages 6 to 12 years) found that the children with DS were more flexible, had more body fat, had lower cardiorespiratory endurance, and had weaker abdominal strength than the mean scores for age-matched children without disabilities.[89] Dichter also found significant relationships among abdominal strength scores and forced vital capacity, forced expiratory volume in 1 second, peak expiratory flow rate, and forced expiratory force values.[89] The findings from the Dichter study suggested that physical fitness activities for children with DS should begin early to prevent a slowing in physical activity and the subsequent tendency toward obesity. However, physical therapists should be aware of the possibility of atlantoaxial instability that is estimated to occur in 12% to 20% of individuals with DS.[11,12] Radiographs are recommended at 2 years of age and periodically administered in childhood and adolescence. Children with asymptomatic instability typically do not require surgery, but should not engage in contact sports, gymnastics, diving, or other fitness activities that might result in injury to the cervical spine.

After the early intervention and preschool period, Kelsey may not require motor-based services other than consultative physical therapy through her school district and adaptive physical education. Kelsey's physical therapist should encourage the family to participate in school- and community-based motor programs that will address fitness and life-long leisure skills for Kelsey.

Functional Training in Self-Care and Home Management and Functional Training in Work, Community, and Leisure Integration or Reintegration

Because of the cognitive deficits associated with DS, Kelsey will be eligible for special education and related services throughout her school years. Individual education plan (IEP) goals during her academic career and eventual vocational goals and training will need to be matched to Kelsey's individual profile of motor abilities. It is anticipated that, as an adult, Kelsey will be able to function in a group home situation unless she remains at home with her parents. She also will be able to attend vocational training and work in a supervised setting within the community or through a work program for adults with developmental disabilities.

Unfortunately, recent studies have documented that many individuals with DS begin to develop dementia as they reach middle age. Cognitive changes in about one third of individuals with DS after age 35 years have been noted.[90] These cognitive changes have been associated with neuropathological changes in the brain of individuals with DS and with signs similar to patterns seen with Alzheimer's disease. Wisniewski and associates[90] identified loss of vocabulary, recent memory loss, impaired short-term visual retention, difficulty in object identification, and loss of interest in surroundings as early cognitive changes. Dalton and Crapper[91] described memory loss in persons with DS ages 39 to 58 years over a 3-year period of time. Four of the 11 subjects deteriorated over the 3 years to the point that they could no longer learn a simple discrimination task. Fenner and coworkers[92] found that the greatest decline in function was in the 45- to 49-year-old group. However, Burt and colleagues in a study of 34 adults with DS, ages 22 to 56 years, found that individuals with DS who had higher cognitive functions at the beginning of the study tended to have less problems as they aged if concrete, simple stimuli were used rather than complex stimuli.[93] Physical therapists and occupational therapists should be aware of early signs of dementia in persons with DS and be prepared to intervene as necessary to retain as much adaptive functioning as possible.

COORDINATION, COMMUNICATION, AND DOCUMENTATION

A coordinated, multidisciplinary approach is important in the management of the patient with DS. Coordination and communication will occur with occupational therapy, speech therapy, and early intervention program personnel (teachers, classroom aides). All elements of the patient's management will be documented following APTA and facility guidelines. Regular communication with the case manager for the early intervention program will occur to provide updates on Kelsey's status.

PATIENT/CLIENT-RELATED INSTRUCTION

The family will receive instruction, education, and training in a home program and updates. The family will be provided with instruction as to how to provide tactile, visual, and vestibular input in working with Kelsey on her perceptual motor, balance, and postural control skills. They will receive information on when it is appropriate to seek additional services. The *Guide* includes home health aides, day care providers, teachers, and educational aides in the definition of caregivers.

THERAPEUTIC EXERCISE

♦ Aerobic capacity/endurance conditioning
  • Games such as "chasing" used when Kelsey is on all-fours to encourage longer periods of movement
  • Holding hands with Kelsey and "dancing" to get movement in standing for longer periods of time

- Pushing a weighted cart or small but heavy baby carriage for increasingly longer distances
- Balance, coordination, and agility training
  - Playing on a small waterbed mattress as a safe environment for work on balance in sitting, all-fours, and kneeling
  - Favorite toys used to motivate Kelsey to move forward
  - Movement from standing to sitting to all-fours position with minimal assistance from physical therapist
  - Movement in environment by climbing over objects, into large box, or onto the sofa during free play
  - Practice standing balance with minimal support given at her pelvis while involved in UE play activities that require trunk rotation
- Body mechanics and postural stabilization
  - Inversion on a therapy ball leading to weightbearing support through Kelsey's arms
  - Sitting and bouncing Kelsey on the therapy ball with the physical therapist assisting in maintaining postural alignment
  - Repetitive tilting while Kelsey sits on an adult's lap; progress to having Kelsey sit on a therapy ball or peanut-shaped bolster
  - Rock back and forth on all-fours while the physical therapist approximates through the head or pelvis
- Gait and locomotion training
  - Place Kelsey in standing at a small table with the physical therapist giving assistance at pelvis to assist with weight shifting and initiation of side stepping for cruising
  - Kelsey participates in UE play activities, such as holding a large ball or toy while the physical therapist approximates through Kelsey's pelvis for correct standing alignment
  - Kelsey standing and playing with toys while the physical therapist gives minimal support at pelvis; support is gradually decreased
  - Encourage Kelsey to propel self on a small riding toy with physical therapist assisting initially with flexing and extending Kelsey's knees while keeping the heels on the floor
- Sensory processing
  - Use of a variety of touching techniques, such as infant massage, joint compression, hugging, vigorous rubbing, and squeezing of limbs to provide Kelsey with more sensory input
  - Introduction of variety of tactile materials to Kelsey during play
    - Encourage her to climb into a bin of dried beans, heavy plastic balls, or into a large cardboard box filled with pillows and blankets

- Pull Kelsey around while she lies on a blanket to increase her tolerance of movement while feeling secure
- Strength, power, and endurance training
  - Kelsey required to assist with lifting her head and flexing trunk when pulled to sitting; stroking or tapping of flexors muscles as needed by physical therapist to help initiate muscle contraction
  - Repetitive tilting of Kelsey while she sits on an adult's lap; progressing to having Kelsey sit on a therapy ball or bolster while being tilted
  - Kelsey maintaining a sitting position while the physical therapist displaces her center of gravity by pushing in various directions
  - Assisted bouncing on extended arms in a hands and knees position on a small trampoline to increase muscle co-activation
  - Kelsey playing tug of war with elastic bands with the physical therapist
  - Use of weighted, resistive toys to improve hand strength, increase sensory input, and upgrade prehension patterns
  - Kelsey required to bat or kick at a suspended balloon while in supported standing to increase UE and LE strength
  - Sitting in a small rocking chair and using legs to rock in a controlled manner

FUNCTIONAL TRAINING IN SELF-CARE AND HOME MANAGEMENT

- Self-care
  - Dressing and undressing skills
    - Putting her arms out for her sleeve during dressing
    - Pulling her sock off on command once her shoe has been removed
  - Feeding skills
    - Bringing her lower lip up and out stabilizing the cup rim during drinking
    - Moving food from the center of her mouth to the side-biting surface for chewing
  - Toileting
    - Pulling down her diaper on command
    - Indicating when she is wet

FUNCTIONAL TRAINING IN WORK, COMMUNITY, AND LEISURE INTEGRATION OR REINTEGRATION

- Play
  - Instruction in balance strategies and positioning related to play activities

- Placement in sitting on the floor for play activities
- Use of small corner chair for play when parents not available for support
- Use of a small bench for Kelsey to sit on during daily activities
- Use of a tray top to help limit throwing of toys

ANTICIPATED GOALS AND EXPECTED OUTCOMES

- ◆ Impact on impairments
  - Apprehension is decreased regarding movement activities.
  - Balance reactions and postural control are improved in all positions.
  - Her lower lip will be used to stabilize under a cup rim, when the cup is presented for drinking with minimal loss of fluid.
  - Only a minimal amount of food will be lost out of her mouth during snack time.
  - Oral motor skills for feeding and sound/speech production tasks are improved.
  - She will be able to reach laterally for a toy while sitting without loss of balance.
  - She will catch herself 50% of the time with loss of balance while on all-fours.
  - Stability is increased in all positions.
  - Strength and endurance are increased for motor activities.
  - Voluntary controlled release and pinch are developed.
- ◆ Impact on functional limitations
  - Goal-directed play is demonstrated.
  - Participation in self-care is increased.
  - She will pick up cereal independently during snack time.
  - While sitting on the floor, she will take off her shoes (laces undone) independently.
- ◆ Impact on disabilities
  - Kelsey is able to participate in home activities with her family.
- ◆ Impact on societal resources
  - Documentation occurs throughout the patient management and across settings and follows APTA's *Guidelines for Physical Therapy Documentation.*[42]
  - Kelsey's parents will have awareness of and use community resources.
  - The resources available to Kelsey and her family are maximally utilized.
- ◆ Patient/client satisfaction
  - Care is coordinated with family and any other caregivers.

- Kelsey's parents will understand the anticipated goals and expected outcomes.
- Parents and caregivers will have increased awareness of the impact of Kelsey's diagnosis across her life span.

REEXAMINATION

It is anticipated that patients placed in this pattern will require multiple episodes of care over the lifetime. Periodic reexamination and initiation of new episodes of care should occur as the patient's functional limitations or disability change. This will allow the patient to continue to be safe and effectively adapt as a result of changes in multiple factors including her own physical status, caregivers, environment, or task demands.

DISCHARGE

Kelsey is discharged from this physical therapy episode of care after attainment of her goals in a total of 48 physical therapy visits over 21 months. As Kelsey has a condition that may require multiple episodes of care throughout her life span, Kelsey's parents received education regarding factors that may trigger a call to her physical therapist for a reexamination and new episode of physical therapy care.

PSYCHOLOGICAL ASPECTS

Although Kelsey's parents have declined home-based services, education of the parents about activities that are to be stressed at home is important. Reinforcing the activities that the parents are currently doing with Kelsey, such as providing tactile, visual, and vestibular input, would be important in working on her perceptual motor, balance, and postural control skills. Additionally, the physical therapist will be an important source of information for the parents about expectations for the next stage of development and about appropriate play activities.

To address Kelsey's needs as she ages for maintaining or improving her general endurance, following directions and classroom routines, as well as the parents' desire for Kelsey to play with her peers, the physical therapist may propose that Kelsey's class participates in the Courageous Pacers[94] program as it addresses general fitness for kids and is an activity in which Kelsey could participate with the whole class. As Kelsey ages, the parents also will need to consider recreational activities that will be appropriate for her. In particular, participation in Special Olympics through Kelsey's school program should be offered as an option to direct physical therapy services. The physical therapist, however, would be available for consultation in the areas of fitness, mobility, and accessing educational activities and areas.

Case Study #2: Developmental Coordination Disorder, Attention Deficit Hyperactivity Disorder

Raymond is a 5-year-old male born at 32 weeks gestational age with a birth weight of 4 pounds 3 ounces with a diagnosis of developmental coordination disorder and attention deficit hyperactivity disorder.

PHYSICAL THERAPIST EXAMINATION

HISTORY

◆ General demographics: Raymond is a 5-year-old black male. His primary language is English. He attends a half-day, everyday kindergarten program at his neighborhood public school.

◆ Social history: Raymond lives with his mother and father, who are the primary caregivers. He has a 3-year-old younger brother, who the parents describe as doing more in motor skills than Raymond.

◆ Employment/work: Raymond is noted to be "clumsy" and is unable to perform gross and fine motor tasks as well as his peers (eg, he cannot ride a bike without training wheels, he has poor coloring skills).

◆ Growth and development: Raymond is of appropriate size for his stated age of 5 years. He was a premature infant who spent a short time in the neonatal intensive care unit (NICU) before being discharged to home. He was noted to have slightly delayed motor milestones (sat at 9 months of age, walked at 18 months).

◆ Living environment: Raymond lives in an old, two-story farmhouse on a 20-acre farm. He has some responsibilities at home for caring for the family pets (two dogs and three cats). He is to make sure that the pets have fresh water each day.

◆ General health status
 ● General health perception: Raymond has been a healthy child since birth.
 ● Physical function: He has always been considered to be a very active child. However, the parents report that he seems to need more naps than other children his age.
 ● Psychological function: Raymond is easily frustrated with motor tasks, and temper tantrums are frequent.
 ● Role function: Son, brother, grandchild, student, friend.
 ● Social function: Raymond is in a half-day kindergar-

ten program. He did not qualify for special education services but receives accommodations under a 504 plan.

◆ Social/health habits: Raymond likes to play with younger children. His mother reports that he seems to be at a similar skill level when playing with 3- and 4-year-old children.

◆ Family history: Raymond's father reports that he was "clumsy" as a child and that he still has problems with sports.

◆ Medical/surgical history: Due to his problems with coordination, Raymond's pediatrician referred him to a neurologist when he was 3 years old. Magnetic resonance imaging (MRI) was performed and no structural abnormalities of the brain were noted. He recently was evaluated by a developmental pediatrician and neuropsychologist and received dual diagnoses of DCD and ADHD. He has been placed on Ritalin. Other past medical history is noncontributory.

◆ Current condition(s)/chief complaint(s): Raymond's parents are concerned about his coordination in fine and gross motor tasks and in his inability to participate in play activities with children his chronological age. He is receiving occupational therapy and speech therapy (each two times a month) through a private agency.

◆ Functional status and activity level: Raymond has difficulty with ADL, such as dressing, use of utensils during mealtime, tooth brushing, and bathing. He also has difficulty in using a pencil, crayon, and scissors in his kindergarten classroom. He has difficulty using playground equipment and is unable to swing himself or climb up on the stairs of a slide safely. He is unable to run, stop, and turn without falling occasionally when playing on the playground. He is unable to kick or catch a ball.

◆ Medications: Ritalin.

◆ Other clinical tests
 ● The PDMS[79] were used to determine Raymond's degree of gross motor delays. He was found to be functioning at the 28-month level in his stationary skills, at the 26-month level in his locomotor skills, and at the 30-month level in his object manipulation skills. His gross motor quotient was 64 (>2 SD below the mean).
 ● The Sensory Profile[95] was used to determine if Raymond had sensory processing problems particularly related to tactile processing since he disliked having his face washed, his hair washed, or wearing new clothes. Raymond was found to have definite differences (>2 SD below the mean) in his auditory, vestibular, touch, and multisensory processing. He scored probable differences (at or above 2 SD below the mean) in his visual and oral sensory processing.

SYSTEMS REVIEW

- Cardiovascular/pulmonary
  - BP: WNL
  - Edema: None observed
  - HR: WNL
  - RR: WNL
- Integumentary
  - Presence of scar formation: Scars are present on Raymond's arms and legs from past injuries that have occurred when Raymond fell or bumped into objects
  - Skin color: Good
  - Skin integrity: Good
- Musculoskeletal
  - Gross range of motion: Hypermobility is noted in both proximal and distal extremities
  - Gross strength: Decreased strength in trunk and all extremities
  - Gross symmetry: Symmetrical positioning and postures noted
  - Height: 44" (1.12 m)
  - Weight: 40 lbs (18.14 kg)
- Neuromuscular
  - Gross coordinated movements: Raymond appears uncoordinated and "clumsy"
- Communication, affect, cognition, language, and learning style
  - Raymond previously was assessed using the BSID-II,[77] and no mental delays were documented
  - Raymond observes other children his age but does not interact with them, but does play with children who are younger than he is
  - Raymond has age-appropriate receptive language skills but does not retain new information without frequent repetition

TESTS AND MEASURES

- Aerobic capacity/endurance
  - Raymond was able to walk on the treadmill for 5 minutes at a slow speed without incline
  - Endurance for age-appropriate activities, such as soccer, is decreased compared to his peers as noted by participation limited by frequent "rest breaks"
- Anthropometric characteristics: Average height and weight for his age
- Arousal, attention, and cognition
  - Raymond's attention span has improved since he began taking medication
  - He still has difficulty with selective attention and often has to be redirected to task

- Formal IQ testing, by the psychologist, on the Stanford-Binet suggests average intelligence
- Raymond has an expressive language delay, often omitting consonants in words and words in sentences
- Assistive and adaptive devices: None
- Cranial and peripheral nerve integrity: WNL and vision and hearing are normal
- Ergonomics and body mechanics
  - Raymond demonstrates trunk instability during movement, self-care, and play activities
  - He has difficulty maintaining a stable posture when using arms or legs for activities
- Gait, locomotion, and balance
  - Raymond walks independently, but occasionally walks on his toes
  - Raymond tends to walk with stiff legs and decreased arm swing
  - He often leans forward as he walks
  - He can walk with a heel-toe gait when reminded
  - He tends to walk too quickly with poor balance, often bumping into environmental objects or other people
  - He cannot walk a 4-inch balance beam without falling off and can only maintain his balance on each foot for 1 to 2 seconds
- Integumentary integrity: Normal
- Joint integrity and mobility: Normal to hypermobile
- Motor function
  - Raymond does not have an abnormal neurological examination that would indicate impaired motor control, although he is consistently characterized as being "clumsy"
  - He has difficulty varying the speed of movement and coordinating UEs and LEs, such as required when performing jumping jacks
  - He has motor planning problems and has difficulty learning new motor tasks
  - He requires more practice than his peers to master each motor skill
  - Skills are not easily generalized
- Muscle performance
  - Raymond has poor muscle definition throughout his body, particularly noticeable in the shoulders and hips
  - He tends to lock his elbows into extension when in an all-fours position
  - His hands also appear to have decreased palmar arches and his hands are "flat" when he bears weight on his hands
  - UE strength is decreased for his age
    - For example, he has difficulty supporting his

weight on his arms to "wheelbarrow" as he either collapses or locks his elbows then cannot unweight one arm to move the other

♦ Neuromotor development and sensory integration
  • Raymond ambulates independently
  • He can run, although he does so in a poorly coordinated pattern
  • He cannot skip but gallops instead
  • He has difficulty with ball skills (eg, catching, throwing, dribbling) and eye-hand coordination
  • He uses a modified lateral pinch for coloring and printing
  • He occasionally demonstrates signs of tactile defensiveness

♦ Orthotic, protective, and supportive devices: Raymond wears metatarsal pads in his shoes for support for his pes planus

♦ Posture
  • In standing, his pelvis is tilted anteriorly, his knees are in genu recurvatum, and he has pes planus
  • In sitting, his pelvis is tilted posteriorly, he sits on his sacrum, his trunk is kyphotic, his shoulders are rounded, and his neck is hyperextended

♦ Range of motion: UEs and LEs and trunk are WNL

♦ Reflex integrity: Normal

♦ Self-care and home management
  • Raymond has difficulty using utensils during meals and prefers finger foods
  • He is independent in dressing, but has difficulty with buttons, snaps, and zippers
  • He prefers Velcro closures for his shoes, t-shirts, and sweatpants
  • He is independent in toileting, but needs to be monitored to do an adequate job with bathing and tooth brushing

♦ Sensory integrity
  • Testing indicates problems with tactile discrimination, kinesthesia, and stereognosis

♦ Ventilation and respiration/gas exchange: Normal

♦ Work, community, and leisure integration or reintegration
  • Raymond prefers video games to gross motor play
  • He avoids physical activity and group sports
  • His parents have been encouraged to explore community resources for Raymond (eg, swimming, karate classes, T-ball, soccer) and to encourage his participation

EVALUATION

Raymond is a 5-year-old child with medical diagnoses of DCD and ADHD. The examination revealed that Raymond has poor muscle definition throughout his body, particularly noticeable in the shoulders and hips with poor stability in weightbearing positions. He tends to lock his elbows into extension when in an all-fours position. Raymond ambulates independently. He can run, although he does so in a poorly coordinated pattern. He has difficulty with in-hand manipulation when using pencils or eating utensils. He continues to need assistance with ADL (eg, dressing, personal hygiene, and utensil usage at mealtimes).

DIAGNOSIS

Raymond has a medical diagnosis of DCD and ADHD. He has impaired: arousal, attention, and cognition; gait, locomotion, and balance; joint integrity and mobility; motor function; muscle performance; neuromotor development and sensory integration; posture; and sensory integrity. He is functionally limited in self-care and home management and in play, community, and leisure actions, tasks, and activities. Raymond's diagnosis for this episode of care is impaired neuromotor development and sensory integration. These findings are consistent with placement in Pattern B: Impaired Neuromotor Development. The identified impairments and functional limitations will be addressed in determining the prognosis and the plan of care.

PROGNOSIS AND PLAN OF CARE

Over the course of the visits, the following mutually established goals have been determined:
♦ Balance reactions and postural control are improved
♦ Endurance for gross motor activities is improved
♦ Frequency of practice of self-selected motor activities is improved
♦ Motor planning skills are improved
♦ Parents' awareness and use of community resources is increased
♦ Parents' awareness of the impact of Raymond's conditions is increased
♦ Participation occurs with peers in age-appropriate gross motor activities
♦ Self-care activities are completed independently
♦ Speech/sound production skills are improved
♦ Upper and lower body strength is improved

To achieve these goals, the appropriate interventions for this patient are determined. These will include: coordination, communication, and documentation; patient/client-related instruction; therapeutic exercise; functional training in self-care and home management; and functional training in work, community, and leisure integration or reintegration.

Based on the diagnosis and prognosis, it is anticipated that Raymond would complete this episode of care with 24 physical therapy visits over the next 12 months. He will continue to receive occupational therapy and speech therapy (each two times a month) through a private agency. When he enters public school for first grade, he will need to be reassessed by an educational team that includes school therapy staff to determine his level of functioning in the school and needs for special education and related services. Intervention in the school program should be based on his functional needs. It is anticipated that Raymond will need periodic, episodic interventions during his academic career. Raymond may be discharged from private physical therapy services when he enters first grade or when anticipated goals and expected outcomes are met.

INTERVENTIONS

RATIONALE FOR SELECTED INTERVENTIONS

Therapeutic Exercise

The emphasis of Raymond's physical therapy program will be on improving motor planning skills, increasing body strength, increasing endurance for gross motor activities, and improving balance and postural reactions. Recreational activities also will be addressed. The primary mode of intervention will be through direct services plus a home program of activities. When Raymond enters first grade he will be reevaluated to determine if he qualifies for special education and related services. It is anticipated that he may require periodic reexamination and consultative services as he ages.

Improving Motor Planning

Treatment approaches that are used by physical therapists with children with DCD are based on a blending of "bottom-up" and "top-down" approaches. Bottom-up approaches include:

♦ Sensory integration

♦ Process-oriented treatment

♦ Perceptual motor training

♦ A combination of these three approaches[96]

Sensory integration therapy focuses on providing the child with sensory stimulation (tactile, proprioceptive, and vestibular) that is designed to promote motor development and motor learning.[97] Kinesthesia is the important component of process-oriented treatment as designed by Laszlo and Bairstow.[62] Perceptual motor training programs provide children with a wide variety of motor experiences

and opportunities to practice skills. Over the past 15 years, research comparing the effects of sensory integration, perceptual motor training, physical education, and tutoring suggests that sensory integration is as effective as any other intervention in improving motor skills.[98-103] Research on the process-oriented approach is inconclusive with some results indicating that the approach is as effective as sensory integration and cognitive-affective training, while other studies indicate that no benefit was obtained.[104-106]

Top-down approaches include:

♦ Task-specific intervention

♦ Cognitive approaches

These approaches emphasize a problem-solving approach to motor skill acquisition.[96] In task-specific intervention, the child focuses on learning of a specific task. However, Revie and Larkin,[107] in an investigation of teaching a child to perform a specific motor task (ie, throw a ball and hop or to catch and bounce a volleyball and target shoot), found that significant gains occurred in the skill, but transfer to other tasks was not seen. Two cognitive approaches, the Cognitive Motor Approach and the Cognitive Orientation to Daily Occupational Performance (CO-OP), have been proposed.[108,109] In these approaches, the physical therapist acts as a coach by helping the child decide how to improve motor performance for a specific task. Preliminary evidence seems to indicate that CO-OP is effective in enabling skill acquisition in children with DCD and in generalization and transfer of skills.[110,111]

Increasing Body Strength

Although body strength is not thought to be a primary impairment in children with DCD, body strength has been identified as a secondary impairment. Raynor[112] found that children with DCD between the ages of 6 to 10 years produced lower levels of maximal strength and power during knee extension and flexion tasks when compared with normally coordinated age-matched peers. He speculated that the major contributor to this decreased strength and power was an increased level of co-activation that may be related to the lack of movement experience and programming problems. Thus, remediation programs should address strengthening programs as well as the use of bottom-up and top-down approaches in order to possibly alleviate some of the secondary impairments seen in children with DCD.

Functional Training in Self-Care and Home Management and Functional Training in Work, Community, and Leisure Integration or Reintegration

Based on the lack of conclusive evidence that one approach is better than another, most therapists use a combination of approaches and individualize therapy for the child. Revie and Larkin[107] investigated the use of task-specific intervention in teaching specific skills to children with DCD. The task-specific training resulted in significant gains for the children on the task being addressed although transfer to other tasks was not seen. This finding was similar to the findings of Polatajko and associates[104] using a process-oriented approach. Thus, Fisher[113] suggested that functional outcomes must be included in all intervention programs, along with inclusion of current theories of motor learning, since research seems to indicate that the child should practice the specific activity that is to be learned.

COORDINATION, COMMUNICATION, AND DOCUMENTATION

A coordinated, multidisciplinary approach is important in the management of the patient with DCD. Coordination and communication will occur with the private occupational therapist, the speech/language pathology clinician, and the kindergarten staff (teachers, classroom aides). Raymond qualifies for support services in the school under a Section 504 plan that was developed for him. He does not qualify for therapy services under Individuals with Disability Education Act (IDEA) since he did not qualify for special education. All elements of the patient's management will be documented following APTA and facility guidelines.

PATIENT/CLIENT-RELATED INSTRUCTION

The family will receive instruction, education, and training in a home program and updates. They will receive information on when it is appropriate to seek additional services.

THERAPEUTIC EXERCISE

◆ Aerobic capacity/endurance conditioning
  ● Walk on the family's treadmill for 7 minutes and gradually increase time
  ● Walk around the neighborhood with the parents and gradually increase the time spent in walking
  ● Ride a three-wheeler or bicycle with training wheels and increase the time he rides for enhanced endurance
  ● Participate in a swimming program at the local pool
◆ Balance, coordination, and agility training
  ● Walk on a balance beam on the playground; do the walking forward and sideward; start with a 4-inch wide beam and progress to a 2-inch beam
  ● Walk with one foot in front of the other (ie, tandem walk) on the curb in front of his house
  ● Jump on and off a small step repeatedly
  ● Sit on a hippity-hop ball and move across the room; stop and start on command; and change direction when a whistle is blown
  ● Play tag with his younger brother and parents
  ● Carry objects of various sizes and weights while he talks with the physical therapist

● Build a structure out of large blocks and climb over and under areas of the structure
◆ Body mechanics and postural stabilization
  ● Wear a weighted vest for periods of 15 to 20 minutes at a time during gross motor activities, such as walking, running, and jumping, to increase core stabilization
  ● While playing on the playground, wear a weighted "fanny pack" during gross motor activities on the playground to enhance core stabilization
  ● Schedule periodic action breaks during day
    ■ During these breaks, participate in postural stabilization activities, such as jumping in place, jumping on a small trampoline, propelling in sitting on a scooter board
  ● Use a wedged cushion in Raymond's chair and when he sits on the floor to increase extension of the back during sitting with highest part of wedge at his back
  ● Look at a storybook while lying on his stomach and propping on his arms to improve stability around his shoulders
  ● Toss bean bags into a container while standing on a small mat to improve postural stability of the trunk
  ● Participate in rhythmical, sustained movement, such as marching or bouncing
◆ Gait and locomotion training
  ● Walk around the local playground on various terrains (eg, sand, gravel, grass)
◆ Neuromotor development training
  ● Activities to improve oral motor skills
    ■ Blowing activities using musical instruments and blow toys
    ■ Cues given prior to blowing, such as pressure to the anterior chest wall to get greater respiratory depth
    ■ Use blowing bubbles through a wand or blowing a ping pong ball across the table to get more pursing of the lips
    ■ Drink through a straw at each mealtime
    ■ Encourage Raymond to chew on rubber tubing placed on the end of a pencil
  ● Use swings to increase vestibular and tactile input to hands and feet
  ● Play in ball baths and find hidden objects with hands
  ● Allow Raymond to be an artist and have him "paint" pictures on a large mirror using shaving cream or funny foam
  ● Use an upright punching bag to get tactile and proprioceptive input to Raymond's hands and UEs
  ● Wear spandex clothing for short periods of time to increase sensory organization

- Deep massages from mother to Raymond's face, abdomen, and feet prior to play sessions
- Use of "waterless" soap on hands with Raymond deeply massaging his own hands prior to fine motor activities
- Squeeze "fidgets" or balls of play clay prior to use of his hands during fine motor tasks

◆ Strength, power, and endurance training
- Use a scooter board to propel himself either in a prone (using his hands) or sitting position (using his feet or his hands)
- Use an individualized exercise video "starring Raymond" using elastic tubing and small hand weights to increase endurance
- Encourage him to participate in recreational activities, such as karate, bowling, soccer, or T-ball
- Participate in workouts with his father at the local health club using small weights on his arms and legs during the exercises
- Push/carry heavy objects, such as books, moving chairs, and play equipment, to strengthen arms, legs, and trunk
- Swing himself on a swing on the playground using his arms for pumping and his legs for pushing
- Climb up the ladder while wearing 2-pound weights around his ankles to get to the top of the slide on the playground
- Participate in play activities, such as tug of war using a rope or elastic tubing

FUNCTIONAL TRAINING IN SELF-CARE AND HOME MANAGEMENT

◆ Self-care
- Feeding skills: Use of utensils during meals instead of his fingers to manipulate food items
- Independent brushing of teeth with parental supervision
- Dressing and undressing activities to include buttoning of shirt and pants
- Toileting activities to include unzipping and zipping pants, use of appropriate hygiene

FUNCTIONAL TRAINING IN WORK, COMMUNITY, AND LEISURE INTEGRATION OR REINTEGRATION

◆ Play
- Instruction in balance strategies and positioning related to play activities, such as during T-ball, soccer, and karate.

ANTICIPATED GOALS AND EXPECTED OUTCOMES

◆ Impact on impairments
- As Raymond's performance improves, small group work with other boys with similar impairments and interests are utilized to improve motor and social skills.
- Balance reactions and postural control are improved.
- Endurance for gross motor activities is increased.
- Frequency of practice of self-selected motor activities is increased.
- Motor planning skills are improved.
- Speech/sound production skills are improved.
- Upper and lower body strength is increased.

◆ Impact on functional limitations
- Both hands are used to throw and catch a 10-inch diameter ball.
- Independent buttoning and unbuttoning large buttons on a shirt is achieved.
- Independent walking with changing speeds and directions as needed on even and uneven terrain without falling is achieved.
- Independent zipping and unzipping the zipper on his jacket after being assisted to engage the zipper is achieved.
- Self-care is completed independently.
- Utensils are used during mealtime to stab food (fork) and butter bread (knife).[42]

◆ Impact on disabilities
- Participation in community activities is achieved.
- Participation in home and family activities is achieved.
- Participation in school activities is achieved.
- Play with others on the playground is achieved.

◆ Impact on health, wellness, and fitness
- Parents encourage Raymond's participation in recreational activities, such as the community swimming program, gymnastics, soccer, or karate.
- Participation in physical activity with his peers for 15 to 20 minutes without undue fatigue is achieved.
- Participation with peers in age-appropriate gross motor activities is enhanced.
- Riding his bike (with training wheels) for 5 miles during family bike trips is achieved.

◆ Impact on societal resources
- Available resources are maximally utilized.
- Documentation occurs throughout the patient management and across settings and follows APTA's *Guidelines for Physical Therapy Documentation.*[42]
- Parents carry out Raymond's home program that will include suggestions for vestibular and proprioceptive activities.

♦ Patient/client satisfaction
  • Care is coordinated with family and any other caregivers.
  • Parents and caregivers will have increased awareness of the impact of Raymond's diagnosis.
  • Raymond's parents will have awareness of and use community resources.

REEXAMINATION

Reexamination is performed throughout the episode of care. It is anticipated that patients placed in this pattern may require multiple episodes of care over the lifetime. Periodic reexamination and initiation of new episodes of care should occur as the patient's functional limitations or disability change. This will allow the patient to continue to be safe and effectively adapt as a result of changes in multiple factors including his own physical status, caregivers, environment, or task demands.

DISCHARGE

Raymond is discharged from physical therapy after a total of 18 physical therapy visits over 12 months and attainment of his goals. As Raymond has a condition that may require multiple episodes of care throughout his life span, Raymond's parents received education regarding factors that may trigger a call to his physical therapist for a reexamination and new episode of physical therapy care.

PSYCHOLOGICAL ASPECTS

Numerous studies reveal that children with DCD are at risk for psychological problems.[114-117] Children with DCD have been noted to perceive themselves as less competent than their coordinated peers in athletic competence, scholastic competence, physical appearance, and social acceptance.[114-117] Skinner and Piek[117] suggested that this perception of incompetence may reduce the motivation of a child with DCD to participate in social and other activities at school. Psychological issues seen in the young child and adolescent with DCD must be given consideration during the goal-setting phase of any physical therapy intervention. Additionally, efforts must be made during the physical therapy intervention to protect and improve the self-perception and self-worth of the child.

REFERENCES

1. Thompson PM, Hayashi KM, Sowell ER, et al. Mapping cortical change in Alzheimer's disease, brain development, and schizophrenia. *Neuroimage.* 2004;23(Suppl 1):S2-S18.
2. Memoli F, Sapiro G, Thompson P. Implicit brain imaging. *Neuroimage.* 2004;23(Suppl 1):S179-S188.
3. Ballmaier M, Kumar A, Thompson PM, et al. Localizing gray matter deficits in late-onset depression using computational cortical pattern matching methods. *Am J Psychiatry.* 2004;161(11):2091-2099.
4. Pitiot A, Delingette H, Thompson PM, Ayache N. Expert knowledge-guided segmentation system for brain MRI. *Neuroimage.* 2004;23(Suppl 1):S85-S96.
5. Leow A, Yu CL, Lee SJ, et al. Brain structural mapping using a novel hybrid implicit/explicit framework based on the level-set method. *Neuroimage.* 2005;24(3):910-927.
6. Nolte J. *The Human Brain: An Introduction to Its Functional Anatomy.* 4th ed. St. Louis, MO: Mosby; 1999.
7. Leonard CT. *The Neuroscience of Human Movement.* St. Louis, MO: Mosby-Year Book Inc; 1998.
8. Crome L. Pathology of Down's syndrome. In: Hilliard LT, Kirman BH, eds. *Mental Deficiency.* Boston, MA: Little Brown; 1965.
9. Gath A. Cerebral degeneration in Down's syndrome. *Dev Med Child Neurol.* 1981;23:814-817.
10. Diamond LS. Orthopedic disorders in Down syndrome. In: Lott IT, McCoy EE, eds. *Down Syndrome: Advances in Medical Care.* New York, NY: Wiley Liss; 1992:111-126.
11. Cohen WI. Health care guidelines for individuals with Down syndrome. *Down Syndrome Quarterly.* 1996;1(2):1-10.
12. Pueschel SM, Siola PH, Perry CD, et al. Atlantoaxial instability in children with Down syndrome. *Pediatr Radiol.* 1981;10:129-132.
13. American Psychiatric Association. Motor skills disorder 315.40.: developmental coordination disorder. In: *Diagnostic and Statistical Manual of Mental Disorders (DSM-IV).* 4th ed. Washington, DC: American Psychiatric Association; 1994:53-55.
14. Miyahara M, Register C. Perceptions of three terms to describe physical awkwardness in children. *Res Dev Disabil.* 2000;21:367-376.
15. Missiuma C, Polatajko H. Developmental dyspraxia by any other name: are they all just clumsy children? *Am J Occup Ther.* 1995;49:619-627.
16. Hall DMB. The children with DCD. *BMJ.* 1988:296;375-376.
17. National Research Council and Institute of Medicine. From neurons to neighborhoods: the science of early childhood development. Committee on integrating the science of early childhood development. In: Shonkoff JP, Phillips DA, eds. *Board on Children, Youth, and Families, Commission on Behavioral and Social Sciences and Education.* Washington, DC. National Academy Press; 2000.
18. Carey J, ed. *Brain Facts: A Primer on the Brain and Nervous System.* Washington, DC: The Society for Neuroscience; 2002.
19. O'Hare ED, Kan E, Yoshii J, et al. Mapping cerebellar vermal morphology and cognitive correlates in prenatal alcohol exposure. *Neuroreport.* 2005;22;16(12):1285-1290.
20. Riley EP, Thomas JD, Goodlett CR, et al. Fetal alcohol effects: mechanisms and treatment. *Alcohol Clin Exp Res.* 2001;25(5 Suppl ISBRA):110S-116S.
21. Walsh D. *Why Do They Act That Way? A Survival Guide to the Adolescent Brain for You and Your Teen.* New York, NY: Free Press; 2004.

22. Gogtay N, Giedd JN, Lusk L, et al. Dynamic mapping of human cortical development during childhood through early adulthood. *Proc Natl Acad Sci U S A.* 2004;101(21):8174-8179.

23. Sowell ER, Thompson PM, Leonard CM, et al. Longitudinal mapping of cortical thickness and brain growth in normal children. *J Neurosci.* 2004;24(38):8223-8231.

24. Als H, Duffy FH, McAnulty GB, et al. Early experience alters brain function and structure. *Pediatrics.* 2004;113:846-857.

25. Elbert T, Rockstroh B. Reorganization of human cerebral cortex: the range of changes following use and injury. *Neuroscientist.* 2004;10(2):129-141.

26. Dong WK, Greenough WT. Plasticity of nonneuronal brain tissue: roles in developmental disorders. *Ment Retard Dev Disabil Res Rev.* 2004;10(2):85-90.

27. Candia V, Wienbruch C, Elbert T, Rockstroh B, Ray W. Effective behavioral treatment of focal hand dystonia in musicians alters somatosensory cortical organization. *Proc Natl Acad Sci U S A.* 2003;100(13):7942-7946.

28. Kramer AF, Bherer L, Colcombe SJ, Dong W, Greenough WT. Environmental influences on cognitive and brain plasticity during aging. *J Gerontol A Biol Sci Med Sci.* 2004;59(9):M940-M957.

29. Carper J. *Your Miracle Brain.* New York, NY: HarperCollins; 2000.

30. Eriksson PS, Perfilieva E, Bjork-Eriksson T, et al. Neurogenesis in the adult human hippocampus. *Nat Med.* 1998;4(11):1313-1317.

31. Eriksson PS. Neurogenesis and its implications for regeneration in the adult brain. *J Rehabil Med.* 2003;(Suppl 41):17-19.

32. Gage FH. Neurogenesis in the adult brain. *J Neurosci.* 2002;22(3):612-613.

33. Brown J, Cooper-Kuhm CM, Kempermann G, et al. Enriched environment and physical activity stimulate hippocampal but not olfactory bulb neurogenesis. *Eur J Neurosci.* 2003;17(10):2042-2046.

34. Leuner B, Mendolia-Loffredo S, Kozorovitshiy Y, et al. Learning enhances the survival of new neurons beyond the time when the hippocampus is required for memory. *J Neurosci.* 2004;24(34);7477-7481.

35. Schaffer DV, Gage FH. Neurogenesis and neuroadaptation. *Neuromolecular Med.* 2004;5(1):1-9.

36. Lie DC, Song H, Colamarino SA, Ming GL, Gage FH. Neurogenesis in the adult brain: new strategies for central nervous system diseases. *Annu Rev Pharmacol Toxicol.* 2004;44:399-421.

37. Schinder AF, Gage FH. A hypothesis about the role of adult neurogenesis in hippocampal function. *Physiology.* 2004;19:253-261.

38. Nyberg J, Anderson MF, Meister B, et al. Glucose-dependent insulinotropic polypeptide is expressed in adult hippocampus and induces progenitor cell proliferation. *J Neurosci.* 2005;25(17):1816-1825.

39. Miyahara N, Mobs I. Developmental dyspraxia and developmental coordination disorder. *Neuropsychol Rev.* 1995;5:245-268.

40. Chu S. Developmental dyspraxia 1: the diagnosis. *British Journal of Therapy and Rehabilitation.* 1998;5:131-138.

41. Hadders-Algra M. Early brain damage and the development of motor behavior in children: clues for therapeutic intervention? *Neural Plast.* 2001;8:31-49.

42. American Physical Therapy Association. Guide to physical therapist practice. 2nd ed. *Phys Ther.* 2001;81:9-744.

43. VanSant AF. Rising from a supine position to erect stance: description of adult movement and a developmental hypothesis. *Phys Ther.* 1988;68:1330-1338.

44. Hook EB, Lindsjo A. Down syndrome in live births by single year maternal age interval in a Swedish study: comparison with results from a New York State study. *Am J Hum Genet.* 1978;30(1):19-27.

45. Novitski E. *Human Genetics.* New York, NY: MacMillian; 1977.

46. Benda CE. *Down Syndrome.* New York, NY: Grune and Stratton; 1969.

47. Wisniewski KE. Down syndrome children often have brain with maturational delay, retardation of growth and cortical dysgenesis. *Am J Med Genet Suppl.* 1990;7:274-281.

48. Raz N, Torres IJ, Briggs MS, et al. Selective neuroanatomic abnormalities in Down's syndrome and their cognitive correlates. Evidence from MRI morphometry. *Neurology.* 1995;45:356-366.

49. Mann DMA. The pathological association between Down syndrome and Alzheimer disease. *Mech Ageing Dev.* 1988;31:99-136.

50. Wisniewski KE, Wisniewski HM, Wen GY. Occurrence of neuropathological changes and dementia of Alzheimer's disease in Down's syndrome. *Ann Neurol.* 1985;17:278-282.

51. Lai F, Williams RS. A prospective study of Alzheimer disease in Down syndrome. *Arch Neurol.* 1989;46:849-853.

52. Pueschel SM, Louis S, McKnight P. Seizure disorders in Down syndrome. *Arch Neurol.* 1991;48:318-320.

53. Fong C, Brodmer GM. Down's syndrome and leukemia. Epidemiology, genetics, cytogenetics and mechanism of leukemogenesis. *Cancer Genet Cytogenet.* 1987;28:55-76.

54. Murphy M, Epstein LB. Down syndrome (trisomy 21) thymuses have a decreased proportion of cells expressing high level of TCRα, β and CD3: a possible mechanism for diminished T cell function in Down syndrome. *Clinical Immunology and Immunopathology.* 1990;55:453-467.

55. Cuadrado E, Barrena MJ. Immune dysfunction in Down's syndrome: primary immune deficiency or early senescence of the immune system? *Clinical Immunology and Immunopathology.* 1996;78:209-214.

56. Kennedy RL, Cuckle HS. Down's syndrome and the thyroid. *Clin Endocrinol.* 1992;37:471-476.

57. Ayres AJ. *Developmental Dyspraxia and Adult Onset Apraxia.* Torrance, CA: Sensory Integration International; 1985.

58. Hulme C, Smart A, Moran G. Visual perceptual deficits in clumsy children. *Neuropsychologia.* 1982;20:475-481.

59. Hulme C, Biggerstaff A, Moran G, et al. Visual, kinaesthetic and cross-modal judgments of length by normal and clumsy children. *Dev Med Child Neurol.* 1982;24:461-471.

60. Wilson PH, McKenzie BE. Information processing deficits associated with developmental coordination disorder: a meta-analysis of research findings. *J Child Psychol Psychiatry.* 1998;39:829-840.

61. Laszlo JI, Bairstow PJ, Bartrip J, et al. Clumsiness or perceptuo-motor dysfunction? In: Colley AM, Beech JR, eds. *Cognition and Action in Skilled Behaviour.* Amsterdam, The

Netherlands: Elsevier; 1988:293-309.

62. Laszlo JI, Bairstow PJ. Kinaesthesis: its measurement training and relationship to motor control. *Q J Exp Psychol.* 1983;35:411-421.

63. Bairstow PJ, Laszlo JI. Kinaesthetic sensitivity to passive movements in children and adults, and its relationship to motor development and motor control. *Dev Med Child Neurol.* 1981; 23:606-616.

64. Smyth MM, Mason US. Direction of response in aiming to visual and proprioceptive targets in children with and without developmental coordination disorder. *Hum Mov Sci.* 1998;17:515-539.

65. Smyth TR, Glencross DJ. Information processing deficits in clumsy children. *Australia Journal of Psychology.* 1986;38:13-22.

66. Wann JP, Mon-Williams M, Rushton K. Postural control and coordination disorders: the swinging room revisited. *Hum Mov Sci.* 1998;17:491-513.

67. McNab JJ, Miller LT, Polatajko HJ. The search for subtypes of DCD: is cluster analysis the answer? *Hum Mov Sci.* 2001; 20:49-72.

68. Kaplan BJ, Wilson BN, Dewey DM et al. DCD may not be a discrete disorder. *Hum Mov Sci.* 1998;17:471-490.

69. Silver LB. *The Misunderstood Child.* Blue Ridge Summit, PA: Tab Books; 1992.

70. Connolly BH. Pediatric medications. Orthopaedic Physical Therapy, Home Study Course 98-2. Orthopaedic Section, American Physical Therapy Association, 1998.

71. Durstine JL, Moore GE, eds. *ACSM's Exercise Management for Persons with Chronic Diseases and Disabilities.* 2nd ed. Champaign, IL: Human Kinetics; 2003.

72. MTA Cooperative Group. A 14-month randomized clinical trial of treatment strategies for attention-deficit/hyperactivity disorder. *Arch Gen Psychiatry.* 1999;56:1073-1086.

73. Schweitzer JB, Cummins TK, Kant CA. Attention-deficit/hyperactivity disorder. *Med Clin North Am.* 2001;85(3):757-777.

74. American Academy of Child and Adolescent Psychiatry. Practice parameter for the use of stimulant medications in the treatment of children, adolescents, and adults. *J Am Acad Child Adolesc Psychiatry.* 2002;41(2, Suppl):26S-49S.

75. Elia J, Ambrosini PJ, Rapoport JL. Treatment of attention-deficit hyperactivity disorder. *N Engl J Med.* 1999;340(10):780-788.

76. Richards G. Growth charts for Down syndrome. Available at: http://www.growthcharts.com/charts/DS/charts.htm. Accessed June 14, 2005.

77. Bayley N. *Bayley Scales of Infant Development-II (BSID-II).* 2nd ed. San Antonio, TX: The Psychological Corp; 1993.

78. Piper MC, Darrah J. *Motor Assessment of the Developing Infant.* Philadelphia, PA: WB Saunders; 1994.

79. Folio MR, Fewell RR. *Peabody Developmental Motor Scales. Examiner's Manual.* 2nd ed. Austin, TX: Pro-ed; 2000.

80. DeGangie GA, Greenspan SI. *Test of Sensory Function in Infants (TSFI).* Los Angeles, CA: Western Psychological Services; 1989.

81. Melyn M, White D. Mental and developmental milestones of noninstitutionalized Down syndrome children. *Pediatrics.* 1973;52:542-545.

82. Connolly B, Russell FF. Interdisciplinary early intervention program. *Phys Ther.* 1978;56:155-158.

83. Connolly B, Morgan S, Russell FF, et al. Early intervention with Down syndrome children: follow-up report. *Phys Ther.* 1980;60:1405-1408.

84. Ulrich DA, Ulrich BD, Angulo-Kinzler RM, et al. Treadmill training of infants with Down syndrome: evidence-based developmental outcomes. *Pediatrics.* 2001;108:84-90.

85. Connolly CH, Morgan SC, Russell FF, Fulliton WL. A longitudinal study of children with Down syndrome who experienced early intervention programming. *Phys Ther.* 1993;73:171-179.

86. Shea AM. Motor attainments in Down syndrome. In: Lister E, ed. *Proceedings of the II STEP Conference; Contemporary Management of Motor Control Problems.* Alexandria, VA: Foundation for Physical Therapy; 1991:225-236.

87. Shumway-Cook A, Woollacott MH. Dynamics of postural control in the child with Down syndrome. *Phys Ther.* 1985; 65:1315-1322.

88. Spano M, Meruri E. Rando T, et al. Motor and perceptual-motor competence in children with Down syndrome: variation in performance with age. *Eur J Paediatr Neurol.* 1999;3:7-13.

89. Dichter CG, Darbee JC, Effgen SK, Palisano RJ. Assessment of pulmonary function and physical fitness in children with Down syndrome. *Pediatric Physical Therapy.* 1993;5:3-8.

90. Wisniewski K, Howe J, Williams DF, Wisniewski HM. Precocious aging and dementia in patients with Down's syndrome. *Biological Psychiatry.* 1978;13:619-627.

91. Dalton AJ, Crapper DR. Down's syndrome and aging of the brain. In: Mittler P, ed. *Research to Practice in Mental Retardation. Biomedical Aspects.* Vol III. Baltimore, MD: University Park Press; 1977.

92. Fenner ME, Hewitt KE, Torpy DM. Down's syndrome: intellectual and behavioral functioning during adulthood. *Journal of Mental Deficiency Research.* 1987;31:241-249.

93. Burt DB, Loveland KA, Chen YW, et al. Aging in adults with Down syndrome. Report from a longitudinal study. *American Journal of Mental Retardation.* 1995;3:262-270.

94. Erson T. *Courageous Pacers.* Corpus Christi, TX. Pro-Activ Publications; 1993.

95. Dunn W. *Sensory Profile.* San Antonio, TX: The Psychological Corp; 1999.

96. Gentile AM. The nature of skill acquisition: therapeutic implications for children with movement disorders. *Medicine and Sport Science.* 1992;36:31-40.

97. Reeves GD, Cermak SA. Disorders of practice. In: Bundy AC, Lane SJ, Murray EA, eds. *Sensory Integration: Theory and Practice.* 2nd ed. Philadelphia, PA: FA Davis; 2002:71-100.

98. Densem JF, Nuthall A, Bushnell J, et al. Effectiveness of a sensory integrative program for children with perceptual-motor deficits. *J Learn Disabil.* 1989;22(4):221-229.

99. Polatajko HJ, Law M, Miller J, et al. The effect of sensory integration program on academic achievement, motor performance, and self-esteem in children identified as learning disabled: results of a clinical trial. *Occupational Therapy Journal of Research.* 1991;11:155-176.

100. Humphries TW, Wright M, Snider I, et al. A comparison of the effectiveness of sensory integration therapy and perceptual motor training in treating children with learning disabilities. *J Dev Behav Pediatr.* 1992;13:31-40.

101. Wilson BN, Kaplan BJ, Fellowes S, et al. The efficacy of sensory integration treatment compared to tutoring. *Physical and Occupational Therapy in Pediatrics.* 1992;12(1):1-35.

102. Stonefelt LL, Stein F. Sensory integrative techniques applied to children with learning disabilities: an outcome study. *Occup Ther Int.* 1998;5(4):252-272.

103. Vargas S, Camilli F. A meta-analysis of research on sensory integration treatment. *Am J Occup Ther.* 1999;53(2):189-198.

104. Polatajko HJ, McNab JJ, Anstett B, et al. A clinical trial of the process-oriented treatment approach for children with developmental coordination disorder. *Dev Med Child Neurol.* 1995;37:310-319.

105. Sims K, Henderson SE, Hulme C, et al. The remediation of clumsiness: an evaluation of Laszlo's kinaesthetic approach (part 1). *Dev Med Child Neurol.* 1996;38(11):976-987.

106. Sims K, Henderson E, Morton J, et al. The remediation of clumsiness: is kinaesthesis the answer? (part two). *Dev Med Child Neurol.* 1996;38(11):988-997.

107. Revie G, Larkin D. Task-specific intervention with children reduces movement problems. *Adapted Physical Activity Quarterly.* 1993; 10:29-41.

108. Bouffard M, Wall AE. A problem solving approach to movement skill acquisition: implications for special populations. In: Reid F, ed. *Problems in Movement Control.* Amsterdam, The Netherlands: Elsevier Science; 1990.

109. Polatajko HJ, Mandich AD, Miller LJ, et al. Cognitive orientation to daily occupational performance (CO-OP): part II–the evidence. *Physical and Occupational Therapy in Pediatrics.* 2001;20(2/3):83-106.

110. Miller LT, Polatajko HJ, Missiuna C, et al. A pilot trial of a cognitive treatment for children with developmental coordination disorder. *Hum Mov Sci.* 2001;20(1-2):183-210.

111. Martini R, Polatajko HJ. Verbal self-guidance as a treatment approach for children with developmental coordination disorder: a systematic replication study. *Occupational Therapy Journal of Research.* 1998;8:157-181.

112. Raynor AJ. Strength, power, and coactivation in children with developmental coordination disorder. *Dev Med Child Neurol.* 2001;43:676-684.

113. Fisher AG. Utilizing practiced and theory: an occupational therapy framework. *Am J Occup Ther.* 1998;52:509-521.

114. Losse A, Henderson SE, Elliman D, et al. Clumsiness in children–do they grow out of it? A 10-year follow-up study. *Dev Med Child Neurol.* 1991;33:55-68.

115. Piek JP, Dworcan M, Barrett N, et al. Determinants of self-worth in children with the without developmental coordination disorder. *International Journal of Disability, Development and Education.* 2000;47:259-271.

116. Rose B, Larkin D, Berger BG. Coordination and gender influences on the perceived competence of children. *Adapted Physical Activity Quarterly.* 1997;12:210-221.

117. Skinner RA, Piek J. Psychosocial implications of poor motor coordination in children and adolescents. *Hum Mov Sci.* 2001;20:73-94.

CHAPTER THREE

Impaired Motor Function and Sensory Integrity Associated With Nonprogressive Disorders of the Central Nervous System— Congenital Origin or Acquired in Infancy or Childhood (Pattern C)

Patricia C. Montgomery, PT, PhD, FAPTA
Barbara H. Connolly, PT, DPT, EdD, FAPTA
Joanell A. Bohmert, PT, MS

ANATOMY

The anatomy and physiology of the CNS are further detailed in Pattern B: Impaired Neuromotor Development; Pattern D: Impaired Motor Function and Sensory Integrity Associated With Nonprogressive Disorders of the Central Nervous System—Acquired in Adolescence or Adulthood; and Pattern H: Impaired Motor Function, Peripheral Nerve Integrity, and Sensory Integrity Associated With Nonprogressive Disorders of the Spinal Cord. The anatomy and physiology of the PNS are further detailed in Pattern F: Impaired Peripheral Nerve Integrity and Muscle Performance Associated With Peripheral Nerve Injury.

The CNS consists of multiple interacting loops of neurons and interneurons that contribute, along with other structures (eg, sensory receptors, the musculoskeletal system), to the control of functions, such as sensory perception, cognition, and movement.

The CNS is made up of the brain and spinal cord. The brain is composed of the cerebrum, cerebellum, and the brainstem. The cerebrum includes two cerebral hemispheres that are joined by the corpus callosum and the diencephalon. The cerebellum includes two hemispheres joined by the vermis. The brainstem includes the midbrain, pons, and medulla oblongata.[1,2]

The cerebral cortex forms the outermost structure of the brain and surrounds deeper structures of the corpus callosum and diencephalon, which are at the core of the cerebral cortex and sit on top of the brainstem and the cerebellum. The brainstem is located anterior to the cerebellum and continues on as the spinal cord. The brain is encased by the skull and surrounded by layers of tissue (meninges) that provide nutrition and protection. The spinal cord is encased in the vertebral column and is surrounded by the same tissue layers of the brain, thereby forming a continuous enclosed system. Within the brain are several areas of open space called ventricles. These areas, as well as the open space between the brain and skull (subarachnoid space), contain the cerebrospinal fluid (CSF) that bathes the brain and spinal cord.

CEREBRUM

The cerebrum is made up of two hemispheres and the diencephalon. During development the brain folds on itself, forming ridges (gyri), grooves (sulci), and deep grooves (fissures) resulting in further subdivision of the cerebral cortex. This subdivision results in five lobes in each hemisphere: frontal, parietal, occipital, temporal, and limbic.[2,3] The hemispheres are connected by the corpus callosum along the medial, inferior surface.

The frontal lobe is the most anterior lobe and is bordered by the central sulcus and lateral sulcus. Directly posterior to the frontal lobe is the parietal lobe that begins at the central sulcus and extends back to the occipital lobe. The lateral sulcus and temporal lobe form the inferior border of the parietal lobe. There is not a specific sulcus that delineates the parietal and occipital lobes or the posterior portion of the parietal and temporal lobes. The temporal lobe is the most lateral lobe, sitting under the frontal and parietal lobes and extending posteriorly to the occipital lobe. The occipital lobe is the most posterior lobe, located directly behind the parietal and temporal lobes. The limbic lobe is located on the interior of the brain under the frontal, parietal, and occipital lobes and on top of the corpus callosum.

The diencephalon is composed of the thalamus, hypothalamus, epithalamus, and subthalamus. It is located in the center of the cerebrum under the corpus callosum and on top of the brainstem. All sensory information, except olfactory, is processed in the thalamus on the way to the cerebral cortex. Motor and limbic information also is processed in the thalamus.

BRAINSTEM

The brainstem is made up of the midbrain, pons, and medulla oblongata. The midbrain is located under the diencephalon and is the first in the series of three structures of the brainstem. The pons consists of the basal pons and pontine tegmentum and is located under the midbrain, forming the floor of the fourth ventricle that is adjacent to the cerebellum. The medulla oblongata consists of an open and closed portion. The closed portion is most caudal and continues as the spinal cord. All cranial nerves, except cranial nerves I (olfactory) and II (optic), are attached to the brainstem.

BASAL GANGLIA

The basal ganglia are comprised of several bilateral structures located deep within the cerebrum and brainstem. The primary nuclei of the basal ganglia include the putamen, caudate nucleus, and globus pallidus while the substantia nigra and subthalamic nucleus are associated nuclei.[4] The caudate nucleus is a C-shaped structure located along the lateral wall of the lateral ventricle, medial to the internal capsule running through the parietal lobe turning anteriorly and terminating in the temporal lobe at the amygdala. The putamen is attached at the anterior end of the head of the caudate. The globus pallidus is located medial to the putamen, lateral to the internal capsule. The substantia nigra is located in the midbrain of the brainstem. The subthalamic nucleus is located inferior and lateral to the thalamus, medial to the internal capsule.

The nuclei of the basal ganglia are grouped and named as follows: striatum or neostriatum, composed of the caudate and putamen; pallidum or paleostriatum including the globus pallidus; and lentiform nucleus composed of the puta-

men and globus pallidus.[2-4] The basal ganglia are a part of the motor circuits that include the primary motor, premotor, and association areas of the cortex and the thalamus. The basal ganglia in each hemisphere function ipsilaterally.

CEREBELLUM

The cerebellum is located posterior to the brainstem under the occipital lobe. It is attached to the brainstem by three pairs of cerebellar peduncles. It can be divided by its transverse or longitudinal fissures. The transverse divisions result in three lobes: anterior, posterior, and flocculonodular. The longitudinal divisions result in a central vermis and two hemispheres that are further subdivided into an intermediate hemisphere, which is next to the vermis, and a lateral hemisphere.[2,3]

The cerebellum is a complex structure that has more neurons than the cerebrum. It contains the nuclei of many pathways. Each hemisphere controls the ipsilateral side of the body.

SPINAL CORD

The anatomy of the spinal cord is detailed in Pattern H: Impaired Motor Function, Peripheral Nerve Integrity, and Sensory Integrity Associated With Nonprogressive Disorders of the Spinal Cord.

SKULL

The skull provides the external covering of the brain. It is composed of bones that form two main structures: the neurocranium and the facial skeleton. The neurocranium contains the brain and its supporting structures. In the adult, the neurocranium is composed of eight bones and the facial skeleton of 14 bones. The neurocranium has a rounded top, the skullcap or calvaria, and a bottom, the cranial base. At birth the bones of the calvaria are soft and separated by six fontanelles. This allows for the rapid expansion of the brain as it grows.[1] The exterior of the skull is covered by the scalp while the interior of the skull is covered by the dura mater.

MENINGES

Cranial Meninges

The meninges consist of three layers of tissue that protect and support the brain. The outer layer is the dura mater, then the arachnoid, and finally the pia mater. The dura mater is the thickest of the three layers and attaches to the underside of the skull while the arachnoid attaches to the dura mater. The pia mater is a vascular membrane that attaches to the brain. The space between the arachnoid and the pia mater is the subarachnoid space and contains the CSF.[2]

Spinal Meninges

The spinal meninges are a continuation of the cranial meninges, except the dura mater no longer is attached to bone. The dura mater's attachment to bone ends at the foramen magnum of the skull then continues down the vertebral canal forming the dural sac, inferiorly attaching to the coccyx. The subarachnoid space continues in the vertebral canal between the arachnoid and the pia mater.

VENTRICULAR SYSTEM

The ventricular system of the brain consists of four ventricles in the brain, the subarachnoid space that surrounds the brain and spinal cord, and the CSF that bathes the brain and spinal cord.

The first and second ventricles are a pair of lateral ventricles contained in each cerebral hemisphere. The lateral ventricles are C-shaped with a posterior projection and pass through all the lobes of each hemisphere. They connect with the third ventricle through the intraventricular foramen. The third ventricle is contained between the two halves of the diencephalon and connects with the fourth ventricle through the cerebral aqueduct of the midbrain. The fourth ventricle is located posterior of the pons and anterior of the cerebellum. It has four apertures: one that communicates with the third ventricle and three that communicate with the subarachnoid space that includes the central canal of the spinal column.[1,2]

The subarachnoid space is the area between the arachnoid and the pia dura. Subarachnoid cisterns are larger spaces between the arachnoid and pia mater that form in various areas of the brain and provide a space for larger pools of CSF and the roots of the cranial nerves, arteries, and veins.[1]

CSF is produced in the choroid plexus that lines the bottom of the lateral ventricles and the top of the third and fourth ventricles. The total amount of CSF in the CNS is approximately 130 mL, of that only 25 mL is actually contained in the ventricles with the majority in the lateral ventricles.[2] The CSF produced by the ventricles circulates through the ventricular system and around the brain and spinal cord. This fluid is eventually reabsorbed over the surface of the brain and large veins that carry the fluid back to the heart.

VASCULAR SUPPLY

The anatomy of the circulatory system for the brain is detailed in Pattern D: Impaired Motor Function and Sensory Integrity Associated With Nonprogressive Disorders of the Central Nervous System—Acquired in Adolescence or Adulthood. The anatomy of the circulatory system for the spinal cord is detailed in Pattern H: Impaired Motor Function, Peripheral Nerve Integrity, and Sensory Integrity Associated With Nonprogressive Disorders of the Spinal Cord.

PHYSIOLOGY

Brain function is highly specialized based on individual programming or choice of activity. Brain function is interconnected and interdependent on other systems of the body and the environment. Much is unknown about why the nervous system develops the way it does or works the way it does and new information is being developed/discovered every day. Models of neuromotor development and brain function are changing based on new techniques to study and analyze brain function.[5-9] There is a wealth of information available in the literature, on Web sites, and in books that describes in detail the development and function of the brain and nervous system. It is not the intent of this chapter to provide the specifics of brain function but rather an overview. Readers are encouraged to access other resources for more detail.

CEREBRAL CORTEX

Pyramidal Neurons

Pyramidal neurons make up the majority of neurons in the cerebral cortex. Pyramidal neurons are coned shaped, with their dendrites extending horizontally and vertically from the cell body. They range in size from small to large and generally have a long axon that extends outside the cortex to other cortical or subcortical sites with a resultant excitatory synaptic effect.[2,3]

Nonpyramidal Neurons

All other neurons of the cerebral cortex are considered nonpyramidal neurons. Nonpyramidal neurons have a variety of structures and generally are smaller in size, are multipolar stellate or granule cells, and have short axons that remain in the cortex with a resultant inhibitory synaptic effect.[2,3]

Organization of Neurons of the Cortex

The cortex is organized horizontally in layers and vertically in columns. Ninety percent of the neocortex is arranged in six horizontal layers (homotypic areas). The type of cells contained within the layer differentiates the layers. Layers are numbered beginning on the external aspect of the neocortex then moving internally. Layers and cell types are as follows[2,3]:

  I. Molecular layer: Primarily axons and dendrites from cells in other layers

 II. External granular layer: Small granular and pyramidal neurons that mainly project to other cortical areas or laminae (interneurons)

III. External pyramidal layer: Medium and large pyramidal cells

 IV. Internal granular layer: Closely packed granular cells

  V. Internal pyramidal layer: Large pyramidal cells

 VI. Multiform (fusiform) layer: Small nonpyramidal cells with dendrite projections up through layers and axon projection down into white matter

Heterotypic areas of the neocortex are areas that do not contain the six layers, but vary in the type and amount of layers. These areas include the primary motor cortex and the primary sensory areas.

In addition to the horizontal layers, the cortex is organized in vertical columns. These columns appear to access the same body region and appear to respond to the same type of stimulus.[10] While this appears to provide an explanation for function being assigned to a specific area of the cortex, the actual performance of a task involves more than one designated area as the task requires the integration of multiple areas. Mapping of the cortex demonstrates general areas of function. Specific mapping continues to evolve and be refined with improved technology.[5-9] In general terms the brain consists of areas for motor, sensory, association, and limbic functions. The frontal lobe contains the primary motor cortex and the premotor cortex. The somatosensory cortex is contained in the parietal lobe. The general areas of the CNS function are described in Table 3-1.

Afferent fibers that originate in the same hemisphere in which they travel or terminate are called association fibers. Afferent fibers that originate on the contralateral hemisphere are called commissural fibers. Association fibers form large bundles that travel through the hemispheres, interconnecting areas within the hemisphere. Commissural fibers travel to the other hemisphere through the corpus callosum or the anterior commissure. The thalamus is the major source of subcortical afferents.

The organization of the layers and columns of the brain is significant for many reasons. An injury in one area of the brain does not just affect those skills and abilities located there but all those functions that are associated with that area. On the other hand, due to the layers and vertical organization, neurons next to an injured area may be able to take over the action of the affected area.

PLASTICITY

Neuroplasticity refers to the brain's ability to learn and adapt throughout life. It is a dynamic, ongoing process that results in multiple structural changes including synaptogenesis, dendritic sprouting, perforated synapses, and multiple synaptic boutons.[2-4,11]

There are three types of plasticity: experience-independent, experience-expectant, and experience-dependent.[12] Experience-independent plasticity occurs spontaneously in the brain and is not dependent on external input to develop. Experience-expectant plasticity requires or "expects" input in order to develop. If the external input is not provided, that area of the brain will not develop. An example of this is development of vision.[13,14] Experience-dependent plasticity is used to refine or further develop specific areas.[14,15] This is the process that is used for learning and accounts for the wide variation in brain mapping from person to person. It is the process used for motor skill acquisition and recovery following insult.[16-18] It is the idea that the brain can change based on experiences and is not regulated by genetics. It is a circular process in which experience changes brain structure and

function, and brain structure and function influence future experiences.[13] It is a neurobiological process that results in the organization and reorganization of brain maps.

Plasticity can be positive or negative. Positive plasticity occurs when the preferred skill is learned and the neural connections are expanded and refined. Negative plasticity occurs through disuse of neural pathways and the neural connections are degraded or lessened. Merzenich and coworkers reported that brain plasticity underlies perceptual, cognitive, and motor skill learning and is vital for maintenance of the brain's modulatory control and functional maintenance.[19-23] Constraints to neural plasticity include anatomical factors, time constraints, immature or dysfunctional sleeping patterns, myelinization, synaptic competition, and timing of injury and intervention.[11,24]

Plasticity does not just occur. It requires attention and practice. It must be a skilled activity that challenges the individual. It must not be too difficult, must involve the individual's desires and goals, must be highly interesting, and the individual must be committed to learn the skill. The skill must be practiced, but practice without attention or motivation to complete the task will not drive the neural changes.[11,19-23,25-28] Nonskilled activities increase angiogenesis, but not neural structures.[27,28] Once a skill is learned it becomes automatic to the brain and does not require attention to perform. An individual is at risk to degrade or lose a motor map if the skill is not used (negative plasticity).[27,28] It is important to remember that motor patterns are highly dynamic and change based on what is practiced, so if the individual practices movement that is atypical then that is what the brain learns.[11,19-23,25-28]

MOTOR CONTROL, LEARNING, AND DEVELOPMENT

Movement is a complex activity that requires the integration of multiple body systems in a very dynamic process. The nervous system contributes to movement through the control, learning, and development of motor function. VanSant[29] provides definitions of these areas from experts in various fields. Brooks, a neurophysiologist, defines motor control as "the study of posture and movements that are controlled by central commands and spinal reflexes, and is also the name given to the functions of mind and body that govern posture and movement."[30] Schmidt and Lee, who are psychologists and kinesiologists, define motor learning as a set of processes associated with practice or experience that leads to relatively permanent changes in the capacity for producing skilled action.[31] Motor development as defined by Roberton, a physical educator, is the study of life span change in motor behavior.[32] While these areas have discrete definitions, they are not discrete entities and there is interaction and shared themes, beliefs, and structures. VanSant[29] states there are different questions to ask when studying these

Table 3-1

OVERVIEW OF GENERAL FUNCTION OF THE MAJOR STRUCTURES OF THE CENTRAL NERVOUS SYSTEM

Structure	*Function*
Cerebrum	
Left hemisphere	Controls right side of body; speech, writing, language, calculation
Right hemisphere	Controls left side of body; spatial abilities, face recognition in vision, music perception and production
Frontal lobe	Initiation of voluntary movement; production of written and spoken language; personality, insight, foresight; executive functions; higher intellectual functions; regulates emotions
Parietal lobe	Initial processing of somatosensory information; comprehension of language; spatial orientation and perception; attention
Temporal lobe	Hearing; comprehension of language; visual perception; speech, language; memory; emotion
Occipital lobe	Vision
Limbic lobe	Emotions; memory; internal drives; biological rhythms
Corpus callosum	Connects right and left cerebral hemispheres; aids in communication between cerebral hemispheres
Diencephalon	
Thalamus	Receives all sensory information
Hypothalamus	Autonomic nervous system; regulation of pituitary function; regulates sleep and appetite; works with limbic system
Brainstem	Conveys information to/from cerebrum to spinal cord/peripheral system; regulates respiration and heart rhythms; reflexes
Midbrain	Regulation of respiration, HR, pain perception, and movement
Pons	Regulation of respiration, HR, conveys information to/from forebrain to spinal cord/ peripheral system
Medulla oblongata	Regulation of vasomotor, cardiac, respiratory; center for cough, gag, swallow, and vomit
Reticular system	Wakefulness; modify sensory input; emotional overlay of motor control; level of alertness
Basal ganglia	Motor processing and motor learning; executing and completing motor sequences; initiation and control of movement and motor planning; scaling of movement (velocity, amplitude, direction); anticipatory and compensatory postural reactions, protective reactions
Caudate	Establishes motor goals and general motor plans; releases GABA which is inhibitory
Putamen	Initiates motor command; eye-hand coordination, balance; releases GABA which is inhibitory
Globus pallidus	Scaling of motor commands
Substantia nigra	Activates other areas of basal ganglia; provides signal to start movement; produces dopamine which is excitatory
Subthalamus	Comparator of motor plan with actual commands

continued

Structure	Function
Cerebellum	Participates in programming of voluntary movement; feedforward and feedback; motor learning and motor programming; equilibrium; balance; coordination of voluntary movement; muscle tone; execution of movement; regulation of muscle forces; comparator function for movement as occurs to what was intended; sequencing of muscle contraction
Vermis	Postural adjustments; eye movements
Lateral hemispheres	Motor planning; speed, timing, and accuracy of movement; acquisition of skilled movement especially for those that become more rapid and precise; impacts ipsilateral side of the body
Intermediate zone	Adjusting limb movements
Flocculus	Equilibrium; slow coordinated eye movements
Spinal cord	Conductor of neural messages (sensory and motor); reflexive activities include regulation of muscle force and length; releases GABA which is inhibitory, spinal pattern generators produce rhythmic stepping
Skull	Protects the brain
Meninges	Protect and support the brain; support vascular system; encase CNS and hold CSF
Ventricular system	Produces and contains CSF that bathes the brain and spinal cord
Vascular supply	Provides nutrients and oxygen and blood supply for CNS

Table 3-1 (continued)

OVERVIEW OF GENERAL FUNCTION OF THE MAJOR STRUCTURES OF THE CENTRAL NERVOUS SYSTEM

areas. For motor control the question is "How is the control of motor behavior organized?" For motor learning it is "How is motor behavior acquired through practice and repetition?" And, for motor development it is "How does motor behavior change with age?" Another difference between these three areas is the time scale over which they occur, with motor control occurring within milliseconds; motor learning over hours, days, or weeks; and motor development happening over months and years. Table 3-2 provides a comparison of motor control, motor learning, and motor development.

Newton[4] describes the neural systems that underlie motor control as the sensory systems, spinal mechanisms, basal ganglia, cerebellum, and cerebral cortex. The three primary areas believed involved in motor learning are the basal ganglia, cerebellum, and cerebral cortex.[4] Motor behaviors are not housed in a specific area of the brain but are rather an emergent property that is the result of a highly interactive system with extensive interconnections and feedback loops. This model of motor control is considered to be a systems model.

In a systems model, movement is dependent on the interaction of the individual with the environment and the specific task. Sensory input of all types is critical to the selection and learning of movement. The individual's prior

experience and understanding of the requirements and the actual environment modify how the task will be performed. The physical environment and task can act to facilitate or restrain motor behavior as can the individual's musculoskeletal system. A systems model allows movement to be flexible to meet the needs of the individual as he or she controls, learns, and develops movement. A systems model replaces the hierarchical model of the CNS, as well as that of a required developmental sequence. The implications are that physical therapists need to not only evaluate the patient but also the environment and the context in which the movement is to occur.

PATHOPHYSIOLOGY

CEREBRAL PALSY

Cerebral palsy (CP) is a neurodevelopmental disorder of the immature CNS related to nonprogressive defects or lesions in single or multiple locations that occur in the prenatal, perinatal, or neonatal periods. It relates to the functioning of neurons and interneurons within various areas of the CNS. CP is a complex of symptoms that is the result

Table 3-2

MOTOR CONTROL, LEARNING, AND DEVELOPMENT: A COMPARISON

Motor control	Control and organization of processes underlying motor development	Milliseconds
Motor learning	Acquisition of skill through practice and experience	Hours, days, weeks
Motor development	Age-related processes of change in motor behavior	Months, years, decades

Reprinted with permission from VanSant A. Motor control, motor learning, and motor development. In: Montgomery PC, Connolly BH, eds. *Motor Control and Physical Therapy.* 2nd ed. Thorofare, NJ: SLACK Incorporated; 2001.

of heterogeneous etiologies[33] and patterns of brain damage that also are heterogeneous.[34] Several studies have documented areas of brain damage in children with CP.[34-36] In children with spastic diplegia, the periventricular white matter primarily is affected. Periventricular leukomalacia (PVL) typically occurs in premature infants and is characterized by multifocal areas of necrosis in the cortical white matter, often symmetrical and adjacent to the lateral ventricles.[37] One study of children with PVL corroborated the hypothesis that involvement of pyramidal tract fibers is related to motor dysfunction.[35] Children with spastic quadriplegia may have cortico-subcortical lesions and hypoplasia of the corpus callosum. Unilateral brain lesions are typical in children with hemiplegia, who also may have damage to white matter, cortico-subcortical lesions, and congenital brain malformations. Dyskinesias in children with CP are characterized by alterations of the basal ganglia and the thalamus. No clear significant correlations exist between neurological signs and abnormalities with brain imaging in children with ataxia.[36,38] However, in children with abnormalities of the cerebellum, clinical symptoms usually include ataxia and general incoordination. The strongest risk factors for CP include prematurity and low birth weight.[39] In a study of etiologies in 217 children with CP, Shevell and coworkers[33] listed the top five etiologic entities as PVL, intrapartum asphyxia, cerebral dysgenesis, intracranial hemorrhage, and vascular causes. Children with CP may demonstrate a combination of symptoms, such as motor problems (eg, poorly controlled movements, disorders of muscle tone), intellectual impairments (ie, mental retardation or learning disabilities), speech disorders, and sensory problems (eg, visual, auditory, somatosensory, vestibular).

SPINA BIFIDA

Myelodysplasia refers to defective development of any part of the spinal cord.[40] Myelomeningocele relates to the spinal cord, spinal nerves, and their sensory and motor functions, as well as to associated functions of the brain and brainstem. Spina bifida is the common term used to describe various forms of myelodysplasia that are a result of neural tube defects (NTDs). The specific cause of spina bifida is unknown but there appears to be a genetic component, as well as environmental factors. Risk factors for spina bifida include previous NTD-affected pregnancy, insulin-dependent diabetes, antiseizure medications (valproic acid and carbamazapine), medically diagnosed obesity, high temperatures early in pregnancy (hot tubs, high fever), race (more prevalent in white individuals than black and more common in Hispanic individuals than non-Hispanic), and lower socioeconomic status. The lack of folic acid in women also has been identified as a risk factor. The US Public Health Service (USPHS) recommends that 0.4 mg (400 micrograms) of folic acid be consumed daily by all women of childbearing age. Due to NTDs occurring in the first month of pregnancy, the USPHS recommends beginning consumption of folic acid at least 3 months before trying to conceive. The Centers for Disease Control and Prevention (CDC) estimates a decrease in NTDs of at least 50% just through the consumption of recommended amounts of folic acid.[41]

Spina bifida is a NTD that results from failure of the spine to close properly in the first month of pregnancy. Spina bifida occulta occurs when one or more vertebrae are malformed, but are covered by a layer of skin. This is the least serious form of spina bifida. Meningocele occurs when the spinal cord develops normally, but the meninges protrude from a spinal opening. Myelomeningocele is a NTD that usually protrudes dorsally. The protruding sac may contain CSF, blood vessels, nerves, spinal cord, and meninges. Myelomeningoceles are not totally covered by skin and typically are associated with paralysis of spinal nerves. Surgery to close the NTD generally is performed within 24 hours after birth to minimize the risk of infection and to preserve existing function of the spinal cord. Myelomeningoceles result from a failure of neural tube closure ("neurulation") early in embryonic development. Myelocystoceles are the least common type of myelodysplasias.[40] They are separate or septated cysts which are separate from the central canal of the spinal cord and from the subarachnoid space. These usually occur in the low lumbar and sacral area and may or may not be associated with nerve impairment.

Additional neurological problems associated with abnormal neurulation include Arnold-Chiari Type II, mental retardation, cranial nerve palsies, and hydrocephalus. In hydrocephalus, there is a build-up of fluid in the brain that must be treated to avoid injury and possibly death. Shunts placed in the brain channel the fluid from the ventricles to another site, typically into the abdominal cavity (ventricular-peritoneal [VP]) where the fluid is absorbed. Problems with shunts (eg, infections, blockage) may be associated with vomiting, irritability, delay or loss of developmental milestones, and failure to thrive. Arnold-Chiari Type II is a malformation of the brainstem, cerebellum, and upper spinal cord that results in compression of these structures that may also disrupt the flow of CSF and increase intracranial pressure. Symptoms on Arnold-Chiari Type II problems include those of shunt dysfunction and brainstem dysfunction (difficulty breathing, weak sucking response, difficulty feeding, inability to swallow, and weakness or numbness in arms). Interventions include shunt revision and/or decompression surgery. Orthopedic problems may include equinovarus of the ankle (clubfoot), contractures (hip, knee, ankle), and spinal deformities.

Clinical tests for spina bifida may include the following:

♦ A screening blood test for alpha-fetoprotein (AFP) can be administered, as pregnant women carrying babies with NTDs may have high levels of AFP.

♦ Ultrasonography can be used in utero to define cranial malformations associated with myelomeningocele.

♦ Amniotic fluid analysis (from amniocentesis) can be used to detect possible birth defects, including NTDs.

IMAGING

Advances in neuroimaging provide methods to evaluate brain structure, biochemistry, and function.[42,43] Cranial ultrasonography and nuclear magnetic resonance modalities (ie, MRI and diffusion-weighted imaging) are two methods currently used. Computed tomography (CT) scans[36] and electroencephalograms (EEGs)[44] also may be useful in diagnosing brain abnormalities or lesions and detecting the presence of seizure activity.

♦ Computerized axial tomography (CAT, CT)
  • Uses low dose x-rays
  • Allows for accurate analysis of cerebral injury

♦ MRI
  • Uses a magnetic field (no radiation)
  • Gives detailed pictures of the brain

PHARMACOLOGY

CEREBRAL PALSY

Pharmacologic intervention usually is provided to address the symptoms of CP, especially spasticity. Phenol blocks or injections of botulinum A toxin[45] may be used to decrease spasticity in specific muscle groups. Baclofen also is intended to decrease spasticity.[46]

In addition, medications often are indicated in children with CP who have a seizure disorder. Physicians monitor anticonvulsant drug levels in the bloodstream to determine/adjust dosage.

♦ Anticonvulsants
  • Examples: Carbamazepine (Tegretol), clonazepam (Klonopin), ethosuximide (Zarontin), phenobarbital, phenytoin (Dilantin), primidone (Mysoline), valproic acid (Depakene)[47]
    ▪ Physicians monitor drug level in the bloodstream to determine/adjust dosage
  • Actions: Inhibit spread of seizure activity; inhibit spike and wave formation; decrease amplitude, frequency, duration, and spread of discharge in seizures
  • Side effects: Headaches and dizziness; ataxia; skin conditions (dermatitis or rash); very high doses may result in lethargy or drowsiness, interfering with ability to participate in requested activities

♦ Neuromuscular blocking agents
  • Botulinum toxin type A
    ▪ Examples: Botox, Dysport, Myobloc (botulinum toxin type B)
    ▪ Action: A chemodenervator that blocks Ach (acetylcholine) released at the neuromuscular junction to decrease spasticity in a specific muscle group[45]
    ▪ Administered: Injected into the selected muscle
    ▪ Duration of effectiveness: UE 4 to 6 months; LE 6 to 8 months
    ▪ Side effects: Pain with injection, hematoma, transient fatigue, or nausea[48]
  • Phenol blocks
    ▪ Example: Phenol
    ▪ Action: A chemodenervator or neuromuscular blocking agent that destroys the protein to decrease spasticty
    ▪ Administered
      ▸ Injected into the motor points or nerve trunks of the selected muscle
      ▸ Technically difficult to administer; may need local anesthesia during administration
    ▪ Duration of effectiveness: 4 to 12 months
      ▸ Cumulative effect can occur

- Side effects
  - ▸ Transient dysaesthesias (15%) and numbness
  - ▸ Hematomas possible
  - ▸ With large intravascular injection, systemic effects may include muscle tremors, convulsions, and depressed cardiac activity, BP, and respiration
- Intrathecal baclofen
  - Example: Lioresal intrathecal
  - Actions
    - ▸ Inhibits monosynaptic and polysynaptic reflexes at spinal level by decreasing gamma aminobutyric acid (GABA) to decrease spasticity
    - ▸ Mixed outcomes[49]: Some children demonstrated improvements while others demonstrated worsening of speech and decrease in appetite, self-feeding, and saliva control
  - Administered
    - ▸ Continuous infusion pump implanted into abdomen with tube inserted into spinal column with the intent to decrease spasticity[46]
    - ▸ To refill pump, medication injected through skin into pump
  - Side effects
    - ▸ Hypotonia and lethargy were the two most common adverse events to occur with intrathecal baclofen[50]
    - ▸ Dizziness, fatigue, weakness, drowsiness, disorientation, seizures
    - ▸ Bowel movement frequency decreased in some children
    - ▸ Complications associated with pump may include blockage or kinking of catheter, dislodgement, infection, or malfunction of the pump that can result in overdose or withdrawal from baclofen
    - ▸ Signs of overdose include confusion, sedation, hypotonia, weakness, respiratory distress, and coma
    - ▸ Signs of withdrawal include hallucinations, spasticity, tachycardia, hyperthermia, purities, and agitation

SPINA BIFIDA

Medications may be required in relation to a neurogenic bowel (stool softeners, such as Senokot or suppositories). Antiseizure medication also is indicated for some children. Although uncommon, patients with myelomeningocele may develop spasticity. If surgical efforts with untethering of the spinal cord and posterior fossa decompression fail to improve symptoms, intrathecal baclofen administered through a surgically implanted pump may be an option.[51]

Case Study #1: Cerebral Palsy, Spastic Diplegia

Miguel is a 24-month-old male born at 29 weeks gestation with a current medical diagnosis of cerebral palsy with spastic diplegia.

PHYSICAL THERAPIST EXAMINATION

HISTORY

- ◆ General demographics: Miguel is a 24-month-old male of Hispanic descent. Spanish is the primary language in the home, and his older brothers are fluent in both English and Spanish. Miguel speaks a mixture of English and Spanish.
- ◆ Social history: Miguel lives with his mother, father, maternal grandmother, and two older brothers (ages 4 and 8 years).
- ◆ Employment/work: Miguel enjoys age-appropriate play activities.
- ◆ Growth and development: At 6 months of chronological age, marked stiffness was noted in Miguel's LEs. At 10 months of age (7 months corrected age), Miguel was unable to maintain a sitting position when placed and had not yet mastered rolling. By 18 months Miguel was able to sit independently when placed, was able to belly crawl, and was beginning to try to move on his hands and knees.
- ◆ Living environment: Miguel lives in an apartment building on the third floor. There are stairs with a hand rail and an elevator. A small playground and swimming pool are part of the apartment complex.
- ◆ General health status
  - General health perception: Miguel has had several respiratory infections since being discharged from the NICU.
  - Physical function: Miguel does not sleep well during the night. He fatigues quickly. He moves on all-fours, sits independently, and pulls to stand.
  - Psychological function: Miguel generally is a happy child and healthy when he does not have a respiratory infection.
  - Role function: Son, brother, grandchild, toddler.
  - Social function: Miguel enjoys age-appropriate play and communicates well with his siblings. He has had limited opportunities to interact with same-age peers.
- ◆ Social/health habits: His mother smokes approximately half a pack of cigarettes a day, but reported that she did

not smoke during her pregnancy. She does not smoke in the home due to Miguel's respiratory problems. His father is a nonsmoker.

♦ Family history: Noncontributory.

♦ Medical/surgical history: Miguel was born prematurely at 29 weeks gestational age. He was noted on an MRI to have PVL. He was on mechanical ventilation for 1 month after birth and discharged after 3 months in the NICU.

♦ Current condition(s)/chief complaint(s): His parents are concerned about Miguel's difficulty in moving around his environment. They also have expressed concern that he may have difficulty walking. On discharge from the NICU, Miguel was referred for early intervention through his local school district. He has been receiving one visit each week from a teacher, with consultations for his Individual Family Service Plan (IFSP) objectives and intervention with the school occupational, physical, and speech therapists. Miguel also is being followed once a week by a physical therapist from a private agency specifically to address his gross motor delay.

♦ Functional status and activity level: Miguel is able to roll consecutively and to belly crawl (using primarily his UEs). He can move on all-fours by "bunny hopping" (ie, symmetrical pattern). He is beginning to use a reciprocal pattern, but this is more fatiguing for him. Miguel can transition in and out of sitting and on to hands and knees independently. He sits well independently, preferring to "W-sit" to free his hands for play. He can pull to stand with assistance, and attempts to cruise two or three "steps" along furniture.

♦ Medications: None.

♦ Other clinical tests
   ● The BSID-II[52] provides both a mental and a motor scale and is a norm-referenced test with high inter-rater reliability (motor r=0.75; mental r=0.96). The BSID-II indicated cognitive abilities within age expectations.
   ● The Gross Motor Function Measure (GMFM)[53] was selected to measure change in gross motor function over time and has been demonstrated to be a valid measure of change in children with CP. The GMFM indicated major deficits in crawling and kneeling (Dimension C) and standing (Dimension C) and inability to complete any items in walking, running, and jumping (Dimension E).
   ● The BSID-II and the GMFM were selected by the NICU staff as part of a protocol for following children discharged from the NICU until they reached 3 years (adjusted age).
   ● The PDMS[54] was administered by school staff to provide additional information to determine needs for special education and physical therapy and occu-

pational therapy services. The PDMS provides measures of gross and fine motor skills from birth to 6 years of age, is norm-referenced with high interrater reliability (r=0.96 to 0.99), and can be administered in 45 to 60 minutes depending on the age of the child. Based on the school's criteria of receiving a score >2.0 SD below the mean on the total motor quotient, Miguel qualified for special education and demonstrated need for physical and occupational therapy services.

♦ The Pediatric Evaluation of Disability Inventory (PEDI)[55] was administered by the physical therapist from the private agency, documenting significant delays in gross motor, self-care, and mobility skills for the third-party payer. The PEDI was selected because it provides information on functional skills, the amount of caregiver assistance needed by the child, and modifications that need to be made to enable the child to perform functional tasks. Miguel received raw scores of 19 in the Self-Care domain, 9 in the Mobility domain, and 31 in the Social domain on the PEDI. Standard scores placed him >2.0 SD below the mean for his age group in Self-Care and Mobility. His standard score on the Social domain was WNL (-1.0 SD).

SYSTEMS REVIEW

♦ Cardiovascular/pulmonary
   ● BP: 85/55 mmHg
   ● Edema: None observed
   ● HR: 120 bpm
   ● RR: 24 bpm

♦ Integumentary
   ● Presence of scar formation: None
   ● Skin color: Good
   ● Skin integrity: Good

♦ Musculoskeletal
   ● Gross range of motion
     ▪ WNL in UEs
     ▪ Tightness in LEs at end range of hips, knees, and ankles
   ● Gross strength
     ▪ Good in UEs: Miguel is able to support his body weight on his arms during creeping; uses his arms during pull to stand and lifts age-appropriate toys during play
     ▪ Moderate stiffness in LEs generally noted throughout the legs with all movement, but does not prevent movement
   ● Gross symmetry: Symmetrical positioning and postures noted
   ● Height: 34" (0.864 m)

- Weight: 28 lbs (12.7 kg)
♦ Neuromuscular
  - Gross coordinated movements
    ▪ UE movements appear well coordinated
    ▪ Problems with LE movements (stiffness, symmetrical movements rather than isolated movements, poor voluntary control)
♦ Communication, affect, cognition, language, and learning style
  - Miguel speaks a mixture of Spanish and English
  - Parents speak primarily Spanish at home but do speak English
  - Older brothers speak fluent English and serve as translators when necessary during treatment sessions, primarily when the grandmother (who does not speak English) is present during sessions
  - Miguel enjoys watching and interacting with his brothers
  - Parents prefer home programming suggestions and activities in which all of the boys may participate

TESTS AND MEASURES

♦ Aerobic capacity/endurance
  - Miguel fatigues easily and breathiness is noted during vigorous physical activities
♦ Anthropometric characteristics
  - Miguel is noted to have very well-developed UEs, but his LEs are thinner than those of same-aged peers
  - He is in the lower 10th percentile for height and weight for his age
♦ Arousal, attention, and cognition
  - Testing on BSID-II (administered by staff in the follow-up clinic in the NICU) measured Miguel's cognition at 85, which is within the average range (85 to 115)
  - He does have periods of inattentiveness, but probably within expectations for his age
  - Results of the PEDI, Social Function domain, indicate difficulty with expressive communication
♦ Assistive and adaptive devices
  - Miguel's family owns a stroller and supine stander with tray
  - A forward and reverse type walker have been tried to assist him in standing balance
♦ Cranial and peripheral nerve integrity: Vision and hearing are normal
♦ Environmental, home, and work barriers
  - None in apartment: Apartment building has elevator and three flights of stairs with a hand rail
  - Playground at apartment has raised borders (railroad ties) and wood chips under the equipment. Miguel has trouble accessing playground, moving on wood chips, and accessing equipment
  - Requires stroller when in community
  - Parents either carry Miguel or use the stroller as he does not walk independently
♦ Gait, locomotion, and balance
  - Results of PEDI indicate that Miguel has difficulty with all transfers (eg, on and off furniture, in and out of bathtub), indoor and outdoor locomotion, and ascending and descending stairs
♦ Integumentary integrity: Normal
♦ Motor function
  - Miguel is able to initiate movement, but is not well coordinated in moving in and out of positions, maintaining ring or tailor sitting positions, or pulling to stand
  - He demonstrates marked LE stiffness in all positions and activities
♦ Muscle performance
  - Weakness is evident in all LE muscles, although formal muscle testing is not done due to inability to isolate movements
  - UE strength is good as observed in performance of functional tasks
  - Abdominal weakness noted as needs moderate assistance to pull to sit from supine
  - Weakness noted in respiratory muscles as he has a weak cough and has difficulty effectively clearing his lungs when he has a respiratory infection
♦ Neuromotor development and sensory integration
  - Gross motor skills on clinical tests scatter up to 12 months with all standard scores >2.0 SD below the mean
♦ Orthotic, protective, and supportive devices
  - LE orthotics are being considered for Miguel
♦ Pain: None reported
♦ Posture
  - In prone and supine
    ▪ Miguel tends to keep both LEs extended
  - In standing
    ▪ Miquel tends to crouch with hip and knee flexion and mild plantarflexion at the ankles
    ▪ His legs typically are adducted with hip internal rotation
♦ Range of motion
  - WNL for passive movement in UEs
  - Limitations at end ranges in hip, knee, and ankle joints
  - Muscle length

- Hip flexors: R=-10 degrees, L=-15 degrees
- Hamstrings (popliteal angle): R=40 degrees, L=35 degrees
- Gastrocnemius (ankle flexion with knee extension): R=5 degrees, L=0 degrees

♦ Reflex integrity
  ● Hyperactive stretch reflexes are present to tendon tap at the ankles (plantarflexors) and knees (quadriceps)
  ● Normal stretch reflexes noted in UEs

♦ Self-care and home management
  ● Results of PEDI indicate difficulty with dressing and toileting
  ● Miguel is starting to assist with dressing but does not yet show interest in toilet training

♦ Sensory integrity
  ● Miguel appears to have appropriate sensory appreciation to tactile and pressure input
  ● Hearing and vision are noted to be normal

♦ Ventilation and respiration/gas exchange
  ● Miguel demonstrates shortness of breath and shallow breathing when moving
  ● He has breathy sounds when singing and difficulty sustaining air flow when blowing through a straw or blow toy
  ● He has difficulty producing an effective cough to clear secretions
  ● Additional ventilation and respiration/gas exchange examinations are scheduled to be completed during his next follow-up visit at the hospital

♦ Work, community, and leisure integration or reintegration
  ● Miguel enjoys age-appropriate play activities and demonstrates typical behaviors for a 24-month-old child when his brothers are present
  ● Parents report difficulty with mobility in apartment complex playground and other community settings

EVALUATION

Miguel is a 24-month-old child with a medical diagnosis of CP with spastic diplegia. The physical therapy examination revealed that Miguel has difficulty moving in his environment and weakness in the LEs. He has stiffness and tightness at terminal ends in the LEs. His overall endurance for vigorous physical activity is limited. His gross motor, functional mobility, and self-care skills are delayed. He is able to initiate movement but has difficulty moving in and out of and maintaining positions. Cognition is within average range, but he has difficulties with expressive communication.

DIAGNOSIS

Miguel has a medical diagnosis of CP with spastic diplegia. He has impaired: aerobic capacity/endurance; gait, locomotion, and balance; motor function; muscle performance; neuromotor development and sensory integration; posture; range of motion; and reflex integrity. He is functionally limited and has disability limitations in self-care and home management and in work, community, and leisure actions, tasks, and activities. Miguel is in need of assistive, adaptive, supportive, and orthotic devices and equipment. These findings are consistent with placement in Pattern C: Impaired Motor Function and Sensory Integrity Associated With Nonprogressive Disorders of the Central Nervous System—Congenital Origin or Acquired in Infancy or Childhood. The identified impairments and functional limitations will be addressed in determining the prognosis and the plan of care.

PROGNOSIS AND PLAN OF CARE

Over the course of the visits, the following mutually established outcomes have been determined:

♦ Balance is improved
♦ Endurance for motor activities is increased
♦ Equipment for mobility and daily cares is explored
♦ Miguel assists with dressing and undressing
♦ Miguel tolerates a variety of sitting positions for play activities
♦ Mobility skills are improved
♦ Muscle length is increased
♦ Muscle performance (strength) of legs is increased
♦ Parents are aware of how CP may impact Miguel as he ages
♦ Parents are provided information on accessing public school services
♦ Parents are provided information on community resources
♦ Respiratory status and endurance are improved
♦ ROM is maintained or increased
♦ Transitions in and out of positions will be improved

To achieve these goals, the appropriate interventions for this patient are determined. These will include: coordination, communication, and documentation; patient/client-related instruction; therapeutic exercise; functional training in self-care and home management; functional training in work, community, and leisure integration or reintegration; and prescription, application, and, as appropriate, fabrication of devices and equipment.

Children with CP with Miguel's history and current functional limitations are classified in Level II of the Gross Motor Function Classification System (GMFCS).[56-58] Children at this level initially need an assistive device for ambulation, but typically progress to independent ambulation between 4 to 6 years of age. Several long-term studies of children with CP suggest that because Miguel is able to sit independently with both hands free to play and move on all-fours by 2 years of age, he has a good prognosis for independent ambulation with or without an assistive device.[59-61]

Because repetition is essential for learning new tasks[11,62] emphasis on a home/school/community program incorporating activities and positions into daily routines may produce the best outcomes. Frequency of intervention with children with CP will depend on multiple factors.[63] However, there is evidence that increasing frequency of physical therapy will not necessarily result in a greater rate of improvement or achievement of motor skills.[64] Episodic care, in which children receive several weeks of intervention followed by a "break" in therapy, may produce the same benefits as ongoing intervention.[65] Because there have been few well-designed studies that have supported treatment efficacy in children with CP[66] attainment of individualized functional objectives will be the most relevant measure of progress.[67]

Based on the diagnosis and prognosis it is anticipated that over the course of 20 visits in 12 months, Miguel will demonstrate optimal motor function and sensory integrity and the highest level of function in the home and community within the context of his impairments, functional limitations, and disability. Miguel will receive private physical therapy once a week for 3 months, with family education for his home program. Appropriate equipment for gait training (orthotics and walker) and self-care (bath chair) will be obtained. Then Miguel will be on a schedule of a 2-month break from private physical therapy followed by intervention twice a week for a month. Discharge from private physical therapy services will be when Miguel begins to attend a preschool program at 3 years of age where physical therapy services will be available to address any continued needs. Miguel's family has agreed to the program, and a service agreement has been signed.

INTERVENTIONS

RATIONALE FOR SELECTED INTERVENTIONS

Emphasis in Miguel's physical therapy program will be on strengthening LE muscles; maintaining flexibility and muscle elongation; facilitating ambulation (gait training); obtaining alternative methods of independent mobility; and performing functional activities. Strengthening activities, gait training, and functional activities also will address respiratory status and endurance. The primary mode of intervention will be through a home program of activities and positions to be incorporated into Miguel's daily routines with assistance of his parents and siblings.[68]

Therapeutic Exercise

Flexibility Exercises

Although neuromotor impairments appear to be primary in children with CP, musculoskeletal abnormalities (either primary or secondary) have been documented.[69] Rose and associates[70] performed a histologic and morphometric study of muscle from 10 children with spastic diplegia. When compared to normal control subjects, the children with CP had abnormal variations in the size of muscle fibers and altered distribution of fiber types. A relationship between an energy expenditure index and prolongation of electromyography (EMG) activity during walking with values for variation in fiber area was documented. Tardieu and coworkers[71] examined the passive contribution of a plantarflexion contracture and the active contribution of plantarflexor muscles during push-off in the gait of children with CP. They identified two separate mechanisms for toe walking—one was from overactivity of the triceps surae muscles, and the other was due to excessive passive shortening of the same muscle group. Different intervention strategies would be needed to address these two different mechanisms. Maintaining PROM is important to allow the motor patterns the child is able to produce to be expressed through the musculoskeletal system.

Gait and Locomotion Training

Research in animal models supports the concept of central pattern generators (CPGs) located in the spinal cord that produce coordinated stepping movements. The strongest evidence that CPGs for stepping exist in human infants is the observation of stepping movements in children born with anencephaly.[72] Because the normal process of cell death occurs in early development, the "use it or lose it" principle may be important in maintaining neural networks in the spinal cord to support stepping. Several authors have discussed early stepping as it relates to ambulation in the human infant/child.[73-77] The use of treadmills to promote the early practice of stepping is an area of research in pediatrics.[78-81] Having parents stand and assist their children in "walking" in typical childrearing activities is appropriate and should not be discouraged. The use of infant walkers also should be considered on a case-by-case basis depending on a number of variables (eg, safety issues, motor abilities of the child, opportunities for standing and stepping).[61,82] Anterior and posterior walkers have been designed for use with children with CP.[83] There are a number of variables to consider when determining the most beneficial walker for an individual child (eg, UE control, balance abilities, posture).[84]

Bleck[85] found that the average age for walking (walking 15 meters on a level surface, crutches allowed) in children with spastic diplegia was 47 months. Badell-Ribera[59] completed a longitudinal prospective study of 50 children with spastic diplegia. Four levels of ambulation were described, including exercise ambulation, household ambulation-low endurance, household ambulation-high endurance, and community ambulation. Forty-five of the 50 children achieved some level of ambulation. The group, who achieved independent crutchless walking, did so between 3½ and 6 years of age. Because functional ambulation skills probably will be delayed, it is important to find other methods of independent mobility for Miguel (eg, tricycle, motorized riding toy, walker, wheelchair) to enable him to access various environments as he matures (eg, home, school, community).[86,87]

Strength, Power, and Endurance Training

Fowler and coworkers[88] assessed the effect of effortful strengthening exercises in children with spastic CP. Knee extensor muscle spasticity was measured before and after one session of intense extensor strengthening exercise. There were no changes in spasticity as measured by the pendulum test. Damiano and associates[89] used a resistive exercise program to strengthen leg muscles in children with spastic CP. Strength increased without an associated increase in spasticity. In subsequent studies Damiano and coworkers[90,91] demonstrated improvement in function following strengthening programs. The importance of strengthening programs for children with CP also has been supported by research comparing changes in motor function with physical therapy in children with or without selective dorsal rhizotomy.[92]

Strengthening of ribcage musculature and abdominals should be incorporated into Miguel's program. Singing and sound play activities to produce longer, more varied sounds can be used, as well as activities such as blowing bubbles through a straw and blowing toy horns and pinwheels to improve respiratory function.[93]

Functional Training in Self-Care and Home Management and Functional Training in Work, Community, and Leisure Integration or Reintegration

Focusing on functional tasks in normal environment(s) is important because motor learning literature does not support the transfer of skills.[62] Transfer of one skill to another skill (eg, riding a tricycle to walking) or within one environment to another environment (eg, walking in the therapy room to walking in a crowded school hallway) tends to occur only if the tasks and environments are very similar. Ketelaar and coworkers[94] used a randomized block design to assign children with CP to two groups. One group received "functional" physical therapy and the second group received treatment based on "normalization or quality of movement." The GMFM and self-care and mobility domains of the PEDI were used as pre- and post-tests. Both groups

had improved GMFM and PEDI scores. Improvements as measured by the GMFM did not differ between groups. However, improvements in functional skills in daily situations demonstrated that children in the "functional" physical therapy group improved more than children in the other group. Pellegrino[95] discussed the importance of focusing on promoting the participation of children with CP in a wide variety of societal functions, rather than focusing on achieving motor milestones.

Prescription, Application, and, as Appropriate, Fabrication of Devices and Equipment

Orthotics, particularly ankle-foot orthoses (AFOs), may be helpful to maintain proper biomechanical alignment during standing and walking.[96] Burton and associates[97] compared muscle performance during perturbed stance with no AFOs, solid AFOs, and dynamic AFOs in four children with spastic diplegia and four age-matched control children. The results supported the use of dynamic AFOs to correct skeletal malalignment, although the same muscle-recruitment patterns were used by the children with CP despite the use or design of the AFO. Knott and Held[98] evaluated the effect of orthoses on multiple tests of function in 28 children with CP (5 to 19 years of age). No significant differences were found in the performance on the functional tests with and without orthoses, but 48% of the children reported more feelings of comfort and stability when wearing orthoses.

COORDINATION, COMMUNICATION, AND DOCUMENTATION

Coordination and communication will occur with school district personnel, the physician, and family. All elements of the patient's management will be documented. Appropriate releases will be obtained.

PATIENT/CLIENT-RELATED INSTRUCTION

Miguel and his family will receive instruction and education in a home program and updates. Emphasis will be on positioning and activities to improve his functional motor skills. The family will receive information on how to enroll Miguel in a preschool program through his local school district. They also will receive information regarding appropriate equipment, such as orthotics, walkers, and a bath chair.

Parent compliance with a home program is essential for Miguel's progress. The parents' goals for Miguel should be the focus of therapeutic objectives and activities. Activities that can be incorporated into the daily care routines of the family are most likely to be carried out consistently. Because Miguel enjoys interacting with and is very motivated by his two older brothers, activities in which they can participate also would be beneficial.

THERAPEUTIC EXERCISE

♦ Aerobic capacity/endurance conditioning
  ● While standing in stander do activities that require continuous use of arms, such as catch, balloon volleyball, and basketball
  ● Increase time of continuous activity
  ● Perform singing and sound play activities, blowing bubbles through a straw, blowing through a variety of blowing toys such as horns and pinwheels
  ● While in the pool, play games that involve kicking, jumping, splashing, and throwing, gradually increasing time of continuous activity
  ● While in the pool, do blowing activities such as bubbles in water, water tubes, and straws

♦ Balance, coordination, and agility training
  ● Activities to improve motor control of LEs
    ■ Allow Miguel to problem solve while trying motor tasks (trial and error learning is critical)
    ■ Provide lots of repetition
    ■ Set up environment to encourage movement
    ■ In playground, practice moving over wood chips, select equipment that encourages use of legs independently, such as spring toys, lifting one leg over the toy to sit, ladders for climbing slides, etc
  ● While sitting on floor practice activities that require use of arms and moving trunk off center, such as reaching to place toys in bucket, play catch or other games with balls, sing songs with movement
  ● Set up environment so Miguel has to reach from couch to chair while cruising, increase distance between furniture so he has to move without support
  ● While standing against couch, set up activities to encourage cruising and reaching for toy so Miguel shifts trunk away from center
  ● Standing next to couch reach out for parent or toy encouraging shifting weight off center and holding on with only one hand
  ● While standing in stander do activities that require reaching above head and out to sides

♦ Flexibility exercises
  ● Stretching exercises for younger children should be done after muscles have been warmed through activity or following a bath and using a slow steady stretch and building up to holding up to 30 to 60 seconds as tolerated
  ● Prolonged stretching can be accomplished through use of equipment (standers) or devices (braces or splints)
  ● Stretching of the LEs, particularly hip flexors and adductors, hamstrings, and heel cords
  ● Positioning for stretching to include prone on elbows, long sitting with back against couch

♦ Gait and locomotion training
  ● To facilitate improved mobility skills, focus on practicing activities/tasks that you want Miguel to do (eg, creeping on all-fours, walking with a walker)
  ● Developmental sequence is not used prescriptively; Miguel should focus on learning how to move and to vary movement instead of attaining motor milestones
  ● Set up the environment to allow Miguel to spontaneously explore and try different movement patterns
  ● Provide age-appropriate activities, such as tricycle when young, bicycle with training wheels, scooter with handle

♦ Strength, power, and endurance training
  ● Young children generally do not want to do exercises, so instead use activities or games designed to provide repeated practice of movements for strengthening and enhancing muscle power and endurance of LE muscles
  ● Make a game of placing small items on the floor so Miguel has to squat down to pick up and place items in a bucket
  ● Have him simulate animal walks (eg, crab walk, bear walk)
  ● Use small ankle weights for gross motor activities
  ● Use climbing up and down curbs and stairs as means of enhancing muscle strength, power, and endurance
  ● Use playground equipment
  ● Walk on soft surfaces such as sand, foam cushions, mats
  ● Use scooter board activities where Miguel can push off of walls while on back or stomach

FUNCTIONAL TRAINING IN SELF-CARE AND HOME MANAGEMENT

♦ Self-care
  ● Dressing and undressing skills
    ■ Miguel should pick out clothes to wear
    ■ Practice taking socks or shirt off while sitting on floor with back against bed
    ■ Practice putting arms through sleeves of t-shirt, sweater, and sweatshirt and then over head
  ● Transfer skills
    ■ Practice getting up on couch by placing one cushion on floor, encourage crawling and reaching up with one leg
    ■ Set up cushions to encourage crawling up and kneeling to standing to get into tub, place foam bath cushions in bottom of tub

- ▪ Place bed on floor
- ◆ Devices and equipment use and training
  - • Use of orthotics, supine stander, bath chair, and walker
    - ▪ Instruct parents in application of orthotics, wearing schedule, and what to watch for to maintain appropriate fit and maintain skin integrity
    - ▪ Instruct parents in use of supine stander and give ideas for activities to do while standing (eg, ball throwing and catching, hitting a balloon)
    - ▪ Instruct parents in body mechanics for transfers in and out of bath chair and tub
    - ▪ Instruct parents in use of walker and how to collapse walker for transportation

FUNCTIONAL TRAINING IN WORK, COMMUNITY, AND LEISURE INTEGRATION OR REINTEGRATION

- ◆ Play
  - • Instruction in balance strategies and positioning related to play activities
    - ▪ Show parent how to set up environment to provide natural obstacles to move over or around
    - ▪ Set up play activities on couch, removing cushions to kneel or stand on
    - ▪ Set up a game so Miguel has to walk from one end of the couch to the other to get toys or pick up toys and drop into container
    - ▪ Set up play activities in apartment playground, selecting equipment that encourages motor planning and isolation of legs while moving

ANTICIPATED GOALS AND EXPECTED OUTCOMES

- ◆ Impact on impairments
  - • Balance will be improved so Miguel can move in and out of positions more easily and stand independently.
  - • Endurance for motor activities will increase to allow Miguel to play for longer periods of time with his brothers without fatiguing.
  - • Muscle strength of LEs will be increased to allow Miguel to cruise at furniture and to walk with a walker for longer distances.
  - • Respiratory function will be improved so Miguel can cough more effectively and clear secretions when he has a cold.
  - • ROM will be maintained or improved so Miguel can tailor sit and ring sit comfortably and achieve full LE extension in standing.

- ◆ Impact on functional limitations
  - • Miguel is able to perform assisted dressing and undressing.
  - • Miguel is able to tolerate a variety of sitting positions for play activities.
  - • Mobility skills are improved.
  - • Transitions in and out of positions are improved.
- ◆ Impact on disabilities
  - • Miguel is able to participate in home activities.
  - • Miguel is able to participate in school activities.
  - • Miguel is able to play with others in the playground.
- ◆ Risk reduction/prevention
  - • Family is aware of appropriate body mechanics to use when assisting Miguel so as to prevent injury to themselves.
  - • Parents have an awareness of Miguel's condition and how it may impact his physical abilities as he ages.
  - • The risk of secondary impairments is reduced.
- ◆ Impact on health, wellness, and fitness
  - • Miguel incorporates physical activity within his daily routine.
  - • Miguel's mother understands the impact of her smoking on Miguel's respiratory function and her general health.
- ◆ Impact on societal resources
  - • Decision making is enhanced regarding patient health and use of health care resources by patient, family, and caregivers.
  - • Documentation occurs throughout the patient management and across settings and follows APTA's *Guidelines for Physical Therapy Documentation*.[99]
  - • School physical therapist and private physical therapist coordinate care to optimize services.
  - • Utilization of physical therapy services will result in efficient use of health care dollars.
- ◆ Patient/client satisfaction
  - • Access, availability, and services provided are acceptable to the family.
  - • Awareness of community resources is improved.
  - • Care is coordinated with school educational team.
  - • Miguel's parents will have increased understanding of goals and outcomes and demonstrate his home program independently.

REEXAMINATION

Reexamination is performed throughout the episode of care. It is anticipated that patients placed in this pattern will require multiple episodes of care over the lifetime. Periodic reexamination and initiation of new episodes of care should occur as the patient's functional limitations or disability change. This will allow the patient to continue to be safe and effectively adapt as a result of changes in multiple factors including his own physical status, caregivers, environment, or task demands.

DISCHARGE

Miguel is discharged from physical therapy after a total of 16 physical therapy sessions over 10 months and attainment of his goals and outcomes. These sessions have covered this entire episode of care. He is discharged because he has achieved his goals and outcomes. As Miguel has a condition that may require multiple episodes of care throughout his life span, Miguel's parents received education regarding factors that may trigger a call to his physical therapist for a reexamination and new episode of physical therapy care.

Case Study #2: Myelomeningocele

Jennifer is a 12-month-old female with a medical diagnosis of a repaired L3 myelomeningocele and with a ventricular-peritoneal shunt.

PHYSICAL THERAPIST EXAMINATION

HISTORY

◆ General demographics: Jennifer is a 12-month-old white female.

◆ Social history: Jennifer lives with her single, teenage mother and maternal grandparents. Jennifer's father is not involved in her care.

◆ Employment/work: Jennifer is responsive to social interaction and attends to objects and people in her environment.

◆ Growth and development: Jennifer was a full-term infant, born by cesarean section due to fetal distress and breech presentation. Jennifer's mother did not have ultrasounds during pregnancy that would have identified a myelomeningocele. At birth a large myelomeningocele was noted, was closed surgically, and a VP shunt was inserted. Jennifer had bouts of apnea and was on a respirator for 2 weeks. Jennifer's gross motor development has been delayed due to orthopedic complications (hip flexion contractures and ankle equinovarus—club feet) and sensory and motor deficits associated with her myelomeningocele.

◆ Living environment: Jennifer and her family live in a rambling style one-story home.

◆ General health status
  • General health perception: Jennifer has been healthy since discharge from the hospital, except for two hospitalizations for problems with the VP shunt that required external ventricular drainage and reinsertion.
  • Physical function: Jennifer is alert and interacts appropriately within her home environment.
  • Psychological function: Jennifer generally is happy and tolerates handling by adults.
  • Role function: Daughter, granddaughter, child.
  • Social function: Jennifer interacts well with her family. She has limited opportunities to interact with other children or adults.

◆ Social/health habits: Her mother is 16 years old and attends her local high school. She had limited prenatal care and may have had poor nutrition early in her pregnancy. There may have been a lack of folic acid (a water-soluble B vitamin) that has been linked to NTD. There is no history of drug, alcohol, or tobacco use. Jennifer's grandparents are providing a supportive environment and daycare while Jennifer's mother attends school.

◆ Family history: A cousin of Jennifer's mother on the grandfather's side of the family also was born with myelomeningocele and is now 8 years old.

◆ Medical/surgical history: Surgical closure of Jennifer's myelomeningocele occurred at birth. She had a hernia repair 1 month later. In the first month of life, Jennifer also had a suspected Arnold-Chiari malformation that was treated by surgical release of the posterior fossa. She had equinovarus deformities and underwent serial casting beginning at 1 month of age. She was discharged from the hospital at 3 months of age. She has had two subsequent hospitalizations due to shunt problems (blockage and infections) requiring external ventricular drainage and reinsertion of the shunts.

◆ Current condition(s)/chief complaint(s): Jennifer's mother and her grandparents continue to worry about "handling" Jennifer. They are afraid they will hurt her. They have questions about her potential for walking and attending a "regular" school. When discharged from the hospital, Jennifer was referred for early intervention services through the local school district. A teacher provides a weekly home visit and a physical therapist and occupational therapist provide consultative services related to goals on the IFSP. The school physical therapist sees Jennifer twice a month at home to update her home program.

◆ Functional status and activity level: Jennifer pushes up on extended arms in prone. She is able to roll from prone to her back and from her back to side-lying, but needs some assist to roll from supine to prone. She has good head and upper trunk control in supported sitting.

◆ Medications: Senokot (to achieve soft-formed stools).

◆ Other clinical tests
  • The BSID-II[52] was administered at 6 months of age by staff in the follow-up clinic at the hospital. The BSID-II is a norm-referenced test used to document mental and motor status from birth to 3 years of age. Jennifer's standard scores on the BSID-II (mental scale=-1.5 SD; motor scale=-3.0 SD) and her medical diagnosis were used to qualify her for school services.
  • A functional muscle test was administered by the school physical therapist, and she attempted to document levels of sensory awareness in the LEs. Goniometric measurements of hip ROM were taken.
  • The school physical therapist plans to administer the PEDI[55] to obtain a baseline of functional skills in the areas of self-care and mobility when Jennifer is 18 months of age.

SYSTEMS REVIEW

◆ Cardiovascular/pulmonary
  • BP: 90/42 mmHg
  • Edema: None noted
  • HR: 100 bpm
  • RR: 30 bpm

◆ Integumentary
  • Presence of scar formation
    ▪ Well-healed scar with no thickening of the skin noted on her back over the myelomeningocele closure area
    ▪ No gibbons deformity noted
  • Skin color: Good
  • Skin integrity: Good; palpation of shunt along right side of skull and neck

◆ Musculoskeletal
  • Gross range of motion
    ▪ Right hip flexion contracture of approximately 40 degrees
    ▪ Contractures in both feet and ankles
  • Gross strength
    ▪ UE strength is good as Jennifer can push up on extended arms in prone and lifts toys above her head when supine
    ▪ Weakness and paralysis noted in LEs
  • Gross symmetry: Asymmetry in prone due to right hip flexion contracture
  • Height: 30" (0.762 m), 90th percentile for age[100]
  • Weight: 24 lbs (10.89 kg), 90th percentile for age[100]

◆ Neuromuscular

  • Gross coordinated movements
    ▪ UE movements well coordinated
    ▪ Paralysis and lack of motor function in LEs

◆ Communication, affect, cognition, language, and learning style
  • Jennifer babbles and has several words (eg, "mama," "bye-bye")
  • She enjoys playing with toys, interacting with people, and watching animated videos
  • Parent/grandparents prefer written home programs

TESTS AND MEASURES

◆ Anthropometric characteristics
  • Jennifer is a large child for her age
  • Her head is larger in proportion to her body than expected due to her hydrocephalus

◆ Arousal, attention, and cognition
  • Testing on the BSID-II indicates mild cognitive delays with performance being more typical of a 9-month-old child

◆ Assistive and adaptive devices
  • Jennifer has a stroller and car seat
  • Consideration is being given for a castor cart and manual wheelchair

◆ Cranial and peripheral nerve integrity
  • Jennifer has loss of sensation in her LEs below the level of lesion at L3
  • Her hearing and vision are noted to be normal

◆ Environmental, home, and work barriers
  • None at home or in the community
  • Jennifer is transported in a stroller or a car seat or is carried

◆ Gait, locomotion, and balance
  • Jennifer has limited floor mobility and cannot bear her weight in standing
  • She has difficulty getting in and out of positions
  • She has difficulty getting on and off furniture
  • Jennifer tends to be content to observe vs move and has limited initiation of movement

◆ Integumentary integrity: Skin condition is good with well-healed scars noted over surgical sites for myelomeningocele closure and hernia repair

◆ Joint integrity and mobility
  • Right hip flexion contracture
  • Tightness bilaterally in foot and ankle complex

◆ Motor function
  • Jennifer is able to push up on extended arms and pivots in prone
  • Her mobility is limited to rolling and attempts at

belly crawling due to paralysis of her LEs

- She attempts to get her knees under her and can kneel with support at a surface
- She has good head and upper trunk control in supported sitting

- Muscle performance
  - Jennifer has functional strength to level of lesion at L3 but strength is less than typical for children her age
  - Muscles at L3 include hip flexors, hip adductors, partial knee extensors, and weak hip rotators
  - No muscle function is noted below L3

- Neuromotor development and sensory integration
  - Gross motor skills are at approximately a 6-month level
  - She has marked sensory and motor deficits in the LEs

- Orthotic, protective, and supportive devices
  - A standing frame is being considered for Jennifer

- Pain
  - None reported, but lack of sensory function below L3

- Posture
  - In sitting, Jennifer needs support as she tends to sit with a marked lumbar lordosis
  - In prone, she demonstrates some asymmetry due to her right hip flexion contracture

- Range of motion
  - She has a right hip flexion contracture of 40 degrees limiting hip extension on the right
  - Her feet are contracted (in spite of casting) so that she cannot bear weight on them

- Reflex integrity
  - Absent deep tendon reflexes at the knee and ankle bilaterally
  - Normal stretch reflexes in the UEs

- Self-care and home management
  - Jennifer assists at mealtime by finger feeding some foods and holding with both hands onto a two-handled cup with sipping cover
  - She assists with dressing by placing arms through sleeves, pulling off socks, and the like
  - She is catheterized and wears diapers due to leakage and bowel movements

- Sensory integrity
  - Jennifer reacts to a facial vibrator applied around the knee joint, but not at the ankle
  - Sensory integrity is appropriate above level of lesion

- Ventilation and respiration/gas exchange:
  - No problems noted

- Work, community, and leisure integration or reintegration
  - Jennifer enjoys age-appropriate play activities, but family is hesitant to do gross motor play, as they are afraid she will get hurt
  - She enjoys playing with musical and electronic toys
  - She responds to social interaction with adults

EVALUATION

Jennifer has a medical diagnosis of L3 myelomeningocele with VP shunt. She has motor and sensory loss below the level of lesion. She has contractures in her LEs, specifically hip flexors and feet, and cannot bear weight in standing. Jennifer has difficulty moving in and out of positions, and she does not spontaneously explore her environment. Her gross motor, functional mobility, and self-help skills are delayed and she has mild cognitive and communication deficits. She enjoys play and responds to social interaction with adults. Her family has concerns about "handling" her and about her future. Jennifer has a stroller and car seat and is in need of additional assistive devices. She participates in her local school district's early intervention program.

DIAGNOSIS

Jennifer has a medical diagnosis of L3 myelomeningocele that was repaired at birth and also had a VP shunt placement following birth. She has impaired: arousal, attention, and cognition; cranial and peripheral nerve integrity; gait, locomotion, and balance; motor function; muscle performance; neuromotor development and sensory integration; posture; range of motion; reflex integrity; and sensory integrity. She is functionally limited in self-care and home management and in play, community, and leisure actions, tasks, and activities. She is in need of assistive, adaptive, orthotic, protective, and supportive devices and equipment. These findings are consistent with placement in Pattern C: Impaired Motor Function and Sensory Integrity Associated With Nonprogressive Disorders of the Central Nervous System—Congenital Origin or Acquired in Infancy or Childhood. The identified impairments and functional limitations will be addressed in determining the prognosis and the plan of care.

PROGNOSIS AND PLAN OF CARE

Over the course of the visits, the following mutually established outcomes have been determined:

- Ability to explore environment and initiate movement is improved
- Ability to move in and out of positions is improved
- Equipment for mobility is obtained (standing frame, a

castor cart, and a wheelchair)

♦ Family is aware of how myelomeningocele may impact Jennifer as she ages

♦ Family is aware of potential complications associated with myelomeningocele and recognize warning signs that require intervention

♦ Family is confident handling Jennifer

♦ Family incorporates use of equipment into Jennifer's daily routine

♦ Independence in floor mobility with and without assistive devices is achieved

♦ Muscle length is increased

♦ Muscle strength in arms and trunk is improved

♦ ROM in LEs is improved

♦ Self-care for feeding and simple dressing tasks is improved

♦ Sitting balance is improved

To achieve these outcomes, the appropriate interventions for this patient are determined. These will include: coordination, communication, and documentation; patient/client-related instruction; therapeutic exercise; functional training in self-care and home management; functional training in work, community, and leisure integration or reintegration; and prescription, application, and, as appropriate, fabrication of devices and equipment.

Jennifer's prognosis for obtaining independent floor mobility between 12 to 18 months of age is good. For the current 6-month episode of care, Jennifer will receive physical therapy through her local school district for a total of 12 visits (two visits per month). Because she still has marked deformities at the ankles, she will be undergoing a surgical correction within the next few months so the feet can be positioned in plantigrade for weightbearing. If stretching and positioning are ineffective in decreasing her hip flexion contracture, a surgical release also may be performed. If surgical correction occurs during this episode of care, Jennifer will be reexamined and her diagnosis for therapy and placement in this practice pattern may change. A brief increase in frequency of services is anticipated in a future episode of care when gait training with a reciprocal gait orthosis (RGO) and walker is initiated.

INTERVENTIONS

RATIONALE FOR SELECTED INTERVENTIONS

Therapeutic Exercise

As Jennifer is 12 months of age, opportunities to explore her environment are becoming increasingly important for cognitive and social development. Limited mobility early in life may have negative effects on other aspects of development,[101,102] and therefore emphasis in her program will be on developing independent mobility. Independent mobility through rolling and crawling and transitions of movement, such as in and out of sitting, will be emphasized. In addition, changes in position are important for obtaining sensory/perceptual information from the environment.[103] Changes in position, such as sitting in a wheelchair or standing in a standing frame, will afford Jennifer different perspectives on her environment. A wheelchair and castor cart that she can propel will allow her to initiate movement, be independent, and increase UE strength.

Children with L3 muscle function have intact hip flexion and adduction, but weak hip rotation.[40] Because the quadriceps muscles are innervated by nerve roots L2 to L4, children usually have antigravity knee extension. Young children may begin ambulation training with a RGO and walker. Ambulation (in the house and for short distances) with the least restrictive devices typically requires knee-ankle-foot orthoses (KAFOs) and forearm crutches. A wheelchair is used for long distances.

Williams and associates[104] studied 15 children with lesions at the mid-lumbar level (L3). Nine children walked (with bracing and assistive devices) at an average of 5 years. Of these nine children, three had ceased walking at an average age of 7 years. Therefore, fewer than 50% of the children maintained ambulation skills past 7 years of age. Hunt and Poulton[105] followed individuals with spina bifida from childhood to adulthood. In their sample of 61 individuals (average age of 25 years), there was a correlation between walking ability and sensory level. Of 26 adults with sensory levels above L3, all were wheelchair dependent. Of the 17 adults with sensory levels below L4, all but one were community ambulators. Three subjects were not included due to asymmetrical sensory loss. Of the remaining 15 individuals with sensory loss of L3 or L4, 12 were nonwalkers and only three remained community ambulators. This was a regression from the average age of 18 years when 12 of the 15 individuals were community ambulators. The authors suggested that, in individuals with sensory levels of L3 and L4, factors other than basic neurology may determine walking abilities in adulthood. Bartonek and Saraste[106] documented that balance disturbances, occurrence of spasticity in hip and knee movements, and shunt revisions adversely affected expected ambulation ability based on the level of the lesion.

Physical therapy intervention for children with spina bifida has not changed considerably over the past 30 years. In 1976, Hewson[107] stated that "physiotherapy for children with spina bifida uses very basic techniques which include prophylactic and therapeutic 'stretching', training to walk, supervision of calipers [orthotics], and instructions to the parents. Success or failure of treatment very largely depends on the ability of the physiotherapist to teach and encourage the parents to help the child become as independent as possible in all aspects of living."(p 117) Similarly, Hunt and Poulton[105] concluded that, although medical interventions have greatly reduced mortality in NTDs, the neural defect dictates the level of disability.

Patient/Client-Related Instruction

Physical therapists should provide education to children and their families regarding warning signs of tethering of the spinal cord. Tethering is a complication that occurs as a result of pathological fixation of the spinal cord, resulting in traction on neural tissue.[108] Ischemia and progressive neurologic deterioration will occur unless there is a surgical intervention. In the follow-up study of 71 individuals with myelomeningocele by Bowman and associates,[109] a tethered cord requiring surgical release occurred in 23 individuals, and the average age when symptoms were noted was 10.9 years. Symptoms of a tethered spinal cord can include increased scoliosis, gait changes, increased spasticity in the LEs, back and leg pain, decreased muscle strength, LE contractures, urinary bladder changes, and changes in motor or sensory level in the LEs.[108-111]

Instruction must also be given about the possibility of latex (rubber) allergy.[109] Symptoms include watery eyes, wheezing, rashes or hives, swelling, and in severe cases, anaphylaxis. In the follow-up study by Bowman and coworkers,[109] latex allergy occurred in 32% of the individuals at an average age of 12.5 years. In several cases, the latex allergy was severe with life-threatening anaphylactic reactions.

Work, Community, and Leisure Integration or Reintegration

Children with myelomeningocele and hydrocephalus are at risk for learning disabilities due to malformations of the CNS.[112,113] In a 25-year follow-up study, Bowman and coworkers[109] documented that 85% of the children were attending high school or college. Sixty-three percent attended regular education classes, 14% needed additional assistance, and 23% were in special education. Of the 71 individuals followed, 77% continued to live at home with parents while 4% lived in residential homes and only 15% lived independently in the community. Two young adults were married and lived with their spouses. Similarly, in their follow-up of 61 individuals into adulthood, Hunt and Poulton[105] reported that only 14 (22%) were living independently in the community.

COORDINATION, COMMUNICATION, AND DOCUMENTATION

Coordination and communication will occur with the orthopedic surgeon, durable medical equipment supplier, other members of the school early intervention team, and family regarding adaptive equipment and physical therapy services. All elements of the patient's management, including examination, evaluation, diagnosis, prognosis, and interventions, will be documented.

PATIENT/CLIENT-RELATED INSTRUCTION

Jennifer and her family will receive instruction and education in a home program with periodic updates. Emphasis will be on activities to improve Jennifer's independent mobility and prevent secondary impairments (eg, contractures, skin breakdown). They also will receive information on standing frames, castor carts, and wheelchairs. Parent education regarding complications associated with myelomeningocele will be stressed. Parent education also will include information on skin care and prevention of pressure areas, particularly on the feet.

The goals of Jennifer's mother and grandparents should be considered and incorporated into the home program. Emphasis should be on increasing Jennifer's independence in mobility and play. Family education to make the family comfortable with Jennifer's medical diagnosis, functional limitations and abilities, and potential for participation in typical environments also is essential.

THERAPEUTIC EXERCISE

♦ Balance, coordination, and agility training
  ● Begin using seating device that supports pelvis to waist
  ● Practice sitting while reading a book to Jennifer allowing her to use hands to prop or support trunk
    ▪ Add reaching activities
    ▪ Initially directly in front of her
    ▪ Then move toys or objects off to side, at shoulder level
    ▪ Then above head
    ▪ Have her reach across to opposite side, pick up objects on one side and drop in bucket on other side
  ● Play catch
    ▪ Begin by having Jennifer push ball and roll it back
    ▪ Progress to throwing ball, shifting weight and keeping balance while arm goes above and behind head
  ● Sit on small rocking chair, practice reaching activities as above
  ● Sit on large pillows, practice reaching activities as above
♦ Flexibility exercises
  ● Instruct family in PROM using natural activities, such as changing diapers as opportunities to perform ROM
  ● Position on stomach on wedge using rolled towels to aid in alignment of legs

- Use gentle slow motions holding at the end of the range for sustained stretch of up to 30 to 60 seconds
- Use equipment including orthotics or splints to assist with maintaining appropriate position and prolonged stretch

◆ Gait and locomotion training
- Set up environment to encourage exploration
- Set up environment to have preferred toys or objects out of reach so Jennifer has to initiate movement to obtain toy
- To encourage rolling, begin using a wedge and place Jennifer at top with preferred toy at bottom, alternate sides to roll down, may need to physically prompt at hips due to right hip flexion contracture
- Encourage belly crawling first on smooth surfaces, such as vinyl floor, as she will slide more easily
- Remind family to make sure Jennifer's legs and feet are protected when belly crawling on floor
- To encourage visual perceptual development encourage family to take Jennifer out in her stroller or wheelchair and vary how they move (move fast, slow, change directions quickly, move backward)

◆ Strength, power, and endurance training
- Work on general strengthening activities to improve strength of UEs and trunk for transitions and mobility on floor
  - Holding toys in air, shaking, reaching up and putting on chair/low table
  - Batting at balloons
  - Put cushion from couch on floor in front of couch, place preferred toy on cushion and more on couch, encourage Jennifer to pull herself up on cushions and onto couch
- UE strengthening using mobility activities
  - Position in castor cart
    ‣ Have Jennifer hold onto hoop while family member pulls her around house, increase amount of time and distance pulled
    ‣ Have Jennifer propel castor cart first on smooth surfaces, such as vinyl or tile, then have her propel on carpet or grass, progressing to having her pull a wagon or cart first empty then with added weight
  - Play tug of war and other games where she must push and pull

FUNCTIONAL TRAINING IN SELF-CARE AND HOME MANAGEMENT

◆ Self-care
- Encourage Jennifer to self-feed using finger foods
- Have her begin to use age-appropriate utensils

- Dressing
  - Position Jennifer in a stable position to practice dressing skills
  - Let Jennifer make choices between two items of clothing
  - Practice pulling off socks and putting on a shirt

◆ Devices and equipment use and training
- Activities to achieve independent use of castor cart and wheelchair
  - Begin by placing Jennifer in castor cart and just playing
  - Show her how to propel the cart
  - Set up an environment so that she has the desired toy or activity just out of reach, gradually increasing distances
  - Begin with a small wheelchair appropriate for Jennifer to propel
    ‣ Begin as above
    ‣ As Jennifer gets stronger, show her how to transfer in and out of wheelchair
- Instruct parent in application of orthotics, wearing schedule, and what to watch for to maintain appropriate fit and maintain skin integrity

FUNCTIONAL TRAINING IN WORK, COMMUNITY, AND LEISURE INTEGRATION OR REINTEGRATION

◆ Play
- Instruction in balance strategies and positioning related to play activities
- Instruct family in how to handle Jennifer for general handling and play activities
- Instruct family in how to set up environment to encourage Jennifer to initiate movement and begin to be more independent in moving within rooms and from room to room

PRESCRIPTION, APPLICATION, AND, AS APPROPRIATE, FABRICATION OF DEVICES AND EQUIPMENT

◆ Assist family in obtaining castor cart
◆ Work with family and chosen vendor to try different wheelchairs to determine most appropriate wheelchair for Jennifer and her family
◆ Instruct family in use of castor cart and wheelchair

ANTICIPATED GOALS AND EXPECTED OUTCOMES

◆ Impact on impairments

- Balance and independent sitting with both hands free for play are improved.
- Endurance and ability to roll consecutively to obtain toys are improved.
- Muscle length is improved, and Jennifer is able to wear orthotics.
- Muscle performance is improved, and Jennifer is able to belly crawl through her home environment.
- Posture is improved, and lordosis is not as marked in sitting.
- ROM of the right hip is maintained or improved to allow positioning for play.

◆ Impact on functional limitations
- Ability to feed herself finger foods is achieved.
- Ability to move around her home environment independently by rolling or belly crawling is achieved.
- Floor mobility skills (ie, rolling, crawling) are improved.
- Independent mobility is obtained via a castor cart and a wheelchair.
- Transitions in and out of positions on the floor are improved.

◆ Impact on disabilities
- Jennifer is handled safely and appropriately and is able to assume her role of child in the family.

◆ Risk reduction/prevention
- Risk of secondary impairments is reduced.
- Mother and grandparents have an awareness of Jennifer's condition and how it may impact her physical abilities as she ages.

◆ Impact on health, wellness, and fitness
- Mother is aware of resources in the community to support both her needs and those of Jennifer.
- Physical function is improved.

◆ Impact on societal resources
- Decision making is enhanced regarding patient health and use of health care resources by patient, family, and caregivers.
- Documentation occurs throughout the patient management and across settings and follows APTA's *Guidelines for Physical Therapy Documentation*.[99]
- Utilization of physical therapy services results in efficient use of health care dollars.

◆ Patient/client satisfaction
- Access, availability, and services provided are acceptable to the family.
- Awareness of community resources is improved.
- Care is coordinated with school educational team.
- Family members understand planned surgical procedures and expected outcomes and understand need for and use of adaptive equipment.

- Jennifer's mother and grandparents have an increased understanding of goals and outcomes and independently are able to demonstrate her home program.

REEXAMINATION

Reexamination is performed throughout the episode of care. It is anticipated that patients placed in this pattern will require multiple episodes of care over the lifetime. Periodic reexamination and initiation of new episodes of care should occur as the patient's functional limitations or disability changes. This will allow the patient to continue to be safe and effectively adapt as a result of changes in multiple factors including her own physical status, caregivers, environment, or task demands.

DISCHARGE

Jennifer is discharged from physical therapy after a total of 12 physical therapy visits over 6 months and attainment of her goals. As Jennifer has a condition that may require multiple episodes of care throughout her life span, Jennifer's family received education regarding factors that may trigger a call to her physical therapist for a reexamination and new episode of physical therapy care.

REFERENCES

1. Moore KL, Dalley AF. *Clinically Oriented Anatomy.* 4th ed. Philadelphia, PA: Lippincott Williams & Wilkins; 1999.
2. Nolte J. *The Human Brain: An Introduction to Its Functional Anatomy.* 4th ed. St. Louis, MO: Mosby; 1999.
3. Leonard CT. *The Neuroscience of Human Movement.* St. Louis, MO: Mosby-Year Book Inc; 1998.
4. Newton RA. Neural systems underlying motor control. In: Montgomery PC, Connolly BH, eds. *Motor Control and Physical Therapy.* 2nd ed. Thorofare, NJ: SLACK Incorporated; 2001:53-78.
5. Thompson PM, Hayashi KM, Sowell ER, et al. Mapping cortical change in Alzheimer's disease, brain development, and schizophrenia. *Neuroimage.* 2004;23(Suppl 1):S2-S18.
6. Memoli F, Sapiro G, Thompson P. Implicit brain imaging. *Neuroimage.* 2004;23(Suppl 1):S179-S188.
7. Ballmaier M, Kumar A, Thompson PM, et al. Localizing gray matter deficits in late-onset depression using computational cortical pattern matching methods. *Am J Psychiatry.* 2004; 161(11):2091-2099.
8. Pitiot A, Delingette H, Thompson PM, Ayache N. Expert knowledge-guided segmentation system for brain MRI. *Neuroimage.* 2004;23(Suppl 1):S85-S96.
9. Leow A, Yu CL, Lee SJ, et al. Brain structural mapping using a novel hybrid implicit/explicit framework based on the level-set method. *Neuroimage.* 2005;24(3):910-927.
10. Rijntjes M, Dettmers C, Buchel C, et al. Blueprint for movement: functional and anatomical representations in the human motor system. *J Neurosci.* 1999;19:8043-8048.

11. Byl N. Neuroplasticity: applications to motor control. In: Montgomery PC, Connolly BH, eds. *Motor Control and Physical Therapy.* 2nd ed. Thorofare, NJ: SLACK Incorporated; 2001:79-108.

12. National Research Council and Institute of Medicine. *From Neurons to Neighborhoods: The Science of Early Childhood Development.* Committee on Integrating the Science of Early Childhood Development. Shonkoff JP, Phillips DA, eds. Board on Children, Youth, and Families, Commission on Behavioral and Social Sciences and Education. Washington, DC: National Academy Press; 2000.

13. Als H, Duffy FH, McAnulty GB, et al. Early experience alters brain function and structure. *Pediatrics.* 2004;113:846-857.

14. Elbert T, Rockstroh B. Reorganization of human cerebral cortex: the range of changes following use and injury. *Neuroscientist.* 2004;10(2):129-141.

15. Dong WK, Greenough WT. Plasticity of nonneuronal brain tissue: roles in developmental disorders. *Ment Retard Dev Disabil Res Rev.* 2004;10(2):85-90.

16. Sadato N. How the blind "see" Braille: lessons from functional magnetic resonance imaging. *Neuroscientist.* 2005;11(6):577-582.

17. Hlustik P, Solodkin A, Noll DC, et al. Cortical plasticity during three-week motor skill learning. *J Clin Neurophysiol.* 2004; 21(3):180-191.

18. You SH, Jang SH, Ynn-Hee K, et al. Cortical reorganization induced by virtual reality therapy in a child with hemiparetic cerebral palsy. *Dev Med Child Neurol.* 2005;47:628-635.

19. Merzenich MM, Wright B, Jenkins WM, et al. Cortical plasticity underlying perceptual, motor and cognitive skill development: implications for neurorehabilitation. *Cold Springs Harbor Symposium in Quantitative Biology.* 1996;61:1-8.

20. Merzenich MM, Jenkins WM. Cortical plasticity, learning and learning dysfunction. In: Jules B, Kovacs I, eds. *Maturational Windows and Adult Cortical Plasticity.* New York, NY: Addison-Wesley; 1995:247-272.

21. Merzenich MM. Development and maintenance of cortical somatosensory representations: functional "maps" and neuroanatomic repertoires. In: Barnard KE, Brazelton TM, eds. *Touch, The Foundation of Experience.* Madison, WI: International University Press; 1991:47-71.

22. Merzenich MM, Allard T, Jenkins WM. Neural ontogeny of higher brain function: implications of some recent neurophysiological findings. In: Franzen O, Westman P, eds. *Information Processing in the Somatosensory System.* London, England: McMillan Press; 1991:293-311.

23. Merzenich M. Neural plasticity: basic mechanisms. III STEP Conference, Salt Lake City, UT; July 2005.

24. Risedal A, Jeng J, Johannson BB. Early training may exacerbate brain damage after focal brain ischemia in the rat. *J Cereb Blood Flow Metab.* 1999;19:997-1003.

25. Kleim JA. Neural mechanisms of motor recovery after stroke: plasticity within residual cortical tissue. III STEP Conference, Salt Lake City, UT; July 2005.

26. Kleim JA, Jones TA, Schallert T. Motor enrichment and the induction of plasticity before or after brain injury. *Neurochem Res.* 2003;28(11):1757-1769.

27. Nudo RJ. Translating results between animal and human studies of brain plasticity after neuronal injury. III STEP Conference, Salt Lake City, UT; July 2005.

28. Nudo RJ, Plautz EJ, Frost SB. Role of adaptive plasticity in recovery of function after damage to motor cortex. *Muscle Nerve.* 2001;24:100-119.

29. VanSant A. Motor control, motor learning, and motor development. In: Montgomery PC, Connolly BH, eds. *Motor Control and Physical Therapy.* 2nd ed. Thorofare, NJ: SLACK Incorporated; 2001:25-52.

30. Brooks VB. *The Neural Basis of Motor Control.* New York, NY: Oxford University Press; 1986:5,129-150.

31. Schmidt RA, Lee TD. *Motor Control and Learning: A Behavioral Emphasis.* 3rd ed. Champaign, IL: Human Kinetics; 1999.

32. Roberton MA. Motor development: recognizing our roots, charting our future. *Quest.* 1989;41:213-223.

33. Shevell MI, Majnemer A, Morin I. Etiologic yield of cerebral palsy: a contemporary case series. *Pediatr Neurol.* 2003;28:352-359.

34. Pueyo-Benito R, Vendrell-Gomez P, Bargallo-Alabart N, et al. Neuroimaging and cerebral palsy. *Rev Neurol.* 2002;35:463-469.

35. Staudt M, Pavlova M, Bohm S, et al. Pyramidal tract damage correlates with motor dysfunction in bilateral periventricular leukomalacia (PVL). *Neuropediatrics.* 2003;34:182-188.

36. Gururaj A, Sztriha L, Dawodu A, et al. CT and MR patterns of hypoxic ischemic brain damage following perinatal asphyxia. *J Trop Pediatr.* 2002;48:5-9.

37. Rezaie P, Dean A. Periventricular leukomalacia, inflammation and white matter lesions within the developing nervous system. *Neuropathology.* 2002;22:106-132.

38. Montgomery PC. Achievement of gross motor skills in two children with hypoplasia: longitudinal case reports. *Pediatric Physical Therapy.* 2000;12:68-76.

39. Lawson RD, Badawi N. Etiology of cerebral palsy. *Hand Clin.* 2003;19:547-556.

40. Hinderer KA, Hinderer SR, Shurtleff DB. Myelodysplasia. In: Campbell SK, ed. *Physical Therapy for Children.* Philadelphia, PA: WB Saunders Co; 1994:571-619.

41. CDC. Recommendations for the use of folic acid to reduce the number of cases of spina bifida and other neural tube defects. *Morb Mortal Wkly Rep.* 1992;41(No. RR-14).

42. Hoon AH Jr, Belsito KM, Nagae-Poetscher LM. Neuroimaging in spasticity and movement disorders. *J Child Neurol.* 2003;12(Suppl 1):S25-S39.

43. Debillon T, N'Guyen S, Muet A, et al. Limitations of ultrasonography for diagnosing white matter damage in preterm infants. *Arch Dis Child Fetal Neonatal Ed.* 2003;88:275-279.

44. Okumura A, Hayakawa F, Kato T, et al. Abnormal sharp transients on electroencephalograms in preterm infants with periventricular leukomalacia. *J Pediatr.* 2003;143:26-30.

45. Corry IS, Cosgrove AP, Duffy CM. Botulinum toxin A compared with stretching casts in the treatment of spastic CP: a randomized prospective trial. *J Pediatr Orthop.* 1998;18:304-311.

46. Butler C, Campbell S. Evidence of the effects of intrathecal baclofen for spastic and dystonic cerebral palsy. *Dev Med Child Neurol.* 2000;42:634-645.

47. Connolly BH. Pediatric medications. *Orthopaedic Physical Therapy, Home Study Course* 98-2. Orthopaedic Section, American Physical Therapy Association, 1998.

48. Sisto SA. Evidence of chemodenervation treatment effectiveness for the neurological patient. *Journal of Neurologic Physical Therapy.* 2003; 27:149-159.

49. Bjornson KF, McLaughlin JF, Loeser JD, et al. Oral motor,

communication, and nutritional status of children during intrathecal baclofen therapy: a descriptive pilot study. *Arch Phys Med Rehabil.* 2003;84:500-506.

50. Albright AL, Gilmartin R, Swift D, et al. Long-term intrathecal baclofen therapy for severe spasticity of cerebral origin. *J Neurosurg.* 2003;98:291-295.

51. Bergenheim AT, Wendelius M, Shahdidi S, et al. Spasticity in a child with myelomeningocele treated with continuous intrathecal baclofen. *Pediatr Neurosurg.* 2003;39:218-221.

52. Bayley N. *Bayley Scales of Infant Development-II (BSID-II).* 2nd ed. San Antonio, TX: The Psychological Corp; 1993.

53. Russell D, Rosenbaum P, Gowland C, et al. *Gross Motor Function Measure (GMFM).* Toronto, Canada: Gross Motor Measures Group; 1993.

54. Folio MR, Fewell RR. *Peabody Developmental Motor Scales. Examiner's Manual.* 2nd ed. Austin, TX: Pro-ed; 2000.

55. Haley SM, Costes WJ, Ludlow LH, et al. *Pediatric Evaluation of Disability Inventory (PEDI) PEDI Research Group.* Boston, MA: New England Medical Center Hospitals Inc; 1992.

56. Palisano R, Rosenbaum P, Walter S, et al. Development and reliability of a system to classify gross motor function in children with cerebral palsy. *Dev Med Child Neurol.* 1997;39:214-223.

57. Palisano RJ, Hanna SE, Rosenbaum PL, et al. Validation of a model of gross motor function for children with cerebral palsy. *Phys Ther.* 2000;80:974-985.

58. Rosenbaum PL, Walter SD, Hanna SE, et al. Prognosis for gross motor function in cerebral palsy: creation of motor development curves. *JAMA.* 2002;288:974-985.

59. Badell-Ribera A. Cerebral palsy: predictive value of selected clinical signs for early prognostication of motor function. *Arch Phys Med Rehabil.* 1976;57:153-158.

60. Campos da Paz A Jr, Burnett SM, Braga LW. Walking prognosis in cerebral palsy: a 22 year retrospective analysis. *Dev Med Child Neurol.* 1994;36:130-134.

61. Montgomery PC. Predicting potential for ambulation in children with cerebral palsy. *Pediatric Physical Therapy.* 1998;10:148-155.

62. Schmidt RA, Lee TD, eds. Retention and transfer. In: *Motor Control and Learning. A Behavioral Emphasis.* 3rd ed. Champaign, IL: Human Kinetics; 1999:386-408.

63. Montgomery PC. Frequency and duration of pediatric physical therapy. *Magazine of Physical Therapy.* 1994;March.

64. Bower E, Michell D, Burnett M, et al. Randomized controlled trial of physiotherapy in 56 children with cerebral palsy followed for 18 months. *Dev Med Child Neurol.* 2001;43:4-15.

65. Trahan J, Malouin F. Intermittent intensive physiotherapy in children with cerebral palsy: a pilot study. *Dev Med Child Neurol.* 2002;44:233-239.

66. Siebes R, Winrolls L, Vermeer A. Qualitative analysis of therapeutic motor intervention programmes for children with cerebral palsy: an update. *Dev Med Child Neurol.* 2002;44:593-603.

67. Montgomery PC. Establishing functional outcomes and organizing intervention. In: Connolly BH, Montgomery PC, eds. *Therapeutic Exercise in Developmental Disabilities.* 3rd ed. Thorofare, NJ: SLACK Incorporated; 2004.

68. Craft MJ, Laken JA, Opliger, RA, et al. Siblings as change agents for promoting the functional status of children with cerebral palsy. *Dev Med Child Neurol.* 1990;32:1049-1057.

69. Dietz V, Berger W. Normal and impaired regulation of muscle stiffness in gait: a new hypothesis about muscle hypertonia. *Exp Neurol.* 1983;79:680-687.

70. Rose J, Haskell WL, Gamble JG, et al. Muscle pathology and clinical measures of disability in children with cerebral palsy. *J Orthop Res.* 1994;12:758-768.

71. Tardieu C, Lespargot A, Tabary C, et al. Toe-walking in children with cerebral palsy: contributions of contracture and excessive contraction of triceps surae. *Phys Ther.* 1989;69:656-662.

72. Andres T, Autgaerden S. Locomotion from pre to post-natal life. In: *Clinics in Developmental Medicine.* No 24. London, England: Medical Books Ltd; 1996:1-88.

73. Forssberg H. Ontogeny of human locomotor control. I: infant stepping, supported locomotion, and transition to independent locomotion. *Exp Brain Res.* 1985;57:480-493.

74. Leonard CT, Hirschfeld H, Forssberg H. The development of independent walking in children with cerebral palsy. *Dev Med Child Neurol.* 1991;33:567-577.

75. Leonard CT. Motor behavior and neural changes following perinatal and adult onset brain damage: implications for therapeutic intervention. *Phys Ther.* 1994;8:753-767.

76. Thelen E, Cooke DW. Relationship between newborn stepping and later walking: a new interpretation. *Dev Med Child Neurol.* 1987;29:380-393.

77. Zelazao PR. The development of walking. *J Mot Behav.* 1983;15:99-137.

78. Schindl M, Forstner C, Kern H, et al. Treadmill training with partial body weight support in non-ambulatory patients with cerebral palsy. *Arch Phys Med Rehabil.* 2002;81:301-306.

79. Davis DW, Thelen E, Keck J. Treadmill stepping in infants born prematurely. *Early Hum Dev.* 1994;39:211-223.

80. Vereijken B, Thelen E. Training infant treadmill stepping: the role of individual pattern stability. *Dev Psychobiol.* 1997;30:89-102.

81. Richards CL, Malouin F, Dumas F, et al. Early and intensive treadmill locomotor training for young children with cerebral palsy: a feasibility study. *Pediatric Physical Therapy.* 1997;9:158-165.

82. Cintas HM. The accomplishment of walking: aspects of the ascent. *Pediatric Physical Therapy.* 1993;5:61-68.

83. Greiner BM, Czernichl JM, Deitz JC. Gait parameters of children with spastic diplegia: a comparison of effects of posterior and anterior walkers. *Arch Phys Med Rehabil.* 1993;74:381-385.

84. Bierman J. Developing ambulation skills. In: Connolly BH, Montgomery PC, eds. *Therapeutic Exercise in Developmental Disabilities.* 3rd ed. Thorofare, NJ: SLACK Incorporated; 2004.

85. Bleck EE. Locomotor prognosis in cerebral palsy. *Dev Med Child Neurol.* 1975;17:18-25.

86. Bottos M, Bolcati C, Sciuto L, et al. Powered wheelchairs and independence in young children with tetraplegia. *Dev Med Child Neurol.* 2001;43:769-777.

87. Butler C. Augmentative mobility. Why do it? *Phys Med Rehabil Clin N Am.* 1991;2:801-815.

88. Fowler EG, Ho TW, Nwigwe A, et al. The effect of quadriceps femoris muscle strengthening exercises on spasticity in children with cerebral palsy. *Phys Ther.* 2001;81:1215-1223.

89. Damiano DL, Vaughan C, Abel MF. Muscle response to heavy

resistance exercise in children with spastic cerebral palsy. *Dev Med Child Neurol.* 1995;37:731-739.

90. Damiano DL, Martellotta TL, Sullivan DJ, et al. Muscle force production and functional performance in spastic cerebral palsy: relationship of co-contraction. *Arch Phys Med Rehabil.* 2000;81:895-900.

91. Damiano DL, Abel MF. Functional outcomes of strength training in spastic cerebral palsy. *Arch Phys Med Rehabil.* 1998;79:119-126.

92. McLaughlin JF, Bjornson KF, Astley SJ, et al. Selective dorsal rhizotomy: efficacy and safety in an investigator-masked randomized clinical trial. *Dev Med Child Neurol.* 1998;40:220-232.

93. Alexander R. Respiratory and oral-motor functioning. In: Connolly BH, Montgomery PC, eds. *Therapeutic Exercise in Developmental Disabilities.* 3rd ed. Thorofare NJ: SLACK Incorporated; 2004.

94. Ketelaar M, Vermeer A, Hart H, et al. Effects of a functional therapy program on motor abilities of children with cerebral palsy. *Phys Ther.* 2001;81:1534-1545.

95. Pellegrino L. Cerebral palsy: a paradigm for developmental disabilities. *Dev Med Child Neurol.* 1995;37:834-839.

96. Morris C. A review of the efficacy of lower-limb orthoses used for cerebral palsy. *Dev Med Child Neurol.* 2002;44:205-211.

97. Burton PA, Woolacott MH, Qualls C. Stance balance control with orthoses in a group of children with spastic cerebral palsy. *Dev Med Child Neurol.* 1999;41:748-757.

98. Knott KM, Held SL. Effects of orthoses on upright functional skills of children and adolescents with cerebral palsy. *Pediatric Physical Therapy.* 2002;14:199-297.

99. American Physical Therapy Association. Guide to physical therapist practice. 2nd ed. *Phys Ther.* 2001;81:9-744.

100. CDC. 2000 Growth Charts for the US. Vital and Health Statistics, Series 11, no. 246, 2000.

101. Butler C, Okamoto GA, McKay TM. Motorized wheelchair driving by disabled children. *Arch Phys Med Rehabil.* 1984;65:95-97.

102. Butler C. Effects of powered mobility on self-initiated behaviors of very young children with locomotor disability. *Developmental Medicine and Child Neurology.* 1986;28:325-332.

103. Gibson JJ. *The Ecological Approach to Visual Perception.* Boston, MA: Houghton Mifflin Co; 1979.

104. Williams EN, Broughton NS, Menelaus MB. Age-related walking in children with spinal bifida. *Dev Med Child Neurol.* 1999;41:446-449.

105. Hunt GM, Poulton A. Open spina bifida: a complete cohort reviewed 25 years after closure. *Dev Med Child Neurol.* 1995; 37:19-29.

106. Bartonek A, Saraste H. Factors influencing ambulation in myelomeningocele: a cross-sectional study. *Dev Med Child Neurol.* 2001;43:253-260.

107. Hewson JE. Basic physiotherapy of spinal bifida. *Dev Med Child Neurol Suppl.* 1976;27:117-118.

108. Stiefee D, Stribata T, Meuli M, et al. Tethering of the spinal cord in mouse fetuses and neonates with spina bifida. *J Neurosurg.* 2003;99:206-213.

109. Bowman EM, McLone DG, Grant T, et al. Spina bifida outcome: a 25 year perspective. *Pediatric Neurosurg.* 2001; 34:114-120.

110. Sharif S, Allcutt D, Marks C, et al. "Tethered cord syndrome"—recent clinical experience. *Br J Neurosurg.* 1997;11:49-51.

111. Sarwark JF, Weer DT, Gariei AP, et al. Tethered cord syndrome in low motor level children with myelomeningocele. *Pediatr Neurosurg.* 1996;25:295-301.

112. Yeates KO, Enrile BG, Loss N, et al. Verbal learning and memory in children with myelomeningocele. *J Pediatr Psychol.* 1995;20:801-815.

113. Dennis M, Barnes M. Math and numeracy in young adults with spina bifida and hydrocephalus. *Dev Neuropsychol.* 2002;21:141-155.

CHAPTER FOUR

Impaired Motor Function and Sensory Integrity Associated With Nonprogressive Disorders of the Central Nervous System— Acquired in Adolescence or Adulthood (Pattern D)

Laura Gilchrist, PT, PhD
Marilyn Woods, PT[†]
Lisa Kuehn, PT
Janice B. Hulme, PT, MS, DHSc

ANATOMY

The anatomy of the CNS is further detailed in Pattern B: Impaired Neuromotor Development; Pattern C: Impaired Motor Function and Sensory Integrity Associated With Nonprogressive Disorders of the Central Nervous System— Congenital Origin or Acquired in Infancy or Childhood; and Pattern H: Impaired Motor Function, Peripheral Nerve Integrity, and Sensory Integrity Associated With Nonprogressive Disorders of the Spinal Cord. The anatomy of the PNS is further detailed in Pattern F: Impaired Peripheral Nerve Integrity and Muscle Performance Associated With Peripheral Nerve Injury.

The CNS has two main components: the spinal cord and the brain. The brain is composed of the cerebrum, cerebellum, and brainstem. The cerebrum is comprised of two cerebral hemispheres with the cerebral cortex surrounding deeper structures of the basal ganglia, hippocampus, and amygdaloid nuclei; the white matter tracts ascending and descending from the cortex; and a fluid-filled ventricular system. The cortex consists of the frontal, parietal, temporal, and occipital lobes. The brain connects to the spinal cord at the brainstem that is made up of the midbrain, pons, and medulla. The cerebellum is located behind the brainstem.[1]

The CNS is encased in a variety of structures that provide protection from damage. The cerebrum, cerebellum, and brainstem are surrounded by bones that create the neurocranium. These bones include the frontal, parietal, occipital, temporal, sphenoid, and ethmoid bones.[1] In young children, these bones have not yet fused, and slow increases in brain size or CSF volume can be accommodated. In adults, the suture lines are fused, leaving little room for expansion without increases in intracranial pressure (ICP).[1] There are a variety of openings through the skull bones for the entrance and exit of cranial nerves as well as for the spinal cord.

The brain is also covered by membranes, called the cranial meninges. These membranes lie immediately internal to the

[†]Deceased.

skull bones. The outermost membrane, the dura mater, is a strong fibrous membrane that is fused to the skull bones. It surrounds the entire CNS, including the spinal cord, and has infoldings that divide the two cerebral hemispheres (the falx cerebri) and divide the cerebrum from the cerebellum (the cerebellar tentorium). Within specific portions of the dura are endothelial cell-lined spaces that act as collection sinuses for cerebral venous blood that ultimately drains venous blood into the internal jugular vein.[1]

Below the dura mater are two thinner membranes, the arachnoid mater and the pia mater. The arachnoid mater sits directly below the dura mater, but is not attached to the dura. The pia mater is a delicate membrane that adheres directly to the surface of the brain. Between the arachnoid and pia is the subarachnoid space, which contains CSF, cerebral arteries, and cerebral veins.[1]

CSF fills the ventricles within the brain and surrounds the brain in the subarachnoid space. It is produced by the choroid plexus, which is a modified vascular structure found within the ventricles. CSF flows through the ventricles through foramina and eventually surrounds both the brain and spinal cord. It is reabsorbed through the arachnoid villi and is returned to the venous blood supply in the dural sinuses. CSF serves both as a mechanical cushion to protect the brain from impact with the skull and also provides a consistent external environment for the optimal functioning of the nerve cells and glia.[2]

Blood is supplied to the brain through the internal carotid arteries and the vertebral arteries.[1] The cerebral hemispheres primarily receive blood from the internal carotid artery. In the brain, the internal carotid arteries separate into middle and anterior cerebral arteries. The middle cerebral artery brings a blood supply to the lateral surfaces of the cerebral hemispheres including the frontal, parietal, and temporal lobes. This includes both primary somatosensory cortex and primary motor cortex, specifically in the areas representing control of the UEs more so than the LEs. Along the way, it also has branches that supply subcortical structures: the internal capsule and basal ganglia. The anterior cerebral artery brings circulation to the medial surfaces of the cerebral hemispheres including the frontal, parietal, and temporal lobes. These areas represent control of the LEs. The brainstem and cerebellum receive their blood supply from the vertebral and basilar arteries. Also arising from the basilar artery are 1) the posterior cerebral arteries that supply the thalamus and occipital cortex, which is important for visual processing; and 2) both superior and inferior cerebellar arteries that supply blood to the cerebellum.

Supply of blood to all areas of the brain is important for survival of neurons. There is an extensive network of collateral arteries in the cerebrum that allows for alternate routes of circulation in the case of vessel occlusion. The Circle of Willis at the base of the brain has communicating arteries. The posterior communicating artery connects the posterior and middle cerebral arteries, and the anterior communicating artery connects the bilateral anterior cerebral arteries. Effectively, blood can be shunted between sides of the brain and from one primary supply (either the vertebral or internal carotid) to the other if it becomes necessary due to vascular occlusion.[3]

PHYSIOLOGY

The physiology of the CNS is further detailed in Pattern B: Impaired Neuromotor Development; Pattern C: Impaired Motor Function and Sensory Integrity Associated With Nonprogressive Disorders of the Central Nervous System—Congenital Origin or Acquired in Infancy or Childhood, and Pattern H: Impaired Motor Function, Peripheral Nerve Integrity, and Sensory Integrity Associated With Nonprogressive Disorders of the Spinal Cord. The physiology of the PNS is further detailed in Pattern F: Impaired Peripheral Nerve Integrity and Muscle Performance Associated With Peripheral Nerve Injury.

The spinal cord is important for motor responses that are automatic or instantaneous in response to sensory stimuli. The lower areas of the brain (medulla, pons, midbrain, hypothalamus, thalamus, cerebellum, and basal ganglia) control "subconscious" bodily functions such as respiration, arterial pressure, equilibrium, and postural reflexes. The higher brain or cortical level comprises a large information storage area. This area of the brain functions for storage of past experiences and patterns of motor response. This information is used at will to control motor functions of the body.

Neurons require constant flow of oxygen and nutrients that are supplied by the circulatory system. "The brain is very active metabolically, but has no effective way to store oxygen or glucose. A stable and copious blood supply is therefore required, and the brain, which represents only 2% of the total body weight, uses about 15% of the normal cardiac output and accounts for nearly 25% of the body's oxygen consumption."[4(p 129)] With complete occlusion of circulation in a specific region, there is complete cessation of neuronal activity in minutes.[5] Anaerobic metabolism is insufficient to meet the brain's needs.[3]

Normally, cerebral blood vessels maintain a constant flow through autoregulation. Levels of metabolites, such as carbon dioxide and oxygen, in the bloodstream alter blood flow to maintain adequate levels in metabolically active tissues. There is indication that cerebral vessels are innervated by autonomic fibers and nerve fibers from the brain, but it is not definitive in regards to the complete role of these fibers in controlling blood flow.[4]

A decrease in blood flow can produce irreversible injury to nerve cells. The circulatory system has collateral circulation to help prevent nerve damage in the event of blood vessels becoming narrowed or blocked. An example of this is the Circle of Willis. There is normally little to no blood flow occurring in the Circle of Willis. However, if one of the major vessels comprising this formation becomes occluded proximally or within this area, the communicating arteries allow blood flow and help to prevent damage. Other routes of collateral circulation exist at the arteriolar and capillary levels between terminal branches of the cerebral arteries. They may or may not be sufficient to maintain an area with blood flow.

PATHOPHYSIOLOGY

NEUROPLASTICITY

The capacity of the nervous system to change with experience is often referred to as neuroplasticity. An example of the nervous system's plasticity is the widespread change in neural activity that occurs with acute cerebral damage. While one might expect that the areas close to the injury may be altered by the damage, studies have shown that areas far away from the injury site, such as in the contralateral hemisphere, also undergo major changes in activity and function (see Stein and Hoffman[6] for a review of the literature in this area). Although recovery of injured neurons in the penumbra may account for some of the improvement in function after nervous system insult, it is now widely held that intact portions of the nervous system may take over lost functions, leading to observable changes in behavior.

In the case of stroke, neuronal depolarization in the peri-infarct area may serve as a signal for axonal sprouting in the nondamaged hemisphere.[7] The new synapses created by axonal sprouting can renervate regions of the cerebrum and brainstem denervated due to the infarct, both by intact areas of the ipsilateral cortex and also by the contralateral hemisphere.[7] Thus, the brain undergoes reorganization due to the injury, where regions of the brain alter their connectivity. Additionally, existing synapses can alter their level of activity, either strengthening or weakening the activity of various pathways. Although the injury itself is able to alter the motor maps in the primary motor cortex, Nudo and colleagues[8,9] found that specific training could induce recovery of function and shape the reorganization of the cortex. Thus, it appears that after injury, when the nervous system is substantially altered due to injury, neuroplasticity is a major contributor to recovery. Therefore, the physical therapist and other rehabilitation professionals must use the brain's natural neuroplastic capabilities to facilitate recovery.

Medical Interventions

Medical treatment of patients with acute stroke includes optimizing blood flow to the brain while preventing bleeding. Determination of the nature of the CVA is important to determine the best course. Ischemic stroke is often treated by maintaining BP and oxygenation status, using anticoagulant and thrombolytic therapy,[10] and potentially removing the clot with an intra-arterial catheter with retrieval device.[11] These therapies need to be initiated early after the stroke onset to

be safe, and thus public education of stroke is imperative. Currently only 5% of patients receive tissue plasminogen activator (tPA), because of the narrow therapeutic window (3 hours) and the large numbers of patients for whom this therapy is contraindicated.[10]

Hemorrhagic stroke is treated differently, as the clot-reducing medications are dangerous in these cases. Surgery may be used to repair ruptured aneurysms, if on the cortical surface, or to evacuate blood/clots. Bleeding can also cause irritation and swelling of the nervous tissues, and thus medications to reduce cerebral edema may be used. For patients at high risk for brain surgery or when the location of the rupture makes surgery difficult, embolization, in which a clotting agent is delivered to the hemorrhagic area, may be used. This technique may also be used to treat aneurysms and arteriovenous malformations before they rupture.[12]

STROKE

In the United States stroke is the third leading cause of death and, in those who survive, is a major cause of long-term disability.[13] Stroke, also called cerebrovascular accident (CVA), is an abnormality of brain function caused by disruption of circulation to the brain leading to permanent tissue damage.[3] Transient ischemic attacks (TIAs) are similar to stroke, but in the case of a TIA, there is no permanent damage and rapid, full recovery occurs.[14] The two main types of stroke are ischemic and hemorrhagic. In more than 80% of cases, stroke tissue damage is due to ischemia. In another 12%, brain tissue damage results from cerebral hemorrhage, and in the remaining 8%, there is bleeding into the subarachnoid space.[15]

Ischemic infarction in brain tissues occurs when the blood supply to a region of the brain is restricted due to occlusion of the blood vessel supplying that area. This can be a result of a large or small vessel thrombus or an embolus from the heart. The development of atherosclerosis of arteries supplying the brain is a major cause leading to the blockage of a blood vessel. This degenerative process continues until a thrombus or clot forms. It is more likely to occur where blood vessels turn or divide. Enlargement of the clot may occur at the site of a clogged vessel (cerebral thrombus), or, in about 35% of strokes, the clot loosens and moves downstream to the brain until it can pass no further (cerebral embolism).[16]

Hemorrhagic vascular disease results when a blood vessel to the brain ruptures. "Younger individuals usually suffer hemorrhage as a result of an anatomical abnormality of a cerebral artery such as an aneurysm."[16(p 33)] In older persons, rupture of cerebral arteries (cerebral hemorrhage) is more likely to occur if that individual has HTN, atherosclerosis, or degenerative vascular changes that predispose one to the formation of thrombi and emboli. A subarachnoid hemorrhage occurs when blood vessels on the surface of the brain break, filling the space between the brain and the skull. Some hemorrhage is a result of head trauma.

All strokes result from restriction of blood flow to brain cells. With the complexity of the brain and the circulatory system supplying the brain, there are usually varying levels of tissue involvement. Neurons are damaged by lactic acidosis and the consequences of anaerobic metabolism due to the inability of the vascular system to remove waste products. The immediate area of the brain without adequate blood supply is considered an infarct. This is dead tissue that will not regenerate. Surrounding this initial area is the penumbra that has tissue that may return to normal function through the development of collateral circulation and early intervention.

The location and amount of cerebral tissue involved in the brain injury determines the symptoms, signs, and extent of disability of the stroke. Table 4-1 details common sites of occlusion and their related signs and symptoms. The magnitude of a neurological deficit is not necessarily related to the size of the infarct causing it. "A very small lesion in the brainstem or internal capsule can have a much more devastating effect than damage to certain relatively large areas of the cerebellum or cerebral hemispheres."[4(p 134)]

The majority of strokes occur in the cerebrum usually on one side and not both.[16] Deficits of cerebral injury include levels of paralysis; impairment of vision, touch, or other sensation; loss of communication; and alteration in normal mentation. If the cerebellum is injured due to stroke, changes in postural control, coordination of eye movements, and fine coordination may be affected. Stroke in the deeper brain centers that control heart and lung functions are often fatal. Since brain cells do not regenerate, every effort is made to regain function after a stroke through retraining of cells that have been left undamaged and through the neuroplastic abilities of the human brain.

TRAUMATIC BRAIN INJURY

Damage to the CNS may occur from many types of traumatic experiences. Car accidents, penetrating objects (such as a bullet), or general anoxia may cause damage to a wide variety of brain structures, including all parts of the cortex, the subcortical structures, the brainstem, and the cerebellum. In TBIs, the damage may be both focal and diffuse.

Focal damage occurs at the site of initial trauma, where brain tissue has been damaged from a force applied to the skull, such as in the impact from a car accident. As in the case of motor vehicle accidents, there is often a coup-contrecoup injury that results from one side of the brain hitting the skull (often the frontal lobe), and then the opposite side of the brain being injured from the backward translation of the brain after impact into the opposite side of the skull (in this instance the occipital lobe). Other types of injuries, such as gunshot wounds to the head or displaced skull fractures, also lead to focal lesions at the site of trauma. The reader is referred to Table 3-1 for specific regions of the CNS that may be injured and their specific functions. Micro- and macroscopic vascular damage occurs at the site(s) of impact, leading to hemorrhagic infarctions within the nervous tissue in the region.

Diffuse axonal injury also often occurs in TBI. Under certain circumstances, shear injuries can occur to axons, particularly in white matter tracts. The axons are not prepared to withstand tensile forces, such as occur in shear injuries, and this elongation of axons can result not only in axonal disruption, but also in abnormalities of the cytoarchitecture of the macroscopically intact axons. Specifically, elongation of the axon leads to mechanical damage of sodium channels. A massive influx of sodium then leads to axonal swelling and an additional influx of calcium into the cell. The increase of intracellular calcium leads to proteolysis and an accumulation of axonal transport proteins within the axons, so that axonal transport ceases to function leaving the axon functionally inactive. These microscopic changes occur over hours to days after injury, and particularly affect the deep and subcortical white matter tracts. While often discussed as diffuse injuries in nature, they are often multifocal, impacting the corpus callosum and brainstem tracts.[17]

Diffuse injury can also occur in the absence of shear forces through both hypoxic-ischemic injuries, as well as increased ICP. Systemic hypotension or anoxia as a result of the initial injury leads to a diffuse loss of oxygen to all of the CNS structures. Metabolically active regions of the CNS will be differentially impacted. Cerebral swelling or disruption of the pathways for CSF result in increased ICP. Because the brain is encased in a rigid skull in adults, a build-up of fluids increases the pressure on CNS tissues. With large increases of ICP, herniations of brain tissue may occur across the tentorium or into the foramen magnum. Both of these complications may result in focal pressure on midbrain structures, including the reticular formation, leading to coma.[18] Patients with this complication would be classified in Pattern I: Impaired Arousal, Range of Motion, and Motor Control Associated With Coma, Near Coma, or Vegetative State.

Hemorrhages outside of the brain tissue can occur in TBIs that have a major impact on the CNS. Subdural hematomas can occur from disruption of the cerebral bridging veins. Bleeding from these veins between the arachnoid and the dura often occurs slowly due to the low pressure nature of the venous system. It may clot as it accumulates, slowly increasing pressure and pushing the cerebrum downward.[19] Signs and symptoms of a subdural hemorrhage are thus slow in onset. Subarachnoid hemorrhages arise from bleeding of a cerebral artery into the subarachnoid space, often due to rupture of an aneurysm. The onset of symptoms is much faster for arterial bleeds due to the higher pressure of the arterial system. Extradural hemorrhages also may occur, especially following head trauma to the temporal bone, causing a rupture of the middle meningeal artery.[20] Because this is also an arterial bleed into the neurocranial space, patients

Table 4-1

COMMON SITES OF OCCLUSION WITH RELATED SIGNS AND SYMPTOMS[2,18]

Artery	*Anatomic Region Supplied*	*Signs and Symptoms*
Anterior cerebral	Frontal lobe—medial aspect	
	Primary motor cortex—LE primarily	Contralateral hemiparesis—mainly LE
	Parietal lobe—medial aspect	
	Primary somatosensory cortex—LE primarily	Contralateral hemisensory loss—mainly LE
	Corpus callosum	Bimanual task impairment
	Cingulate gyrus	Emotional control impairments
Middle cerebral	Frontal lobe—lateral aspect	
	Primary motor cortex—UE primarily	Contralateral hemiparesis—UE>LE
	Broca's area on left	Motor speech impairment
	Premotor cortex	Apraxia
	Frontal eye fields	Loss of conjugate gaze
	Parietal lobe—lateral aspect	
	Primary somatosensory cortex—lateral aspect	Contralateral hemisensory loss—UE>LE
	Optic radiations	Homonymous anopsia—inferior quadrant
	Temporal lobe	
	Auditory cortex	Sensorineural hearing loss
	Wernicke's area on left	Receptive speech impairment
	Internal capsule	Loss of axonal connections for motor control and somatosensation
	Optic radiations	Homonymous anopsia—superior quadrant
	Basal ganglia	Motor control impairments
Posterior cerebral	Occipital cortex	Contralateral homonymous hemianopsia
	Temporal cortex	Memory impairment
	Thalamus	Sensory disturbance, thalamic pain syndrome
	Subthalamic nucleus	Movement disorder including tremor and involuntary movement
Superior cerebellar	Cerebellar peduncles; superior and middle	Cerebellar ataxia
	Superior cerebellum	Cerebellar ataxia, vestibular dysfunction
Inferior cerebellar	Cranial nerves	Loss of sensation in face, dysphagia
	Cerebellar peduncles, inferior	Cerebellar ataxia
	Inferior cerebellum	Cerebellar ataxia
Basilar	Pons	Tetraplegia (corticospinal tract), cranial nerve dysfunction (IV to VIII), coma (reticular formation)
Vertebral	Medulla	Hemiplegia (contralateral), cranial nerve dysfunction (IX to XII)

deteriorate quickly and surgical intervention is often necessary.[19] With any of these hemorrhages, bleeding into any of these spaces creates a space-occupying lesion, creating pressure on the brain and brainstem tissues that may lead to brain herniations.

CENTRAL VESTIBULAR DYSFUNCTION

The pathophysiology of vestibular dysfunction, including central dysfunction, is detailed in Pattern F: Impaired Peripheral Nerve Integrity and Muscle Performance Associated With Peripheral Nerve Injury.

IMAGING

One or more of the following imaging tests may be used to find ischemic or hemorrhagic damage to the CNS or alterations in cerebral circulation.

♦ CAT, CT
  ● Uses low dose x-rays and a computer to accurately analyze cerebral injury, including the areas of bleed or infarction that resulted from the CVA
  ● Assists in differentiating ischemic from hemorrhagic stroke for purpose of thrombolytic therapy
♦ CT angiography
  ● Requires injection of contrast dye to demonstrate vascular lesions
♦ Echocardiography
  ● Evaluates heart function
  ● Used to document a cardioembolic source of stroke
♦ Magnetic resonance angiography (MRA)
  ● Used to image blood vessels to the brain, indicating areas of stenosis or anyeurysm
♦ MRI
  ● Uses a magnetic field (no radiation) to give detailed pictures of the brain
  ● Used early in assessment to rule out hemorrhagic stroke for use of tPA
♦ Positron emission tomography scan (PET scan)
  ● Sometimes used for showing utilization of oxygen, glucose, and other nutrients by the brain (metabolism)
  ● Used to identify areas weakened or damaged by the stroke
♦ Single photon emission computed tomography (SPECT)
  ● Uses nuclear isotopes to provide a tomographic image of the brain
  ● Shows perfusion in the brain
♦ Transesophageal echocardiography (TEE)
  ● Used to look for cardioembolic source of infarct
  ● Provides higher accuracy of identifying thrombus from the left atrium

OTHER CLINICAL TESTS

One or more of the following clinical tests may be used to find ischemic or hemorrhagic damage to the CNS or alterations in cerebral circulation.

♦ Carotid duplex and transcranial Doppler ultrasound
  ● Assesses flow of arteries supplying the brain
♦ Electrocardiography (ECG)
  ● Detects embolisms
  ● Evaluates heart function and identifies cardiac arrhythmias
♦ Electroencephalography
  ● Allows an electrical activity assessment of the brain
  ● Identifies seizure activity
  ● Establishes levels of unconsciousness in unresponsive patients

PHARMACOLOGY[21-23]

The following pharmacologic agents may be used for patients with ischemic or hemorrhagic stroke.

♦ Anticoagulant drugs
  ● Examples: Heparin, warfarin (Coumadin), enoxaparin (Lovenox)
  ● Actions: Increase antithrombin III and inhibit clotting through interference with clotting factors and lengthening the time required for a clot to form
  ● Side effects: Increased risk of bleeding
♦ Anticonvulsants
  ● Examples: Carbamazepine (Tegretol), clonazepam (Klonopin), ethosuximide (Zarontin), phenobarbital, phenytoin (Dilantin), primidone (Mysoline), valproic acid (Depakene)
  ● Actions: Inhibit spread of seizure activity; inhibit spike and wave formation; decrease amplitude, frequency, duration, and spread of discharge in seizures
  ● Side effects: Headaches and dizziness; ataxia; skin conditions (dermatitis or rash); very high doses may result in lethargy or drowsiness, interfering with ability to participate in requested activities
♦ Antifungal drugs
  ● Examples: Mycostatin, Mycostatin pastilles, Nystatin ointment
  ● Action: Reduce fungal infections
  ● Side effects: Itching, irritation, burning
♦ Antihistamine drugs
  ● Example: Diphenhydramine (Benadryl, Percogesic, Sudafed, Tylenol)
  ● Actions: Selectively counteracts the pharmacological effects of histamine following its release from the mast cells, thus preventing histamine-triggered reactions

- Side effects: Dry mouth, upset stomach, drowsiness, chest congestion, headache
◆ Antihypertensive drugs
  - Angiotensin-converting enzyme (ACE) inhibitors
    - Example: Lisinopril (Prinivil)
    - Action: Lowers BP by decreasing arterial spasm
    - Side effects: Cough, dizziness, tiredness, diarrhea, tiredness, runny nose
  - Beta-adrenergic blockers
    - Cardioselective
      ▸ Examples: Atenolol (Tenormin), metoprolol (Lopressor, Toprol XL)
      ▸ Actions: Lower HR and vasodilate to lower BP
      ▸ Side effects: Dizziness, drowsiness, fatigue, hypotension, insomnia, and syncope and may mask hypoglycemia
    - Nonselective
      ▸ Example: Propranolol (Inderal, InnoPran XL)
      ▸ Action: Lowers HR and BP
      ▸ Side effects: Fatigue, dizziness, and syncope
  - Calcium channel blockers
    - Examples: Amlodipine (Norvasc), diltiazem (Cardizem, Dilacor), nifedipine (Adalat, Procardia) Verapamil (Calan, Verelan)
    - Actions
      ▸ Inhibit vascular smooth muscle cell proliferation to decrease vascular resistance and vasodilate
      ▸ Prevent influx of calcium through voltage-operated channels with action at both cellular and vascular levels and therefore lowers BP
    - Side effects: Headache, OH, nausea, swelling in ankles, dizziness, drowsiness, flushing
◆ Corticosteroids
  - Example: Dexamethasone
  - Action: Reduces severe cerebral edema
  - Side effects: Upset stomach, vomiting, headache, easy bruising, dizziness, insomnia, depression, anxiety, acne, increased hair growth
◆ Diuretics
  - Loop
    - Example: Furosemide (Lasix)
    - Action: Acts on the ascending loop of Henle in the kidney to decrease fluid volume
    - Side effects: Arrhythmias, dehydration, electrolyte imbalance, impairment of glycemic control
  - Potassium sparing
    - Examples: Amiloride (Midamor), spironolactone (Aldactone)
    - Actions: Decrease fluid volume, spare potassium, and decrease risk of arrhythmias
    - Side effects: Dehydration and impaired glycemic control

  - Thiazides
    - Examples: Chlorthalidone (Clorpres, Tenoretic, Thalitone), hydrochlorothiazide (Aldactazide, Capozide, Dyazide, HydroDIURIL, Lopressor HCT, Maxzide, Vaseretic)
    - Actions: Block reabsorption of sodium in distal tubules of the kidneys and thus decrease fluid volume in vascular system to lower BP
    - Side effects: Dehydration, electrolyte imbalance, glucose intolerance, and increased triglyceride and cholesterol levels
◆ Hypercholesteremic drugs
  - Examples: Simvastatin (Zocor), atorvastatin calcium (Lipitor)
  - Action: Inhibit cholesterol production
  - Side effects: May cause liver damage and rhabdomyolysis
◆ NSAIDs
  - Examples: Ibuprofen (Advil, Motrin)
  - Actions: Relieves pain, tenderness, swelling
  - Side effects: Dizziness, constipation, diarrhea, ringing in ears
◆ Platelet-inhibiting drugs
  - Examples: Aspirin and other platelet anti-aggregant drugs, such as ticlopidine, clopidogrel, dipyridamole
  - Actions: Prevent blood from coagulating by reducing the adhesiveness of platelets
  - Side effects: Nausea, vomiting, stomach pain, heartburn, diarrhea, headache
◆ Stool softeners
  - Examples: Colace, Doxinate, Senokot
  - Action: Stool softening
  - Side effects: Stomach or intestinal cramps, upset stomach
◆ Thrombolytic agents
  - Example: Streptokinase (Abbokinase, Activase, Retavase, Streptase)
    - Actions
      ▸ Injected directly into an occluded or stenotic cerebral artery during angiography to lyze the thrombus
      ▸ Usually done within 6 hours after ischemic stroke onset
    - Side effects: Increased risk of bleeding
  - Example: tPA
    - Actions
      ▸ Intravenous thrombolytic therapy used for acute ischemic strokes to dissolve blood clot
      ▸ Used within 3 hours of the stroke to improve outcome and reverse some neurological deficits

■ Side effects: Increased risk of bleeding

♦ Zolpidem
  ● Example: Ambien
  ● Actions: A sedative-hypnotic drug used to treat insomnia by slowing brain activity to induce sleep
  ● Side effects: Dizziness, drowsiness, headache, balance difficulty, constipation, diarrhea, heartburn, stomach pain, shaking, tingling, muscle aches, joint pain

Case Study #1: Stroke

Mr. Dale Schreiner is a 60-year-old male who sustained a sudden onset of dizziness and left hemiparesis 3 days ago secondary to acute hemorrhagic infarct of the penetrating branches of the middle cerebral artery and is currently medically stable in an acute care hospital.

PHYSICAL THERAPIST EXAMINATION

HISTORY

♦ General demographics: Mr. Schreiner is a 60-year-old male whose primary language is English. He is right handed. He is a college graduate.

♦ Social history: Mr. Schreiner is married and is the father of four grown children, all of whom live nearby. He has five grandchildren. His wife works part-time and is able to work flex hours. She reports that she is healthy and willing to do what is necessary to allow her husband to come home.

♦ Employment/work: He is the manager of the Rural Electric Association.

♦ Living environment: He lives in a large home with five steps to enter in the front or two steps to enter through the back of the house, both with hand rails on both sides. There is one flight of stairs with a single right hand rail to the basement which has a family room, laundry, and half-bath. The main floor has the kitchen, living room, dining room, two bathrooms (one with tub and shower combination and one with just shower), and three bedrooms.

♦ General health status
  ● General health perception: Prior to this episode, his health was generally good.
  ● Physical function: Prior to this episode, his function was normal for his age.
  ● Psychological function: He reports some depression at this time.

● Role function: Son, husband, father, grandfather, manager, community leader.
● Social function: Mr. Schreiner belongs to several professional organizations and is active in his church and community. He loves to read, listen to music, and fish.

♦ Social/health habits: He was a smoker for 30 years, one to two packs per day, and quit 10 years ago. He drinks only socially.

♦ Family history: His mother died at age 72 and had a history of heart disease. His father is 88 years of age and is healthy.

♦ Medical/surgical history: He has HTN and a history of hyperlipidemia. Mr. Schreiner also had a L5 disc herniation (no surgery) 25 years ago.

♦ Current condition(s)/chief complaint(s): Three days ago, Mr. Schreiner sustained a sudden onset of dizziness and left hemiparesis secondary to acute hemorrhagic infarct of the penetrating branches of the middle cerebral artery leading to right basal ganglia and internal capsule. He was admitted to a hospital that specializes in stroke rehabilitation where he underwent CT and MRI testing. He currently complains of numbness and weakness in his left arm and leg, difficulty with speech (dysarthria), decreased memory, hemiparesis, and decreased balance. He is unable to walk, do daily activities, and to work. He wants to return to his home and to his work. He is now medically stable and is able to begin rehabilitation.

♦ Functional status and activity level: He has been unable to ambulate and requires assistance with all mobility since the acute stroke.

♦ Medications (preadmission): Zocor, Prinivil, Norvasc, Colace, Senokot, atenolol, Tylenol.

♦ Other clinical tests: CT and MRI scans show a 2.5-cm right basal ganglia hemorrhage with some extension into the ventricle.

SYSTEMS REVIEW

♦ Cardiovascular/pulmonary
  ● BP: 132/72 mmHg on medications
  ● Edema: None
  ● HR: 74 bpm
  ● RR: 18 bpm
♦ Integumentary
  ● Presence of scar formation: None
  ● Skin color: Normal
  ● Skin integrity: Intact
♦ Musculoskeletal
  ● Gross range of motion: WFL
  ● Gross strength: Right upper and lower extremity

(RUE and RLE) WNL, left upper and lower extremity (LUE and LLE) impaired

- Gross symmetry: Left hemiparesis and facial droop
- Height: 5'10" (1.77 m)
- Weight: 205 lbs (92.99 kg)

◆ Neuromuscular
  - Balance: Impaired sitting and standing balance
  - Locomotion, transfers, and transitions: Needs assistance with all transitions, unable to ambulate

◆ Communication, affect, cognition, language, and learning style
  - Communication, affect, and cognition
    ▪ Mild dysarthria
    ▪ Left neglect
    ▪ No aphasia
  - Learning style
    ▪ Memory WFL but new learning moderately impaired (per speech pathology evaluation)
    ▪ Able to follow two-step commands

TESTS AND MEASURES

◆ Aerobic capacity/endurance
  - Mr. Schreiner has been on bedrest for 2 days
  - Anticipate loss of aerobic capacity and endurance due to deconditioning
  - Note elevated HR and RR following attempts at moving and transfers
  - Prior to stroke, he reports no problems with being short of breath or having difficulty completing physical tasks

◆ Arousal, attention, and cognition
  - Oriented x3 but sleepy
  - Follows verbal commands
  - Communication
    ▪ Appears to understand verbal commands but has delays in responding
    ▪ Need to give him time to respond
  - Cooperative and motivated

◆ Assistive and adaptive devices
  - None currently
  - Will need assistive device for any ambulation and may benefit from bracing to provide improved ankle stability and knee control during weightbearing activities given LLE weakness
  - Will initially need manual wheelchair for all mobility and for a few months for community mobility
  - Will need to evaluate home for rails in bathroom, bath or shower chair, and stool for self-care in bathroom and kitchen

◆ Cranial and peripheral nerve integrity
  - Right gaze preference

- Can track target to approximately 30 degrees left of midline at slow speeds with verbal cues

◆ Environmental, home, and work barriers
  - Home has five steps to enter in front, two steps in back, and one flight of steps to basement
  - Can live on main floor
  - Laundry in basement
  - Floors are mostly carpeted
  - Mrs. Schreiner believes they will be able to accommodate the wheelchair in the house, but it may be tight getting into the bathroom
  - Work
    ▪ Within walking distance but drives to work, two blocks to bus stop, has coworkers who could transport
    ▪ Needs to use keyboard, phone, talk to customers and clients, file
    ▪ One step into building, everything on one level, tiled floors, standard doors, no handicap-accessible features for doors, standard handicap-accessible bathroom stall (bar, raised toilet)

◆ Gait, locomotion, and balance
  - Sitting balance
    ▪ Requires moderate assistance sitting upright at edge of bed due to significant left lean
    ▪ Does not spontaneously put left arm out to support self, can put partial weight on arm if hand is positioned by physical therapist
  - Standing balance
    ▪ Maximal assist needed to maintain static balance due to left lean, contact guarding at left knee required to prevent buckling
    ▪ Unable to use balance strategies (ankle, hip, stepping)
    ▪ Unable to sway in standing, tends to lean to left and freeze
    ▪ Unable to ambulate due to poor balance, inability to weight shift, inability to advance LLE
    ▪ Sit to stand with moderate assist of two people

◆ Integumentary integrity
  - Skin integrity intact

◆ Motor function
  - Observation reveals decreased awareness of left side
  - Unable to perform pinch with left hand, has weak grasp
  - Fine motor skills of LUE severely limited, difficulty with bimanual tasks
  - Coordination limited in LLE movements due to hemiparesis
  - Decreased muscle tone in left extremities distally, stiffness in left hamstring
  - Difficulty initiating movement of left arm and leg

- Difficulty varying speeds, start, stop, or change directions of movement, overshoots endpoint with movements of the LLE
- Difficulty recruiting muscles for spontaneous support of limb, leg in standing and arm when sitting or standing
- Appears to understand motor command but difficulty accessing motor program

◆ Muscle performance
  - Manual muscle testing (MMT) revealed the following deviations from normal:
    ■ LUE: 2/5 at shoulder, 3-/5 at elbow, 2/5 at forearm, 3-/5 at wrist, 1/5 at fingers
    ■ LLE: Hip flex 3-/5; knee flexion and extension 3+/5; ankle dorsiflexion and plantarflexion 1/5; eversion and inversion 0/5
  - Endurance: Patient fatigues as evidenced by increased left lean with greater than 5 minutes of unsupported sitting

◆ Orthotic, protective, and supportive devices
  - Will need assistive device for initial ambulation to provide improved ankle stability and knee control during weightbearing
  - Will need a wheelchair for transport and use in the community and/or home
  - Will need bathroom equipment and adaptive devices to assist with ADL (to coordinate with occupational therapy)

◆ Pain
  - No pain reported

◆ Posture
  - Left lean in sitting and standing
  - Unable to correct with visual cues

◆ Range of motion
  - PROM: WFL throughout
  - AROM: WFL on right
  - AROM
    ■ LLE: Limited to approximately 85% of range in the hip and knee and <50% in ankle
    ■ LUE: Limited to approximately 30% of normal range in the shoulder, 50% at the elbow, and 10% in the wrist and hand
  - Mild tightness in hamstrings bilaterally

◆ Reflex integrity
  - Deep tendon reflexes present throughout
    ■ 3+ left patella and Achilles tendon on the left
    ■ 2+ right
  - Positive Babinski, indicates abnormal response on the left
  - Positive Hoffman's sign on the left

◆ Self-care and home management
  - Transfers/transitions
    ■ Sit to/from supine with moderate assist for trunk and LLE, maximal assist for LUE
    ■ Bed to/from wheelchair with moderate assist
  - Observed able to brush teeth and comb hair with right hand once set up
    ■ Demonstrates left neglect with these tasks
    ■ Needs to be sitting to perform these tasks
  - All other self-care tasks are dependent

◆ Sensory integrity
  - Poor sensory appreciation of left limbs to tactile and somatosensory
    ■ Decreased sensation to pinprick and light touch on left
    ■ Extinguishes on left to double simultaneous stimulation
    ■ Proprioception mildly impaired in left foot and ankle
  - Reports numbness of left lower arm and lower leg

◆ Work, community, and leisure integration or reintegration
  - Unable to work
  - Job requires Mr. Schreiner to come into office, use computer and phone to contact customers and employees, conduct meetings, direct employees, and oversee general management of company
  - Unable to access community activities
  - Unable to read due to visual problems

EVALUATION

Mr. Schreiner's history indicates that he was an active, right-handed male employed as the manager of the Rural Electric Association. His risk factors for stroke were HTN and history of smoking. He is 3 days post hemorrahagic infarct of the right middle cerebral artery including damage to right basal ganglia and internal capsule resulting in left hemiparesis and is currently medically stable in the acute care facility. He has primary impairments in strength, balance, sensation, proprioception, and cognition. These have led to functional limitations of being unable to sit or stand without assistance, being unable to ambulate, and requiring assistance with all bed mobility, transfers, and self-cares. Mr. Schreiner also is at risk due to his decreased awareness of his left side. He is at high risk for falls and, if early mobility is not initiated, he will be at risk for skin breakdown. He is unable to manage independently or with assistance from family at home or participate in his previous roles in church and community.

Diagnosis

Mr. Schreiner had a right hemorrhagic stroke, resulting in left hemiparesis. He has impaired: arousal, attention, and cognition; cranial and peripheral nerve integrity; gait, locomotion, and balance; motor function; muscle performance; posture; range of motion; reflex integrity; and sensory integrity. He is functionally limited in self-care and home management and in work, community, and leisure actions, tasks, and activities. He has environmental, work, and community barriers that will need adaptation. He is also in need of devices and equipment. These findings are consistent with placement in Pattern D: Impaired Motor Function and Sensory Integrity Associated With Nonprogressive Disorders of the Central Nervous System—Acquired in Adolescence or Adulthood. The identified impairments, functional limitations, barrier adaptation, and device and equipment needs will be addressed in determining the prognosis and the plan of care.

Prognosis and Plan of Care

Over the course of the visits, the following mutually established outcomes have been determined:

♦ Ability to move in bed is improved

♦ Bed mobility is independent

♦ Gait, locomotion, and balance are improved

♦ Motor function is improved

♦ Muscle performance is improved

♦ Perceptual information is integrated into function

♦ Plan for transition and management, including plan for falls, is in place

♦ Posture is improved

♦ Relevant community resources to meet his discharge needs are identified

♦ Risk of falls is reduced

♦ Standing with single UE support is achieved

♦ The extent to which the decreased awareness of left side interferes with function is limited

♦ Toileting is independent

♦ Transfers from car, chair, toilet, bed, to/from wheelchair with supervision are attained

♦ Unsupported sitting without loss of balance is achieved

♦ Visual attending to left is improved

♦ Wheelchair mobility in household is independent

To achieve these outcomes, the appropriate interventions for this patient are determined. These will include: coordination, communication, and documentation; patient/client-related instruction; therapeutic exercise; functional training in self-care and home management; functional training in work, community, and leisure integration or reintegration; manual therapy techniques; and prescription, application, and, as appropriate, fabrication of devices and equipment.

It is anticipated that Mr. Schreiner will have an episode of care that takes him from the acute care setting to home with home-based physical therapy and then transition to outpatient physical therapy for intense rehabilitation. It is anticipated that he will need 18 to 20 visits over 12 days in the hospital and then a further six to nine visits over 3 to 4 weeks after discharge to home. It is anticipated that he would begin an intense outpatient program that would initially focus on achieving ambulation at a higher level and independence in self-care and begin to address transition back to work. It is anticipated he will need 20 to 30 visits over 4 to 6 weeks. It is also anticipated that when his left wrist and hand function improve to meet criteria for participation in constraint-induced movement therapy (CIMT) he would need 10 visits over 14 days.

Mr. Schreiner is expected to have a good prognosis and has a strong family support system at home.

Interventions

RATIONALE FOR SELECTED INTERVENTIONS

Clinical practice guidelines (CPGs) for management of adult stroke rehabilitation care have been developed by the Veterans Affairs/Department of Defense and endorsed by the American Heart Association (AHA) and the American Stroke Association.[24] The CPGs recommend starting therapy as early as possible after stroke reporting evidence that earlier starting leads to higher functional abilities. No specific guidelines were provided for intensity of therapy due to the individuality of each patient and readiness or appropriateness for therapy. Clinicians are encouraged to access the full guidelines for greater detail.

Coordination, Communication, and Documentation

The CPGs recommend use of a rehabilitation facility that includes a multidisciplinary team that provides coordinated care in an organized manner. Better outcomes were found when patients participated in a rehabilitation program in a setting in which there was a coordinated multidisciplinary team that had experience in working with acute and subacute strokes.[25] Team members may include a physician, nurse, physical therapist, occupational therapist, kinesiotherapist, speech and language pathologist, psychologist, recreational therapist, patient, and family/caregivers. Family/caregiver involvement should begin as soon as possible and include participation in decision making and treatment planning.[24] In addition to communication regarding the current therapy program, families/caregivers need information regarding community resources so they may begin planning for services following discharge.[24]

Planning needs to include transition to home, return to work, driving, and social activities as these are difficult areas reported by stroke survivors.[26] Social services and vocational counseling should be consulted to assist with appropriate planning and support for return to community living and work. Support systems for families/caregivers should also be provided.[24,26]

Patient/Client-Related Instruction

Studies have demonstrated that patient and caregiver knowledge can be improved through educational strategies that are not passive.[24] Just providing the material or information did not improve knowledge. While specific education did improve the patient and caregiver knowledge, it did not transfer to better long-term outcomes, such as improved health or well-being.[24] Jette and colleagues[27] found that patient/caregiver education is included 84% of the time as an intervention by the physical therapist. Transfer activities, advanced gait activities, and community mobility activities were the most common areas of education. Maeshima and coworkers[28] demonstrated that families were able to be educated in both a home program that progressed the patient and in an inpatient rehabilitation program with higher patient satisfaction. Consideration needs to be given to the patient's and caregivers' emotional status, ability to process information in relation to all that is happening, and the preferred way of receiving information.

Therapeutic Exercise

The AHA has developed recommendations for physical activity and exercise for stroke survivors.[29] These recommendations stress the importance of being active, recognize the improvements in function, and stress the need to prevent secondary complications post stroke. They encourage the use of physical activity and structured exercise to prevent complications of inactivity common to stroke, decrease risk factors for a second stroke, and increase aerobic capacity.[29] Studies have demonstrated that chronic stroke survivors can benefit from participation in exercise routines[30-34] in the clinic, community, or home.

Aerobic Capacity/Endurance Conditioning

Energy expenditure following stroke may be increased due to deconditioning, spasticity, weakness, poor motor programming, decreased mechanical efficiency, and bracing.[29] Costs during ambulation have been reported to be up to two times higher than nondisabled individuals.[35] Aerobic exercise has been shown to be effective in improving aerobic capacity, submaximal exercise systolic BP response,[36] and more efficient energy expenditure and cardiovascular function.[37] Treadmill training with[38-40] and without body weight support[37,39] are effective in providing a cardiovascular workout

while also improving gait. HR should be monitored while walking, as Hesse and colleagues[41] found that energy costs may be higher with slower gait speeds.

The AHA recommends graded exercise testing prior to beginning an exercise program.[29] A pre-exercise evaluation to determine the physical readiness for exercise and the impact of medications on exercise is important, as there is a high incidence of coexisting heart disease in patients with stroke.[29] The following are recommendations from the AHA Guidelines[29]:

♦ Target heart rate (THR): Using 200 bpm–age=maximum heart rate (MHR)
- Graded exercise test has been performed: 50% to 80% of MHR
- No graded exercise test performed: 40% to 70% of MHR
- Use these methods only if the individual is not taking beta blockers or calcium channel blockers as these medications lower resting and working HRs

♦ Perceived exertion
- More reliable to use perceived exertion scales with individuals on beta blockers or calcium channel blockers
- Using the Borg rate of perceived exertion (RPE) scale, CR 10[42] target range would be 3 to 4 on scale of 0 to 10 or 11 to 14 on scale of 6 to 20

♦ Aerobic
- Any large muscle activity
- 40% to 50% peak oxygen uptake
- 40% to 70% HR reserve
- 11 to 14 (6 to 20 scale) Borg RPE
- 3 to 7 days per week
- 20 to 60 min/session or multiple 10 min sessions/day

♦ Strength
- Circuit training, weight machines, free weights, isometric exercises
- One to three sets of 10 to 15 repetitions
- 8 to 10 exercises involving major muscle groups
- 2 to 3 days a week

♦ Flexibility
- Stretching
- Before or after aerobic and strength training
- 2 to 3 days a week
- Hold each stretch for 10 to 30 seconds

♦ Neuromuscular
- Coordination and balance activities
- 2 to 3 days a week

Balance, Coordination, and Agility Training

Following stroke with hemiparesis, patients consistently

demonstrate an asymmetry with weightbearing in both sitting and standing. This is due to unilateral weakness and decreased postural control of the involved limb.[43] When standing posture and weightbearing are asymmetrical, patients are unable to perform normal reciprocal ambulation or other tasks that require good dynamic balance. Therefore, instructing patients in techniques to improve symmetry with weightbearing should result in improved quality, efficiency, and safety with balance and ambulation. Many approaches have been used to achieve this end, including the use of biofeedback force plate platforms. Comparisons of these approaches with physical therapy interventions that included early initiation of gait and balance tasks in a functional context have shown that, while these "high tech" approaches showed gains in the specific skills trained, they did not result in any additional benefit in functional outcomes over functional, task-specific gait training.[43-47] In addition, including visual deprivation (eyes closed) in a balance reeducation program has been shown to lead to greater gains in dynamic balance than that done only with free vision.[45] Bonan and associates[45] hypothesized that restricting visual input forces patients to use somatosensory and vestibular information more, rather than being dependent on vision as the sole source of sensory input.

The presence of visual neglect, most common in patients following right hemisphere stroke, presents an additional challenge to rehabilitation. Patients with neglect typically have greater functional disability and longer recovery time than patients with only motor deficits.[48] To date, research that has examined the impact of therapeutic interventions on visual neglect has shown that, regardless of technique used, improvements tend to be short term and specific to training tasks with little carryover to improvements in general functional tasks.[48,49] However, using task-specific training principles to improve left side awareness may be somewhat effective if family members are available to consistently reinforce the techniques.

Motor Function and Control

Many different treatment techniques to improve functional outcomes are used in stroke rehabilitation, including Bobath/NDT (neurodevelopmental treatment) approach, proprioceptive neuromuscular facilitation (PNF), Brunnström, and biofeedback. For these techniques, research demonstrates no difference between these techniques in outcomes for most measures of function.[44-47,50-53] However, the motor learning principle of task specificity, practicing or training a task that is specific to the desired outcome,[54] has been demonstrated repeatedly in the literature[43,46,47,51,55-59] to improve function, whereas treatment focused on a particular component of a task results in gains specific to the task taught with no consistent carryover into other functional tasks. Thus, the more functional and desirable the treatment task can be designed to be, the greater the impact on desired functional outcomes.

Another principle of motor learning—random vs blocked practice—has also been examined with patients who sustained a stroke. Hanlon[60] compared the retention of tasks taught in a blocked (ie, repetitive, drill-style) pattern of practice with those taught in a random practice pattern, where the target tasks were interspersed with other unrelated tasks. He found that, while the rate of initial skill acquisition may be slower with random practice, this technique results in better retention and true learning of the skill. This finding is something the physical therapist should try to incorporate into the organization of each treatment session.

For this patient, motor function and control principles of task-specificity practice variables will be incorporated into appropriate interventions.

Neuromotor Development Training

Neuromotor development training for this patient with a stroke will be aimed at regaining motor skills either through recovery or compensation. Massed practice doing task-specific activities with the impaired limb has been found to be an effective intervention for improved UE use[61] and is being investigated for LE use.[62,63]

Constraint-Induced Movement Therapy

CIMT is an intervention that requires the focused use of the involved UE to improve motor skills. It is a task-focused therapy that has been shown to improve motor function following stroke even in chronic stroke and is a recommended intervention in the stroke CPG.[24] There are several theories about how this improvement in motor function works. These theories include learned nonuse,[64] compensatory learning,[65] and structural and psychological factors.[66] The actual mechanism for improvement in cortical reorganization is not known but studies using transcranial magnetic stimulation[67-70] and functional MRI[38,71-74] have demonstrated changes in brain activity and representation (neural excitability). There are several variations of CIMT in which the intensity, location, and type of practice vary. "Forced use" is intervention in which the patient practices functional tasks at home with the involved limb, while the non-involved limb is placed in a sling or mitten.[75,76] CIMT in the clinic incorporates a very intense daily schedule of 6 hours and variation in task practice, including repetitive and adaptive practice.[65,77] Modified CIMT is a combination of home and clinic setting using distributed practice.[78-80] The specific dosage and structure of the training program has been and continues to be studied.[81] Patient motivation, ability to attend to task, and adherence to the intense practice schedule are factors that need to be considered when using CIMT as an intervention for the patient.[82] Fritz and coworkers[81] found the most significant impairment predictor for CIMT is self-initiated finger extension. Richards and colleagues used 10 degrees of wrist extension and 10 degrees of finger and thumb extension as inclusion criteria for CIMT in their study.[80] Muscle weakness of the UE[83] and decreased grip strength[84] have been identified as predictors of use. Underwood and associates[82] found that the intensity of practice did not increase pain or fatigue.

Taub and colleagues identified three components for CIMT: 1) repetitive, task-oriented training or function following shaping principles for several hours a day for 10 or 15 consecutive weekdays, 2) use of the impaired extremity or function during all waking hours and may restrain unimpaired extremity, and 3) use of behavioral methods that aid transfer of skills from clinic to the real world.[77] In another study, Fritz and colleagues[61] attempted to determine if there were specific patient characteristics that would predict which patients with a stroke would benefit from CIMT. They found that only age was predictive of improved functional ability 6 months post CIMT. This was an inverse relationship in that the younger the patient, the better the outcomes. They also found that other patient characteristics, such as side of stroke, chronicity, hand dominance, sex, and ambulation status, were not predictive of success at follow-up. CIMT is an intense intervention program that requires commitment from the patient to complete the therapy and continued practice at home. Robotic assistive devices continue to be studied.[85]

This patient with an acute stroke and limited movement of the wrist against gravity and minimal to no finger extension of the involved hand may be a candidate for CIMT as muscle strength and volitional movement improve as part of spontaneous recovery and results of therapy. Mr. Schreiner should be reexamined for potential inclusion of CIMT as part of his episode of care.

Gait and Locomotion Training

Impaired walking is a common functional limitation following stroke that may lead to disability due to an inability to participate in community and work environments. Weakness, deconditioning, spasticity, and incoordination of movement contribute to decreased speed of walking. Gait speed has been shown to correlate with higher function and better prognosis following stroke.[86,87] There are tests that have been shown to be effective in determining walking speed.[88] However, it is felt that these tests may overestimate true walking ability[89] and do not accurately reflect the level attained by the patient as ambulation in the community involves more than being able to walk at a higher level of speed. There are also classification systems for determining ambulation[87,90] ability that are functionally relevant to the patient. Perry and colleagues[87] identified a classification system for ambulation post stroke that includes six categories. Table 4-2 lists the categories with general descriptors of the tasks and speed of walking required for each level. Perry and colleagues[87] also identified four variables that needed to be mastered for independent community ambulation: 1) changes in level and terrain irregularities, 2) obstacle avoidance, 3) increased distance, and 4) manual handling of loads. While full community walkers, according to the classification

system, need to be walking at 0.8 m/s it should be recognized that typical adults without disability walk at 1.33 m/s.[91] Schmid and coworkers[86] studied the clinical usefulness of gait velocity as related to Perry's classification based on gait speed. They found that a velocity-based classification was meaningful to measure changes in levels of ambulation.

Body Weight Supported Treadmill Training

Body weight supported treadmill training (BWSTT) is a task-specific locomotor training program that has been shown to be effective in improving walking in acute, subacute, and chronic stroke. Treadmill training without support has been shown to be as effective at improving gait as standard rehabilitation,[50,52,92] and BWSTT has been shown to be more effective than treadmill training without support.[93] BWSTT has been shown to improve lower limb kinematics, postural abilities,[94] weightbearing on the involved lower limb, symmetry of gait pattern, LE strength,[54] and walking speed.[38,54,95] It has also been shown to decrease spasticity while walking[95] and oxygen consumption.[40,41]

BWSTT requires a supportive harness system, treadmill, and at least two therapists to assist the patient in attaining proper alignment and limb kinematics while walking. By providing body weight support with a harness system, as needed in the presence of absent or weak LE muscles, the patient's steps can be facilitated manually with maximized sensory cues from the treadmill. Components of BWSTT include upright trunk alignment, weight shift, weightbearing through the lower limbs, appropriate limb kinematics for stance and swing, coordinated stride characteristics between the limbs, and reciprocal arm swing.[38] UE support may be used initially for balance, and patients are encouraged to not hold on with their hands so loading occurs through the lower limbs instead of through the upper limbs. Orthotics are not used during the training so as to allow maximal sensory input, loading, and dorsiflexion of the foot. The initial amount of body weight that is supported varies, should not exceed 30% to 40%,[95] and is determined by the amount of support while performing appropriate limb kinematics. The initial speed also varies with early studies starting at very slow speeds (0.16 to 0.5 mph)[96] and more recent studies suggesting beginning speeds at 0.5 mph[95] or higher.[38,54] As the patient improves, body weight support is decreased and speed is increased. Sullivan and colleagues[38] found that BWSTT at speeds that were closer to normal walking velocity (2.0 mph) were more effective in improving self-selected walking velocity for overground walking. In another study, Sullivan and coworkers[54] used a high-intensity locomotor program in which participants walked body weight supported (BWS) on the treadmill at speeds in the range of 1.5 to 2.5 m/s. This program resulted in increased walking speed, distance, and LE strength. These studies suggested that patients with chronic stroke need to be challenged to walk at faster rates when using BWSTT to more effectively

Table 4-2

CLASSIFICATION OF FUNCTIONAL AMBULATION IN STROKE SURVIVORS[87]

Category	Characteristics	Velocity (meters/second)
Physiological walker	Walks for exercise only Uses wheelchair for bathroom and bedroom mobility	0.1 m/s
Limited household walker	Uses walking for some home activities Requires assistance to walk Uses wheelchair for bathroom or bedroom mobility	0.23 m/s
Unlimited household walker	Walks for all home activities Walks for bathroom and bedroom mobility Can enter/exit home without wheelchair but needs supervision Difficulty with stairs, uneven terrain Needs supervision with curbs	0.27 m/s
Most-limited community walker	Independent enter/exit home, curbs Assistance in local store and shopping centers, may use wheelchair	0.4 m/s
Least-limited community walker	Moderate community activities without wheelchair Assistance in crowded shopping center No assistance in local store or uncrowded shopping center	0.58 m/s
Community walker	Independent home and moderate community activities Manages uneven terrain Negotiates crowded shopping centers	>0.8m/s

improve walking outcomes for transfer to typical speeds for functional community ambulation.[38,54] Lamontagne and Fung[39] found supported treadmill fast walking and overground fast walking were both beneficial in low- and high-functioning patients with a stroke. However, low-functioning patients benefited more from treadmill BWS walking than overground walking. While Perry and coworkers[87] classified speeds for community ambulation as walking velocity of 0.58 m/s and unlimited community ambulation as walking velocity of 0.8 m/s (see Table 4-2), most adults without disability walk at speeds of 1.2 m/s (2.7 mph). At this time there are no standard protocols for the use of progression of patients using BWSTT. Chen and Patten[97] provided a review of parameters as presented in the literature and provided suggestions for training, and Sullivan and colleagues[54] provided the parameters used in the STEPS randomized clinical trial. Robotic gait orthoses are also being used as an alternative to the labor-intense therapist-assisted BWSTT and as a method to provide BWSTT to more severely impaired patients.[98-100]

This patient with an acute stroke would benefit from treadmill BWS ambulation to improve postural control and LE strength and coordination and to facilitate regaining of his walking pattern. As strength and balance improve, the amount of BWS would be reduced and the speed of the treadmill would increase.

Strength, Power, and Endurance Training

Muscle weakness[29,101] and decreased cardiovascular endurance[29,102,103] are common following stroke. LE muscle strength has been shown to be an indicator of function at discharge,[28,104] correlates with gait speed,[105] and inversely correlates with risk of falling.[24] Studies have demonstrated that strength can be improved with training.[33,36,37,103,106] Strengthening and endurance training programs are important interventions for improving impairments and reducing functional limitations and disability and should be included in the post-stroke plan of care.[24,29,107,108]

Strengthening programs have varied in type of exercise, muscle groups to strengthen, frequency, and duration.[32,101,109] Morris and colleagues,[32] in a systematic review of progressive resistance strength training following stroke from 1998 to 2002, found the following: strength in the UEs and LEs significantly improved with training; no significant change in spasticity, flexibility, or depression; walking ability improved; mixed results in improving speed and symmetry of sit-to-stand and speed of climbing stairs; and improvement in upper limb activities. Sullivan and colleagues[54] combined a LE strengthening program with BWSTT on alternating days for adults post stroke and found that the added strengthening did not improve walking ability. There appeared to be an overtraining effect since adults post stroke who did not perform strength training but did perform BWSTT did improve walking ability. Physical therapists need to consider the summative effects of exercise when developing an exercise program.

Strengthening programs for stroke survivors have included progressive resistive exercise,[32,110,111] high-intensity resistance training,[107] circuit training,[109] pedaling against resistance,[34] high-intensity locomotor program using BWSTT,[54] strengthening and conditioning programs,[30,33,103] and yoga.[31] The AHA has recommended guidelines for strengthening programs. In addition, the American College of Sports Medicine and the AHA have recommendations for physical activity and public health in older adults that provide additional information that may be helpful for clinicians.[112] The reader is encouraged to review Pattern A: Primary Prevention/Risk Reduction for Loss of Balance and Falling for additional information and intervention strategies. For additional information on strengthening the reader is encouraged to review Musculoskeletal Pattern C: Impaired Muscle Performance in the *Musculoskeletal Essentials: Applying the Preferred Physical Therapist Practice Patterns*[SM].[113]

Prescription, Application, and, as Appropriate, Fabrication of Devices and Equipment

The use of assistive and adaptive devices and equipment is common for individuals with stroke, especially in the early stages.[24] These devices should be used for safety and to provide more independence in completion of tasks while the patient is learning to perform the task. The CPGs stress that devices and equipment should only be supplemental and not replace mastery of the task.[24] Laufer[114] found that use of a quad cane did decrease postural sway and improve postural stability as the weight was shifted onto the cane. While this is important for immediate safety, use of a device provides a different motor program and does not allow the patient to practice weight shifting just onto the involved leg for standing or walking without the device. LE orthotics must also be considered when working on balance and gait as they may interfere with joint ROM, balance strategies, and sensory input and may restrict muscles. BWSTT protocols[38,41,54,98] and task-specific training programs[54,62,109] recommend orthotics not be used during training sessions.

This patient with limited balance, mobility, and ADL skills will need to use an assistive device for mobility and independence in ADL and in future IADL. Both assistive and orthotic devices may increase mobility and stability and reduce risk of falls. Use of equipment and devices will be based on the purpose of the task.

COORDINATION, COMMUNICATION, AND DOCUMENTATION

Communication will occur with Mr. Schreiner, family members, and all members of the multidisciplinary rehabilitation team. All elements of the patient's management will be documented. Interdisciplinary teamwork will be demonstrated in patient-family conferences and patient care rounds. Discharge needs will be determined, and discharge planning will be coordinated with all concerned.

PATIENT/CLIENT-RELATED INSTRUCTION

The patient and family will be instructed in the current condition and reasons for the patient's impairments and functional limitation. Information will also be provided to them regarding recovery and community resources for additional support. Mr. Schreiner and his family will also be involved in the development of the plan of care. They will be taught techniques to enhance the patient's attention to and awareness of his left side and, when safe, techniques to assist the patient with his mobility. They will also be taught how to work with Mr. Schreiner at home during his ADL, IADL, and exercise program.

THERAPEUTIC EXERCISE

◆ Aerobic capacity/endurance conditioning
  ● Patient needs to be medically cleared for activity
  ● Monitor HR and exertion during activities
  ● Mode
    ■ Aerobic using UE and LE muscles
    ■ Any large muscle activity
    ■ Continuous or for prolonged period
  ● Examples
    ■ Initially performance of ADL, basic movements, transfers, repetitive activities (eg, rolling, supine to sit, sit to stand)
    ■ UE exercises, moving arms (hold together) overhead, out to side, rotating
    ■ Progress to aerobics while sitting, upper body ergometer with strap/mitt to hold left hand on pedal
    ■ Progress to leg equipment, such as assistive devices, BWS treadmill, stationary bicycle with toe clip

or foot strap
- Duration
  - Begin with 2 minutes of continuous activity followed by 2 minutes rest, 2 minutes of activity, progressing to 5 to 10 minutes of continuous activity
  - Goal is to work up to 20 to 60 minutes a day or multiple 10-minute sessions a day
  - Increase duration progressively, increasing intensity and resistance of activity
- Intensity
  - 40% to 50% peak oxygen uptake
  - 40% to 70% HR reserve
  - 11 to 14 (6 to 20 scale) Borg RPE
- Frequency
  - Start with daily low intensity activities and movements
  - Progress to specific aerobic activities three to seven times per week

◆ Balance, coordination, and agility training
- Activities to promote left side awareness, such as visual scanning, reaching across midline to left side of body
  - Practice finding specific items or persons in room, select those to the left of the patient
  - Set up environment to require reaching across body to pick up items (eg, remote control, book, water)
  - Select tasks that require use of two hands
  - Practice weight shifting while sitting using hands on side to support
  - Practice activities in front of a mirror and have patient verbalize what he sees (eg, postural asymmetry)
  - Therapist should approach patient from left side whenever possible and seek eye contact
- Balance challenges
  - Goal is for patient to do a functional task without physical or verbal cues, only supervision
  - Begin with task that patient can do (eg, sitting on edge of bed)
  - Practice swaying trunk forward, backward, and to the side
  - Increase difficulty of the task (eg, increase distance swayed, do faster/slower, stop, change directions)
  - Do with hand support then without hand support
  - Progress to reaching (sideward, forward, overhead) and vary speed and direction
  - Add reach and pick up object, move across body, and set down
  - Play catch in sitting and standing (increase difficulty, catch off to side, overhead, by legs, throw fast/slow, use different balls/balloons)
  - Play hitting items in sitting and standing (increase difficulty, hit to side, overhead, by legs, throw fast/slow, use different objects)
  - Practice sitting and standing, does not have to wait to achieve normal sitting before starting standing
  - Practice stepping (begin with support, forward, backward, sideward) and increase difficulty of the task (increase distance stepped, speed of step, stop, change directions)
  - Practice moving from sitting to standing (increase difficulty, do fast/slow, different chairs/surfaces, with/without hand support)
  - Once walking, practice starting, stopping, changing directions, reaching for object, turning head while walking to visually scan environment or to talk to someone
  - BWSTT begin with 30% to 40% weight supported, decrease support, practice taking weight, shifting weight

◆ Flexibility exercises
- Tilt table or standing frame to introduce partial weightbearing with protection of joint integrity of the hip, knee, ankle, and foot and to provide prolonged stretch to LEs (progress to standing for 20 to 30 minutes, full upright position)
- Instruct patient in active assistive range of motion (AAROM) using right to assist left
- Instruct patient in long sitting stretch, sitting in chair with back and arms, place both legs on another chair in front, sit with knees straight for 1 minute then slowly try to lean as far forward as he can while keeping knees straight; hold for 1 to 2 minutes

◆ Gait and locomotion training
- Gait training should begin with standing balance tasks, incorporating weight shifting both laterally and forward onto the LE that is advanced
- Both forward and backward steps should be taught to allow safe stand to sit transition
- BWSTT should begin early and include the following components
  - Suspended harness initially supporting 30% to 40% body weight
  - Physical therapist behind patient to monitor/assist trunk alignment and weight shifting
  - Physical therapist at impaired leg to assist with kinematics for gait if robotic gait orthoses not available
  - No orthotics while on treadmill to allow appropriate kinematics and sensory input

- Initial speed of 0.5 mph and increase to challenge patient
- Walk for 2 minutes then rest; walk a total of four times (2 minutes each time with rest between) and increase timed walked and decrease rest time
- Instruction in proper use and sequencing of assistive devices with ambulation should begin when the patient is ready to progress outside of parallel bars
- Wheelchair propulsion should utilize RUE and RLE until left side is strong enough to assist and should focus on avoidance of obstacles through continued visual scanning to the left of midline

◆ Neuromotor development training
- Activities that demand integration of sides and visual scanning (eg, carrying laundry basket, hitting balloon with tennis racket [grip assisted by therapist], sprinkling powder with one hand, smoothing over body with the other hand [assisted initially])
- Practice specific tasks needed for daily routine
  - Begin to encourage use of left hand for tasks (patient is right-hand dominate so will naturally use right hand before left), may need to begin use of mitt for right to allow practice by left
  - Grip on walker, hold onto sink to brush teeth and hair, pull slacks up, pick up book, hold book to read, grip light weights
  - Practice functional mobility as a whole routine (eg, out of bed, stand, walk to bathroom)
  - Make tasks purposeful and meaningful to patient, ask patient to select two tasks he would like to work on

◆ Relaxation
- Mental imagery
  - Practice visualization of specific tasks two times per hour during the intervals between therapy sessions (ie, visualizing using the left hand for tasks, such as brushing teeth, combing hair, holding a book, or visualizing a mobility skill, such as walking as performed prior to the CNS injury)[115]

◆ Strength, power, and endurance training
- Initially strengthening will occur through performance in physical therapy sessions and functional activities
  - Standing activities that promote weightbearing through the involved (left) side once midline awareness has improved
  - UE weightbearing for joint compression and strong proprioceptive input into a properly aligned joint and limb
  - Progress to adding light weights to left ankle during functional tasks, removing weight periodically to change proprioceptive input

- PREs should begin focusing on right side and core strengthening
  - Closed chain and functional tasks, such as bridging and repeated sit to/from stand, can be done initially with assistance to increase weightbearing and functional use of the extremities; gradually reducing assistance and progressing to resistance as motor function improves
  - Use combinations of assistive and manual resistance to work on UE exercises (shoulder shrugs, rows, shoulder press, elbow flexion/extension, wrist flexion/extension) and progress to moving limb with resistance through functional movements (eg, reaching forward, overhead, across body, pushing down, pulling up)
  - Use containers with weights or use functional items
    ► Practice picking up and setting down (vary heights, weights, shapes)
    ► Hold items close to body initially using those items that require bimanual manual function (such as laundry basket)
    ► Progress to items that can be manipulated unilaterally
  - Variable resistance machines
    ► Use mitt with Velcro strap to assist with grasp on left
    ► Start with large muscle groups (eg, hip flexors, knee extensors/flexors, ankle dorsiflexors/plantarflexors, shoulder flexors/extensors, shoulder elevators, back extensors)
    ► Start with light weights to learn motor program then increase weights, repetitions (one to three sets of 10 to 15 repetitions)
- Core strengthening
  - Begin abdominal strengthening with wedge behind back while supine providing assistance as necessary and eventually progress to sit-ups while flat or in dynamic situation on a ball
  - Work on extension exercises using prone on elbows and assisting at left shoulder
- Wheelchair propulsion
  - Use only left extremities
  - Use just legs, pulling with heels, first bilaterally then reciprocally, for excellent strengthening of hamstrings and gastrocnemius (do without AFO)
  - Increase challenges as endurance and strength improve (add inclines, carpet, outdoor terrains and surfaces)
- Muscular endurance training can be accomplished by decreasing rest time during therapy sessions, increasing repetitions, and increasing sets

FUNCTIONAL TRAINING IN SELF-CARE AND HOME MANAGEMENT

- ◆ Self-care and home management
  - Reinforce self-care and home management actions, tasks, and activities to include ADL training and use of assistive and adaptive devices and equipment (obtained through occupational therapy) during ADL
  - Many of the therapeutic exercises described in the previous section will help support ADL training (ie, sit to/from stand from lower surfaces will help with toilet transfer technique, bridging will assist with bed mobility, seated and standing reaching exercises will help with grooming/hygiene tasks)
  - Patient to begin practicing ADL performed at natural time in the hospital, and physical therapist may provide interventions in the patient's room to facilitate these activities
  - A home evaluation would be ideal, providing the most task-specific assessment of the layout of the house and readiness of the patient and family to manage at home
- ◆ Injury prevention or reduction
  - Instruct Mr. Schreiner and his family in injury prevention
    - Provide family with opportunities for return demonstration in performing safe techniques to assist with ambulation and stair climbing
  - Create task-specific environment
    - Ambulation is performed on both firm and carpeted surfaces
    - Number of stairs and set-up of railings (and the like) mirror those at his home as closely as possible
  - Important to ensure that interventions include changing environment or task so the activities are not always the same, since many falls are from not being able to anticipate or react to unexpected things
  - For fall prevention, see Pattern A: Primary Prevention/ Risk Reduction for Loss of Balance and Falling

FUNCTIONAL TRAINING IN WORK, COMMUNITY, AND LEISURE INTEGRATION OR REINTEGRATION

- ◆ Functional training programs
  - Mr. Schreiner will be instructed in strategies for safe and efficient travel in the community and at work using appropriate assistive devices
  - Transfer training in and out of car to prepare Mr. Schreiner for home visits and discharge to home
  - Begin task-specific practice of work activities and

have Mr. Schreiner select two work required activities to train in task-focused practice

MANUAL THERAPY TECHNIQUES

- ◆ PROM
  - Use of early mobilization to promote ROM and prevent joint contracture in both left extremities[116]

PRESCRIPTION, APPLICATION, AND, AS APPROPRIATE, FABRICATION OF DEVICES AND EQUIPMENT

The physical therapist will select the most appropriate assistive device based on Mr. Schreiner's impairments throughout the episode of care. He will be instructed in the use and care of the device including the indications for each type. Instructions in use and care of the assistive device and/or wheelchair will be provided to the patient and family when issued for home use.

In addition, the physical therapist will assess the need for an AFO to provide ankle and knee stability for standing activities. The therapist will coordinate care with the orthotist to fabricate an AFO based on the physical therapist's recommendations. If an AFO is needed, Mr. Schreiner and his family will be given instructions for donning and doffing the orthotic and how to monitor his skin. In addition, suggestions will be provided on the type of shoe to fit over the AFO.

- ◆ AFO should initially be used only if needed for safety or to protect the joints
- ◆ An articulated AFO is preferred to allow ankle movements for balance strategies and more appropriate gait pattern
- ◆ AFO would not be worn during strengthening, BWS treadmill or overground training, or standing balance activities
- ◆ ADL should be practiced with and without devices
- ◆ The goal is to not need an orthotic device

ANTICIPATED GOALS AND EXPECTED OUTCOMES

- ◆ Impact on impairments
  - Ambulation with appropriate assistive device for 50 feet with contact guard assistance on firm and carpeted surfaces is achieved.
  - Awareness of left side is improved as demonstrated by spontaneous use of the involved limb for bimanual activities.
  - Knee control at stance phase and clearing of foot during swing phase of LLE with ambulation on firm and carpeted surfaces is achieved.

- LLE strength is improved to 4-/5 in hip flexion, 4/5 in knee flexion and extension, and 2/5 in ankle dorsiflexion and plantarflexion.
- Postural sway is controlled, and balance strategies when standing unsupported are used.
- Standing with single UE support for 5 minutes is achieved.
- Transfer from bed to/from chair with supervision is achieved.
- UE strength is improved to 3+ in wrist extension and 2 in finger and thumb extension.
- Weight is borne on left arm to support self when leaning to side in sitting and standing.

♦ Impact on functional limitations
- Climbing up and down one flight of stairs with a rail and contact guard assistance from family member is achieved.
- Independent bed mobility is achieved.
- Independent standing with single UE support for 5 minutes to perform daily grooming tasks (eg, shave with electric razor, brush teeth, comb hair) is achieved.
- Involved UE is used for functional tasks by wearing a mitt on non-involved hand.
- Toileting is performed with stand-by assistance for transfers.
- Unsupported sitting is achieved without loss of balance for 30 minutes in order to perform simple hygiene and ADL tasks (eg, able to reach and shift weight to either side for donning socks or shifting to put on a button front shirt) independently.

♦ Impact on disabilities
- Access of community settings and activities is attained through ability to transfer in/out of car with moderate assistance.
- Attendance at church services is achieved.
- Independent wheelchair mobility is achieved in his household to ensure safe mobility when unsupervised.
- Involvement in social activities with his grandchildren is achieved.
- Rehabilitation services, his employer, and the patient will determine feasibility of returning to work, ability to modify job requirements, and any needed accommodations.

♦ Risk reduction/prevention
- Patient and family are able to demonstrate appropriate techniques to increase patient's awareness of the left side.
- Patient and family are aware of need for devices and equipment to provide safety and improve independence with function.

- Patient and family are aware of personal risk factors for recurrence of stroke and have developed a plan to address them.
- Patient and family have a plan to handle falls if they should occur, including strategies for getting up if medically approved.
- Patient and family know how to practice activities without devices and equipment and still remain safe.
- Safety of patient and family is improved through demonstration by patient and family of safe techniques for assisted ambulation and stair climbing.

♦ Impact on health, wellness, and fitness
- Patient will participate in home exercise program to improve muscle strength, endurance, and flexibility.
- Patient will perform cardiovascular activities using DVD of commercially available programs for fitness programs done while sitting.

♦ Impact on societal resources
- Available resources are maximally utilized.
- Care is coordinated with patient, family, and other professionals.
- Documentation occurs throughout patient management in all settings and follows APTA's *Guidelines for Physical Therapy Documentation*.[117]
- Interdisciplinary collaboration occurs through patient care rounds and patient family meetings.
- Patient will be able to identify relevant community resources to meet his discharge needs.
- Referrals are made to other professionals or resources whenever necessary and appropriate.

♦ Patient/client satisfaction
- Admission data and discharge planning are completed.
- Care is coordinated with patient, family, and other professionals.
- Discharge needs are determined.
- Patient and family understanding of anticipated goals and expected outcomes is increased.
- Patient and family will verbalize an awareness of the diagnosis, prognosis, interventions, and anticipated goals/expected outcomes.

REEXAMINATION

Reexamination is performed throughout the episode of care with adjustments to the plan of care as needed.

DISCHARGE

Mr. Schreiner is discharged from physical therapy after a total of 18 visits over 9 days in the hospital and attainment of his goals and expectations. These sessions have covered his inpatient services. Mr. Schreiner's discharge plan includes a home program developed with the physical therapist that outlines his daily routine, needs, and how the family can assist him. He has a plan for preventing falls and how to get up if he does fall. Mr. Schreiner has selected five activities and five exercises that he will work on until he has his first visit and examination from his home care physical therapist. Mr. Schreiner is motivated to return to home and work and has strong family support for his transition to home. His focus for home care is to be functional in self-care and mobility skills with minimal assistance. Once Mr. Schreiner is able to access the community and transfer in and out of care with minimal assistance, he is planning to begin an intense outpatient rehabilitation program. He made significant gains with BWSTT and would like to continue the program with a clinic that provides high-intensity programming. His priorities are to increase independence in self-care and home activities, improve walking and mobility skills, and increase strength and endurance with the ultimate goal of accessing the community and returning to work.

Case Study #2: Traumatic Brain Injury

Mr. Ben Foster is a 23-year-old male who sustained a traumatic brain injury resulting in tetraparesis as a result of a motor vehicle accident 7 weeks ago.

PHYSICAL THERAPIST EXAMINATION

HISTORY

♦ General demographics: Ben is a 23-year-old white male whose primary language is English. He is left handed.

♦ Social history: Ben is single. His parents live nearby. They are very supportive and concerned about Ben's physical and emotional well-being and future. He has a college education with a degree in criminal justice.

♦ Employment/work: Ben is a police officer and had been on the force for 1 year prior to his accident.

♦ Living environment: He lives in a rented duplex, two-story home with two steps to enter with hand rails on the right when ascending. The flight of stairs to the second floor has one railing on the left when ascending. There is one flight of stairs with a single right hand rail

from the first floor to the basement, which has a laundry room. His home has an eat-in kitchen, living room, and a lavette on the first floor. There are two bedrooms and one bathroom on the second floor. An elderly husband and wife live in the other side of the duplex.

♦ General health status
  ● General health perception: Prior to this episode, his health was excellent.
  ● Physical function: Prior to this episode, his physical function was better than average for his age.
  ● Psychological function: There were no issues prior to the injury according to family report.
  ● Role function: Son, brother, grandson, friend, police officer, community leader.
  ● Social function: Ben's primary social activities have been with his friends. He participates in many fund-raising and educational programs related to his job. He loves to read, listen to music, play basketball, ski, and play golf. He enjoyed going out with friends and was taking ballroom and line dancing lessons. He belongs to a book club that meets monthly. A few of his professional colleagues and friends have been very supportive and visit regularly.

♦ Social/health habits: He has never smoked. He drinks only socially.

♦ Family history: His mother is 54 years of age, and his father is 57 years of age. Both are healthy and live nearby. He has two grandmothers who are both in their late 70s and are generally in good health. Ben's medical history is positive for myocardial infarction in his maternal grandfather and chronic obstructive pulmonary disease in his paternal grandfather.

♦ Medical/surgical history: Ben's past medical history is unremarkable according to the family. He has a history of acne and had been using Accutane for this for about 1½ months prior to his accident. He has no known allergies.

♦ Current condition(s)/chief complaint(s): Ben sustained a TBI resulting in tetraparesis, when he apparently lost control of his car 7 weeks ago. He was unresponsive with a Glasgow Coma Scale of 3 (verbal 1, eye opening 1, motor 1)[118,119] and required intubation at the scene before being airlifted to the acute care hospital. During his acute care stay he had a pericutaneous tube inserted and a tracheostomy performed, which is now plugged. He had a right VP shunt put in place. A peripherally inserted central catheter (PICC) line was inserted in his RUE and is still in place. Percutaneous endoscopic gastrostomy tube was inserted in the left abdomen and is still in place. Compression garments were applied for deep venous thrombophlebitis prophylaxis, and he was given multipodus boots. An altered level of consciousness with cognitive deficits persisted for about 3 weeks, when there was an emergence of restlessness and agitation and his Glasgow Coma Scale was upgraded to 9 (verbal 3, eye opening 2, motor 4).[118,119] At this time 7 weeks later, he has been admitted to a rehabilitation facility, and he is dependent in all mobility and ADL skills. The family is extremely supportive and their goal is to have Ben return home as appropriate.

♦ Functional status and activity level: He requires assistance with all mobility since the brain injury.

♦ Medications (preadmission to rehabilitation facility): Lovenox, valproic acid elixir, ferrous sulfate, Zantac, Afrin, Nystatin swish, nasal saline, Ambien, Tylenol, Motrin elixir, Nystatin powder, Benadryl.

♦ Other clinical tests
  ● Imaging studies revealed a large frontal/basal ganglion hemorrhage with associated hydrocephalus and effacement of the lateral ventricle with a midline shift.
  ● Temperature: 100.4°F rectally.
  ● Neuropsychological evaluation of cognition
    ▪ Above average psychometric intellect premorbid based on background history described by family.
    ▪ Nonverbal sections of the Wechsler Abbreviated Scale of Intelligence (WASI) indicate current function in low average range of general adaptive abilities with a performance IQ of 89.
    ▪ Working memory is mildly impaired.
    ▪ Recognition memory significantly impaired.
    ▪ Mild to moderate mental slowing evident on tasks of processing, mental flexibility, and psychomotor speed.
    ▪ No significant perseveration, impulsivity, or confusion documented.
  ● Speech pathology evaluation
    ▪ Unable to read or communicate functionally.
    ▪ Understands simple commands inconsistently.
    ▪ Right visual field cut and/or neglect.
    ▪ Oral and verbal apraxia.
    ▪ Profound deficits in verbal expression.
    ▪ Minimal deficits in auditory comprehension.

SYSTEMS REVIEW

♦ Cardiovascular/pulmonary
  ● BP: 125/80 mmHg
  ● Edema: None
  ● HR: 80 bpm
  ● RR: 34 bpm
♦ Integumentary
  ● Presence of scar formation

    ▪ Healed scars on his scalp
    ▪ Midline plugged tracheostomy
    ▪ Right chest tube scar
    ▪ Percutaneous endoscopic gastrotomy tube present in the left abdomen
    ▪ PICC line in the RUE proximal to the elbow anteromedially
  ● Skin color: Normal
  ● Skin integrity: History of acne otherwise intact, warm, and dry
♦ Musculoskeletal
  ● Gross range of motion: PROM was WNL except bilateral wrist extension and ankle dorsiflexion
  ● Gross strength: Tetraparesis involving right greater than left
  ● Gross symmetry: Some asymmetry in postural alignment noted secondary to imbalance of motor control
  ● Height: 5'10" (1.77 m)
  ● Weight
    ▪ 205 lbs (92.99 kg) prior to the accident
    ▪ Weight at this time approximately 180 lbs (82 kg)
♦ Neuromuscular
  ● No functional movement of right hand and UE
  ● Generally slightly more movement proximally than distally in the left extremities
  ● Bilateral foot drop
  ● Balance, locomotion, transfers, and transitions: Needs assistance with all transitions, unable to maintain upright in any position without assistance, unable to ambulate
♦ Communication, affect, cognition, language, and learning style
  ● Communication, affect, and cognition are impaired
  ● Ben's expressive language skills are more significantly impaired than language comprehension
  ● He is pleasant and cooperative
  ● He is very motivated, but does admit to periods of frustration
  ● Learning style: Unknown at this time

TESTS AND MEASURES

♦ Aerobic capacity/endurance
  ● Unable to sit without assistance, requires rest after approximately 8 minutes of assisted sitting balance activities by patient request due to fatigue, no evidence of dyspnea
  ● Borg RPE: Patient indicates exertion as 17 on scale of 6 to 20[42]
♦ Anthropometric characteristics

- BMI=705 x (body weight [in pounds] divided by height^2 [in inches])[120]
- Ben's BMI=25.89
- BMI values between 25 and 29.9 are considered overweight[121]

◆ Arousal, attention, and cognition
  - Arousal, attention, and memory
    - Appears to be oriented and alert WFL, however speech and language problems make it difficult to accurately assess
    - Glasgow Coma Scale upgraded to 14 (verbal 4, eye opening 4, motor 6)[118,119]
    - Imitates nonverbal communication gestures with 100% accuracy given a visual demonstration
    - Able to focus on tasks, basic attention is low to average
    - Able to follow simple directions without confusion
  - Cognition: See Other Clinical Tests
  - Communication
    - Significant dysphasia
    - Verbal praxis, decreased verbal initiation, and articulation
    - Understands simple verbal commands inconsistently, dysnomia, and poor fluency
    - Cooperative and motivated

◆ Assistive and adaptive devices
  - Will need assistive device for any ambulation
  - May benefit from bilateral orthotics to provide improved ankle stability and knee control during weightbearing activities given bilateral LE weakness and drop foot
  - Will need a wheelchair for transport and use in the community and/or home
  - Will need bathroom equipment and adaptive devices to assist with self-care, feeding, and homemaking skills

◆ Circulation
  - Circumferential measurements and palpation did not indicate edema in either LE

◆ Cranial and peripheral nerve integrity
  - Left gaze preference
  - Difficulty diverting his eyes to the right of midline
  - Able to visually track target to approximately 30 degrees left of midline at slow speeds with verbal cues

◆ Environmental, home, and work barriers
  - Potential barriers include the inability to make significant modifications to his home secondary to the fact that it is a rental property
  - Will need home modifications

- Discharge to his parents' home presents the following barriers
  - Steps to the entrance
  - Stairs to bedroom/bathroom on the second floor
  - Carpeting
  - Potential barriers for eventual return to work include the need to drive to work and during work, communication, fine motor skills, manual dexterity, and physical endurance

◆ Ergonomics and body mechanics
  - Assistance required to maintain upright sitting
  - Asymmetrical use of trunk during attempts at self-care activities and reaching in sitting secondary to muscle imbalances
  - Leans primarily to right and attempts to self-correct with cues

◆ Gait, locomotion, and balance
  - Sitting balance
    - Moderate assistance to come to sitting from supine
    - Requires moderate assistance sitting upright at edge of bed
  - Standing balance
    - Sit to stand with moderate assistance of two people
    - Moderate assist of two to maintain static standing balance primarily due to poor trunk control and inability to actively weightbear through right extremities
  - Ambulates in parallel bars with maximum assistance for two steps
  - Maximal assistance to advance LLE, unable to assist in advancing RLE
  - Wheelchair mobility needs assistance and moderate cues to propel 20 feet on level indoor surface without turns

◆ Integumentary integrity
  - Overall skin integrity intact
    - History of acne
    - Healed scars on his scalp, right chest from tube, and anterior throat from plugged tracheostomy
  - Percutaneous endoscopic gastrotomy tube present in the left abdomen
  - PICC line in the RUE proximal to the elbow anteromedially
  - Skin color: Normal

◆ Motor function
  - No motor abilities in RUE
  - Fine motor skills of LUE severely limited
  - Mildly slowed repetitive action and dexterity of dominant left hand

- Smooth coordinated movements impaired in LLE secondary to weakness
- Muscle tone
  - Generally flaccid with emerging flexor tone in RUE, distally emerging extensor tone throughout RLE
  - No increase in tone in left extremities
  - Modified Ashworth Scale: 1 right extremities[119,122,123]
- Muscle performance
  - MMT and observation reveal the following deviations from normal
    - RUE and RLE
      - No functional movement of right hand and upper extremity, muscle activity noted inconsistently in the extensors of the RLE and in the elbow and wrist flexors of the RUE
      - Right foot drop
    - LUE
      - 2+/5 to 3/5 throughout, greater gross motor movement than fine motor
      - Mildly slowed repetitive action with dominant left hand
      - Manual dexterity slowed
    - LLE
      - Generally 2+/5 to 3/5 movement proximally in the left extremities and 2-/5 distally
      - Able to move the leg in bed with effort
      - Left foot drop
  - Muscle endurance
    - Patient fatigues as evidenced by increased loss of trunk control/balance with greater than 2 minutes of sitting bedside with assist
- Neuromotor development and sensory integration
  - Unable to functionally assume and/or maintain posture in any position without assistance
- Orthotic, protective, and supportive devices
  - Assessment of joint mobility and motor function indicates the need for orthotic devices and equipment to increase/maintain mobility and provide stability (eg, multipodus boots, LE AFOs, hand splint)
- Pain
  - Using numeric pain rating scale (NPS)[18] (0=no pain and 10=worst possible pain) complains of pain of 2/10 with PROM right shoulder near end of range
- Posture
  - Asymmetrical weightbearing; Bears weight left>right
- Range of motion
  - PROM WFL throughout except
    - Right shoulder: External rotation 0 to 10 degrees

and abduction 0 to 50 degrees by goniometric measurement
    - Wrist extension: 0 to 10 degrees on the right and 0 to 35 degrees on the left by goniometric measurement
    - Ankle dorsiflexion: 0 degrees on the right and 0 to 5 degrees on the left by goniometric measurement
    - Mild hamstring tightness bilaterally
- Reflex integrity
  - Deep tendon reflexes
    - Present and normal in the LLE
    - Increased on right 3+ patella and Achilles tendons
  - Bilateral positive Babinski
- Self-care and home management
  - Overall functional status using the Barthel Index: 0 which indicates that he is completely dependent in all feeding, self-care, and mobility skills.[116,119,124]
  - Bed mobility/transfers/transitions
    - Rolls to right using his left leg to initiate rolling and using his left arm minimally on the bed rail
    - Moderate cues and moderate assistance needed when rolling to the left since unable to use his right arm to assist with rolling to the left
    - Sit to/from supine with moderate assist for trunk and both LEs, able to assist minimally with the LUE
    - Bed to/from wheelchair with maximal assist and moderate cues
  - All self-care tasks require moderate to maximal assist with set-up
- Sensory integrity
  - Unable to accurately test secondary to lack of communication abilities
  - Responds to noxious stimulus in all extremities
  - Appears to have diminished sensation to light touch on RUE and RLE
  - Sensation appears to be intact on the left
- Work, community, and leisure integration or reintegration
  - Unable to live independently upon discharge
  - Unable to access community activities independently

EVALUATION

Ben's history indicates that he was an active, 23-year-old, left-handed male employed as a police officer. He suffered a TBI as the result of a motor vehicle accident 7 weeks ago. He was in a coma for approximately 1 month with a Glasgow Coma Scale of 4. He was healthy prior to the accident with above average intelligence. He was just recently transferred to a rehab facility where he will be receiving physical therapy twice a day along with occupational, speech, and recreational therapy. Discharge is anticipated in 7 weeks to his parents' home.

Ben has primary impairments in trunk and motor control, strength, balance, and cognition. These have led to functional limitations, including inability to sit or stand without assistance, inability to ambulate, and required assistance with all bed mobility, transfers, and self-care. Ben is unable to manage independently or with assistance only from his family. He will need continued services, equipment, and home modifications on discharge. He will not be able to resume his social or work roles at the time of discharge. He is motivated and cooperative, has a good insurance plan, and has an extremely supportive family.[125,126] Ben has made considerable progress since the time of his accident. These factors are thought to be positive prognostic indicators to maximize his outcome in therapy.[127,128]

DIAGNOSIS

Ben had a TBI, resulting in tetraparesis. He has impaired: arousal, attention, and cognition; anthropometric characteristics; cranial and peripheral nerve integrity; gait, locomotion, and balance; motor function; muscle performance; neuromotor development and sensory integrity; posture; range of motion; reflex integrity; and sensory integrity. He is functionally limited in self-care and home management and in work, community, and leisure actions, tasks, and activities. He has environmental, social, and work barriers that will require adaptation for Ben to achieve a satisfactory level of participation.[129] He is also in need of devices and equipment. These findings are consistent with placement in Pattern D: Impaired Motor Function and Sensory Integrity Associated With Nonprogressive Disorders of the Central Nervous System—Acquired in Adolescence or Adulthood. These impairments, functional limitations, barriers, and device and equipment needs will be addressed in determining the prognosis and the plan of care.

PROGNOSIS AND PLAN OF CARE

Over the course of the stay in the rehabilitation facility, the following mutually established outcomes have been determined:

♦ Ability to move in bed is improved
♦ Endurance is improved
♦ Gait, locomotion, and balance are improved
♦ Independence is achieved in wheelchair mobility in household
♦ Independent bed mobility is achieved

♦ Motor function is improved
♦ Muscle performance is improved
♦ Postural control is improved
♦ Relevant community resources are identified to meet his discharge needs
♦ Sitting unsupported without loss of balance is achieved
♦ Standing with single UE support is achieved
♦ Transfer from bed to/from chair is independently performed

To achieve these outcomes, the appropriate interventions for this patient are determined. These will include: coordination, communication, and documentation; patient/client-related instruction; therapeutic exercise; functional training in self-care and home management; functional training in work, community, and leisure integration or reintegration; manual therapy techniques; and prescription, application, and, as appropriate, fabrication of devices and equipment.

It is anticipated that Ben will need 105 physical therapy visits over 7 weeks in the rehab facility and then continue with physical therapy home services three to five times a week after discharge.[130] It is projected that Ben will return home initially with therapy services, with a home health aide, and with family assistance 24 hours per day. His transition to home care physical therapy will occur when the above outcomes have been met. Ben is extremely motivated and has good family support to facilitate his rehabilitation program.

INTERVENTIONS

RATIONALE FOR SELECTED INTERVENTIONS

Therapeutic Exercise

TBI, even a mild injury, can cause life-long deficits that affect and limit an individual's ability to perform ADL and to return to home, school, and work.[131-133] Secondary complications, including infections from catheters or feeding tubes, pressure sores, contractures, respiratory complications, and heterotopic ossificans,[134-136] may also occur, not as a result of the primary impairments, but as a result of treatment rendered, bedrest, and altered mobility.[115] Because of the complex nature of the problems associated with TBI, the role of the physical therapist is not just to improve functional abilities, but to improve functional deficits that are compounded by physical, sensory, visual-spatial, cognitive, emotional, and behavioral constraints, as well as secondary complications. Therapeutic exercise in rehabilitation is used not only to treat the existing impairments and functional limitations, but to prevent other impairments as well.[115,137,138]

The treatment plan for Ben is targeted toward those impairments associated with TBI that have been identified in the physical therapist's examination. The efficiency and effectiveness of treatment can be improved by multitasking, working on the biomechanical and movement components and skills needed to accomplish a specific task in combination with other interventions.[139-141] For example, when the patient's heel cords are stretched in bed by the physical therapist that is all that is accomplished. But if the heel cords are stretched by increasing their ROM through weightbearing activities, which also incorporate strengthening as a result of the closed-chain movement and skill improvement as a result of practicing a functional activity, then changes will have been made not only in the impairment but also in function and carryover tasks.[115,142,143] As another example, the practice of sit to stand with appropriate handling and cues can be used to increase hip and ankle ROM, LE strength, and postural control all in the context of functional mobility.[140,144] While the therapeutic activities listed for Ben are itemized and categorized, the skill in treatment of this patient with complex problems is the ability to combine treatment of impairments and functional deficits simultaneously in a nonlinear program that promotes variability in movement.[144] Most functional treatment activities can be initiated at a very low level and progress to a level in which the demands for movement, balance, and control are greater. Within the context of rolling, functional retraining can occur on a bed with a slightly raised head using the side rails, which then may be progressed to resisted upper body or lower body initiation, and then to rolling unsupported by the bed holding midway, and then to rolling a small amount back and forward repeatedly. Transitions do not have to be linear; they can vary according to the active engagement of the patient within the environment.[145]

Of equal importance in the choice of treatment interventions is the amount, type, and method of feedback provided. Appropriate feedback, including the practice schedule and relative frequency of feedback, will facilitate behavioral changes that are permanent with carryover outside the treatment room.[115,146] Learning should be an active process to promote long-term retention. Learning best occurs when task-oriented strategies are used to organize motor behavior.[143,147] Strategies to promote learning will be incorporated in all treatment interventions and will ensure that:

♦ Participation is active

♦ Actions are goal directed

♦ Sessions include both repetition and problem solving

♦ Practice occurs in meaningful contexts

♦ Performance is enhanced by assuming an optimal state of readiness[148]

People with TBI have been shown to be significantly more deconditioned than sedentary people without disability.[149] Aerobic exercise has been shown to increase endurance.[150] Aerobic exercise combined with neuromuscular training has also been shown to increase efficiency in locomotion and

endurance.[151] Participation in cardiovascular/pulmonary aerobic conditioning programs in rehabilitation and after discharge should be part of the physical therapy program to prevent secondary disability.[149] The type, intensity, and duration of aerobic exercise for each patient is based on the patient's ability, tolerance, and cardiac status. With Ben, because of the low level of function, low-level activities will be used initially.[152] His aerobic exercise regime can be progressed to include use of a recumbent bicycle, since this type of aerobic exercise is something that he can transfer to home use.

Impaired muscle strength has many implications, but for patients with neurologic deficits the most significant is the impact on function, specifically gait.[122,139,147] To become stronger, a muscle must be progressively challenged to develop tension.[139] Both manual and mechanical resistance can be used for therapeutic strengthening exercise. There are advantages and disadvantages to both. Manual resistance provided by the physical therapist is useful for exercising in functional patterns, but the amount of resistance cannot be quantified. Mechanical resistance can be quantified, but is often nonfunctional.[139] Both forms of exercise will be used in Ben's treatment plan, depending on the phase of his program and the specific activities being addressed.

Postural control, the ability to control the body's position in space, is fundamental to all activities one does in daily life, whether they be movement, functional and self-care skills, or work, community, and leisure activities. Postural control is complex and involves the interaction of multiple systems organized to perform tasks within diverse environments. Postural control, or balance, integrates sensory information to maintain, anticipate, or react as necessary to maintain a position or move.[143,147,153] If changes occur in the complex body systems responsible for coordinating controlled movements and balance is impaired functionally, then significant changes in walking and balance can occur.[154]

Following TBI, ongoing assessment of the impairments contributing to walking and balance is needed to recognize changes.[154] Intensive task-specific training is an important component of rehabilitation.[152] The effectiveness of only retraining impairments of gait to improve performance may not be enough to ensure recovery of ambulation skills. Treatment interventions aimed at improving gait strategies and functional performance are also essential.[147] Techniques to improve ambulation should be goal oriented and task specific.[141] Most literature indicates that treadmill training may be of benefit for people with limited or no walking ability,[155] however some researchers have found conventional overground gait training to be more effective than BWSTT for improving gait symmetry.[156,157] Utilization of both methods is appropriate at different stages in long-term rehabilitation. Rehabilitation programs for people with TBI must progress to include practice of ambulation strategies in natural and complex environments.[158] Changing the environment so activities are not always the same is critical to teach appropriate strategies to increase functional independence and prevent falls.[147]

COORDINATION, COMMUNICATION, AND DOCUMENTATION

Communication will occur with the patient and family in both verbal and written formats. Communication will also occur with other members of the health care team and other members of the multidisciplinary rehabilitation team (medical director, occupational therapist, and speech therapist as appropriate).[159,160] All elements of the patient's management will be documented. Discharge needs will be determined, and discharge planning will be coordinated with all concerned.

PATIENT/CLIENT-RELATED INSTRUCTION

Ongoing education and education in preparation for discharge must be a major focus of interventions when working with patients with disabilities.[161] The patient and family will be educated regarding the injury to the brain and reasons for the patient's current impairments and functional limitations. They will participate in the development of the plan of care. The family and nursing staff will be instructed on mobility skills and in methods to enhance Ben's performance. When appropriate, Ben will also be instructed in exercises that he can perform independently.

In preparation for discharge, information will also be provided to them regarding community resources for additional support. In the initial stages, they will be taught ways to touch and move Ben and activities to do when he is up in a chair. As Ben progresses, they will be taught techniques to assist Ben with mobility skills using safe body mechanics and to eventually assist him with ambulation. Prior to discharge, they will have learned how to safely transport and get Ben in and out of the house. The patient and the family will understand the importance of his home exercise program. Use of a written and pictorial home program will be used to maximize compliance and help to circumvent barriers because of cognitive problems. Ben's family will have an understanding of:

- ♦ How to communicate effectively with Ben
- ♦ Techniques of sensory stimulation to improve arousal
- ♦ Ways to encourage Ben in his rehab program
- ♦ Ways to actively participate in Ben's exercise and eventual walking program

THERAPEUTIC EXERCISE

- ♦ Aerobic capacity/endurance conditioning
  - In addition to the mode of exercise, frequency, intensity, and duration, factors such as fatigue, increases in tone, sensory changes, and balance disturbances need to be considered in the design of aerobic capacity interventions
  - Vital signs and symptoms of exertion need to be monitored regularly during and after exercise[18,150,162,163]
  - Mode of exercise
    - Initially repetitive activities (rolling, supine to sit, sit to stand) may be used to enhance aerobic capacity
    - BWSTT
    - Recumbent bicycle
  - Intensity
    - Maximum: 60% to 75% peak MHR
    - Continuous activity with monitoring RPE
    - Work at an RPE of fairly light (Borg scale 11) increasing to moderately hard (Borg scale 13)[42]
  - Duration
    - 1 to 2 minutes cycling
    - Begin with assisted movements, gradually increasing duration as tolerated
    - Long-term goal 20 minutes
  - Frequency
    - Daily
    - Circuit training may be optimal
- ♦ Balance, coordination, and agility training
  - Reaching with UE while maintaining sitting balance and progressing to include weight shift with reach
  - Progress to reaching and weight shifting in standing
  - Progress from kneeling to high kneeling activities, including static balance and eventually reaching and weight shifting
  - Sitting on rolling chair/stool and moving with feet in varying directions
  - Improve standing balance through tasks that require trunk stability while moving the LEs[164]
    - Sitting bedside or on the mat marching in place
    - While sitting and eventually standing, alternate stepping up to a low stool[152]
    - Stand with one foot on the floor and one foot on a low stool/step while reaching
    - Standing weight shifting, stepping to the side, stepping across, and braiding
  - Use of Biomechanical Ankle Platform System (BAPS) and/or balance boards for balance and coordination, beginning in sitting and progressing to standing with UE support[139]
  - Focus on maintaining trunk stability while moving limbs (arm and legs), while physical therapist provides manual resistance
  - Exercise ball activities for balance
    - Maintaining balance sitting on the ball while

therapist moves ball

- Sitting on the ball, bouncing gently, and maintaining balance
- Progress to inclusion of UE and hand activities (eg, clapping, catching a ball, moving arms in a variety of directions, first one arm at a time and progress to bilateral as in jumping jack movements)

♦ Body mechanics and postural stabilization
- Postural control activities[136,143]
  - Sitting at edge of bed with visual feedback from a mirror (as tolerated) and/or verbal feedback, practice weight shifts with upper and lower trunk initiation
  - Sitting at edge of bed without back support for a set amount of time and increase as tolerated
  - Incorporate reaching and ADL activities as tolerated utilizing bedside items, sheets, and pillow
  - Incorporate postural control with basic functional activities, such as sit to stand
  - Progress level of difficulty, not necessarily in a linear fashion, of the task as his trunk control, balance, and strength improve (eg, postural control with transfers)[154]
  - Challenge trunk control through developmental sequencing and changing base of support activities by increasing the demands on the trunk
    - ► Alter the base of support (eg, firm support sitting, sitting on a squishy surface, standing on the floor, standing on a floor mat)
    - ► Alter the height of the center of mass using developmental sequence positions (eg, raise and lower the bed height, side-lying, kneeling, standing)
  - Postural control while holding, carrying, and moving objects in front of body, overhead, and out to side
  - Postural control on an exercise ball
    - ► Sitting on the ball, moving with lower trunk initiated movements in all directions
    - ► Maintaining sitting stability on the ball while therapist moves ball
    - ► Postural control while pushing (eg, sled, shopping cart, weighted wheelchair, ultrasound machine) done from sitting initially and progress to postural control while standing[136]

♦ Flexibility exercises
- Stretching exercises should be done after warming up, using a slow and steady stretch accompanied by deep breathing, and building hold up to 30 to 60 seconds
- Improve ROM and prevent contractures by means of manual stretching in bed, on tilt table, and when

standing from high plinth
- Teach family appropriate stretching exercises
- Weightbearing through wrists (supine to sit)
- Sit to stand (varying foot position)
  - Move from sit to stand with arms supported on the arm rests of a chair or on a table
  - The physical therapist assists with foot and ankle position to increase dorsiflexion range by maintaining foot flat on the floor[165]

♦ Gait and locomotion training
- A tilt table or standing frame can be utilized early in the rehabilitation process to gradually introduce weightbearing while protecting joint integrity at the hip, knee, ankle, and foot
- Partial weightbearing permits posture, equilibrium, movement, and weightbearing components of gait to occur concurrently[141]
- Locomotion training should be goal oriented and task specific
- Pre-gait activities in parallel bars stressing all components of gait
  - Standing weight shifts in all directions
  - Forward, lateral, and backward steps
- Instruction in proper use and sequencing of assistive devices with ambulation should begin when the patient is ready to progress outside of parallel bars (quad cane, straight cane, no assistive device)
- Stepping in standing, changing position of feet, and changing the surface
- BWSTT
- Step stance
  - One leg remains in stance, while the other leg swings forward and backward
  - Stand and weight shift onto RLE in a forward direction then taking a step forward with the LLE
  - Followed by shift of weight onto the left leg without stepping with the right
  - Then reverse the procedure: Shift back to the RLE, step back with the LLE and shift weight onto the LLE (without lifting the RLE)
  - Weight shifting, foot position, and hip and knee alignment can be assisted/facilitated as needed by the physical therapist
- Step up/down to low step, forward, backward, sideways
- Progressive ambulation training to include ambulation outdoors, on uneven terrain, stairs, and curbs as able[158]
- Change temporal-distance requirements of gait
- Manage doorways and other environmental barriers
- Carry things while walking

- Push weighted objects (eg, wheelchair, sled, wheeled machines) while walking[136]
- Wheelchair propulsion should utilize LUE and LLE until right side is strong enough to assist and should focus on avoidance of obstacles through continued visual scanning to the left of midline
- ◆ Neuromotor development training
  - Tactile, verbal, and visual cues and weight shifting to improve midline awareness
  - Balance exercises sitting on a ball with head turning
- ◆ Strength, power, and endurance training
  - Elastic band for primarily LUE and LLE strengthening
    - UE: Securing one end of elastic band and move the arm through all ranges (eg, flexion, extension, abduction, etc) as able
    - LE: Secure elastic band and loop onto leg and move leg through all ranges as able
    - Assistance may be provided as needed initially
  - Isokinetic strengthening of the LEs with focus initially on the left iliopsoas, hamstrings, tibialis anterior, medial gastrocnemius
  - Functional strengthening
    - Bridging/rolling
    - Repeated sit to stand and stand to sit[152]
    - Marching in place and toe and heel walking
    - Wheelchair propulsion changing how wheelchair is propelled
  - Muscle endurance can be augmented by decreasing rest time during physical therapy sessions

FUNCTIONAL TRAINING IN SELF-CARE AND HOME MANAGEMENT

- ◆ Functional mobility
  - All activities done with appropriate handling/cues/feedback to meet demands of the task, safety in performance, quality of movement, and reduction of long-term movement complications[136,139]
    - Bridging[116]
    - Rolling in bed
    - Supine to sit
    - Reaching
    - Sit to stand[152]
    - Transfers (bed, chair, toilet, shower, dining room chair, car)
  - Practice functional activities, such as putting on/off shoes and socks[166]
- ◆ Self-care and home management
  - Proper bed positioning to prevent skin breakdown

and prevent other impairments
- Reinforce self-care and home management actions, tasks, and activities to include ADL training and use of assistive and adaptive devices and equipment during ADL[159]
- Many of the therapeutic exercises described previously will help support ADL training (eg, sit to stand and stand to sit to and from lower surfaces will help with toilet transfer technique, bridging will assist with bed mobility, seated and standing reaching exercises will help with grooming/hygiene tasks)
- Practice exercises in context of self-care and home management
- ◆ Injury prevention or reduction
  - Home evaluation for the assessment of readiness of the patient and family to manage at home and predict areas of difficulty[167]
  - Appropriate recommendations will be made
    - Remove throw rugs
    - Sit while changing clothes
    - Rearrange furniture for safe mobility
    - Use a shower bench
    - Use grab bars for shower, tub, and toilet
  - Instruct, demonstrate, and practice safe techniques to assist with ambulation and stair climbing
  - Create task-specific environment
    - Ambulation is performed on both firm and carpeted surfaces
    - Practice elevation activities that mirror as closely as possible the number of stairs and set up of railings at patient's home

FUNCTIONAL TRAINING IN WORK, COMMUNITY, AND LEISURE INTEGRATION OR REINTEGRATION

- ◆ Functional training programs
  - Instruct patient and his family in strategies for safe community ambulation using appropriate assistive devices
  - Transfer training in and out of car
- ◆ Focus community reentry programs on development of higher level motor, social, and cognitive skills to prepare the person with a brain injury to return to independent living and potentially to work
- ◆ Focus on safety in the community, interacting with others, initiation and goal setting, and money management skills
- ◆ Vocational evaluation and training may also be a component of this program[168]
- ◆ Recommendations for support systems

- Brain Injury Association of America: 800-444-6443, www.biausa.org[169]
- Brain Injury Source: www.biausa.org/Pages/source_abstracts.html
- National Association of State Head Injury Administrators: 301-656-3500, www.nashia.org
- National Brain Injury Research Treatment and Training Foundation: www.nbirtt.org
- National Center for Medical Rehabilitation Research: 800-370-2943, www.nichd.nih.gov/about/ncmrr
- National Institute of Neurological Disorders and Stroke: 800-352-9424, www.ninds.nih.gov
- Local chapters of the Brain Injury Association, Office of Rehabilitation Services/Vocational Rehabilitation

MANUAL THERAPY TECHNIQUES

- ◆ Direct manual therapy treatment will be used to reduce neuromusculoskeletal imbalances improving motor control by strengthening and increasing ROM
- ◆ Indirect manual therapy will be used to improve functional skills through intervention targeted at static and dynamic postural control and movement patterns providing for variability, repetition, and carryover in motor learning[115]

PRESCRIPTION, APPLICATION, AND, AS APPROPRIATE, FABRICATION OF DEVICES AND EQUIPMENT

- ◆ Adaptive devices
  - Adaptive devices and equipment for the bathroom (eg, raised toiled seat, tub seat, grab bars in the shower, and grab bars along side of the toilet)
  - Adaptive devices and equipment for the kitchen (eg, reacher, Dycem to keep eating and cooking items from sliding, equipment to allow function with one hand, such as a can opener, bottle/jar opener, adapted cutting board, etc) as he will be functioning initially primarily with the LUE
- ◆ Assistive devices
  - Upon completion of a home assessment, recommendations are made for equipment, including purchase price and ordering information
  - Assistive devices and equipment for mobility to enhance performance and independence in ADL and IADL (eg, wheelchair, cane, AFO)
    - Wheelchair will be needed for long-distance activities
    - Coordinate wheelchair assessment, documentation, fitting, and ordering of the chair with appropriate vendor
    - A tilt-in-space wheelchair will be optimal during

the early stage of rehabilitation to provide the ability to change position for proper pressure relief
  - Assistive devices and equipment to increase stability and reduce risk of falls (eg, cane, grab bars for the shower, additional rails at the stairs, night lights, marking on stairs to distinguish one from the other)
- ◆ Orthotic devices
  - Orthotic devices and equipment to increase stability and mobility
    - Multipodus boots to position the feet to prevent foot drop and skin breakdown[18]
    - AFO, bilateral if appropriate, to provide ankle and knee stability for standing activities and ambulation[170]
      - ▶ Coordinate care with the orthotist to fabricate the AFO based on the physical therapist's recommendations
      - ▶ Provided instructions to patient and family in donning and doffing the AFO and how to monitor skin
      - ▶ Establish a wearing schedule and instructions for patient and family
  - Appropriate shoes to accommodate the AFOs
- ◆ Supportive devices
  - Use of a splint is common in the management of adults with TBI
    - Goal is to prevent contracture and structural deformities that would affect functional skills,[143,153] however its use may restrict movement and could contribute to muscle shortening, stiffness, and weakness as a result of nonuse[136,143,147,171,172]
    - Determine necessity of splint in collaboration with occupational therapy and if deemed necessary, monitor schedule of use, duration, and impact on function

ANTICIPATED GOALS AND EXPECTED OUTCOMES

Given the long-term nature of TBI and the variability among individuals, it is often difficult to determine short- and/or long-term prognoses for individuals post TBI.[137,173] The following outcomes presented are based on the examination completed and information provided by the family. The goals and outcomes will be modified as necessary if Ben's progress does not proceed as anticipated.

- ◆ Impact on impairments
  - Aerobic capacity and endurance is increased so that patient can function throughout the day, including management of self-care and ADL and participation in therapy and family activities with only short rests.
  - Ascending and descending stairs with the hand rail and AFO is independently achieved.

- Balance and postural control are improved, and patient is able to sit, lean, and reach out of his base of support without falling; he is able to let go of the cane in standing to reach, open a door, and move small items in the kitchen and bathroom without falling.
- Balance is improved so that Ben is able to ambulate functional distances (eg, to the car, into therapy) using an orthotic and assistive device with the assist of one person.
- Balance is improved so that the patient is able to perform dynamic sitting balance independently for dressing and bathing.
- Gait is improved so that patient is able to ambulate household distances with a cane on level indoor surfaces without assistance and stand with single UE support for 5 minutes.
- Independent bed mobility is achieved, and he can align himself in bed.
- Muscle performance is increased so that patient is able to demonstrate hip and knee control on the right knee during stance phase and clear foot during swing phase of RLE with ambulation on firm and carpeted surfaces.
- Patient is independent in his home exercise program.
- Transfer from bed to/from chair without assistance is achieved.

◆ Impact on functional limitations
- Ability to perform activities related to mobility, such as bed mobility and climbing stairs, is increased.
- Ability to perform ADL and IADL is increased.
- Performance of these activities with equipment and adaptive devices is improved.

◆ Impact on disabilities
- Ability to assume or resume required self-care and home management roles is improved.
- Ability to be independent in wheelchair mobility in places where the distance is too great to walk, such as in the mall or hospital, is improved.
- Performance levels in community or leisure activities are improved.

◆ Risk reduction/prevention
- Level of supervision to perform a task is decreased.
- Risk factors are reduced.
- Risk of secondary impairments is reduced and safety is improved during performance of self-care activities and home exercise program.
- Safety of patient and family is improved.

◆ Impact on health, wellness, and fitness
- Behaviors that foster healthy habits, wellness, and

prevention are acquired.
- Physical function is improved.

◆ Impact on societal resources
- Available resources are maximally utilized.
- Community resources to meet his discharge needs are identified.
- Documentation occurs throughout patient management and follows APTA's *Guidelines for Physical Therapy Documentation*.[117]
- Referrals are made to other professionals or resources whenever necessary and appropriate.

◆ Patient/client satisfaction
- Admission data and discharge planning are completed.
- Case is managed throughout the episode of care.
- Clinical proficiency and interpersonal skills of the physical therapist are acceptable to patient/client.
- Communication and interdisciplinary collaboration occurs across settings through case conferences, patient care rounds, patient family meetings, and documentation.
- Family Satisfaction Scale developed for families of TBI survivors to measure satisfaction with family cohesion and adaptability indicates satisfacation.[174]
- Patient and family knowledge and awareness of the diagnosis, prognosis, interventions, and anticipated goals and expected outcomes are increased.

REEXAMINATION

Reexamination is an ongoing part of the plan of care and will be performed throughout the episode of care with adjustments to the plan of care as needed.

DISCHARGE

Ben is discharged from physical therapy and the rehabilitation facility after a total of 105 physical therapy visits over 7 weeks and attainment of his goals.[128] These sessions have covered his inpatient rehabilitation services. It is further anticipated that he will require home physical therapy for 12 visits after discharge to home and then 20 to 30 outpatient physical therapy visits.

Case Study #3: Stroke—Central Vestibular Dysfunction

Mr. Jeremy Smith is a 67-year-old male, who is 1-week post brainstem stroke and has just been admitted to a rehabilitation unit due to complaints of severe dizziness and disequilibrium.

PHYSICAL THERAPIST EXAMINATION

HISTORY

♦ General demographics: Mr. Smith is a 67-year-old white male who was born and raised in the United States, speaks English, and is right handed. He is a college graduate.

♦ Social history: Mr. Smith is married and has one daughter who is 35 years old.

♦ Employment/work: Mr. Smith recently retired from an electrical engineering position at a local consulting firm.

♦ Living environment: He lives in a two-level home with his wife. There are three steps with a rail to enter the house. His bedroom is on the second floor. The stairs to the second floor have a hand rail on the right. His daughter lives within 20 miles of his house.

♦ General health status
  ● General health perception: Mr. Smith reported that he had been in fairly good health until the admission to the hospital.
  ● Physical function: Prior to the hospitalization, he was independent with all ADL and IADL. He had been walking 20 minutes a day, 3 days a week during the year, and in the summer months he would walk the golf course.
  ● Psychological function: Normal and he appears to be coping with recent events in a positive, upbeat manner.
  ● Role function: Father, husband, retiree, volunteer, recreational golfer.
  ● Social function: Prior to admission, he regularly attended church and volunteered delivering meals to the elderly in the community. During the summer months he was in a golf league and played two to three times a week.

♦ Social/health habits: He is a nonsmoker and occasionally drinks socially.

♦ Family history: Noncontributory.

♦ Medical/surgical history: Mr. Smith has a medical history that includes a recent diagnosis of diabetes mellitus, HTN, and elevated lipids. All are controlled with medication with the exception of his diabetes, which is currently diet controlled.

♦ Current condition(s)/chief complaint(s): Prior to admission to the hospital, he awoke with symptoms of vertigo and disequilibrium. His wife attempted to help him out of bed, but together they were unable to get him mobilized safely. His wife called 911, and he was taken to the hospital via ambulance. He was diagnosed with an acute infarct in the lateral pontine and medullary regions of the brainstem. (Brainstem or cerebellar lesions may result in central vestibular problems.) Initially his dizziness was so severe that he kept his eyes closed when he attended therapy. One week after his stroke, he was admitted to a rehabilitation unit. His dizziness is now less severe, and he is able to keep his eyes open about 90% of the time during his therapy sessions. Mr. Smith's primary obstacles are his feelings of dizziness and disequilibrium. He reports an increase in symptoms with head movement from side to side.

♦ Functional status and activity level: His mobility varies between needing minimal to moderate assist with all his transfers and ambulation. He walks with a wheeled walker. He leans to the left in sitting and standing. If he shifts his weight out of his base of support, he is unable to self-recover.

♦ Medications: Prior to his hospitalization and rehab admission, Mr. Smith was on medication for HTN and elevated cholesterol. After his stroke and subsequent hospitalization he continued on all of his medications. In addition, a blood thinner and sleeping pill were added. His current medications include Coumadin, lisinopril, and Lipitor.

♦ Other clinical tests: MRI revealed an acute infarct in the lateral pontine and medullary regions of the brainstem. Lesions in this area depending on the size could affect a number of structures including the vestibular nerve, the vestibular nuclei, and the tracts/pathways that travel through this area of the brain.

SYSTEMS REVIEW

♦ Cardiovascular/pulmonary
  ● BP: 132/54 mmHg
  ● Edema: None noted
  ● HR: 80 bpm at rest
  ● RR: 18 bpm

♦ Integumentary
  ● Presence of scar formation: None noted
  ● Skin color: Good

- Skin integrity: Intact
- Musculoskeletal
  - Gross range of motion: WNL
  - Gross strength: Appears to be between 4/5 and 5/5 throughout all extremities and trunk
  - Gross symmetry: Leans to left in sitting and standing
  - Height: 5'11" (1.8 m)
  - Weight: 190 lbs (86.18 kg)
- Neuromuscular
  - Balance: Poor sitting and standing balance
  - Locomotion, transfers, and transitions
    - Ambulates with a wheeled walker and moderate assist of one for 40 feet exhibiting a wide base of support and leaning to the left
    - Transitions including sit to/from stand, supine to/from sit, bed to/from chair vary and at times trigger strong sways and loss of balance that he is unable to self-recover
- Communication, affect, cognition, language, and learning style
  - Mr. Smith is oriented x3
  - His speech is intact and is able to communicate appropriately with staff and family
  - His cognition appears to be at his baseline per evaluation by a speech pathologist
  - He reports he learns easily through verbal instruction

TESTS AND MEASURES

- Aerobic capacity/endurance
  - Able to perform continuous movement for only 2 to 3 minutes before needing a seated rest break
  - Patient reports a RPE of 13
- Anthropometric characteristics
  - BMI=705 x (body weight [in pounds] divided by height [in inches][120]
  - Mr. Smith's BMI=28.8
  - BMI values between 25 and 29.9 are considered overweight[121]
- Assistive and adaptive devices
  - Two-wheeled walker
  - Hospital bed with side rails
  - Transfer belt
- Circulation
  - Orthostatic BP: BP tested in supine, sitting, and standing with minimal change
- Cranial and peripheral nerve integrity
  - Eye tests (see Pattern F: Impaired Peripheral Nerve Integrity and Muscle Performance Associated With

Peripheral Nerve Injury, Other Clinical Tests, Vestibular Dysfunction)
  - Nystagmus
    - Characteristics of a central nystagmus include the following[175-177]
      - The nystagmus is found in one direction (ie, torsional, vertical, or horizontal)
      - It can change direction
      - It is unable to be suppressed with visual fixation
    - Initially Mr. Smith had spontaneous vertical nystagmus present
    - Visual fixation did not change nystagmus
  - Saccades: Intact
  - Smooth pursuit: Occasional corrective saccades noted
  - Vestibular-ocular reflex (VOR): Impaired with decreased VOR gain
  - VOR cancellation: Intact
  - Reports an increase in dizziness symptoms with head turns when his eyes are open
- Gait, locomotion, and balance
  - Walks with a two-wheeled walker provided by rehab unit and moderate physical help from the physical therapist to control the walker due to lean to left and feelings of dizziness
  - Walks with a wide base of support and lean to the left
  - Shows decreased awareness of where his LEs are during mobility
  - Able to statically sit with supervision of the physical therapist, but as he fatigues, leans left
  - Reports the lean as a feeling of being pulled
  - Unable to perform standing Romberg test with eyes open or shut
  - Tinetti Balance and Gait Assessment[178]
    - Including assessment of sitting balance, rising, attempt to rise, immediate standing balance, being nudged, eyes closed, turning 360 degrees, sitting down, initiation of gait, step length and height, step symmetry, step continuity, path, trunk, and walking stance
    - Score: 14/28 which indicates he has a high risk for falls
- Motor function
  - Coordination: Heel to shin test
    - Patient supine and instructed to place right heel on left shin and slide heel up/down shin
    - Result: Abnormal since was unable to complete at a normal pace and accuracy of placement was poor secondary to poor proprioception

- Normal UE movements
- See Gait, Locomotion, and Balance

◆ Muscle performance: Between 4/5 and 5/5 throughout trunk and extremities

◆ Posture
  - Sitting
    - Shoulders rounded and forward head
    - Uses hands to widen base of support on edge of bed
    - Leans to left
  - Standing
    - Stands with wide base of support
    - Leans to the left
    - Shoulders rounded

◆ Self-care and home management
  - Prior to the stroke was independent in all ADL and IADL
  - Current difficulty with ADL that require balance in standing including brushing teeth, shaving, washing dishes, and getting dressed
  - IADL: Unable to shop, drive, or mow lawn

◆ Sensory integrity
  - Difficulty with interpretation of sensory input for balance
  - Unable to use feedback of position in space to realign body
  - Sitting and standing balance poor with or without vision due to left lean
  - Proprioception impaired in LEs

◆ Work, community, and leisure integration or reintegration
  - Currently in rehabilitation facility so Mr. Smith is unable to drive or participate in community or leisure activities
  - He has difficulty moving in standing and walking with walker in stable and unstable environments

EVALUATION

Mr. Smith had an acute infarct in the lateral medullary and pontine regions of the brainstem affecting how his brain processes information related to balance. Mr. Smith has dizziness, a left lean, dysphagia nausea, nystagmus, disequilibrium, and sensation or sensory changes. Because of his constant dizziness that varies in intensity and is affected by head movements and his lean, he is showing functional deficits in his ambulation and transfers and is dependent with many of his daily cares. He can no longer ambulate without assistance from another person and is dependent on a walker for support and balance. He is unable to ambulate community distances or drive. Mr. Smith is at high risk for falls.

DIAGNOSIS

Mr. Smith sustained an acute infarct in the lateral pontine and medullary regions of the brainstem resulting in findings consistent with a lesion in the brainstem. He has impaired: aerobic capacity/endurance; cranial and peripheral nerve integrity; gait, locomotion, and balance; motor function; muscle performance; posture; and sensory integrity. He is functionally limited in self-care and home management and in work, community, and leisure actions, tasks, and activities. He is in need of devices and equipment. These findings are consistent with placement in Pattern D: Impaired Motor Function and Sensory Integrity Associated With Nonprogressive Disorders of the Central Nervous System— Acquired in Adolescence or Adulthood. The identified impairments, functional limitations, and device and equipment needs will be addressed in determining the prognosis and the plan of care.

PROGNOSIS AND PLAN OF CARE

Over the course of the visits, the following mutually established outcomes have been determined:

◆ Ability to perform self-care activities is improved

◆ Aerobic capacity and endurance are increased

◆ Balance while standing and walking is increased

◆ Fitness is improved

◆ Functional independence in ADL and IADL is increased

◆ Muscle performance is increased

◆ Physical capacity is improved

◆ Physical function is improved

◆ Posture is improved

◆ Risk factors are reduced

◆ Self-management of symptoms is improved

To achieve these outcomes, the appropriate interventions for this patient are determined. These will include: coordination, communication, and documentation; patient/client-related instruction; therapeutic exercise; functional training in self-care and home management; functional training in work, community, and leisure integration or reintegration; and prescription, application, and, as appropriate, fabrication of devices and equipment.

Based on the diagnosis and prognosis, Mr. Smith is expected to require 36 visits over a 3-week period of time in the rehabilitation facility. Mr. Smith has good social support, is motivated, and will follow through with his exercise program. Although he has physical impairments, he is generally healthy.

INTERVENTIONS

RATIONALE FOR SELECTED INTERVENTIONS

Therapeutic Exercise

After a stroke an individual will demonstrate a decrease in endurance secondary to relative inactivity or bedrest as compared to prior to the stroke.[18] Early intervention can decrease the effect of inactivity.[18] This patient is in an inpatient rehabilitation unit. Initially, functional mobility during therapy can be used to increase endurance and cardiovascular fitness level.[18] As the patient progresses in the setting or even at discharge from this setting, he would benefit from a continued type of cardiovascular program to improve his fitness level. Because a high percent of stroke patients also have cardiac disease, it is recommended that the patient undergo cardiac testing.[179]

Other factors common after stroke include impaired sensation, impaired proprioception, visual impairments, abnormal tone, abnormal synergy patterns, abnormal reflexes, apraxia, postural control, balance, cognitive dysfunction, and perceptual dysfunction.[18] Any or all of these may contribute to impairments in mobility. Rehabilitation facilitating normal patterns of movement and progressing the level of difficulty will assist in promoting maximal independence.

Involvement of the central vestibular system may also occur in patients who have sustained a stroke. Injury to the central vestibular system can impair balance, impair gaze stabilization, and cause nausea and/or dizziness. The central vestibular system as defined by Furman and Whitney includes the vestibular nuclei, vestibulo-ocular pathways, vestibulospinal pathways, vestibulocolic pathways, vestibulo-autonomic pathways, vestibulocerebral pathways, vestibulocerebellum, and perihypoglossal nuclei.[180] Individuals with damage in the central part the vestibular system have benefited from vestibular rehabilitation.[181,182] Patients will show improved functional status but not full recovery, and the progress tends to be slower when compared with patients who have vestibular rehabilitation for peripheral vestibular problems.[181]

COORDINATION, COMMUNICATION, AND DOCUMENTATION

Communication will occur with the patient and his wife both in verbal and written format. Communication will also occur with other members of the health care team. All elements of the client's management will be documented.

PATIENT/CLIENT-RELATED INSTRUCTION

Mr. Smith and his wife will be educated regarding the injury to the brain and the effects on the rest of his body.

They will participate in the development of the plan of care. Mr. Smith will be instructed during treatment on mobility skills and instructed in methods to enhance his performance. When appropriate, he will also be instructed in balance exercises that he can perform independently. His wife will be instructed in how to assist Mr. Smith and how to provide appropriate cues to him during ADL tasks.

THERAPEUTIC EXERCISE

♦ Aerobic capacity/endurance conditioning
  • Note: Always check to determine if any cardiac precautions exist before beginning an aerobic exercise program and clear aerobic exercise with physician
  • Mode: Initial walking with a walker
  • Intensity
    ▪ Continuous activity with monitoring of perceived exertion
    ▪ To work at an RPE of fairly light (11 on the Borg scale) working up to moderately hard (13 on the Borg scale)[42]
  • Duration
    ▪ At this time he tolerates 3 minutes
    ▪ Long-term goal is 20 to 30 minutes increasing duration as tolerated
  • Frequency: Daily

♦ Balance, coordination, and agility training
  • Sitting at edge of bed without back support for a set amount of time, increase as tolerated
  • Reaching with UE while maintaining sitting balance and progressing to include weight shift with reach
  • Kneeling activities including static hold and progress to reaching and weight shifting
  • Static stance with UE support on walker and assist from physical therapist
  • Progress to reaching and weight shifting in standing

♦ Body mechanics and postural stabilization
  • Sitting at edge of bed with visual feedback from a mirror (if he tolerates it) or verbal feedback, ask questions about weightbearing on hips and how his body position feels
  • Scapular and chin tuck exercises in sitting to decrease rounded shoulders and forward head
  • Correct lean in sitting with physical therapist assist or cues if appropriate

♦ Gait and locomotion training
  • Start with the basics (sit to stand) and as his skill improves increase the skill of the task (pivot transfers)
  • Perform pre-gait activities in parallel bars to encourage weight shift, reciprocal steps, and heel strike when gait is initiated
  • Use appropriate assistive device and progress as less

assistance needed (parallel bars → walker → quad cane → single-end cane → no assistive device)

- Progress to walking outdoors, walking on uneven terrains, and climbing stairs
- Progress to four-wheeled walker to be used in community

◆ Neuromotor development training
  • Vestibular training
    ▪ Tolerance to having eyes open in different positions (supine, sitting, standing) and in different environments
    ▪ Start in an environment with minimal stimulation and increase as tolerated
    ▪ Exercises to enhance the VOR for adaptation
      ▸ VOR gain is defined as eye velocity/head velocity and is equal to 1 in a normal vestibular system so that when the head turns to the right, the eyes move in an equal and opposite direction to the left to maintain gaze stability[176,183]
      ▸ Gaze stabilization exercises are used for this patient, who has a decreased VOR gain
      ▸ Note: Some patients with cerebellar lesions have an enhanced VOR, and in that case these exercises would not be appropriate[182]
  • Vestibular stimulation exercises[175,183]
    ▪ Patient begins sitting facing a wall with a plain background and focuses on a target taped on the wall that can be clearly seen or read
    ▪ Patient turns head from side to side for 30 seconds and gradually progresses to duration of 2 minutes of head turns while focusing on the target
    ▪ As patient progresses, the exercise is advanced by increasing the speed of head turns, putting the target on a busy background, or having him stand or march in place while turning the head
    ▪ Exercises may also be done with the head moving up and down
◆ Advance to other motion-tolerance activities if or when patient progresses (turning head, watching others moving, scanning while walking)

FUNCTIONAL TRAINING IN SELF-CARE AND HOME MANAGEMENT AND FUNCTIONAL TRAINING IN WORK, COMMUNITY, AND LEISURE INTEGRATION OR REINTEGRATION

◆ ADL training
  • Transfer training into/out of bed and in the bathroom

- Perform repetition of functional tasks
- Injury prevention or reduction
  ▪ Remove throw rugs
  ▪ Patient to sit while changing clothes
  ▪ Put frequently used items in kitchen, bathroom, and bedroom at trunk level
  ▪ Use a shower bench
  ▪ Use grab bars for shower, tub, and toilet
- Home evaluation to work on mobility in simulation of patient's own environment

◆ Device and equipment use training
  • Training on how to use walker during daily activities
◆ IADL training
  • Transfer in and out of car
  • Rest of IADL training will be done when he is an outpatient and when he is at a higher level of functioning

PRESCRIPTION, APPLICATION, AND, AS APPROPRIATE, FABRICATION OF DEVICES AND EQUIPMENT

◆ Walker to assist with ambulation
  • Mr. Smith will be fitted with a four-wheeled walker prior to discharge
  • He and his wife will be educated on appropriate height of walker
  • Since the walker chosen for him will be a folding walker for easy transport, he and his wife will be instructed in proper use of this feature

ANTICIPATED GOALS AND EXPECTED OUTCOMES

◆ Impact on impairments
  • Ability to get from car to house, into house, and up stairs is improved.
  • Aerobic capacity and endurance are increased so that he can tolerate a 10-minute activity without complaints of fatigue.
  • Balance is improved so that Mr. Smith can perform static sitting balance independently in order to get dressed.
  • Gait is improved so that Mr. Smith is able to ambulate household distances with walker and contact guard assist of his wife.
  • Postural control is improved, and Mr. Smith is able to sit at edge of bed independently.
  • Sensation of dizziness is decreased.
◆ Impact on functional limitations
  • Ability to perform and functional independence in

ADL and IADL is increased.
- Ability to perform physical actions, tasks, and activities is improved.
- Ability to turn head symptom free during ADL is achieved.
- Level of supervision for task performance is decreased.

◆ Impact on disability
- Ability to assume or resume required self-care and home management roles is improved.

◆ Risk reduction/prevention
- Level of supervision to perform a task is decreased.
- Risk factors are reduced.
- Safety of patient and family is improved.
- Self-management of symptoms is improved.

◆ Impact on health, wellness, and fitness
- Behaviors that foster healthy habits, wellness, and prevention are acquired.
- Physical capacity is improved.
- Physical function is improved.

◆ Impact on societal resources
- Available resources are maximally utilized.
- Documentation occurs throughout patient management and follows APTA's *Guidelines for Physical Therapy Documentation.*[117]

◆ Patient/client satisfaction
- Access, availability, and services provided are acceptable to patient/client.
- Case is managed throughout the episode of care.
- Clinical proficiency and interpersonal skills of the physical therapist are acceptable to patient/client.
- Communication and interdisciplinary collaboration occurs across settings through case conferences, patient care rounds, patient/family meetings, and documentation.
- Coordination of care is acceptable to patient/client.
- Intensity of care is reduced.
- Patient and family understand and participate in determining goals and outcomes.
- Patient's and wife's knowledge and awareness of diagnosis, prognosis, interventions, and anticipated goals and outcomes are increased.
- Sense of well-being is improved.

REEXAMINATION

Reexamination is performed throughout the episode of care.

DISCHARGE

Mr. Smith is discharged from physical therapy and the rehabilitation facility after a total of 36 physical therapy visits over 3 weeks and attainment of his goals. As Mr. Smith has a condition that may require multiple episodes of care throughout his life span, he received education regarding factors that may trigger a call to his physical therapist for a reexamination and new episode of physical therapy care. Some of those factors may include an increase in dizziness, an increase in lean, or a decrease in functional mobility that becomes unsafe or persists.

REFERENCES

1. Moore KL, Dalley AF. *Clinically Oriented Anatomy.* 5th ed. Philadelphia, PA: Lippincott Williams & Wilkins; 2006.
2. Kandel ER, Schwartz JH, Jessell TM. *Principles of Neural Science.* 4th ed. New York, NY: McGraw Hill; 2000.
3. Weinberger J. *Contemporary Diagnosis and Management of Stroke.* Newton, PA: Handbooks in Health Care Co; 1999.
4. Nolte J. *The Human Brain.* 4th ed. St. Louis, MO: Mosby; 1999.
5. Sharp FR, Swanson RA, Honkaniemi J, et al. Neurochemistry and molecular biology. In: Barnett HJM, Mohr JP, Stein BM, Yatsu FM, eds. *Stroke: Pathophysiology, Diagnosis, and Management.* 3rd ed. New York, NY: Churchill Livingstone; 1998.
6. Stein DG, Hoffman SW. Concepts of CNS plasticity in context of brain damage and repair. *J Head Trauma Rehabil.* 2003; 18:317-341.
7. Komitova M, Johansson BB, Eriksson PS. On neural plasticity, new neurons and the post-ischemic milieu: an integrated view on experimental neurorehabilitation. *Exp Neurol.* 2006; 199:42-55.
8. Nudo RJ, Milliken GW. Reorganization of movement representations in primary motor cortex following focal ischemic infarcts in adult squirrel monkeys. *J Neurophysiol.* 1996;75: 2144-2149.
9. Nudo RJ, Wise BM, SiFuentes F, Milliken GW. Neural substrates for the effects of rehabilitative training on motor recovery after ischemic infarct. *Science.* 1996;272:1791-1794.
10. Weinberger JM. Evolving therapeutic approaches to treating acute ischemic stroke. *J Neurol Sci.* 2006;249:101-109.
11. Xavier AR, Farkas J. Catheter-based recanalization techniques for acute ischemic stroke. *Neuroimaging Clin N Am.* 2005;15: 441-453.
12. US Multicenter, Randomized Controlled Study Comparing the Performance of Onyx (EVOH) and TRUFILL (n-BCA) in the Presurgical Embolization of Brain Arteriovenous Malformations (BAVMs). Washington DC: Georgetown University Hospital; 2003.
13. Kochanek KD, Smith BL. Deaths: preliminary data for 2002. *Natl Vital Stat Rep.* 2004;54:1-6.
14. Goodman CC, Boissonault WG, Fuller KS. *Pathology: Implications for the Physical Therapist.* New York, NY: WB Saunders; 2003.

15. Marsden CD, Fowler T. *Clinical Neurology*. 2nd ed. New York, NY: Oxford University Press; 1998.

16. Foley C, Pizer HF. *The Stroke Fact Book*. Golden Valley, MN: Courage Press; 1990.

17. Smith DH, Meaney DF, Shull WH. Neuroplasticity. *J Head Trauma Rehabil*. 2003;18(4):307-316.

18. O'Sullivan SB, Schmitz TJ. *Physical Rehabilitation: Assessment and Treatment*. 5th ed. Philadelphia, PA: FA Davis; 2007.

19. Kiernan JA. *Barr's The Human Nervous System: An Anatomical Viewpoint*. 8th ed. Philadelphia, PA: Lippincott Williams & Wilkins; 2005.

20. Purves D, Augustine GJ, Fitzpatrick D, et al. *Neuroscience*. 3rd ed. Sunderland, MA: Sinauer Associates; 2004.

21. Medline Plus Drug Information. Available at: http://www.nlm.nih.gov/medlineplus/druginfo/medmaster/a684001.html. Accessed September 28, 2007.

22. Centre for Neuro Skills (CNS), Pharmacology Guide. Available at: http://www.neuroskills.com. Accessed September 28, 2007.

23. RXList: The Internet Drug Index. Available at: http://www.rxlist.com/script/main/hp.asp. Accessed September 30, 2007.

24. Duncan PW, Zorowitz R, Bates B, et al. Management of adult stroke rehabilitation care: a clinical practice guideline. *Stroke*. 2005;36:e100-e143.

25. Organized inpatient (stroke unit) care for stroke. Stroke Unit Trialists' Collaboration. *Cochrane Database Syst Rev*. 2002;(2): CD000197. [Update in: *Cochrane Database Syst Rev*. 2002;(1): CD000197.]

26. Rittman M, Faircloth C, Boylstein C, et al. The experience of time in the transition from hospital to home following stroke. *J Rehabil Res Dev*. 2004;41:xi-xii.

27. Jette DU, Latham NK, Smout RJ, et al. Physical therapy interventions for patients with stroke in inpatient facilities. *Phys Ther*. 2005;85:238-248.

28. Maeshima S, Ueyoshi A, Osawa A, et al. Mobility and muscle strength contralateral to hemiplegia from stroke: benefit from self-training with family support. *Am J Phys Med Rehabil*. 2003;82:456-462.

29. Gordon NF, Gulanick M, Costa F, et al. Physical activity and exercise recommendations for stroke survivors: an American Heart Association scientific statement from the Council on Clinical Cardiology, Subcommittee on Exercise, Cardiac Rehabilitation, and Prevention; the Council on Cardiovascular Nursing; the Council on Nutrition, Physical Activity, and Metabolism; and the Stroke Council. *Stroke*. 2004;35:1230-1240.

30. Olney SJ, Nymark J, Brouwer B, et al. A randomized controlled trial of supervised versus unsupervised exercise programs for ambulatory stroke survivors. *Stroke*. 2006;37:476-481.

31. Bastille JV, Gill-Body KM. A yoga-based exercise program for people with chronic poststroke hemiparesis. *Phys Ther*. 2004; 84:33-48.

32. Morris SL, Dodds KJ, Morris ME. Outcomes of progressive resistance strength training following stroke: a systematic review. *Clin Rehabil*. 2004;18:27-39.

33. Teixeira-Salmela LF, Olney SJ, Nadeau S, Brouwer B. Muscle strengthening and physical conditioning to reduce impairment and disability in chronic stroke survivors. *Arch Phys Med Rehabil*. 1999;80:1211-1218.

34. Brown DA, Kautz SA. Increased workload enhances force output during pedaling exercise in persons with poststroke hemiplegia. *Stroke*. 1998;29:598-606.

35. Roth EJ, Harvey RL. Rehabilitation of stroke syndromes. In: Braddom RL, ed. *Physical Medicine and Rehabilitation*. 2nd ed. Philadelphia, PA: WB Saunders; 2000:1117-1163.

36. Potempa K, Braun LT, Tinknell T, Popovich J. Benefits of aerobic exercise after stroke. *Sports Med*. 1996;21:337-346. Review.

37. Macko RF, DeSouza CA, Tretter LD, et al. Treadmill aerobic exercise training reduces the energy expenditure and cardiovascular demands of hemiparetic gait in chronic stroke patients: a preliminary report. *Stroke*. 1997;28:326-330.

38. Sullivan KJ, Knowlton BJ, Dobkin BH. Step training with body weight support: effect of treadmill speed and practice paradigms on poststroke locomotor recovery. *Arch Phys Med Rehabil*. 2002;83:683-691.

39. Lamontagne A, Fung J. Faster is better: implications for speed-intensive gait training after stroke. *Stroke*. 2004;35:2543-2548.

40. Danielsson A, Sunnerhagen KS. Oxygen consumption during treadmill walking with and without body weight support in patients with hemiparesis after stroke and in healthy subjects. *Arch Phys Med Rehabil*. 2000;81:953-957.

41. Hesse S, Werner C, Paul T, et al. Influence of walking speed on lower limb muscle activity and energy consumption during treadmill walking of hemiparetic patients. *Arch Phys Med Rehabil*. 2001;82:1547-1550.

42. Borg G. *Borg's Perceived Exertion and Pain Scales*. Champaign, IL: Human Kinetics; 1998.

43. Aruin AS, Hanke T, Chaudhuri G, et al. Compelled weight bearing in persons with hemiparesis following stroke: the effect of a lift insert and goal-directed balance exercise. *J Rehabil Res Dev*. 2000;37:65-72.

44. Cheng PT, Wu SH, Liaw MY, et al. Symmetrical body-weight distribution training in stroke patients and its effect on fall prevention. *Arch Phys Med Rehabil*. 2001;82:1650-1654.

45. Bonan IV, Yelnik AP, Colle FM, et al. Reliance on visual information after stroke. Part II: effectiveness of a balance rehabilitation program with visual cue deprivation after stroke: a randomized controlled trial. *Arch Phys Med Rehabil*. 2004;85: 274-278.

46. Geiger RA, Allen JB, O'Keefe JO, Hicks RR. Balance and mobility following stroke: effects of physical therapy interventions with and without biofeedback/forceplate training. *Phys Ther*. 2001;81:995-1005.

47. Walker C, Brouwer BJ, Culham EG. Use of visual feedback in retraining balance following acute stroke. *Phys Ther*. 2000;80: 886-895.

48. Kalra L, Perez L, Gupta S, Wittink M. The influence of visual neglect on stroke rehabilitation. *Stroke*. 1997;28:722-728.

49. Baily MJ, Riddoch MJ, Crome P. Treatment of visual neglect in elderly patients with stroke: a single-subject series using either a scanning and cueing strategy or a left-limb activiation strategy. *Phys Ther*. 2002;82:782-789.

50. da Cunha Filho IT, Lim PAC, Qureshy H, et al. A comparison of regular rehabilitation and regular rehabilitation with supported treadmill ambulation training for acute stroke patients. *J Rehabil Res Dev*. 2001;38:37-47.

51. Gelber DA, Josefczyk PB, Herman D, et al. Comparison of two therapy approaches in the rehabilitation of the pure motor

hemiparetic stroke patient. *Journal of Neurologic Rehabilitation.* 1995;9:191-196.

52. Nilsson L, Carlsson J, Danielsson A, et al. Walking training of patients with hemiparesis at an early stage after stroke: a comparison of walking training on a treadmill with body weight support and walking on the ground. *Clin Rehabil.* 2001;15:515-527.

53. Hesse SA, Jahnke MT, Bertelt CM, et al. Gait outcome in ambulatory hemiparetic patients after a 4-week comprehensive rehabilitation program and prognostic factors. *Stroke.* 1994; 25:1999-2004.

54. Sullivan KJ, Brown KA, Klassen T, et al. Effects of task-specific locomotor and strength training in adults who were ambulatory after stroke: results of the STEPS randomized clinical trial. *Phys Ther.* 2007;87(12):1580-1602.

55. Mudie H, Winzcher-Mercay U, Radwan S, Lee L. Training symmetry of weight distribution after stroke: a randomized control pilot study comparing task-related reach, Bobath, and feedback training approaches. *Clin Rehabil.* 2002;16:582-592.

56. Chun C, Cheng P, Chen CL, et al. Effects of balance training on hemiplegic stroke patients. *Chang Gung Med J.* 2002;25:583-589.

57. Sunnerhagen KS, Brown B, Kasper CE. Sitting up and transferring to a chair: two functional tests for patient with a stroke. *J Rehabil Med.* 2003;35:180-183.

58. Dean CM, Shepherd RB. Task-related training improves performance of seated reaching tasks after stroke. *Stroke.* 1997; 28:722-728.

59. Langhammer B, Stanghelle JK. Bobath or motor relearning programme? A comparison of two different approaches of physiotherapy in stroke rehabilitation: a randomized controlled study. *Clin Rehabil.* 2000;14:361-369.

60. Hanlon RE. Motor learning following unilateral stroke. *Arch Phys Med Rehabil.* 1996;77:811-815.

61. Fritz SL, Light KE, Clifford SN, et al. Descriptive characteristics as potential predictors of outcomes following constraint-induced movement therapy for people after stroke. *Phys Ther.* 2006;86:825-832.

62. Fritz SL, George SZ, Wolf SL, Light KE. Participant perception of recovery as criterion to establish importance of improvement for constraint-induced movement therapy outcome measures: a preliminary study. *Phys Ther.* 2007;87:170-178.

63. Fritz SL, Pittman AL, Robinson AC, et al. An intense intervention for improving gait, balance, and mobility for individuals with chronic stroke: a pilot study. *Journal of Neurologic Physical Therapy.* 2007;31:71-76.

64. Taub E, Uswatte G, Elbert T. New treatments in neurorehabilitation founded on basic research. *Nat Rev Neurosci.* 2002;3:228-236.

65. Sunderland A, Tuke A. Neuroplasticity, learning and recovery after stroke: a critical evaluation of constraint-induced therapy. *Neuropsychological Rehabilitation.* 2005;15(2):81-96.

66. Wolf SL. Revisiting constraint-induced movement therapy: are we too smitten with the mitten? Is all nonuse "learned"? and other quandaries. *Phys Ther.* 2007;87:1212-1223.

67. Liepert J, Bauder H, Wolfgang HR, et al. Treatment-induced cortical reorganization after stroke in humans. *Stroke.* 2000;31:1210-1216.

68. Liepert J, Miltner WH, Bauder H, et al. Motor cortex plastic-

ity during constraint-induced movement therapy in stroke patients. *Neurosci Lett.* 1998;250:5-8.

69. Ro T, Noser E, Boake C, et al. Functional reorganization and recovery after contraint-induced movement therapy in subacute stroke: case reports. *Neurocase.* 2006;12:50-60.

70. Butler AJ, Wolf SL. Putting the brain on the map: use of transcranial magnetic stimulation to assess and induce cortical plasticity of upper-extremity movement. *Phys Ther.* 2007;87: 719-736.

71. Schaechter JD, Kraft E, Hilliard TS, et al. Motor recovery and cortical reorganization after constraint-induced movement therapy in stroke patients: a preliminary study. *Neurorehabil Neural Repair.* 2002;16:326-338.

72. Kim YH, Park JW, Ko MH, et al. Plastic changes of motor network after constraint-induced movement therapy. *Yonsei Med J.* 2004;45:241-246.

73. Dong Y, Dobkin BH, Cen SY, et al. Motor cortex activation during treatment may predict therapeutic gains in paretic hand function after stroke. *Stroke.* 2006;37:1552-1555.

74. Levy CE, Nichols DS, Schmalbrock PM, et al. Functional MRI evidence of cortical reorganization in upper-limb stroke hemiplegia treated with constraint-induced movement therapy. *Am J Phys Med Rehabil.* 2001;80:4-12.

75. Ostendorf CG, Wolf SL. Effect of forced use of the upper extremity of a hemiplegic patient on changes in function: a single-case design. *Phys Ther.* 1981;61:1022-1028.

76. Wolf SL, Lecraw DE, Barton LA, Jann BB. Forced use of hemiplegic upper extremities to reverse the effect of learned non-use among chronic stroke and head-injured patients. *Exp Neurol.* 1989;104:125-132.

77. Taub E, Uswatte G. Constraint-induced movement therapy: answers and questions after two decades of research. *NeuroRehabilitation.* 2006;21:93-95.

78. Page SJ, Sisto SA, Levine P, et al. Modified constraint induced therapy: a randomized feasibility and efficacy study. *J Rehabil Res Dev.* 2001;38:583-590.

79. Page SJ, Sisto SA, Levine P. Modified constraint-induced therapy in chronic stroke. *Am J Phys Med Rehabil.* 2002;81:870-875.

80. Richards L, Gonzalez Rothi LJ, Davis S, et al. Limited dose response to constraint-induced movement therapy in patients with chronic stroke. *Clin Rehabil.* 2006;20:1066-1074.

81. Fritz SL, Light KE, Patterson TS, et al. Active finger extension predicts outcomes after constraint-induced movement therapy for individuals with hemiparesis after stroke. *Stroke.* 2005;36: 1172-1177.

82. Underwood J, Clark PC, Blanton S, et al. Pain, fatigue, and intensity of practice in people with stroke who received constraint-induced movement therapy. *Phys Ther.* 2006;86: 1241-1250.

83. Wagner JM, Lang CE, Sahrmann SA, et al. Sensorimotor impairments and reaching performance in subjects with post-stroke hemiparesis during the first few months of recovery. *Phys Ther.* 2007;87:751-765.

84. Harris JE, Eng JJ. Paretic upper-limb strength best explains arm activity in people with stroke. *Phys Ther.* 2007;87:88-97.

85. Frick EM, Alberts JL. Combined use of repetitive task practice and an assisted robotic device in a patient with subacute stroke. *Phys Ther.* 2006;86:1378-1386.

86. Schmid A, Duncan PW, Studenski S, et al. Improvements in

speed-based gait classifications are meaningful. *Stroke.* 2007; 38:2096-2100.

87. Perry J, Garrett M, Gronley JK, Mulroy SJ. Classification of walking handicap in the stroke population. *Stroke.* 1995; 26:982-989.

88. Eng JJ, Chu KS, Dawson AS, et al. Functional walk test in individuals with stroke: relation to perceived exertion and myocardial exertion. *Stroke.* 2002;33:756-761.

89. Lord SE, Rochester L. Measurement of community ambulation after stroke: current status and future developments. *Stroke.* 2005;36:1457-1461.

90. Kollen B, Kwakkel G, Lindeman E. Time dependency of walking classification in stroke. *Phys Ther.* 2006;86:618-625.

91. Perry J. *Gait Analysis: Normal and Pathological Function.* Thorofare, NJ: SLACK Incorporated; 1992.

92. Kosak MC, Reding MJ. Comparison of partial body weight-supported treadmill gait training versus aggressive bracing assisted walking post stroke. *Neurorehabil Neural Repair.* 2000; 14:13-19.

93. Visintin M, Barbeau H, Korner-Bitensky N, et al. A new approach to retrain gait in stroke patients through body weight support and treadmill stimulation. *Stroke.* 1998;29:1122-1128.

94. Barbeau H, Visintin M. Optimal outcomes obtained with body-weight support combined with treadmill training in stroke subjects. *Arch Phys Med Rehabil.* 2003;84(10):1458-1465.

95. Hesse S, Werner C, von Frankenberg S, Bardeleben A. Treadmill training with partial body weight support after stroke. *Phys Med Rehabil Clin N Am.* 2003;14:S111-S123.

96. Hesse S, Bertelt C, Jahnke MT, et al. Treadmill training with partial body weight support compared with physiotherapy in nonambulatory hemiparetic patients. *Stroke.* 1995;26:976-981.

97. Chen G, Patten C. Treadmill training with harness support: selection of parameters for individuals with poststroke hemiplegia. *J Rehabil Res Dev.* 2006;43:485-498.

98. Hesse S, Uhlenbrock D, Werner C, et al. A mechanized gait trainer for restoring gait in non-ambulatory subjects. *Arch Phys Med Rehabil.* 2000;81:1158-1161.

99. Hesse S, Werner C, Uhlenbrock D, et al. An electomechanical gait trainer for restoration of gait in hemiparetic stroke patients: preliminary results. *Neurorehabil Neural Repair.* 2001; 13:157-165.

100. Husemann B, Muller F, Krewer C, et al. Effects of locomotion training with assistance of a robot-driven gait orthosis in hemiparetic patients after stroke: a randomized controlled pilot study. *Stroke.* 2007;38:349-354.

101. Patten C, Lexell J, Brown HE. Weakness and strength training in persons with poststroke hemiplegia: rationale, method, efficacy. *J Rehabil Res Dev.* 2004;41:293-312.

102. Dean CM, Richards CL, Malouin F. Walking speed over 10 metres overestimates locomotor capacity after stroke. *Clin Rehabil.* 2001;15:415-421.

103. Duncan P, Studenski S, Richards L, et al. Randomized clinical trial of therapeutic exercise in subacute stroke. *Stroke.* 2003; 34:2173-2180.

104. Andrews AW, Bohannon RW. Discharge function and length of stay for patients with stroke are predicted by lower extremity muscle force on admission to rehabilitation. *Neurorehabil*

Neural Repair. 2001;15:93-97.

105. Bohannon RW, Walsh S. Nature, reliability, and predictive value of muscle performance measures in patients with hemiparesis following stroke. *Arch Phys Med Rehabil.* 1992;73:721-725.

106. Rimmer JH, Riley B, Creviston T, Nicola T. Exercise training in predominantly African-American group of stroke survivors. *Med Sci Sports Exerc.* 2000;32:1990-1996.

107. Ouellette MM, LeBrasseur NK, Bean JF, et al. High-intensity resistance training improves muscle strength, self-reported function, and disability in long-term stroke survivors. *Stroke.* 2004;35:1404-1409.

108. Studenski S, Duncan PW, Perera S, et al. Daily functioning and quality of life in a randomized controlled trial of therapeutic exercise for subacute stroke survivors. *Stroke.* 2005;36: 1764-1770.

109. Dean CM, Richards CL, Malouin F. Task-related circuit training improves performance of locomotor tasks in chronic stroke: a randomized, controlled pilot trial. *Arch Phys Med Rehabil.* 2000;81:409-417.

110. Moreland JD, Goldsmith CH, Huijbregts MP, et al. Progressive resistance strengthening exercises after stroke: a single-blind randomized controlled trial. *Arch Phys Med Rehabil.* 2003;84:1433-1440.

111. Thielman GT, Dean CM, Gentile AM. Rehabilitation of reaching after stroke: task-related training versus progressive resistive exercise. *Arch Phys Med Rehabil.* 2004;85:1613-1618.

112. Nelson ME, Rejeski J, Blair SN, et al. Physical activity and public health in older adults. Recommendations from the American College of Sports Medicine and the American Heart Association. *Circulation.* 2007;116. Available at: http://cir. ahajournals.org. Accessed August 23, 2007.

113. Babyar SR, Krasilovsky G. Impaired muscle performance. In: Moffat M, Rosen E, Rusnak-Smith S, eds. *Musculoskeletal Essentials: Applying the Preferred Physical Therapist Practice Patterns.*[SM] Thorofare, NJ: SLACK Incorporated; 2006:55-98.

114. Laufer Y. The effect on walking aids on balance and weight-bearing patterns of patients with hemiparesis in various stance positions. *Phys Ther.* 2003;83:112-122.

115. Umphred D. *Neurological Rehabilitation.* 4th ed. St. Louis, MO: Mosby; 2001.

116. Cameron MH, Monroe LG. *Physical Rehabilitation: Evidenced Based Examination, Evaluation and Intervention.* St. Louis, MO: WB Saunders; 2007.

117. American Physical Therapy Association. Guide to physical therapist practice. 2nd ed. *Phys Ther.* 2001;81:9-744.

118. Teasdale G, Jennett B. Assessment of coma and impaired consciousness. *Lancet.* 1974;ii:81-83.

119. Herndon RM. *Handbook of Neurologic Rating Scales.* 2nd ed. New York, NY: Demos Med Pub; 2006.

120. Oatis C. *Kinesiology: The Mechanics and Pathomechanics of Human Movement.* Philadelphia, PA: Lippincott Williams & Wilkins; 2004.

121. USDA Center for Nutrition Policy and Promotion. Body mass index and health. *Nutrition Insight.* 2000; March. www. cnpp.usda.gov/Publications/NutritionInsights/Insight16.pdf. Accessed September 3, 2007.

122. Bohannon RW, Smith MB. Interrater reliability of a modified Ashworth scale of muscle spasticity. *Phys Ther.* 1987;67(2):206-

207.

123. Blackburn M, vanVliet P, Mockett SP. Reliability of measurements obtained with the modified Ashworth Scale in the lower extremities of people with stroke. *Phys Ther.* 2002;82:25-34.

124. Lewis C, McNerney PT. *The Functional Toolbox.* Washington, DC: Learn Publications; 1994.

125. Perlesz A, Kinsella G, Crowe S. Impact of traumatic brain injury on the family: a critical review. *Rehabilitation Psychology.* 1999;44(1):6-35.

126. Kolakowsky-Hayner, SA, Miner, KD, Kreutzer, JS. Long-term life quality and family needs after traumatic brain injury. *J Head Trauma Rehabil.* 2001;16(4):1-15.

127. Powell JM, Machamer JE, Temkin NR, Dikmen SS. Self-report of extent of recovery and barriers to recovery after traumatic brain injury: a longitudinal study. *Arch Phys Med Rehabil.* 2001;82:1025-1030.

128. Chan L, Doctor J, Temkin N, et al. Discharge disposition from acute care after traumatic brain injury: the effect of insurance type. *Arch Phys Med Rehabil.* 2001;82:1151-1154.

129. Whiteneck GG, Gerhart KA, Cusick CP. Identifying environmental factors that influence the outcomes of people with traumatic brain injury. *J Head Trauma Rehabil.* 2004;19:191-204.

130. Cifu DX, Kreutzer JS, Kolakowsky-Hayner MA, et al. The relationship between therapy intensity and rehabilitative outcomes after traumatic brain injury: a multicenter analysis. *Arch Phys Med Rehabil.* 2003;84:1441-1448.

131. Langlois JA, Rutland-Brown W, Thomas KE. *Traumatic Brain Injury in the United States: Emergency Department Visits, Hospitalizations, and Deaths.* Atlanta, GA: Centers for Disease Control and Prevention, National Center for Injury Prevention and Control; 2004.

132. Finkelstein E, Corso P, Miller T. *The Incidence and Economic Burden of Injuries in the United States.* New York, NY: Oxford University Press; 2006.

133. Johnstone B, Vessell R, Bounds T, et al. Predictors of success for state vocational rehabilitation clients with traumatic brain injury. *Arch Phys Med Rehabil.* 2003;84:161-167.

134. Bruno-Petrina A. *Posttraumatic heterotopic ossification.* Available at: http://www.emedicine.com/pmr/topic112.htm. Last updated: December 6, 2006. Accessed September 3, 2007.

135. Hurvitz EA, Mandac BR, Davidoff G, et al. Risk factors for heterotopic ossification in children and adolescents with severe traumatic brain injury. *Arch Phys Med Rehabil.* 1992;73(5): 459-462.

136. Davies PM. *Starting Again.* New York, NY: Springer-Verlag; 1994.

137. Bush BA, Novack TA, Malec JF, et al. Validation of a model for evaluating outcome after traumatic brain injury. *Arch Phys Med Rehabil.* 2003;84:1803-1807.

138. Gordon WA, Sliwinski M, Echo J, et al. The benefits of exercise in individuals with traumatic brain injury: a retrospective study. *J Head Trauma Rehabil.* 1998;13(4):58-67.

139. Huber FE, Wells CL. *Therapeutic Exercise: Treatment Planning for Progression.* St. Louis, MO: Saunders Elsevier; 2006.

140. Sullivan KJ, Klasses T, Mulroy S. Combined task-specific training and strengthening effects on locomotor recovery post-stroke: a case study. *Journal of Neurologic Physical Therapy.* 2006;30(3):130-141.

141. Seif-Naraghi AH, Herman RM. A novel method for locomotion training. *J Head Trauma Rehabil.* 1999;14(2):146-162.

142. Winstein C. Knowledge of results and motor learning: implications for physical therapy. In: *Movement Science, A Monograph of the American Physical Therapy Association.* Alexandria, VA: APTA; 1991.

143. Howle JM. *Neuro-Developmental Treatment Approach: Theoretical Foundations and Principles of Clinical Practice.* Laguna Beach, CA: NDTA; 2002.

144. Mudie H, Winzcher-Mercay U, Radwan S, Lee L. Training symmetry of weight distribution after stroke: a randomized control pilot study comparing task-related reach, Bobath, and feedback training approaches. *Clin Rehabil.* 2002;16:582-592.

145. Stergiou N, Harbourne RT, Cavanaugh JT. Optimal movement variability: a new theoretical perspetive for neurologic physical therapy. *Journal of Neurologic Physical Therapy.* 2006;30(3):120-129.

146. Schmidt RA, Lee TD. *Motor Control and Learning: A Behavioral Emphasis.* 3rd ed. Champaign, IL: Human Kinetics; 1999.

147. Shumway-Cook A, Woollacot, M. *Motor Control: Translating Research into Clinical Practice.* 3rd ed. Baltimore, MD: Lippincott Williams & Wilkins; 2007.

148. Goodgold-Edwards S. Principles for guiding action during motor learning. *Physical Therapy Practice.* 1993;2(4):30-39.

149. Mossberg KA, Ayala D, Baker T, et al. Aerobic capacity after traumatic brain injury: comparison with a nondisabled cohort. *Arch Phys Med Rehabil.* 2007;88(3):315-320.

150. Vitale AE, Jankowski LW, Sullivan SJ. Reliability for a walk/run test to estimate aerobic capacity in a brain-injured population. *Brain Inj.* 1997;11(1):67-76.

151. Jankowski LW, Sullivan SJ. Aerobic and neuromuscular training: effect on the capacity, efficiency, and fatigability of patients with traumatic brain injuries. *Arch Phys Med Rehabil.* 1990;71(7):500-504.

152. Canning CG, Shepherd RB, Carr JH, et al. A randomized controlled trial of the effects of intensive sit-to-stand training after recent traumatic brain injury on sit-to-stand performance. *Clin Rehabil.* 2003;17(4):355-362.

153. Ryerson S, Levit K. *Functional Movement Reeducation: A Contemporary Model for Stroke Rehabilitation.* New York, NY: Churchill Livingston; 1997.

154. Basford JR, Chou L, Kaufman KR, et al. An assessment of gait and balance deficits after traumatic brain injury. *Arch Phys Med Rehabil.* 2003;84:343-349.

155. Moseley AM, Stark A, Cameron ID, Pollock A. Treadmill training and body weight support for walking after stroke. *Cochrane Database Syst Rev.* 2003;(3):CD002840. DOI 10.1002/14651858.CD002840.

156. Brown TH, Mount J, Rouland BL, et al. Body weight-supported treadmill training versus conventional gait training for people with chronic traumatic brain injury. *J Head Trauma Rehabil.* 2005;20(5):402-415.

157. Ada L, Dean CM, Hall JM, et al. A treadmill and overground walking program improves walking in persons residing in the community after stroke: a placebo controlled randomized trial. *Arch Phys Med Rehabil.* 2003;84:1486-1491.

158. Moseley AM, Lanzarone S, Bosman JM, et al. Ecological validity of walking speed assessment after traumatic brain injury: a pilot study. *J Head Trauma Rehabil.* 2004;19(4):341-348.

159. Chard SE. Community neurorehabilitation: a synthesis of current evidence and future research directions. *Neuro Rx.* 2006; 3(4):525-534.

160. Kalb R. *Multiple Sclerosis: A Focus on Rehabilitation.* New York, NY: National Multiple Sclerosis Society; 2004.

161. Serio CD, Kreutzer JS, Gervasio AH. Predicting family needs after brain injury: implications for intervention. *J Head Trauma Rehabil.* 1995;10(2):32-45.

162. Costello E, Curtis CL, Sandel IB, Bassile CC. Exercise prescription for individuals with multiple sclerosis. *Neurology Report.* 1996;20:24-30.

163. Mulcare J. Multiple sclerosis. In: American College of Sports Medicine. *ACSM's Exercise Management for Person's with Chronic Disease and Disabilities.* Champaign, IL: Human Kinetics; 1997.

164. Smedal T, Lygren H, Myhr KM, et al. Balance and gait improved in patients with MS after physiotherapy based on the Bobath concept. *Physiother Res Int.* 2006;11(2):104-116.

165. Ford-Smith CD, VanSant AF. Age differences in movement patterns used in to rise from bed in subjects in the third through fifth decades of age. *Phys Ther.* 1988;68(2):185-192.

166. Black K, Zafonte R, Millis S, et al. Sitting balance following brain injury: does it predict outcome? *Brain Inj.* 2000; 14(2):141-152.

167. Rapport LJ, Hanks RA, Millis SR, Dehpande SA. Executive functioning and predictors of falls in the rehabilitation setting. *Arch Phys Med Rehabil.* 1998;79:629-633.

168. Ryan TV, Sautter SW, Capps CF, et al. Utilizing neuropsychological measures to predict vocational outcome in a head trauma population. *Brain Inj.* 1992;6(2):175-182.

169. Brain Injury Association of America. Available at: http://www.biausa.org/treatmentandrehab.htm#icu. Accessed September 8, 2007.

170. Mount J, Dacko S. Effects of dorsiflexor endurance exercises on foot drop secondary to multiple sclerosis: a pilot study. *NeuroRehabil.* 2006;21(1):43-50.

171. Lannin NA, Horsley SA, Hebert R, et al. Splinting the hand in the functional position after brain impairment: a randomized, controlled trial. *Arch Phys Med Rehabil.* 2003;84(2):297-302.

172. Carr JH, Shepherd RB. *Movement Science: Foundations for Physical Therapy in Rehabilitation.* 2nd ed. Gaithersburg, MD: Aspen Publishers; 2000.

173. Grasso MG, Troisi E, Rizzi F, et al. Prognostic factors in multidisciplinary rehabilitation treatment in multiple sclerosis: an outcome study. *Mult Scler.* 2005;11:719-724.

174. Underhill AT, LoBello SG, Fine PR. Reliability and validity of the family satisfaction scale with survivors of traumatic brain injury. *J Rehabil Res Dev.* 2004;41(4):603-610.

175. Herdman SJ. *Vestibular Rehabilitation.* Philadelphia, PA: FA Davis Co; 2000.

176. Solomon D. Distinguishing and treating causes of central vertigo. *Otolaryngol Clin North Am.* 2000;33:579-601.

177. Baloh RW. Differentiating between peripheral and central causes of vertigo. *Otolaryngol Head Neck Surg.* 1998;119(1):55-59.

178. Tinnetti ME. Performance oriented assessment of mobility problems in the elderly patients. *J Am Geriatr Soc.* 1986; 34:119-126.

179. Gordon NF, Gulsnick M, Fernando C, et al. Physical activity and exercise recommendations for stroke survivors: an American Heart Association scientific statement from the Council on Clinical Cardiology, Subcommittee on Exercise, Cardiac Rehabilitation, and Prevention; the Council on Cardiovascular Nursing; the Council on Nutrition, Physical Activity, and Metabolism; and Stroke Council. *Circulation.* 2004;109:2031-2041.

180. Furman JM, Whitney SL. Central causes of dizziness. *Phys Ther.* 2000;80(2):179-187.

181. Whitney SL, Metzinger RM. Efficacy of vestibular rehabilitation. *Otolaryngol Clin North Am.* 2000;33:659-672.

182. Gill-Body K. Current concepts in the management of patients with vestibular dysfunction. *PT-Magazine of Physical Therapy.* 2001;9:40-58.

183. Herdman SJ. Assessment and treatment of balance disorders in the vestibular-deficient patient. In: Duncan P, ed. *Balance: Proceedings of the APTA Forum.* Alexandria, VA: American Physical Therapy Association; 1990:87-94.

CHAPTER FIVE

Impaired Motor Function and Sensory Integrity Associated With Progressive Disorders of the Central Nervous System (Pattern E)

Rose Wichmann, PT

Janice B. Hulme, PT, MS, DHSc

ANATOMY

PARKINSON'S DISEASE

The basal ganglia, also known as the extrapyramidal system of the brain, are a group of gray matter structures deep within the cerebral hemispheres and ventral midbrain. The extrapyramidal system is comprised of the caudate nucleus and putamen (striatum), globus pallidus, subthalamic nucleus, substantia nigra, and intralaminar nuclei of the thalamus.[1] The basal ganglia serve a number of important roles in movement control, including maintenance of purposeful motor activity, suppression of unwanted movement, and assistance in monitoring posture, body support and skeletal muscle tone achieved through sustained contractions. These structures are also associated with a variety of other functions including learning, control of emotions, and cognition.[2]

MULTIPLE SCLEROSIS

The anatomy and physiology of the CNS are detailed in Pattern B: Impaired Neuromotor Development, Pattern C: Impaired Motor Function and Sensory Integrity Associated With Nonprogressive Disorders of the Central Nervous System—Congenital Origin or Acquired in Infancy or Childhood, and Pattern D: Impaired Motor Function and Sensory Integrity Associated With Nonprogressive Disorders of the Central Nervous System—Acquired in Adolescence or Adulthood.

Myelin Sheaths

White and gray matter of the brain and spinal cord are distinguished by the presence or absence of myelin sheaths wrapped around the axons.[3] The presence of myelin enables the normal impulse in the nerve cells to go between the brain and other parts of the body.[4,5] Myelin is formed by specialized supporting glial cells that are known as oligodendrocytes in the CNS and Schwann cells in the PNS.[6-8] These glial cells, which are composed of lipids and proteins, wrap the layers of their own plasma membrane tightly around the axonal membrane creating the myelin sheath.[8] This sheath insulates the axonal membrane, limits the amount of current that can leak from it, and thus increases the rate at which an action potential can be conducted.[8] The myelin sheath is interrupted at regular intervals leaving short lengths of exposed axonal membrane called the nodes of Ranvier.[8] It is at these nodes that the action potentials are generated.

Corticospinal Tracts

Two major groups of pathways, the lateral and ventromedial, are responsible for communication between the brain and the motor neurons of the spinal cord. The lateral pathways are involved in voluntary movement of the distal musculature, and the ventromedial pathways are involved in control of posture and locomotion.[9] The descending spinal tracts provide a mechanism for the brain to influence reflex pathways and afferent inputs to the spinal cord, regulate somatic motor activity, and manage some visceral activities.[10]

The corticospinal tract, or pyramidal tract, is the most clinically significant of the lateral descending pathways,[9,10] since it is the only direct pathway from the cortex to the spine and is the main pathway for control of voluntary movement.[11]

The corticospinal tract is composed of over one million fibers (700,000 are myelinated) and is the largest and most important descending tract.[12] About two thirds of the fibers originate in the motor cortex from neurons in the precentral gyrus (Brodmann area 4), premotor area (area 6), postcentral gyrus (areas 1, 2, 3, and 3b), and adjacent parietal cortex (area 5). Only a small part of the corticospinal tract fibers originate from the large pyramidal cortical neurons in each hemisphere (Brodmann area 4), but most of these are the large fibers.[12] Other fibers originate from the somatosensory areas of the parietal lobe pyramidal tract. A small number of fibers originate from the red nucleus of the midbrain forming the rubrospinal tract. Most of the fibers of the corticospinal tract cross over to the opposite side of the body as they descend through the brainstem and then continue to descend through the spine, terminating at the appropriate spinal levels.[11]

Optic Nerve

Unmyelinated optic nerve fibers emerge from the retinal ganglion cells, exiting through the back of the eye at the optic disc where they become myelinated and form the optic nerve.[7,9,13] The optic nerve from each eye proceeds medially and posteriorly, enters the cranial cavity through the optic foramen, and unites to form the optic chiasm.[7] The axons from the temporal side of the eye continue on the same side, while those on the nasal side of the eye cross. At this point the optic nerve becomes the optic tract.[13]

PHYSIOLOGY

PARKINSON'S DISEASE

The pertinent physiology for Parkinson's disease (PD) relates to the function of the substantia nigra, which contains approximately 400,000 nerve cells. Substantia nigra cells manufacture dopamine, a chemical neurotransmitter responsible for sending signals to the striatum. The dopamine that is released by the neurons from the substantia nigra has excitatory effects on D1 receptors and inhibitory effects on D2 receptors. Hence, both excitatory and inhibitory signals are received by the caudate, which innervates different areas of the putamen. Dopamine is transported and released onto receptors in the putamen, causing either excitatory or inhibitory currents within those cells.[2] These currents are the signals responsible for producing normal patterns of smooth and coordinated movement. The basal ganglia also receives input from the cerebral cortex, producing an information loop that functions in the selection and initiation of voluntary movements.[14]

MULTIPLE SCLEROSIS

The anatomy and physiology of the CNS are detailed in Pattern B: Impaired Neuromotor Development, Pattern C: Impaired Motor Function and Sensory Integrity Associated With Nonprogressive Disorders of the Central Nervous System—Congenital Origin or Acquired in Infancy or Childhood, and Pattern D: Impaired Motor Function and Sensory Integrity Associated With Nonprogressive Disorders of the Central Nervous System—Acquired in Adolescence or Adulthood.

In a myelinated axon, the nodes of Ranvier are the specific points at which an action potential can be elicited. If the entire surface of an axon were insulated by myelin, there would be no place for current to flow out of the axon for action potentials to be generated.[8] With the existence of the nodes, active excitation is restricted to small areas of the axonal plasma membrane. As a result, metabolic energy is conserved and action potentials travel faster.[8] Action potentials propagate from node to node along the myelinated axons through a process called saltatory conduction.[8] Because the myelin inhibits electrical charge leakage through the membrane and the cytoplasm of the axon is electrically conductive, there is sufficient depolarization at each node of Ranvier to bring the voltage at the next node to the threshold necessary to generate an action potential. As a result, action potentials in myelinated axons do not propagate as waves or a flow, but "jump" along the axon, traveling faster than they would otherwise.[15]

Action potential conduction is compromised by the loss of the myelin sheath surrounding many axons with resultant abnormal patterns of nerve conduction.[8]

MRI studies have shown the most common sites of optic nerve involvement in optic neuritis. There are five segments attributed to optic nerve involvement, including the anterior segment adjacent to the optic disc, the mid-intraorbital section, the intracanalicular portion, the intracranial prechiasmatic segment, and the chiasmatic segments. Occasionally more than one site is involved.[16]

PATHOPHYSIOLOGY

PARKINSON'S DISEASE

PD occurs when substantia nigra cells in the basal ganglia area of the midbrain degenerate at an accelerated rate, resulting in a chemical deficit of dopamine. It is estimated that approximately 60% to 80% of the substantia nigra cells of a patient with PD are depleted before the first clinical symptoms of the disease become evident. At autopsy, sectioning of the brain reveals decreased pigmentation of the substantia nigra. Histological changes also occur within the remaining substantia nigra neurons. Rounded pathological inclusions, called Lewy bodies, are frequently seen during post mortem microscopic evaluation of PD brain tissue.

Although PD is primarily a disease of the nigrostriatal pathway and not the entire extrapyramidal system, loss of dopaminergic neurons in the substantia nigra leads to dysregulation of the extrapyramidal system.[17] Since this system regulates posture and skeletal muscle tone, a result is the characteristic bradykinesia of PD. With the loss of dopamine-producing neurons, the globus pallidus becomes overactive, resulting in inhibition of the ventral lateral nucleus of the thalamus and consequently there is reduced excitation of the cortex. This leads to a condition called hypokinesia.[18]

The impact of exercise on the brain is still unclear. Recent studies in a rodent model of Parkinson's indicated that regular treadmill exercise in the first 10 days following chemically induced nigrostriatal damage in these animals ameliorated the neurochemical deficits and related motor symptoms.[19]

PD is classified as a movement disorder. The primary symptoms of PD include resting tremor, muscle rigidity, bradykinesia, and postural instability. A wide variety of secondary symptoms, including low voice volume, depression, seborrhea, micrographia, gait changes, constipation, and dysphagia, may also occur. It should be noted that each individual's course of Parkinson's symptoms and progression is unique and that all symptoms are not present in every patient.

The Hoehn and Yahr scale[20] is a commonly used system for describing how the symptoms of PD progress. The scale delineates stages from 0 to 5 that indicate the relative level of disability as follows:

◆ Stage 1: Symptoms on one side of the body only

◆ Stage 2: Symptoms on both sides of the body, no impairment of balance

◆ Stage 3: Balance impairment, mild to moderate disease, physically independent

◆ Stage 4: Severe disability, but still able to walk or stand unassisted

◆ Stage 5: Wheelchair bound or bedridden unless assisted

The Unified Parkinson's Disease Rating Scale[21] (UPDRS) is a rating scale used to follow the longitudinal course of PD. It is made up of six sections according to the following:

1. Mentation, behavior, and mood

2. ADL

3. Motor

4. Complications of therapy

5. Hoehn and Yahr stage

6. Schwab and England Activities of Daily Living Scale

These are evaluated by interview and clinical observation. Some sections require multiple grades assigned to each extremity. Clinicians and researchers use the UPDRS (and the motor section in particular) to follow the progression of a person's PD.

MULTIPLE SCLEROSIS

Multiple sclerosis (MS) is a chronic inflammatory process that damages the myelin insulating the axons[4,22] throughout the nervous system.[23] The disease is characterized by numerous plaques or lesions[3,24-26] that are most numerous in the white matter of the cerebrum, brainstem, cerebellum, and spinal cord[3,10] and in the optic nerves.[10,26] These lesions cause anatomical and tissue disruption that results in impaired neurotransmission[27,28] and that is responsible for the progression of the disease and the irreversible clinical disability.[5] The PNS is not affected.

The exact cause of MS is unknown at this time. However, many theories exist regarding its etiology, most commonly involving the immune system. There are two mechanisms by which the immune system attacks and destroys antigens: cellular immunity and humoral immunity. Cellular immunity involves a response by macrophages and T cells, while humoral immunity involves a response by B cells and antibodies. Evidence suggests that cellular immunity contributes to demyelinization.[29] In patients with MS, the immune response activates T lymphocyte and immunoglobulin production.[30] This production activates an antigen, which produces autoimmune cytoxic effects within the CNS. The blood-brain barrier fails allowing the myelin-sensitized T lymphocytes to enter and attack the myelin sheath that surrounds the nerve.[30]

In MS the effects of loss of myelination are dramatically demonstrated when myelin sheaths in some regions of the CNS are randomly destroyed. When this happens the propagation of nerve impulses is greatly slowed, often with a variety of serious neurological consequences.[8] The locations of the affected regions dictate the signs and symptoms of MS. Problems that are predominant are monocular blindness, motor weakness or paralysis, abnormal somatic sensations, double vision, and dizziness. These problems are due to lesions of the optic nerve, corticospinal tracts, somatic sensory pathways, medial longitudinal fasciculus, and vestibular pathways, respectively.[8]

The involvement of the corticospinal tracts produces an atypical upper motor neuron syndrome: spasticity, muscle weakness, hyperreflexia, and positive Babinski response. Commonly seen paresthesias, numbness, and loss of proprioception can be attributed to involvement of the spinal sensory tracts, especially in the posterior columns.[10] In many cases, the cerebellum and its connections with the brainstem are involved begetting nystagmus, dysarthria, ataxia, and considerable disability.

A bias exists for involvement of the optic nerve and its chiasms that creates an array of visual disturbances, including blurred vision and abnormal visual fields. The inflammation of the optic nerve is due to demyelination and can be idiopathic and isolated. Optic neuritis, the most common initial symptom of MS, occurs in 15% to 20% of cases. Between

38% and 50% of people with MS develop optic neuritis at some point during the course of their disease. The risk of developing MS within 5 years of an episode of isolated optic neuritis is reported to be 30%. MRI studies have shown five common sites that can be attributed to optic nerve involvement in optic neuritis seen in patients with MS. These segments are the anterior segment adjacent to the optic disc, the mid-intraorbital section, the intracanalicular portion, the intracranial prechiasmatic segment, and the chiasmatic segments. Occasionally more than one site is involved.[16] The most valuable predictor for the development of subsequent MS is the presence of abnormalities in the white matter.[16]

Urinary bladder dysfunction that results from disturbances of autonomic function may be present at the onset of the disease or may develop in the later stages. The development of these problems is frequently a major source of patient distress and social disability. Urgency, or frequency of urination, a spastic bladder with incontinence, and/or a spastic bowel causing severe constipation are seen most often. Sexual dysfunction, impaired cognition and memory, emotional changes, and depression are common neurobehavioral problems associated with MS.[10]

Correlation of anatomically established lesions with clinical symptomatology is not always possible.[10] The variability of anatomical locations, the number of plaques, and the time frame and sequence in which they occurred are factors in the presentation of clinical symptoms.[27] The most common symptoms are optic neuritis, visual disturbances, sensory abnormalities, pain, unsteady gait, weakness of one or more extremities, incoordination, tremor, speech impairment (dysarthria), swallowing problems (dysphagia), emotional changes, cognitive impairment, and bowel and/or bladder problems.[10,25-27] Fatigue is the most common complaint and usually occurs early and persists throughout the course of the disease.[10]

Risk Factors

Although a few factors associated with an increased probability of acquiring MS have been identified, generally it is not possible to foresee who will acquire the disease and what the course and severity will be. MS is the most common progressive neurological disease of young adults.[4,25] It affects people most often between the ages of 20 and 40 years and occurs three times more often in women than men.[25,31]

The distribution of this disease is not totally random. The incidence of MS has definitely been linked with latitude. MS has been found to be most prevalent in moderate climates, with the incidence increasing significantly for people living further from the warm climates near the equator.[10,25,26,31] Epidemiologic studies and migration patterns have shown that the risk of acquiring MS is associated with the risk level of one's home for the first 15 years suggesting that exposure to some environmental agent before puberty may play a part in the disease.[25,31]

Although MS is not contagious or hereditary, the risk of

acquiring MS is about 2% to 3% greater for children and siblings if a family member has MS. An identical twin of a person with MS has a 31% chance of also developing the disease.[25,32] Pregnancy does not influence the prognosis of the disease as was once thought. Extensive studies have shown that in pregnancy the relapse rate remains similar to that of the pre-pregnancy year. Women who do have greater disease activity in the year before pregnancy and during pregnancy have a higher risk of relapse in the first trimester following delivery.[33-36] Between 20% and 40% of pregnant women with MS do have a relapse in these months. However, there is no evidence that the overall course of the disease is affected, negatively or positively, by pregnancy or childbirth. Although MS poses no significant risks to the fetus, physical limitations can make child care more difficult and should be closely considered in family planning.[37]

Countless attempts have been made to identify viral, socioeconomic, trauma, dietary, and environmental factors that predict the onset of MS.[10] There is still consideration that an unidentified infectious agent (viral or bacterial) may be responsible.[26] The results of many studies for these and other factors have been contradictory and have not explicitly linked any of these factors to the onset of the disease.[10]

Categorizing the disease serves both as a tool for the development of clinical research and as a guide to treatment options. The classification system used to describe the disease patterns in MS was the result of an international survey done by Lublin and Reingold in 1991, who put forth the following four categories[10,25-27,38]:

1. Relapsing-remitting multiple sclerosis (RRMS)
2. Secondary progressive multiple sclerosis (SPMS)
3. Primary progressive multiple sclerosis (PPMS)
4. Progressive-relapsing multiple sclerosis (PRMS)

Since MS is a variable and unpredictable disease, a particular person with MS may not fit exactly into one of the categories.[26] Approximately 85% of people are diagnosed with RRMS. This course of the disease is characterized by clearly defined episodes of acute worsening of symptoms followed by recovery and a period without disease progression. After an exacerbation, recovery may be full or there may be some residual deficits. The degree of residual disability increases over time.[23,26,30,39]

An initial course of relapsing-remitting disease followed by progression at a variable rate with or without occasional relapses is associated with SPMS. Although this category may include occasional relapses and plateaus, the rate of progression of the disease is steady. Of the 85% of people who start with RRMS, more than 50% will develop SPMS within 10 years. Ninety percent will develop SPMS within 25 years.[25,26]

People with PPMS exhibit a steady progression of disability from onset without plateaus or remissions or with only occasional temporary minor improvements. Approximately

10% of the people with MS have PPMS.[23,30,39] The least common disease course, PRMS, is characterized by a progression from onset with acute relapses with or without recovery. However, between relapses there is progressive worsening of the disease. PRMS accounts for only 5% of the people who have MS[27] and is most commonly seen in people with an onset of MS after the age of 40.[30]

There is no single test to diagnose or rule out MS. A clinical diagnosis is made on the basis of medical history, a neurologic exam, and symptoms reported by the patient. A definitive diagnosis of MS requires all of the following conditions[25,26]:

♦ Evidence of plaques in two distinct areas of the CNS

♦ Evidence that the plaques occurred at discrete points in time

♦ No explanation other than MS for the plaques in the white matter of the CNS

The time between episodic events may range from months to years making the diagnostic process long and frustrating. The symptoms are variable and subjective, and often the symptomatology has been ignored by the person who has been exhibiting them.[26]

MS is treated primarily using three separate, but parallel, means: disease modification, symptomatic treatment, and rehabilitation. Disease-modifying agents treat the underlying disease to lessen the number of exacerbations and slow the progression of physical disability.[40] Symptom management targets the clinical manifestations of MS.[41] Rehabilitation is aimed at strategies to reduce impairments and promote functional mobility and independence.[30]

MEDICAL AND SURGICAL INTERVENTIONS

PARKINSON'S DISEASE

As PD progresses, medications become less efficacious, and patients tend to develop a number of side effects including motor fluctuations and involuntary movements called dyskinesia. For some patients with PD experiencing these complications, deep brain stimulation may be a treatment option. Electrodes are surgically implanted into specific areas of the brain. The wires from these electrodes are connected to a battery pack placed into the chest wall or abdomen, and electrical signals are delivered to the brain on a constant basis to stimulate the brain. Most surgical interventions are performed at the level of the thalamus, globus pallidus, and subthalamic nucleus, aiming at the disruption of the pathological activity. With this abnormal neuronal activity neutralized, normal movements can in many cases be restored.[42]

Deep brain stimulation has been proven to be effective in reducing such symptoms as tremor, slowness, and stiffness.

Deep brain stimulation is not a cure for PD and has not been found to be helpful for symptoms such as postural instability, freezing, or cognitive changes. Patients considering surgery must be closely evaluated prior to the procedure to determine if they are appropriate candidates, and then they usually require ongoing follow-up to achieve optimal programming of the implanted stimulator.

MULTIPLE SCLEROSIS

Fatigue, muscle weakness, and spasticity in the form of increased tone in the muscle or intermittent spasms can compromise ADL.[43] Before any treatment is considered, a thorough assessment of the impact of spasticity on function must be done. All decisions regarding the treatment plan must be specifically chosen for the individual.[44]

Medications are available to treat spasticity. Most of these medications, such as baclofen and diazepam, reduce spasticity through muscle relaxation. While these medications can be effective, side effects, including drowsiness or toxicity, can limit their value.[45]

When spasticity is not controlled effectively by oral medications, another option is to infuse baclofen, a muscle relaxant, through a pump surgically implanted near the spinal cord. Without additional surgery the pump can be refilled using a syringe. A baclofen pump generally provides relief from spasticity with fewer side effects, because the medication goes only into the spinal area. Infection and dislocation of the pump or the tubing can occur.[45]

When spasticity is severe and other methods of treatment have failed, surgical treatment is available.[46] Spasticity is sometimes alleviated by surgical release of the tendons of spastic muscles to help relieve pain and muscle contractions. The objective of this type of surgery is to eliminate the cause of the spasticity by interrupting the spinal reflex. The tendon of the spastic muscle may be cut or lengthened, or nerves innervating the spastic muscle may be severed. Surgery is invasive and surgical changes are often irreversible. Although it can be an effective way to treat spasticity, surgery should be considered only after carefully weighing the alternatives.[45,47]

IMAGING

PARKINSON'S DISEASE

It is not possible to visualize dopamine changes in the brain of a patient with PD through MRI. However, an MRI scan may be ordered during the diagnostic process in order to rule out other potential sources of reported neurological symptoms (eg, stroke, tumor).[48] Reduction of fluorodopa uptake within the striatum can be visualized through PET scans. PET scans are typically used in research only and are not currently used as part of the routine diagnostic process.[49]

MULTIPLE SCLEROSIS

♦ MRI has greatly assisted the process of diagnosis in MS, however, MRIs of the brain are abnormal in 95% of persons, thus they can only be used to confirm evidence of the disease[27]

   ● It is the most sensitive diagnostic tool for MS

   ● MRI is able to discriminate between active and inactive disease activity in more than 90% of patients based on the appearance and number of plaques[41]

   ● MRI uses the signal from hydrogen protons to form anatomic images, distinguishing the properties of that region from those of surrounding regions

♦ Magnetic resonance spectroscopy (MRS) is also used to confirm a diagnosis

   ● It makes routine direct clinical diagnosis that was previously unavailable by radiologic or clinical tests possible

   ● MRS complements MRI as a way to characterize tissue non-invasively

   ● MRS provides information about the chemistry of the involved region by determining the concentration of brain in the tissue examined

   ● The clinical application of MRS has been extensive in the evaluation of CNS disorders[50,51]

   ● It also has diagnostic value for the evaluation and monitoring of the progression of MS[6]

OTHER CLINICAL TESTS

MULTIPLE SCLEROSIS

♦ Visual evoked potentials

   ● Are used to confirm diagnosis and/or rule out other problems in MS by detecting pre- and post-chiasmal lesions and asymptomatic optic neuritis[2,26]

♦ Somatosensory evoked potentials

   ● Are used to identify clinically silent lesions in the sensory pathways, particularly through detection of plaques in the spinal cord[52]

♦ CSF analysis through lumbar puncture

   ● Is used as a diagnostic tool in MS to detect increased amounts of immunoglobulin or oligoclonal bands[41]

PHARMACOLOGY

PARKINSON'S DISEASE[53-55]

♦ First line pharmacological agents

   ● Levodopa (carbidopa/levodopa)

      ■ Examples: Sinemet, Stalevo, Parcopa

   ■ Actions

      ► When absorbed, levodopa crosses the blood-brain barrier and is converted into dopamine

      ► It is typically paired with carbidopa to minimize side effects of nausea and vomiting

      ► May be less effective when ingested with foods high in protein

      ► Available in several strengths and in both immediate and controlled release forms

         ○ Parcopa is an orally disintegrating tablet

         ○ Stalevo combines carbidopa/levodopa with the drug entacapone (see below)

   ■ Side effects: Nausea, dyskinesia, confusion, sleep disturbances, hallucinations, and OH

   ● Dopamine agonists

      ■ Examples: Apomorphine, bromocriptine, pramipexole, rotigotine, ropinirole

      ■ Actions

         ► Act directly on dopamine receptors in the brain and frequently given as first line treatment for younger or healthier patients in attempts to delay use of levodopa

      ■ Side effects: Nausea, sleep disturbances, hallucinations, confusion, OH, dyskinesia, and dizziness

      ■ Each dopamine agonist comes in a variety of tablet strengths

         ► Apomorphine is an injectable drug, usually prescribed as "rescue therapy" for patients experiencing sudden off periods

         ► Rotigotine is administered via a transdermal patch

♦ Adjunctive pharmacological agents

   ● Catecholamine-o-methyltranferase (COMT) inhibitors

      ■ Examples: Entacapone, tolcapone

      ■ Actions

         ► Block levodopa breakdown by the enzyme COMT, thus allowing more levodopa to enter the brain with each dose of medication, but is only effective when used in conjunction with levodopa

         ► Help to increase the duration of effect of each levodopa dose

         ► Available in individual tablets or in a combination form with carbidopa/levodopa (Stalevo)

      ■ Side effects

         ► Severe diarrhea, hallucinations, and urine discoloration

         ► Side effects can also occur due to increased dopamine activity when taking these medications, and levodopa dosages may need to be adjusted accordingly

- ▸ Tolcapone is more rarely used due to potential side effects of liver toxicity, and thus requires regular blood testing to monitor effects
- ● Amantadine (was originally developed as an antiviral medication for treatment of influenza)
  - ■ Actions
    - ▸ Mild symptomatic benefit as an anti-Parkinson medication
    - ▸ Often used to help control dyskinesia (involuntary movements experienced as a side effect of levodopa and dopamine agonists)
  - ■ Side effects: Ankle/foot edema, livedo reticularis (reddish blotching of skin on legs), anxiety, dizziness, urinary retention, and hallucinations
- ● Anticholinergics
  - ■ Examples: Benztropine mesylate, biperidin HCl, trihexyphenidyl HCl, procyclidine
  - ■ Actions
    - ▸ Block the chemical actions of Ach in the brain, thus creating a more "normalized" dopamine balance
    - ▸ Used to help control tremor and for other mild anti-Parkinson benefits
  - ■ Side effects: Dry mouth, confusion, blurred vision, constipation, urinary retention, sedation, and hallucinations, especially in the elderly population
- ● Monoamine oxidase B inhibitors
  - ■ Examples: Azilect, Eldepryl, selegiline, Zelapar
  - ■ Actions
    - ▸ Reduce totals of needed levodopa dosage in some patients
    - ▸ As adjunctive therapy for patients experiencing a decreased quality response to their dopaminergic medications
  - ■ Available in tablet form or orally disintegrating tablets (Zelapar)
  - ■ Shown in animal research to prevent dopamine brain cell degeneration produced by MPTP, a man-made toxic chemical, suggesting a possible neuroprotective effect[56]
  - ■ Side effects
    - ▸ Recommended twice daily dosage be taken in the morning and noon due to potential side effects of insomnia
    - ▸ Eldepryl should never be given with meperidine (Demerol) due to potential for serious or fatal drug interaction
- ◆ Contraindicated (dopamine-blocking) drugs in PD
  - ● Examples
    - ■ Neuroleptics used as anti-emetics, such as prochlorperazine or Reglan
    - ■ Neuroleptics used as sedatives, such as Haldol,

Melleril, Navane, and Thorazine
  - ■ Antihypertensive drug reserpine
  - ● Actions: Dopamine-blocking properties within the brain and can lead to the exacerbation of existing PD symptoms or the development of drug-induced Parkinsonism

MULTIPLE SCLEROSIS

Immunomodulatory and/or immunosuppressant drugs are usually the drugs of choice in MS therapy at this time. These drugs are not a cure for the disease, nor are they designed to make people feel better. They have been shown to slow the disease process and/or modify the course of the disease.[26] However, they have limited efficacy, so they are usually restricted to the early phases of the disease when inflammation is more predominant, rather than in the later phases when inflammation is less evident and neurological damage is considerable. Five drugs have been approved by the FDA at this time for treating MS.[25,26,57-59] When treatment has not been effective, other FDA-aproved treatments that are not specifically for MS are used to try to slow the progression of the disease. These include intravenous immunoglobulin (IVIg) therapy, methotrexate, azathioprine (Imuran), cyclophosphamide (Cytoxan), and cladribine (Leustatin).[26]

- ◆ Immunomodulators[25,26,57-65]
  - ● Example: Glatiramer acetate injection (Copaxone)
    - ■ Action: Reduces episodes of symptoms in patients with RRMS by stopping myelin damage
    - ■ Side effects: Pain, swelling, redness at injection site; weakness, flushing, back and neck pains, headache, weight gain, upset stomach; depression, confusion, nervousness
  - ● Example: Interferon beta-1a intramuscular injection (Avonex)
    - ■ Actions: Decreases the frequency of clinical exacerbations, slows the number of episodes, and decreases the progression of physical disability in patients with RRMS
    - ■ Side effects[26,59,60]: Lymphopenia, injection site reaction; flu-like symptoms following injection; dizziness, excessive tiredness; headache, pain, depression
  - ● Example: Interferon beta-1b injection (Betaseron)
    - ■ Action: Reduces the frequency of clinical exacerbations in patients with RRMS
    - ■ Side effects[59]: Injection site reactions (swelling, redness, discoloration, or pain), flu-like symptoms, depression
  - ● Example: Interferon beta-1a subcutaneous injection (Rebif)
    - ■ Actions: Prevents or lowers relapse rate, prolongs time to first relapse, reduces MRI lesion activity and area

- Side effects[59]: Flu-like symptoms following injection, injection site reaction, depression, liver problems, blood abnormalities

♦ Immunosuppressant[26,57,59]

- Example: Mitoxantrone IV infusion (Novantrone)[57]
  - Actions
    - ▶ Used in SPMS or PRMS or worsening RRMS,[26,59] but not indicated for PPMS
    - ▶ Suppresses the activity of T cells, B cells, and macrophages that are thought to lead the attack on the myelin sheath[57]
    - ▶ Reduces neurologic disability and/or frequency of clinical relapses
  - Side effects: Cardiotoxicity, nausea, hair loss, sterility, liver toxicity, changes in menstrual cycle, fever or chills, lower back or side pain, bladder infections, painful or difficult urination, swelling of feet and lower legs, cough or shortness of breath, sores in mouth and on lips, stomach pain, diarrhea, constipation, and black, tarry stools[57]
- Example: Tysabri (natalizumab)
  - Actions[59]
    - ▶ Hampers movement of potentially damaging immune cells from the bloodstream across the blood-brain barrier into the brain and spinal cord
    - ▶ Impedes the ascent of physical disability
    - ▶ Reduces the frequency of exacerbations in patients with relapsing types of MS
  - Side effects[59]: Headache, pain in arms or legs, joint pain, feeling tired, diarrhea, pain in the stomach area, depression, allergic reactions (hives, itching, trouble breathing, chest pain, dizziness, chills, rash, nausea, flushing of skin, low BP), pneumonia, urinary tract infection, gastroenteritis, vaginal infection, tooth infection, and other infections

Pharmacological agents used to treat the symptoms of MS include the following drugs[25,26,57-59]:

♦ Antispasticity drugs

- Examples: Baclofen (Lioresal), tizanidine (Zanaflex), diazepam (Valium), intrathecal baclofen pump, botulinum toxin injections into individual muscles
- Actions: Decrease the number and severity of muscle spasms, relieve pain, improve muscle movement
- Side effects: Seizures, difficulty breathing, fatigue, weakness, dizziness, confusion, upset stomach

♦ Antitremor drugs

- Examples: Propranolol (Inderal), clonazepam (Klonopin), primidone (Mysoline), isoniazid, buspirone (BuSpar), ondansetron (Zofran)
- Actions

  - Depress CNS and therefore slows down the nervous system
  - Enhance the activity of GABA, the major inhibitory neurotransmitter in the CNS
  - Used in MS primarily for the treatment of tremor, pain, and spasticity
- Side effects: Fatigue, dizziness, weakness, dry mouth, diarrhea, upset stomach, changes in appetite, restlessness, constipation, difficulty or frequent urinating, blurred vision, changes in sex drive or ability, seizures, shuffling walk, fever, difficulty breathing or swallowing, severe skin rash, yellowing of the skin or eyes, irregular heartbeat, and persistent, fine tremor or inability to sit still

Other pharmacological agents used for patient with MS may include any of the following drugs:

♦ Anti-anxiety

- Examples: Benzodiazepines, such as alprazolam (Xanax)
- Actions: Used to relieve nervousness and tension or improve sleep disturbances by decreasing abnormal brain excitation
- Side effects: Drowsiness, lightheadedness, fatigue, irritability, dry mouth, weight changes

♦ Anticholinergic agents[26]

- Examples: Oxybutynin (Ditropan), tolterodine (Detrol), hyoscyamine sulfate, propantheline bromide (Pro-Banthine)
- Actions: Antispasmodic agents used in bladder disorders of urgency, frequency, incontinence, and nocturia aimed at achieving scheduled voiding and avoidance of use of diuretics by decreasing muscle spasms of the bladder[26]
- Side effects: Constipation, decreased sweating, drowsiness, blurred vision, decreased flow of breast milk, decreased sexual ability, difficulty swallowing, headache, increased light sensitivity, nausea or vomiting, trouble sleeping, unusual tiredness or weakness, and dryness of mouth, nose, and throat[57]

♦ Antidepressants

- Example: Escitalopram (Lexapro)
- Actions: A selective serotonin reuptake inhibitor that increases the levels of brain serotonin to maintain mental balance
- Side effects: Nausea, diarrhea, constipation, drowsiness, dizziness, dry mouth

♦ Antifatigue agents

- Examples: Amantadine (Symmetrel), modafinil (Provigil), pemoline (Cylert), fluoxetine (Prozac)
- Actions: Reduce fatigue and lassitude, decrease depression, improve sleep
- Side effects: Anxiety, headache, nausea, nervousness,

trouble sleeping, decrease in appetite, diarrhea, dryness of mouth, flushing or redness of skin, muscle stiffness, stuffy or runny nose, tingling, vomiting, burning, trembling, and shaking

◆ Antivertigo agents[26]
  ● Examples: Meclizine (Antivert)
  ● Actions: Decreases symptoms of nausea, vomiting, and dizziness
  ● Side effects: Changes in mood, drowsiness, blurred vision, constipation, difficult or painful urination, dizziness, fast heartbeat, headache, loss of appetite, nervousness or restlessness, trouble sleeping, skin rash, upset stomach, and dryness of mouth, nose, and throat[57]

◆ Bronchodilators
  ● Examples: Albuterol, Proventil-HFA, Ventolin HFA
  ● Actions: Relax and open air passageways to make breathing easier
  ● Side effects: Nervousness, shaking, headache, nausea, cough

◆ Corticosteroids[26]
  ● Example: Clonzepam (Klonopin)
  ● Action: Decrease symptoms of optic neuritis, diplopia, and nystagmus
  ● Side effects: Changes in mood, fatigue

Case Study #1A: Stage 1 Parkinson's Disease

Mr. Anthony Barris is a 63-year-old male who has recently been diagnosed with Parkinson's disease.

PHYSICAL THERAPIST EXAMINATION

HISTORY

◆ General demographics: Mr. Barris is a 63-year-old white male whose primary language is English. He is a college graduate.

◆ Social history: He is married with one adult daughter who lives in another state.

◆ Employment/work: Mr. Barris works full time as a bank manager. His typical work schedule is 50 hours per week. His work duties consist of frequent client, staff, and community meetings; telephone calls; financial management; and computer work.

◆ Living environment: He lives in a two-level home in suburban Chicago. There are four stairs to enter his home. The floor surfaces are carpeted and hardwood. He has a large yard on lakeside property.

◆ General health status
  ● General health perception: Mr. Barris reports his current general health to be "good." He expresses fear of the unknown future, since he has been diagnosed with a chronic, progressive illness.
  ● Physical function: He has been noting tremor and stiffness in his left extremities, with additional stiffness in his neck and trunk noted when seated at his desk or playing golf.
  ● Psychological function: Mr. Barris describes high stress levels at work that are exacerbated by the fact that many of his clients and staff have not been informed of his diagnosis of PD.
  ● Role function: Husband, father, bank manager, participant in many local service organizations, treasurer of his church.
  ● Social function: Mr. Barris is socially active. He and his wife attend many church and community events, and they entertain and travel frequently. They enjoy attending theater, movies, and concerts. He volunteers at the local community theater and at his church two to three times a week.

◆ Social/health habits: He is a nonsmoker and drinks alcohol almost daily with a typical consumption of one to two cocktails a day.

◆ Family history: Both of his parents are deceased. There are no known family members with PD or related movement disorders.

◆ Medical/surgical history: Mr. Barris was diagnosed with PD 1 year ago, but reports noting first onset of symptoms approximately 8 months prior to that time. Previously he had a left patellar fracture at the age of 20 as a result of a sports injury, and he had an appendectomy at the age of 36.

◆ Prior hospitalizations: He has been hospitalized only once for his appendectomy at the age of 36 years.

◆ Preexisting medical and other health-related conditions: He has degenerative joint disease (DJD) of his left knee. There is no prior history of cardiovascular/pulmonary conditions, and he denies any shortness of breath.

◆ Current condition(s)/chief complaint(s): Since his recent diagnosis of PD, he has noted general stiffness in his neck and shoulders and difficulty turning his head when attempting to move his car in reverse. Mr. Barris reports balance imprecision when walking on the golf course and getting in and out of his boat. He states that his family and coworkers have recently commented on changes in his posture and slowing of his walking speed.

◆ Functional status and activity level: He ambulates without assistive devices and plays golf and tennis one or two times a week in warm weather months. He does yard work and enjoys fishing and boating.

◆ Medications: Pramipexole 0.75 mg tid, ibuprofen prn for control of left knee pain.

◆ Other clinical tests: The results of an MRI of his brain done 3 weeks ago were negative.

SYSTEMS REVIEW

◆ Cardiovascular/pulmonary
  ● BP
    ▪ Sitting: 130/68 mmHg
    ▪ Standing: 128/64 mmHg
  ● Edema: None noted
  ● HR: 72 bpm and regular
  ● RR: 16 bpm

◆ Integumentary
  ● Presence of scar formation: Well-healed incisional scar from appendectomy
  ● Skin color: WNL
  ● Skin integrity: WNL

◆ Musculoskeletal
  ● Gross range of motion: Limitations in left knee and neck rotation and hamstring tightness
  ● Gross strength: No functional deficit
  ● Gross symmetry
    ▪ Holds left shoulder lower than right in sitting and standing positions
    ▪ Increased forward head and thoracic kyphosis
  ● Height: 5'10" (1.78 m)
  ● Weight: 180 lbs (81.65 kg)

◆ Neuromuscular
  ● Balance
    ▪ Notes occasional left leg imprecision and tripping on uneven terrain, especially when carrying golf bag on golf course
    ▪ Denies freezing, retropulsion, festination, or falls
  ● Locomotion, transfers, and transitions
    ▪ Independent ambulation without assistive device
    ▪ Hypokinesia evident, resulting in reduced stride length and arm swing in left extremities
    ▪ Turns en bloc, with greater reduction in step size noted while turning
    ▪ Reports independent transfers from all surfaces, but notes he has increased difficulty with rolling in bed at night

◆ Communication, affect, cognition, language, and learning style
  ● Communication, affect, and cognition

    ▪ Mildly decreased voice volume and facial expression
    ▪ Appears pleasant, alert, and oriented with no cognitive deficits
  ● Learning style
    ▪ He has had many questions relating to his diagnosis of PD and has been seeking information through reading books and on the Internet
    ▪ He expresses an interest in speaking to others diagnosed with PD
    ▪ He prefers to have written material

TESTS AND MEASURES

◆ Aerobic capacity/endurance
  ● Is able to ambulate in community with no complaints or evidence of dyspnea or fatigue
  ● Tolerates leisure activities with no complaints or evidence of dyspnea or fatigue
  ● 6-Minute Walk Test (6MWT)=600 meters

◆ Environmental, home, and work barriers
  ● Four steps to enter house with sturdy hand rail and large landing on exterior
  ● Floors are hardwood, thresholds are flat for interior doorways, and half-inch thresholds for exterior doors and patio doors
  ● Area rugs have nonskid padding
  ● No bars are in the tub/shower, but the bottom of the tub has a nonskid surface

◆ Gait, locomotion, and balance
  ● Berg Balance Score (BBS)[66]: 52/56 (the BBS is a performance-oriented measure of balance in elderly individuals, consisting of 14 items scored on a scale of 0 to 4 with a maximum total score of 56)
    ▪ Sitting to standing: 4=able to stand without using hands and stabilize independently
    ▪ Standing unsupported: 4=able to stand safely for 2 minutes
    ▪ Sitting unsupported: 4=able to sit safely and securely 2 minutes
    ▪ Standing to sitting: 4=sits safely with minimal use of hands
    ▪ Transfers: 4=able to transfer safely with minor use of hands
    ▪ Standing unsupported with eyes closed: 4=able to stand 10 seconds safely
    ▪ Standing unsupported with feet together: 4=able to place feet together independently and stand 1 minute safely
    ▪ Reaching forward with outstretched arm: 4=can reach forward confidently 25 cm (10 in)
    ▪ Pick up object from floor: 4=able to pick up slip-

per safely and easily

- Turn to look behind/over left and right shoulders: 4=looks behind from both sides and weight shifts well
- Turn 360 degrees: 4=able to turn 360 degrees safely in 4 seconds or less
- Alternating steps on stool: 4=able to stand independently and complete eight steps in 20 seconds
- Standing unsupported, one foot in front: 2=able to take small step independently and hold 30 seconds
- Stand on one leg: 2=able to lift leg independently and hold more than 3 seconds
- Percent probability of falling based on BBS and fall history=7% (based on the equation developed by Shumway-Cook for calculating probability of falling based on the BBS and the number of falls a patient had taken within the past 6 months[67])

- Gait speed timed over a 10-meter course
  - Result: 0.98 meters/second (3.2 feet/second)
  - Comfortable gait speed for males between the ages of 60 to 69 years is 1.36 meters/second[68]
- Timed Up and Go[69-71]
  - Result: 10.1 seconds (the Timed Up and Go test measures the time in seconds taken by an individual wearing his or her regular footwear and using his or her regular assistive device if needed to stand up from a standard arm chair [approximate seat height of 46 cm and arm height 65 cm], walk a distance of 3 meters [9.84 feet], turn, walk back to the chair, and sit down again with no physical assistance provided)
  - Norms for 60- to 69-year-olds were shown to be 8.1 seconds (with a range of 7.1 to 9.0)[72,73]
- Gait analysis through observation revealed
  - Reduced stride length affecting foot clearance in LLE
  - Absent arm swing in LUE
  - Hypokinesia with reduced rotation of trunk or head noted when turning
  - Step size further reduced with attempts to turn
  - Forward trunk lean during stance and ambulation

◆ Motor function
- UPDRS[21] motor section scores
  - Speech: Grade 1=slight loss of expression, diction, and/or volume
  - Facial expression: Grade 2=slight but definitely abnormal diminution of facial expression
  - Tremor at rest
    ▸ RUE: Grade 0=absent
    ▸ RLE: Grade 0=absent
    ▸ LUE: Grade 2=mild in amplitude and persis-

tent or moderate in amplitude but only intermittently present
    ▸ LLE: Grade 1=slight and infrequently present
    ▸ Action or postural tremor of hands: Grade 0=absent
- Rigidity
  ▸ Judged on passive movement of major joints with patient relaxed in a sitting position, with cogwheeling ignored
  ▸ RUE: Grade 1=slight or detectable only when activated by mirror or other movements
  ▸ RLE: Grade 0=absent
  ▸ LUE: Grade 2=mild to moderate
  ▸ LLE: Grade 1=slight or detectable only when activated by mirror or other movements
- Finger taps
  ▸ Patient taps thumb with index finger in rapid succession with widest amplitude possible, each hand separately
  ▸ Results: Grade 1=mild slowing and/or reduction in amplitude (11 to 14/5 seconds)
- Hand movements
  ▸ Patient opens and closes hands in rapid succession with widest amplitude possible, each hand separately
    ○ RUE: Grade 1=mild slowing and/or reduction in amplitude
    ○ LUE: Grade 1=mild slowing and/or reduction in amplitude
- Rapid alternating movements of hands (pronation and supination movements of hands vertically or horizontally, with as large an amplitude as possible, both hands simultaneously
  ▸ Result: Grade 2=moderately impaired with definite and early fatiguing and with occasional arrests of movement
- Leg agility
  ▸ Patient taps heel on ground in rapid succession with knee bent and picking up entire leg—amplitude should be about 3 inches
    ○ RLE: Grade 1=mild slowing and/or reduction in amplitude
    ○ LLE: Grade 2=moderately impaired with definite and early fatiguing and with occasional arrests of movement
- Arising from chair
  ▸ Patient attempts to arise from a straight back wood or metal chair with arms folded across chest
  ▸ Result: Grade 0=normal
- Posture
  ▸ Result: Grade 1=not quite erect, slightly

stooped posture
  ▸ Could be normal for an older person
- Gait
  ▸ Result: Grade 1=walks slowly, may shuffle with short steps, but no festination or propulsion
- Postural stability
  ▸ Response to sudden posterior displacement produced by pull on shoulders while patient is erect with eyes open and feet slightly apart (Note: Patient is prepared)
  ▸ Result: Grade 0=normal
- Body bradykinesia and hypokinesia
  ▸ Combines slowness, hesitancy, decreased arm swing, small amplitude, and poverty of movement in general
  ▸ Result: Grade 2=mild degree of slowness and poverty of movement which is definitely abnormal or some reduced amplitude
- Observation of patient performance of bed mobility/rolling
  - Exhibits limited rotation of trunk during this task with lack of dissociation between head, upper trunk, and lower trunk
- Sleeps on two or three pillows at night
- Performs independent transfers from all surfaces including hard and soft chairs, chairs with and without arms, tub without rail, in and out of car, and up from ground

◆ Muscle performance
- Five Times Sit to Stand test
  - Patient is asked to perform sitting to standing five times consecutively with arms folded across chest
  - Score of >15 seconds for older adults considered abnormal and is indicative of LE weakness[74,75]
  - Result: 11 seconds
- MMT revealed grades of 5/5 in all extremities

◆ Pain
- NPS[76,77] (0= no pain and 10=worst possible pain)
  - Pain of 3/10 on the NPS in the left knee with stair climbing, kneeling, or prolonged walking
  - Downie and associates[76] described a high degree of agreement between the visual analog scale (VAS), NPS, and the simple descriptive scale (SDS) although they reported that the NPS performed better; Jensen et al found the NPS to be the most practical tool[77]

◆ Posture
- Photographic assessment of sitting and standing postures revealed
  - Significant forward head and increased thoracic kyphosis

- Reduced lumbar curve in sitting and standing

◆ Range of motion
- Active neck rotation exhibits mild limitations at end ranges: Lacks 5 degrees of left rotation and 10 degrees of right rotation
- Mild changes noted in trunk flexibility at end ranges of rotation bilaterally
- Lacks 15 degrees of terminal extension in left knee with significant joint crepitus noted
- Lacks 5 degrees of terminal extension in right knee
- Hamstring tightness noted in both left and right knees

◆ Self-care and home management
- Mr. Barris reports no difficulty with dressing, toileting, or other self-care or home management skills other than turning in bed

◆ Ventilation and respiration/gas exchange
- Denies episodes of dyspnea, chest pain, or excessive fatigue

◆ Work, community, and leisure integration or reintegration
- Observation of patient work environment
  - Uses low desk chair with poor lumbar support
  - Frequently sits with telephone cradled between neck and shoulder
- Able to carry out all activities related to work, community, and leisure at this time with slight balance imprecision when walking on the golf course and getting in and out of his boat
- Concerned about emergence of tremor and other visible Parkinson's symptoms during work-related activities
- Reports noting changes in walking speed during community ambulation

EVALUATION

Mr. Barris' history and risk factors previously outlined indicated the he is a 63-year-old male with a medical diagnosis of Stage 1 PD based on the Hoehn and Yahr rating scale.[20] Results of his physical therapist examination on this date revealed him to demonstrate impairments in postural alignment, gait, muscle rigidity/stiffness, and bed mobility relating to this diagnosis. The patient also experiences left knee pain as the apparent result of DJD. Mr. Barris reported significant amounts of stress in his daily life. He expressed limited knowledge of PD and would like more information.

DIAGNOSIS

Mr. Barris is a patient with a diagnosis of PD and has pain in his left knee. He has impaired: gait, locomotion, and balance; motor function; muscle performance; posture; and range of motion. He is minimally functionally limited in work, community, and leisure actions, tasks, and activities. Both he and his wife exhibit knowledge deficits related to PD. These findings are consistent with placement in Pattern E: Impaired Motor Function and Sensory Integrity Associated With Progressive Disorders of the Central Nervous System. The identified impairments will be addressed in determining the prognosis and the plan of care.

PROGNOSIS AND PLAN OF CARE

Over the course of the visits, the following mutually established outcomes have been determined:

♦ Ability to move in bed is improved

♦ Gait is improved

♦ Motor function is improved

♦ Pain is decreased

♦ Patient and wife have knowledge regarding PD and the impact of associated impairments of functional tasks and activities

♦ Posture is improved

♦ ROM is improved

To achieve these outcomes, the appropriate interventions for this patient are determined. These will include: coordination, communication, and documentation; patient/client-related instruction; therapeutic exercise; functional training in self-care and home management; and functional training in work, community, and leisure integration and reintegration.

The *Guide* takes into consideration that patients placed in this pattern have progressive conditions that may have ongoing impairments, functional limitations, and disabilities. The result of this is that the stated prognosis for this pattern is to have optimal function within a variety of settings "within the context of the impairments, functional limitations, and disabilities."[78] Mr. Barris is expected to require eight visits over 4 weeks. Mr. Barris has good social support, is motivated, and will follow through with his home exercise program. He is not severely impaired and is healthy.

INTERVENTIONS

RATIONALE FOR SELECTED INTERVENTIONS

Numerous studies have indicated the efficacy of physical therapy treatment in the management of patients with PD.[79,80] A multidimensional exercise routine has been shown to be most effective at addressing deficits in balance, mobility, and fall risk.[81] Exercise programs for those with PD should include stretching activities due to the primary symptom of muscle rigidity and its accompanying potential for flexibility loss. Inclusion of exercises promoting spinal flexibility appears to be particularly needed in the early stages of PD.[82] Movement enhancement strategies with attention to making motions more mindful and complete can further enhance exercise performance.[83] Patients should also receive cueing and instruction in exercises focusing on amplitude-based large scale movements that have been shown to result in improved speed-amplitude scaling relation across both UEs and LEs.[84]

It appears that bradykinetic movement combined with muscle rigidity may contribute to the patient's perceptions of lessened muscle strength. No significant strength deficits were found between individuals with PD and normal subjects, with the exception of abdominal strength.[85] This seems to suggest a need for particular attention to strengthening core muscles of stability when designing the exercise program.

Regular conditioning exercises are incorporated in a comprehensive routine to maintain activity tolerance and cardiovascular fitness. It has been found that individuals with PD benefit from aerobic exercise just as much as those without PD.[86] A variety of conditioning exercise activities or fitness equipment can be used depending on availability and patient preferences. Upper body supported treadmill training has been shown to allow ambulation at increased rate and for longer distances. Some studies have suggested that treadmill training may produce greater improvements than conventional physical therapy approaches, with improvements in stride length and gait speed maintained up to 4 months after conclusion of treatment.[87,88] Mood and subjective reports of well-being also were shown to improve in individuals with PD through participation in sports activities in the early to medium stages of the disease.[89]

Developing self-awareness of posture and gait is often advantageous to individuals with early to mid-stage PD. Performing frequent "posture checks" throughout the day promotes postural awareness and good alignment.[90] Use of lumbar and/or cervical pillows helps to improve sitting and sleeping postures. Exercises promoting trunk strength, axial extension, pelvic mobility, and back/abdominal strength also are helpful in posture training.[91,92] Instruction in self-monitoring skills and attentional strategies have been found to be helpful in minimizing hypokinesia and regulating stride length, especially during complex movement sequences and situations that provide balance challenges.[93,94]

COORDINATION, COMMUNICATION, AND DOCUMENTATION

Communication will occur with the patient, his wife, and his physician during the course of treatment. Mr. Barris will be introduced to the benefits of a comprehensive interdisciplinary team, and he will be provided with resources on how to access appropriate team members as needs are identified. Appropriate referrals will be made, including referral to a speech pathologist to assess reduced voice volume and to a social worker to discuss patient/spouse questions relating to support groups and educational resources in the community. He will be provided with appropriate information on exercise groups, stress management classes, and complementary therapy providers. Interdisciplinary teamwork will occur through information exchange at team rounds. All elements of the patient's management will be documented.

PATIENT/CLIENT-RELATED INSTRUCTION

Education regarding his current condition, impairments, and functional limitations will be discussed. In addition, instruction will be provided in the following areas:

♦ Education and training for Mr. Barris and his wife relating to his current condition (impairments, functional limitations, and disabilities)

♦ Enhancement of performance through compensatory movement and attentional strategies to improve bed mobility/rolling

♦ Enhancement of performance through compensatory strategies for ambulation and balance safety during ADL and work, community, and leisure actions, tasks, and activities

♦ Risk factors regarding primary symptoms of PD and their potential impact on physical mobility

Maintenance of a regular exercise program must be instilled in this patient. These tips may be included in part of the patient-related instruction and may include any or all of the following:

♦ Add exercise to one's daily schedule (walk during lunch break at work, do stretches while seated at desk)

♦ Aerobic and endurance conditioning (walking or swimming) for follow through of home exercise program several times per week

♦ Find activities that may be done after work (walking or swimming)

♦ Flexibility exercises/stretching with emphasis on neck, anterior chest, trunk, and hamstring musculature

♦ Gait training with emphasis on self-cueing strategies and compensation techniques to be used on uneven terrain

♦ If a scheduled exercise time is missed, work into schedule at another time during the day or week

♦ Relaxation/stress management techniques including deep breathing and performance of Tai Chi[95]

♦ Strengthening training/exercise with emphasis on core muscles

A long-range health and wellness program must also be part of the instruction given to Mr. Barris. Instruction in

his home exercise program will be provided so that he may independently follow through with the program.

THERAPEUTIC EXERCISE

♦ Aerobic capacity/endurance conditioning
  - Treadmill training
    - Upper body supported treadmill training allows patients with PD opportunities to ambulate at increased rate and for longer distances
    - Research studies have used a protocol of 45-minute training sessions three times a week for 4 weeks with resultant improvements in gait speed and stride length[87,88]
  - At conclusion of the treatment program, patient will progress to a home exercise program of community ambulation, with emphasis on attentional strategies and auditory cueing to minimize hypokinesia

♦ Balance, coordination, and agility training
  - Amplitude-based exercises
    - Place concentrated emphasis on "moving big" during exercise and activities to improve relations between speed and amplitude scaling
    - Practice walking on a variety of surfaces, focusing on self-cueing strategies to maintain large steps with adequate foot clearance
  - Provide instruction in balance safety strategies for use when reaching overhead, carrying objects, or performing other multitasking activities
  - Introduce options for complementary exercise programs, including Tai Chi, for emphasis on weight shift and balance training

♦ Body mechanics and postural stabilization
  - Body mechanics training
    - Appropriate sitting posture for work and leisure actions, tasks, and activities
    - Appropriate use of body mechanics while working at the computer and answering telephone calls
    - Appropriate lifting and carrying instructions
    - Appropriate bending instructions
  - Postural control training
    - Instruct in proper alignment of head, cervical and thoracic spines, and shoulders
    - Axial extension through prone on elbows and press-ups
    - Chin tucks
    - Hip rocks and hip clocks
    - "Mad cat" stretch (on all fours and round back up)
    - Scapula retraction and depression
    - Chicken wing position (hands behind head, horizontal abduction of shoulders)
    - Corner stretch

- Transition of positions from supine to sitting, standing, and walking
- Weight shifting drills and activities
  - Postural stabilization activities
    - Bridging
    - Unilateral bridging
    - Arm raises unilateral and then bilateral in prone progressing to quadruped and then over the exercise ball
    - Leg raises over the exercise ball
    - Alternate opposite arm and leg
    - Challenge patient out of center of gravity/base of support
  - Postural awareness training
    - Use of mirror for visual input of appropriate alignment
    - Increase awareness through instruction in frequent "posture checks" throughout the day
    - Use of visual reminders or notes in strategic locations around home, car, and office
- Flexibility exercises
  - Stretching exercises should be done after warming up, using a slow and steady stretch accompanied by deep breathing, and building hold up to 30 to 60 seconds
  - Cervical ROM in all directions
  - Shoulder ROM in all directions
  - Scapula ROM in all directions including diagonals
  - Anterior chest wall stretching
  - Trunk rotation through hip rolls with arms moving in opposite direction
  - Thoracic extension
  - Focused attention on amplitude of movement during exercise
  - Aquatic exercises for flexibility
  - Complementary exercise programs, including Tai Chi and yoga for flexibility
- Gait and locomotion training
  - Attentional strategies
  - Compensate for hypokinesia or reduced step size through self-awareness and auditory cueing
- Relaxation
  - Instruct in deep breathing for relaxation with emphasis on diaphragmatic breathing
  - Introduce appropriate relaxation techniques, including guided imagery and/or progressive relaxation
  - Provide information on complementary programs, such as music therapy, massage therapy, spiritual care, involvement in hobbies and the creative arts
- Strength, power, and endurance training
  - Active exercise, including repeated sit to stand from varying chair heights, core strengthening exercises for

trunk and abdominal muscles, bilateral and unilateral toe raises for calf strengthening, and step up/step down stair climbing
- Resistive exercise, including use of elastic band for UE diagonals and scapular retraction exercises, progressing home program to include use of free weights for UE and LE strengthening two to three times per week
- Aquatic exercises provide options for UE and LE strengthening exercises that reduce excessive joint stress on left knee, allow variability in exercise program, and enhance maintainance of interest in home program
- Complementary exercise programs, including Tai Chi and yoga for core and extremity strengthening activities

FUNCTIONAL TRAINING IN SELF-CARE AND HOME MANAGEMENT

- Self-care and home management
  - ADL training (bed mobility)
    - Instruct in attentional strategies, that is, breaking the movement sequence into a series of steps, providing focused attention on each movement, and incorporating mental rehearsal of movement prior to performing task
    - Emphasize focusing on large amplitude movements throughout the movement sequence
    - Offer practical strategies, such as use of satin-based drawsheet or pajamas to help movements when rolling in bed and/or use of a lightweight comforter/duvet to reduce constriction during bed motion
    - Use of cervical pillow when sleeping

FUNCTIONAL TRAINING IN WORK, COMMUNITY, AND LEISURE INTEGRATION OR REINTEGRATION

- Work
  - Devices and equipment use and training
    - Readjust work chair
    - Establish system and routine for regular "posture checks" at work incorporating chin tucks, shoulder shrugs, scapular retractions, standing trunk extension, and wall push-ups into "mini stretch breaks" throughout the day
    - Use of lumbar pillow when sitting in desk chair
    - Use of telephone headset at work
  - Functional training program for work activities
    - Simulated work tasks, including use of telephone and computer while sitting at work station

- Leisure
  - Instruction in balance safety related to yardwork (reaching, carrying items, stooping, etc)
  - Instruction in balance safety strategies on golf course and use of cart for golf clubs
  - Balance safety when climbing in and out of his boat

ANTICIPATED GOALS AND EXPECTED OUTCOMES

- Impact on impairments
  - Patient accurately demonstrates awareness of good postural alignment and body mechanics and of methods of self-correction for incorporation during home and work activities.
  - Patient correctly demonstrates self-cueing strategies performed during ambulation on flat and uneven terrain.
  - Patient demonstrates home exercise program correctly.
  - Patient exhibits full cervical/trunk ROM in all planes.
  - Patient tolerates 8 hours of work activities with reported decrease in episodes of neck and trunk stiffness during workday.
- Impact on functional limitations
  - Patient demonstrates improved ease in bed mobility and rolling through use of attentional strategies and adaptation of bed linens and nightwear.
- Impact on disabilities
  - Patient continues to tolerate regular performance levels of self-care, home chores, work schedule, yard work, golfing, boating, and community service and volunteer activities.
- Risk reduction/prevention
  - Patient accurately identifies challenging balance tasks and uses safety strategies to reduce falls risk.
  - Patient accurately verbalizes understanding of PD impact on mobility, along with strategies for risk reduction/prevention of potential mobility changes through regular exercise and activity.
- Impact on health, wellness, and fitness
  - Patient identifies appropriate behaviors that foster healthy habits, wellness, and prevention.
  - Patient incorporates relaxation strategies into daily routine.
- Impact on societal resources
  - Decision making is enhanced regarding patient health and the use of health care resources by patient, family, significant others, and caregivers.
  - Documentation occurs throughout patient management and follows APTA's *Guidelines for Physical Therapy Documentation.*[78]
- Patient/client satisfaction
  - Access, availability, and services provided are acceptable to patient.
  - Care is coordinated with patient, family, and other health care professionals.
  - Patient and family knowledge and awareness of the diagnosis, prognosis, interventions, and anticipated goals and expected outcomes are increased.
  - Referrals are made to other professionals or resources whenever necessary and appropriate.

REEXAMINATION

Reexamination is performed throughout the episode of care. It is anticipated that patients placed in this pattern will require multiple episodes of care over the lifetime. Periodic reexamination and initiation of new episodes of care should occur as the patient's functional limitations or disability changes.

DISCHARGE

Mr. Barris is discharged from this episode of care after a total of six physical therapy visits over 4 weeks and attainment of his goals. As Mr. Barris has a condition that may require multiple episodes of care throughout his life span, Mr. Barris and his wife received education regarding factors that may trigger a call to his physical therapist for a reexamination and new episode of physical therapy intervention.

Case Study #1B: Stage 3 Parkinson's Disease

Mr. Barris is now a 67-year-old male who has been referred to home physical therapy for a new episode of care due to generalized weakness and low endurance post hospitalization for bowel obstruction surgery 5 days ago.

PHYSICAL THERAPIST EXAMINATION

Note: Only changes from his first episode are included in this case.

HISTORY

- General demographics: Mr. Barris is now a 67-year-old male.
- Employment/work: He retired from full-time employ-

ment as a bank manager 1 year ago.

◆ General health status
  • General health perception: Mr. Barris recognizes the physical changes that have occurred since his hospitalization.
  • Physical function: He also notes weakness and gait/balance changes since the recent surgery. He has noted occasional difficulty initiating motion when starting to walk and is concerned with episodic dizziness during transitional movements.
  • Psychological function: Mr. Barris is motivated to return to pre-surgery level of function.
  • Social function: He is currently sedentary due to low endurance post hospitalization.

◆ Medical/surgical history: His PD was diagnosed 4 years ago. Mr. Barris had a bowel obstruction requiring surgery 5 days ago. He was discharged from hospital 2 days ago to his home.

◆ Current condition(s)/chief complaint(s): He has generalized weakness and low endurance post hospitalization and reports fatigue and shortness of breath with mild exertion since the hospitalization. He was discharged to home with support from his wife and home health services. Mr. Barris previously received physical therapy services for assessment and management of PD and for periodic updating of his home program. He has been participating in a Parkinson's clinic program.

◆ Functional status and activity level: He has not participated in community ambulation or leisure activities since his surgery. Normally he plays golf one or two times a week in warm weather months, and he had one fall on the golf course 3 months ago without injury. He also attends movies, concerts, or the theater one or two times a week and travels frequently with his wife. He stopped playing tennis 1 year ago after experiencing difficulty with his serve and problems performing quick stops and starts on the tennis court. Typically he had been performing his home exercise program of stretching, strengthening, and conditioning exercises three to four times per week, but he stopped approximately 1 month prior to this hospitalization. The patient has also begun to experience the onset of motor fluctuations with decreased motor ability occurring as he nears the end of each carbidopa/levodopa dose.

◆ Medications: Carbidopa/levodopa, pramipexole, Celebrex, Miralax.

SYSTEMS REVIEW

◆ Cardiovascular/pulmonary
  • BP
    ▪ Sitting: 122/64 mmHg
    ▪ Standing: 100/52 mmHg

◆ Integumentary
  • Presence of scar formation: Healing abdominal surgical incision from bowel surgery
  • Skin color: Good, mild redness around incision
  • Skin integrity
    ▪ Seborrhea noted on nose, ears, and at hairline
    ▪ Small healing abrasion on left elbow

◆ Musculoskeletal
  • Gross range of motion
    ▪ Decreased neck and spinal flexibility
    ▪ Hamstring and heel cord tightness noted bilaterally
  • Gross strength: Generalized weakness
  • Gross symmetry: When standing reduced lumbar lordosis and hip/knee flexion
  • Weight: 173 lbs (78.47 kg)

◆ Neuromuscular
  • Balance
    ▪ Balance imprecision noted when ambulating to bathroom or kitchen since hospitalization
    ▪ Has noted several episodes of start hesitation, reporting one fall since arriving home from hospital (lost balance when turning in bathroom resulting in a small healing abrasion on left elbow and no other injury)
    ▪ Reports lightheadedness upon rising from bed, toilet, and chair
  • Locomotion, transfers, and transitions
    ▪ He still ambulates without assistive devices, but he tends to reach out for objects in walking path for added stability
    ▪ Hypokinesia is more prominent with reduction noted bilaterally in stride length and arm swing
    ▪ Occasional start hesitation is evident
    ▪ He requires arm rest support upon rising from the chair and notes difficulty with reduced step size as he approaches the chair to sit down that affects proper body alignment as he moves from standing to sitting

◆ Communication, affect, cognition, language, and learning style
  • Communication, affect, and cognition: His voice volume is decreased with mild facial masking
  • Learning style: He is motivated, asks many questions, and has been using his home written program with diagrams from previous episode of care

TESTS AND MEASURES

◆ Aerobic capacity/endurance

- 6MWT measures the distance that a patient can walk on a flat, hard surface in a period of 6 minutes
  - Mean scores for males age 60 to 69 for this test was found to be 497.7 meters[96-98]
  - Result: 282 meters
- He currently notes shortness of breath after household ambulation of greater than 2 minutes

◆ Assistive and adaptive devices
  - Trial use of a single-end cane produced increased stability when walking
  - Needs side rail on bed to assist with coming to sitting

◆ Circulation
  - OH observed
    - Sitting BP: 122/64 mmHg
    - Standing BP: 100/52 mmHg
  - Patient describes "lightheadedness" upon rising, but denies visual disturbance or "blackout"
  - Patient reports lightheadedness is worse upon rising in the morning and after meals

◆ Ergonomics and body mechanics
  - Body mechanics
    - Exhibits difficulty when approaching chair to sit down
    - Has significant reduction in step size as he approaches the target, reaching too far forward for arm rest, and beginning to turn and sit before achieving good body alignment that results in uncontrolled descent as he moves from standing to sitting
    - Mrs. Barris (who is 6 inches shorter than her husband) is unsure how to assist with transfers, does not position herself to allow good body mechanics when providing transfer assistance, tends to speak too rapidly, and offers frequent verbal input and commands as patient attempts to move

◆ Gait, locomotion, and balance
  - Timed Up and Go Test: 14 seconds[69-71]
  - Observation of gait revealed
    - Reduced stride length and foot clearance secondary to hypokinesia
    - Start hesitation
    - Turns using multiple short, shuffling steps with balance instability noted
  - BBS[66]: 48/56
    - Sitting to standing: 3=able to stand independently using hands
    - Standing unsupported: 4=able to stand safely for 2 minutes
    - Sitting unsupported: 4=able to sit safely and securely 2 minutes
    - Standing to sitting: 2=uses back of legs against chair to control descent

- Transfers: 3=able to transfer safely with definite use of hands
- Standing unsupported with eyes closed: 4=able to stand 10 seconds safely
- Standing unsupported with feet together: 4=able to place feet together independently and stand 1 minute safely
- Reaching forward with outstretched arm: 4=can reach forward confidently 25 cm (10 in)
- Pick up object from floor: 4=able to pick up slipper safely and easily
- Turn to look behind/over left and right shoulders: 4=looks behind from both sides and weight shifts well
- Turn 360 degrees: 4=able to turn 360 degrees safely in 4 seconds or less
- Alternating steps on stool: 4=able to stand independently and complete eight steps in 20 seconds
- Standing unsupported, one foot in front: 2=able to take small step independently and hold 30 seconds
- Stand on one leg: 2=able to lift leg independently and hold more than 3 seconds
- Percent probability of falling based on BBS and fall history[67]: 69%

◆ Motor function
  - UPDRS[21] motor section scores
    - Speech: Grade 2=slurred but understandable, moderately impaired
    - Facial expression: Grade 2+=slight but definitely abnormal diminution of facial expression
    - Tremor at rest
      ▶ RUE: Grade 1=slight and infrequently present
      ▶ RLE: Grade 0=absent
      ▶ LUE: Grade 2=mild in amplitude and persistent or moderate in amplitude but only intermittently present
      ▶ LLE: Grade 2=mild in amplitude and persistent or moderate in amplitude but only intermittently present
    - Action or postural tremor of hands: Grade 0=absent
    - Rigidity
      ▶ RUE: Grade 2=mild to moderate
      ▶ RLE: Grade 2=mild to moderate
      ▶ LUE: Grade 2=mild to moderate
      ▶ LLE: Grade 2=mild to moderate
    - Finger taps: Grade 2=moderately impaired with definite and early fatiguing and may have occasional arrests of movement (7 to 10/5 sec)
    - Hand movements: Grade 2=moderately impaired with definite and early fatiguing and may have occasional arrests of movement (7 to 10/5 sec)

- Rapid alternating movements of hands: Grade 2=moderately impaired with definite and early fatiguing and may have occasional arrests of movement
- Leg agility
  - RLE: Grade 2=moderately impaired with definite and early fatiguing and may have occasional arrests of movement
  - LLE: Grade 3=severely impaired with frequent hesitation in inititating movements or arrests in ongoing movement
- Arising from chair: Grade 2=pushes self up using arms of seat
- Posture: Grade 2=moderately stooped posture, definitely abnormal, can be slightly leaning to one side
- Gait: Grade 2=walks with difficulty but requires little or no assistance and may have some festination, short steps, or propulsion
- Postural stability: Grade 2=absence of postural response and would fall if not caught by examiner
- Body bradykinesia and hypokinesia: Grade 3=moderate slowness and poverty or small amplitude of movement

◆ Muscle performance
  - Exhibits significant effort and difficulty when rising from chairs and getting legs into bed
  - LE muscle testing
    - Hip flexors=4-/5
    - Hip extensors=3-/5
    - Knee extensors=4-/5
    - Knee flexors=4/5
    - Ankle dorsiflexors=4+/5
    - Ankle plantarflexors=4-/5
  - Standing tolerance approximately 6 minutes

◆ Pain: 4/10 on the NPS[76,77] in the left knee with stair climbing, kneeling, or prolonged walking

◆ Posture: Increased trunk flexion noted in stance and ambulation with guarded posture related to abdominal incision

◆ Range of motion
  - Cervical motions exhibit mild limitations at end ranges and lacking 10 degrees of rotation bilaterally
  - Left knee lacks 15 degrees of active extension
  - Right knee lacks 7 degrees of active extension
  - Patient reports "pull" in posterior thighs and knees when attempting to bend forward
  - Hamstring tightness noted bilaterally

◆ Self-care and home management
  - Physical Performance Test[99,100]

- Is a timed test administering a series of simulated functional activities performed during ADL
- Score is based on total time to perform all items
- Patient may be given up to two chances to complete each item and may use assistive devices for tasks 6 through 9
- Results
  - Write a sentence ("Whales live in the blue ocean."): 16.5 seconds (score 2=between 15.5 to 20 seconds)
  - Simulated eating: 13.5 seconds (score 3=between 10.5 to 15 seconds)
  - Sitting with feet on floor, lift a book (eg, *Physician's Desk Reference* or similar book weighing 5.5 lbs) from bed height of 19 cm and put it on a shelf of 118 cm height: 3 seconds (score 3=between between 2.5 to 4 seconds)
  - In standing, put on and remove a jacket (may use a bathrobe, button-down shirt, or hospital gown): 14 seconds (score 3=between 10.5 to 15 seconds)
  - Pick up a penny from the floor: 3 seconds (score 3=between 2.5 to 4 seconds)
  - Turn 360 degrees: 5 seconds (score 4=continuous steps and steady)
  - 50-foot walk test (started sitting for instructions): 23 seconds (score 2=between 20.5 to 25 seconds)
  - Cimb one flight of stairs: 13.5 seconds (score 2=between 10.5 to 15 seconds)
  - Climb stairs (number of flights up and down, max score 4): 1
  - Total score: 23/36, which places this patient in the category of moderately frail

● Occasionally needs minimal assistance of wife with transfers since hospital discharge, especially as medication levels wear off near end of dosage

● During this time, he often requires assistance to rise from chair, exhibiting difficulty scooting to edge of chair and poor foot placement when attempting to stand

● Wife is also providing physical assistance to lift patient's legs in and out of bed

● Receiving home health services for assistance with bathing and shower three times a week for 2 weeks post hospital discharge

● Wife currently provides standby to minimal assistance with morning and evening routine

◆ Work, community, and leisure integration or reintegration
  - Mr. Barris has not participated in any activities outside the home since surgery

- He anticipates difficulty participating in community and leisure activities due to difficulty getting in and out of the home because of the stairs, transferring into and out of the car, and walking and participating in activities because of decreased endurance
- He currently needs to rest or nap after being up for 2 hours

EVALUATION

Mr. Barris' history and risk factors previously outlined indicate he is a 67-year-old male with a diagnosis of PD and recent hospitalization and surgery for bowel obstruction. Results of his physical therapist examination on this date revealed his PD has progressed to Stage 3 (based on the Hoehn and Yahr rating scale),[20] and he demonstrates impaired endurance associated with deconditioning related to his recent hospitalization and surgery. Deconditioning is currently affecting his gait, transfer ability, ability to move safely in his home, and ability to participate in community and leisure activities. OH is also noted as well as continued pain in his left knee from DJD.

DIAGNOSIS

Mr. Barris has a diagnosis of Stage 3 PD with pain in his left knee. He has impaired: aerobic capacity/endurance; circulation; ergonomics and body mechanics; gait, locomotion, and balance; motor function; muscle performance; posture; and range of motion. He is functionally limited in self-care and home management and in work, community, and leisure actions, tasks, and activities. He is in need of devices and equipment. These findings are consistent with placement in Pattern E: Impaired Motor Function and Sensory Integrity Associated With Progressive Disorders of the Central Nervous System and also in Cardiovascular/Pulmonary Pattern B: Impaired Aerobic Capacity/Endurance Associated With Deconditioning in the APTA's *Guide to Physical Therapist Practice*.[78]

In this aspect of Mr. Barris' case, it is his impaired endurance related to his recent hospitalization and surgery for bowel obstruction that will drive his interventions for this episode of care along with all of the other needs identified during the examination. The physical therapist needs to take into consideration the impact of the PD on the systems and how that may alter selection and application of the intervention plan. The identified impairments and functional limitations will be addressed in determining the prognosis and the plan of care.

PROGNOSIS AND PLAN OF CARE

Over the course of the visits, the following mutually established outcomes have been determined:

- Endurance is improved
- Mr. and Mrs. Barris are aware of importance of frequent movement and exercise
- Mrs. Barris uses appropriate body mechanics when assisting her husband
- Participation in community activities is restored
- Safety is improved
- Transfers are improved

To achieve the identified outcomes, the appropriate interventions for this patient are determined. These will include: coordination, communication, and documentation; patient/client-related instruction; therapeutic exercise; functional training in self-care and home management; functional training in work, community, and leisure integration or reintegration; and prescription, application, and, as appropriate, fabrication of devices and equipment.

The *Guide* takes into consideration that patients placed in this pattern have progressive conditions that may have ongoing impairments, functional limitations, and disabilities. The result of this is that the stated prognosis for this pattern is to have optimal function within a variety of settings "within the context of the impairments, functional limitations, and disabilities."[78] Mr. Barris is expected to need 8 to 10 visits (two home visits and six to eight visits in the clinic) over a 10-week period of time.

INTERVENTIONS

RATIONALE FOR SELECTED INTERVENTIONS

It is typical to see symptoms in patients with PD exacerbate during times when a patient is under significant physical or emotional stress.[101] In the event of acute illness, surgery, or hospitalization, a physical therapy referral should be initiated as soon as the patient with PD is medically stable. Bedrest or inactivity significantly impairs mobility and complicates the rehabilitation process.[102] Early physical therapy intervention allows timely mobilization and reduces the risk of complications. It should be noted that there is an increased likelihood of postoperative complications and that the rehabilitation process after illness or injury might be slowed significantly for a patient with PD.[103,104] Expected outcomes should take this into consideration, and interventions should be designed accordingly. Family caregiver instruction should also be included, as the deconditioned patient with PD may require more assistance upon discharge to home post hospitalization.

Physical therapy interventions in this case will focus on building endurance and enhancing mobility post hospitalization. Bergen and associates found that aerobic exercise improved both aerobic capacity and movement initiation in patients with PD.[86] The presence of OH in patients with PD may be related to the disease process and further exacerbated by the side effects of common PD medications.[105] Exercises for flexibility and strengthening may initially be best performed in supine and sitting positions due to lowered BP in standing, which adds to the risk of dizziness or falls. Several of the national Parkinson's organizations have appropriate seated exercise programs available for patient follow through and home programming following discharge from physical therapy.[92,106]

Patients also require instruction in safety precautions to be used during transitional movements and transfers. Additional suggestions for transfer training using attentional strategies and self-cueing (eg, breaking down movement components of the transfer into a step-by-step sequence and performing mental rehearsal of movements prior to intiating movement) are outlined by Morris for physical therapy in PD.[90]

There is also a continued need for gait training focusing on strategies for normalizing stride length and enhancing balance. Instruction in the use of visual and auditory cues has been found to improve gait velocity, cadence, and stride length in patients with PD.[107] Evaluation and training in the use of appropriate gait assistive devices should also be included in the physical therapy plan of care.

See Case Study #1A for further rationale for selected interventions.

COORDINATION, COMMUNICATION, AND DOCUMENTATION

Communication will occur with the patient, his wife, and his physician during the course of treatment. Mr. Barris will receive information about the benefits of a comprehensive interdisciplinary team approach to management of PD, and he will be provided with resources on how to access appropriate team members as needs are identified. Appropriate referrals will be made to his physician and home care nursing to address the patient's low standing BP. He may also be referred to occupational therapy. Interdisciplinary teamwork will occur through information exchange at team rounds. All elements of the patient's management will be documented.

PATIENT/CLIENT-RELATED INSTRUCTION

Education regarding his current condition (PD complicated by recent surgery) will be discussed. In addition, he and his wife will receive instruction regarding the plan of care including:

♦ Enhancement of performance through compensatory movement strategies during bed and chair transfers

♦ Enhancement of performance through compensatory strategies for safety during transitional movements related to OH

♦ Instruction in appropriate home exercise program

♦ Gait training with assistive device

THERAPEUTIC EXERCISE

♦ Aerobic capacity/endurance conditioning
  ● Endurance reconditioning through reintroduction of walking program
♦ Balance, coordination, and agility training
  ● Practice safe turning strategies for use in bathroom and other small, cramped spaces
  ● Practice balance strategies (eg, with and without support, stand on both legs, stand on one leg, change arm positions)
♦ Body mechanics and postural stabilization
  ● Body mechanics training for wife when providing assistance during transfers
  ● Postural control training including practice standing and weight shifting while performing reaching activities in the home environment
♦ Flexibility exercises
  ● Stretching exercises should be done after warming up, using a slow and steady stretch accompanied by deep breathing, and building hold up to 30 to 60 seconds
  ● Exercises initially performed sitting to reduce risk of OH and progress to standing as patient improves and standing BP becomes more stable
  ● Neck: Seated rotation, lateral flexion, chin tucks
  ● Trunk
    ▪ Seated rotation, extension, sidebending with opposite arm overhead
    ▪ Supine full body stretch
  ● Shoulders
    ▪ Wand exercises including flexion, diagonals, and circles
    ▪ Shoulder shrugs
    ▪ Scapular retraction
  ● LEs
    ▪ Seated hamstring stretch and calf stretch using towel or belt under sole of foot
    ▪ Ankle circles
♦ Gait and locomotion training: Use single-end cane for gait
♦ Relaxation: Focused deep breathing exercises to reduce abdominal discomfort during transitional movements and to reduce stress reaction when attempting to initiate motion for walking
♦ Strength, power, and endurance training: All considering knee pain
  ● Initial strengthening exercise program to be completed in supine and seated positions due to lightheaded-

ness and low endurance with gradual progression to supported standing exercises

- Supine LE AROM progressing to progressive resistive exercises
- Unilateral and bilateral bridging
- Hip rolls
- Seated UE AROM progressing to progressive resistive exercises
- Chair push-ups
- Standing at kitchen counter toe raises, marching, hip abduction, hip extension, and knee bends

FUNCTIONAL TRAINING IN SELF-CARE AND HOME MANAGEMENT

- Self-care
  - Transfer training of sit to supine and supine to sit emphasizing breaking down each movement sequence into a series of steps
    - Use log rolling technique to reduce incisional discomfort
    - Use adaptive equipment and half side rail to assist during transfer
  - Transfer training of sit to stand and stand to sit with emphasis on proper body alignment, attentional strategies, and controlled descent
- Home management
  - Safety awareness training during common ADL including precautions to minimize OH (pause before moving after transitional movements, perform several repetitions of isotonic LE exercise prior to rising from chair, avoid exercise or excessive activity immediately after meals, maintain adequate hydration throughout day)

FUNCTIONAL TRAINING IN WORK, COMMUNITY, AND LEISURE INTEGRATION OR REINTEGRATION

- Leisure
  - Safety awareness training using cane for added stability initially during leisure activities in the community
  - Gradually progress to walking stick or hiking pole for use on golf course or uneven terrain on lake property as endurance allows return to more active leisure pursuits

PRESCRIPTION, APPLICATION, AND, AS APPROPRIATE, FABRICATION OF DEVICES AND EQUIPMENT

- Adaptive devices

- Obtain and install half side bed rail
- Assistive devices
  - Obtain single-end cane
  - Consider obtaining walking stick or hiking pole for more active leisure pursuits as endurance improves
- Supportive device
  - Assess ability to don and wear LE compression garments to aid in control of OH (may not be feasible as these are often difficult for patients with PD to manage due to reduced manual dexterity)

ANTICIPATED GOALS AND EXPECTED OUTCOMES

- Impact on impairments
  - Ambulation throughout home environment is possible without fatigue or complaints of dizziness.
  - Home exercise program is performed correctly with improvements in LE strength to 4/5 in all muscle groups.
  - Patient tolerates being up for 4 to 6 hours without rest.
  - Safe, independent ambulation is achieved throughout home environment using single-end cane with eventual progression to ambulation without assistive devices at home (using hiking pole or walking stick during active leisure pursuits).
- Impact on functional limitations
  - Bed and chair transfers are independently performed.
  - Self-cueing strategies are exhibited to minimize start hesitation during ambulation.
  - Strategies to reduce risks related to OH are accurately verbalized and utilized.
- Impact on disabilities
  - Community ambulation for attendance at church and social functions is achieved.
  - Cueing strategies are properly used to improve gait and balance safety during community activities.
- Risk reduction/prevention
  - Fall risk is reduced through patient education and use of safety compensatory strategies.
  - Patient and wife demonstrate proper postural alignment and body mechanics for use during assisted transfers.
  - Risk of secondary impairment is reduced through patient awareness of mobility enhancement strategies and home exercise program.
- Impact on societal resources
  - Communication enhances risk reduction and prevention through awareness and use of an interdisci-

plinary team.

- Decision making is enhanced regarding patient health and the use of health care resources by patient, family, significant others, and caregivers.
- Documentation occurs throughout patient management and follows APTA's *Guidelines for Physical Therapy Documentation.*[78]

◆ Patient/client satisfaction

- Access, availability, and services provided are acceptable to patient.
- Care is coordinated with patient, family, and other health care professionals.
- Patient and family knowledge and awareness of the diagnosis, prognosis, interventions, and anticipated goals and expected outcomes are increased.
- Referrals are made to other professionals or resources whenever necessary and appropriate.

REEXAMINATION

Reexamination is performed throughout this second episode of care.

DISCHARGE

Mr. Barris is discharged from physical therapy after a total of eight physical therapy visits over 10 weeks and attainment of his goals. As Mr. Barris has a condition that may require multiple episodes of care throughout his life span, Mr. Barris and his family received education regarding factors that may trigger a call to his physical therapist for a reexamination and new episode of physical therapy care.

Case Study #1C:
Stage 4 Parkinson's Disease

Mr. Barris is now a 72-year-old male who is returning to physical therapy for a new episode of care due to increased incidents of falling and loss of balance.

PHYSICAL THERAPIST EXAMINATION

Note: Only changes from his previous two episodes are included in this case.

HISTORY

◆ General demographics: Mr. Barris is now a 72-year-old male.

◆ Living environment: He recently moved into a one-level townhouse in suburban Chicago. The floor surfaces are either carpeted or linoleum. Yard work and outdoor maintenance are taken care of by the development association.

◆ General health status

- General health perception: Mr. Barris notes progression of his PD symptoms and indicates additional loss of manual dexterity, increasing muscle stiffness and rigidity, greater postural changes, and decline in stability and gait.
- Physical function: Mr. Barris notes declining balance with increasing falls.
- Psychological function: He reports feeling depressed, is frustrated by changes in physical function, and is becoming more isolated.
- Role function: He continues to manage his own personal finances, although his wife occasionally assists with writing and signing checks due to the patient's micrographia.
- Social function: He has stopped community volunteer work as of last year due to balance instability and feelings of depression. His participation in leisure interests (theater, movies, and concerts) has been limited in the recent past due to balance loss and episodes of freezing. He is becoming less active in community activities. He still enjoys traveling (though feels his destination options are more limited due to declining balance) and attends monthly Parkinson's support group meetings.

◆ Medical/surgical history: His PD was diagnosed 9 years ago. He had a left total knee replacement (TKR) 4 years ago.

◆ Preexisting medical and other health-related conditions: He now has DJD in his right knee. He has a history of OH.

◆ Current condition(s)/chief complaint(s): Mr. Barris has noted increasing balance imprecision with three falls within the past month and six falls over the past year. One fall occurred as he attempted to lift an item down from an overhead shelf. The second fall occurred as he attempted to carry a grocery bag from his car to the door of his home. The third fall was related to a freezing episode, which occurred as he attempted to move through the doorway at a movie theater. In addition, he notes a tendency for backward balance loss when standing in the shower. He has received physical therapy services following his surgeries and for periodic updating of his home program.

◆ Functional status and activity level: He is independent in most ADL, although he reports increasing difficulty with dressing (buttoning, tying shoes, donning jackets) and bathing. He stopped playing golf last summer due to balance changes. He performs his stretching and strengthening home exercise program five times per week. He walks 20 minutes three to four times per week using a walking stick for added support on a paved outdoor walking trail in summer and in a nearby shopping mall in winter.

♦ Medications: Carbidopa/levodopa, pramipexole, Celebrex, fludrocortisone acetate.

SYSTEMS REVIEW

♦ Cardiovascular/pulmonary
  ● BP
    ▪ Sitting: 138/68 mmHg
    ▪ Standing: 128/64 mmHg
  ● HR: 68 bpm and regular
  ● No dyspnea
♦ Integumentary
  ● Presence of scar formation: Well-healed abdominal incision and incisional scar on left knee from TKR
♦ Musculoskeletal
  ● Gross range of motion
    ▪ Left knee ROM WNL
    ▪ Right knee ROM lacks 10 degrees terminal extension, with joint crepitus evident
  ● Gross strength: No functional deficits
  ● Weight: 183 lbs (83 kg)
♦ Neuromuscular
  ● Balance: Increasing balance imprecision with three falls within the past month
  ● Locomotion, transfers, and transitions
    ▪ He ambulates with narrow base of support without assistive devices in the home environment and uses a walking stick for longer distance community ambulation
    ▪ He exhibits significant hypokinesia, episodes of festination, freezing, and retropulsion
    ▪ Motor fluctuations cause patient's skills to change throughout the day, and wife provides occasional assistance during "off" periods for bed and chair transfers
♦ Communication, affect, cognition, language, and learning style
  ● Communication, affect, and cognition
    ▪ His voice volume is decreased, and he is occasionally asked to repeat himself during conversation
    ▪ He has moderate facial masking and reduced eye blink
    ▪ He notes bradyphrenia, mild decrease in short-term memory, and reduced executive function skills
    ▪ He reports feelings of depression and frustration with mobility changes and falling
  ● Learning style

■ He is open and responsive to participation in physical therapy and follows through with the home programs that have been provided to him from previous episodes of care

■ He attends the PD support group and enjoys speaking with others who have similar concerns, though notes occasional difficulty "keeping up" in conversation during group discussions due to slowing of thought processes

TESTS AND MEASURES

♦ Assistive and adaptive devices
  ● While he had a single-end cane that he used after past hospitalizations to assist with balance, he reports that it does not provide adequate support now
  ● He is becoming more fearful during his community walking program while using the walking stick and reports episodes of uncontrolled walking speed and inadequate support with the device
  ● He was evaluated for the need of a rolling walker and was found to exhibit improved stability, larger step size, and more constant gait velocity with this device
  ● He was also able to operate the walker's hand brakes effectively when festination started to occur
  ● Mr. Barris reports that he still uses the half side bed rail to get in and out of bed
  ● He has recently purchased a lounge chair with a stable base and firm cushions to facilitate standing
  ● He has no adaptive equipment for either the shower or tub
♦ Ergonomics and body mechanics
  ● Observations of assisted transfers showed the wife's body mechanics to be good when assisting patient with bed or chair transfers, but poor with attempts to assist him from the floor
  ● She was observed attempting to bend forward and pull up on his extended arms in an attempt to lift him off the floor
  ● She reports that she sustained back and shoulder stiffness after helping patient off the floor following his last fall
♦ Gait, locomotion, and balance
  ● Timed Up and Go Test[69-71]: 17.8 seconds
  ● BBS[66]: 43/56
    ▪ Sitting to standing: 4=able to stand without using hands and stabilize independently
    ▪ Standing unsupported: 4=able to stand safely for 2 minutes
    ▪ Sitting unsupported: 4=able to sit safely and securely 2 minutes
    ▪ Standing to sitting: 3=controls descent with minimal use of hands

- Transfers: 4=able to transfer safely with minor use of hands
- Standing unsupported with eyes closed: 4=able to stand 10 seconds safely
- Standing unsupported with feet together: 4=able to place feet together independently and stand 1 minute safely
- Reaching forward with outstretched arm: 4=can reach forward confidently 25 cm (10 in)
- Pick up object from floor: 4=able to pick up slipper safely and easily
- Turn to look behind/over left and right shoulders: 4=looks behind from both sides and weight shifts well
- Turn 360 degrees: 2=able to turn 360 degrees safely but slowly
- Alternating steps on stool: 2=able to complete four steps without aid with supervision
- Standing unsupported, one foot in front: 0=loses balance while stepping or turning
- Stand on one leg: 0=unable to try or needs assist to prevent fall
- Percent probability of falling based on BBS and fall history[67]: 88%
- Gait speed test: 0.95 m/sec
- Gait observation revealed
  - He ambulates with narrow base of support without assistive devices in the home environment, using walking stick for longer distance community ambulation
  - Exhibits significant hypokinesia, with reduced stride length and absent arm swing noted bilaterally
  - Episodes of festination are noted during ambulation as step size declines while walking
  - Freezing occurs occasionally in door thresholds, when turning, and during approach to chair when going to sit down
  - Retropulsion is evident as patient reaches into overhead cupboards or attempts to pull open the front door of his home
  - He has required consistent assistance from his wife to rise from the floor after falling
  - Further gait decline noted during attempts at multitasking with both added cognitive and motor tasks and around potential environmental barriers
- Motor function
  - UPDRS[21] motor section scores
    - Speech: Grade 2=slurred but understandable, moderately impaired
    - Facial expression: Grade 3=moderate hypomimia

with lips parted some of the time
- Tremor at rest
  - RUE: Grade 1=slight and infrequently present
  - RLE: Grade 0=absent
  - LUE: Grade 3=moderate in amplitude and present most of the time
  - LLE: Grade 2=mild in amplitude and persistent or moderate in amplitude but only intermittently present
- Action or postural tremor of hands: Grade 2=moderate in amplitude and present with action
- Rigidity
  - RUE: Grade 2=mild to moderate
  - RLE: Grade 2=mild to moderate
  - LUE: Grade 3=marked but full ROM easily achieved
  - LLE: Grade 2=mild to moderate
- Finger taps: Grade 2=moderately impaired with definite and early fatiguing and may have occasional arrests of movement (7 to 10/5 sec)
- Hand movements: Grade 2=moderately impaired with definite and early fatiguing and may have occasional arrests of movement (7 to 10/5 sec)
- Rapid alternating movements of hands: Grade 2=moderately impaired with definite and early fatiguing and may have occasional arrests of movement
- Leg agility
  - RLE: Grade 3=severely impaired with frequent hesitation in initiating movements or arrests in ongoing movement
  - LLE: Grade 3=severely impaired with frequent hesitation in initiating movements or arrests in ongoing movement
- Arising from chair: Grade 3=tends to fall back and may have to try more than one time, but can get up without help
- Posture: Grade 2=moderately stooped posture, definitely abnormal, and can be slightly learning to one side
- Gait: Grade 2=walks with difficulty but requires little or no assistance, may have some festination, short steps, or propulsion
- Postural stability: Grade 3=very unstable and tends to lose balance spontaneously
- Body bradykinesia and hypokinesia: Grade 3=moderate slowness and poverty or small amplitude of movement
- Needs minimal assistance of wife with bed and chair transfers when in "off state," which means that the PD medications are not working at peak level, and the patient exhibits increased motor impairment and

more prominent PD symptoms during these "off" times

- Usually independent with significant effort and difficulty when in "on state," which means that the PD medications are working at peak level, and the patient exhibits decreased motor impairment and maximized control of PD symptoms during these "on" times
- Motor fluctuations occur throughout the day
- Mild to moderate resting tremor noted in UEs and LLE when "off"
- Mild dyskinesia noted in trunk and LEs when "on"

♦ Muscle performance
- Five Times Sit to Stand[74,75]
  - Result: 16 seconds
  - Mean speed on timed sit to stand scores to be 11.6 seconds in males aged 70 to 79[98]

♦ Posture
- Increased forward head
- Increased kyphosis
- Decreased lumbar lordosis

♦ Range of motion
- Right knee lacks 15 degrees of active extension
- Lacks 10 degress of active extension bilaterally due to tight hip flexors
- Significant reduction in active trunk extension

♦ Self-care and home management
- Parkinson's Activity Scale[108] tests ability to perform functional activities (such as chair transfers, ambulation, and bed mobility) and scoring performed during both on and off states to account for variability in functional performance
  - Getting up on: Without arms and with mild difficulty
  - Getting up off: Dependent on physical assistance
  - Sitting down on: With arms and abrupt landing or ending in an uncomfortable position
  - Sitting down off: With arms and abrupt landing or ending in an uncomfortable position
  - Gait akinesia on: Hesitation or short festination
  - Gait akinesia off: Unwanted arrests of movement with or without festination lasting 5 seconds or less
  - Turning 360 degrees on: Unwanted arrests of movement with or without festination lasting more than 5 seconds
  - Turning 360 degrees off: Unwanted arrests of movement with or without festination lasting more than 5 seconds
  - Bed mobility
    - Lying down on: Two difficulties with lifiting legs or moving trunk or reaching adequate end position

    - Lying down off: Dependent on physical assistance
    - Rolling on to side on: Two difficulties with turning, shifting trunk, or reaching adequate end position
    - Rolling on to side off: Three difficulties with turning, shifting trunk, or reaching adequate end position
    - Rising on: Two difficulties with moving legs or trunk to meet adequate end position
    - Rising off: Dependent on physical assistance
  - Bed mobility with cover
    - Lying down with cover on: Two difficulties with moving body, adjusting cover, or reaching adequate end position
    - Lying down with cover off: Dependent on physical assistance
    - Rolling on to side with cover on: Three difficulties with moving body, adjusting cover, or reaching adequate end position
    - Rolling on to side with cover off: Dependent on physical assistance
    - Rising with cover on: Two difficulties with turning body, adjusting cover, or reaching adequate end
    - Rising with cover off: Dependent on physical assistance
- Safety concerns with loss of balance when performing self-care and home living activities
  - Needs to sit while dressing and undressing
  - Reports falling backward when showering
  - Has difficulty rising from low chairs or those without arm rests
  - Skills vary dependent on motor fluctuations
  - At times achieves independent bed mobility and transfers using the half side rail on bed, and at other times requires wife's assistance
  - Requires consistent assistance to rise from floor after falling, and his wife provides this assistance

♦ Work, community, and leisure integration or reintegration
- Safety concerns with loss of balance and freezing episodes when in community or participating in leisure activities
- He has limited activities in community due to concerns about falling

EVALUATION

Mr. Barris' history and risk factors previously outlined indicate he is a 72-year-old male with a diagnosis of PD. Results of his physical therapist examination on this date revealed his PD has progressed to Stage 4 based on the Hoehn and Yahr[20] rating scale, and he demonstrates increasing difficulties with balance and gait and has difficulty negotiating in both home and community environments. OH is noted, as well as pain in his right knee from DJD.

DIAGNOSIS

Mr. Barris has a diagnosis of Stage 4 PD with pain in his right knee. He has impaired: ergonomics and body mechanics; gait, locomotion, and balance; motor function; muscle performance; posture; and range of motion. He is functionally limited in self-care and home management and in work, community, and leisure actions, tasks, and activities. He is in need of devices and equipment. These findings are consistent with placement in Pattern E: Impaired Motor Function and Sensory Integrity Associated With Progressive Disorders of the Central Nervous System and also in Pattern A: Primary Prevention/Risk Reduction for Loss of Balance and Falling.

In this aspect of Mr. Barris' case, it is his impaired balance and risk of falling that will drive the primary interventions for this episode of care along with all of the other needs identified during the examination. The physical therapist needs to take into consideration the impact of PD on the systems and how that may alter selection and application of the intervention plan. The identified impairments, functional limitations, and device and equipment needs will be addressed in determining the prognosis and the plan of care.

PROGNOSIS AND PLAN OF CARE

Over the course of the visits, the following mutually established outcomes have been determined:

♦ Ability to resume safe home, community, and leisure roles is improved

♦ Gait, locomotion, and balance are improved

♦ Risk of falling is reduced through use of compensatory balance safety strategies in high-risk situations and consistent use of a gait assistive device

♦ Risk of secondary impairments is reduced

♦ Safety is improved

♦ Self-management of symptoms is improved

To achieve these outcomes, the appropriate interventions for this patient are determined. These will include: coordination, communication, and documentation; patient/client-related instruction; therapeutic exercise; functional training in self-care and home management; functional training in work, community, and leisure integration or reintegration; and prescription, application, and, as appropriate, fabrication of devices and equipment.

The *Guide*[78] takes into consideration that patients placed in these patterns have progressive conditions that may have ongoing impairments, functional limitations, and disabilities. Mr. Barris is expected to need eight visits over 10 weeks,

five visits in the clinic and three home or community visits. He continues to have good social support, is motivated, and will follow through with his home exercise program. He is increasingly impaired, but is still relatively healthy.

INTERVENTIONS

RATIONALE FOR SELECTED INTERVENTIONS

Postural instability is the primary symptom of PD that appears least responsive to available medications.[109] Decreases in flexibility and weakness caused by inactivity or a sedentary lifestyle combined with a narrowed base of support and decreased postural righting reflexes produce balance changes. Gait changes in PD include hypokinesia, reduced stride length, narrowed base of support, and difficulty turning. It has been shown that patients experience increased gait difficulties when attempting to multitask, with added cognitive or motor tasks shown to be equally demanding.[110] Many patients report frequent episodes of significant balance loss or falling. A multidimensional exercise routine has been shown to be most effective at addressing deficits in balance, mobility, and fall risk.[81]

Retropulsion, festination, and freezing are frequently seen in PD, requiring gait training to effectively cope with these alterations. Identification of common "triggers" helps to determine where a patient is most likely to freeze. Visual, audio, tactile, and kinesthetic cues have all been found to be helpful strategies to use during freezing episodes.[94,107,111] Appropriate environmental modifications are also helpful. Retropulsion results in involuntary backward balance loss that is worsened with attempts to reach overhead, open a door, or carry objects up against the body. Festination usually causes loss of forward balance, as the patient experiences uncontrolled increases in gait velocity with decreases in stride length.

Many patients with PD find it necessary to use a gait assistive device to maximize safety when ambulating. Assistive devices such as four-post walkers or quad canes interrupt the flow of movement and require divided attention or multitasking that further contributes to balance instability. Many patients benefit from the use of specialty walkers available with swivel casters and hand brakes that offer more options for controlling walker speed and turning stability. Patients also require gait training in order to use assistive devices safely in both home and community environments.

As the PD progresses, patients often begin to develop motor fluctuations and varying response to PD medications. These on/off periods may be cyclical correlating with each medication dose or may be unpredictable throughout the day. These motor fluctuations may significantly affect the patient's functional levels, and physical therapy interventions may need to be modified to account for the variations in functional performance throughout the day. Examination and intervention should occur within both phases of the cycle if possible, and strategies should be developed for patients' functional abilities in both on and off states.

COORDINATION, COMMUNICATION, AND DOCUMENTATION

Communication will occur with the patient, his wife, and his physician during the course of treatment. The patient will receive information about the benefits of a comprehensive interdisciplinary team approach to management of his PD, and he will be provided with resources on how to access appropriate team members as needs are identified. Appropriate referrals will be made, including referral to an occupational therapist to assess current difficulties with dressing and bathing and to a music therapist who specializes in management of patients with neurologic dysfunction for instruction in techniques of rhythmic auditory facilitation[112,113] to assist during ambulation and freezing episodes. Interdisciplinary teamwork will occur through information exchange at team rounds, including discussion about and referral for consultation for his depression and its impact on his quality of life. All elements of the patient's management will be documented.

PATIENT/CLIENT-RELATED INSTRUCTION

Education will continue regarding his current condition (decreasing balance and increasing falls). In addition, he and his wife will receive instruction regarding the plan of care including:

♦ Enhancement of performance through compensatory movement strategies to initiate motion when freezing

♦ Enhancement of performance through compensatory strategies for balance during ADL and leisure activities

♦ Instruction, education, and training regarding proper body mechanics during floor-to-stand transfers

♦ Risk factors and situations that commonly trigger retropulsion or freezing episodes

THERAPEUTIC EXERCISE

♦ Balance, coordination, and agility training
  • Gait drills
    ▪ Stepping around and over obstacles
    ▪ Side stepping
    ▪ 180-degree turns
  • Practice balance challenges
    ▪ Standing on foam
    ▪ Reaching activities
    ▪ Seated activities on exercise ball
  • Task-specific, high-risk balance activities that cause retropulsion
    ▪ Carrying items

▪ Opening doors
▪ Reaching overhead
▪ Divided attention tasks (ie, searching in pocket or purse for key to unlock and open door)
▪ Turning to move away from bathroom sink or kitchen counter

♦ Body mechanics and postural stabilization
  • Body mechanics training for his wife when providing assistance after patient falls
  • Instruct patient and wife in safest technique for getting up from ground
  • Instruct wife in use of a transfer belt
  • Postural control training and continued stress on thoracic extension

♦ Flexibility exercises
  • Stretching exercises for hamstring and heel cord musculature should be done after warming up, using a slow and steady stretch accompanied by deep breathing, and building hold up to 30 to 60 seconds

♦ Gait and locomotion training
  • Gait training using wheeled walker, including practice of safe turning, backing up, and walking on outdoor surfaces and inclines with wheeled walker
  • Instruction and practice in use of walker hand brakes to assist during episodes of festination
  • Instruction in safe transfers on and off walker bench seat
  • Use of sensory enhancement cues (visual, audio, tactile, and kinesthetic) to improve walking pattern and for reduction or "breakout" of freezing episodes
    ▪ Use of portable metronome for use as auditory cue to allow consistency in stride length and gait speed during ADL
    ▪ Instruct wife in appropriate use of cueing strategies (eg, breaking down movement components into a step-by-step sequence) to assist patient when he freezes
  • Design separate sets of compensatory and attentional strategies for gait use during "on" and "off" states[90]

♦ Relaxation
  • Shift focus from attempting to force movement when freezing to relaxation
  • Visualization strategies to enhance relaxation and assist in initiating movement

♦ Strength, power, and endurance training
  • Modification of current strengthening program to provide increased emphasis on standing and LE weightbearing exercises
    ▪ Hip rocks/clocks
    ▪ Toe raises
    ▪ One leg stand

- Hip abduction and extension
- Continued core strength training for trunk musculature for greater ability to recover from postural perturbations or disturbances

FUNCTIONAL TRAINING IN SELF-CARE AND HOME MANAGEMENT

- Self-care
  - ADL training for bed mobility and transfer training
  - Safety awareness training during common ADL and leisure tasks
  - Sit down when dressing
  - Use counterbalancing strategies when performing overhead reach, opening doors, or carrying items
- Home management
  - Safety awareness training during common ADL and IADL
  - Use taped lines on floor in door thresholds as a visual cue to decrease freezing episodes in this area
  - Mark floor in front of bed, chair, and toilet with taped X to facilitate movement and decrease freezing upon approach to target when moving to sit down

FUNCTIONAL TRAINING IN WORK, COMMUNITY, AND LEISURE INTEGRATION OR REINTEGRATION

- Community
  - Ambulation and participation in the community with use of devices or equipment
  - Arrive early at community events and stay until crowds have left to minimize ambulation in crowded areas
  - Schedule appointments and community activities to coincide with "on" times as able
  - Consider use of knee or elbow pads for added joint protection
- Leisure
  - Safety awareness training during common leisure tasks
    - How to carry items during travel to preclude falls
    - Request of accessible rooms or facilities at travel destination
    - Use walker or other adaptive equipment during leisure activities

PRESCRIPTION, APPLICATION, AND, AS APPROPRIATE, FABRICATION OF DEVICES AND EQUIPMENT

- Obtain and install safety grab bar and bench seat in shower

- Obtain specialized swivel walker with hand brakes and bench seat
- Install safety grab bar at door frame of front door to minimize backward balance loss due to retropulsion

ANTICIPATED GOALS AND EXPECTED OUTCOMES

- Impact on impairments
  - Patient demonstrates improved gait stability and safety during community ambulation with use of wheeled walker.
  - Patient demonstrates modified home exercise program correctly.
  - Patient utilizes appropriate compensatory strategies designed for use in "on" and "off" stages of motor fluctuations.
- Impact on functional limitations
  - Patient demonstrates improved safety and reduced balance loss when turning, reaching, carrying items, and opening doors.
- Impact on disabilities
  - Patient and wife verbalize awareness of compensatory strategies for use when traveling away from home.
  - Performance levels in self-care, home management, work, community, and leisure actions, tasks, and activities are improved.
  - Wife demonstrates understanding of appropriate verbal cueing strategies to use when assisting patient.
- Risk reduction/prevention
  - Fall risk is reduced through patient understanding and use of compensatory strategies to minimize freezing, festination, and retropulsion.
  - Patient and wife are able to identify potential risk situations that increase freezing and/or retropulsion, as well as environmental modifications to reduce risks.
  - Patient and wife demonstrate improved safety and good body mechanics during patient transfers off floor.
  - Patient utilizes joint protection equipment to reduce fall injury risk.
- Impact on societal resources
  - Communication enhances risk reduction and prevention.
  - Decision making is enhanced regarding patient's health and the use of health care resources by patient, family, significant others, and caregivers.
  - Documentation occurs throughout patient management and follows APTA's *Guidelines for Physical Therapy Documentation.*[78]

♦ Patient/client satisfaction
  • Access, availability, and services provided are acceptable to patient.
  • Care is coordinated with patient, family, and other health care professionals.
  • Patient and family knowledge and awareness of the diagnosis, prognosis, interventions, and anticipated goals and expected outcomes are increased.
  • Referrals are made to other professionals or resources whenever necessary and appropriate.

REEXAMINATION

Reexamination is performed throughout this third episode of care.

DISCHARGE

Mr. Barris is discharged from physical therapy after a total of eight physical therapy visits and attainment of his goals. As Mr. Barris has a condition that may require multiple episodes of care throughout his life span, Mr. Barris received education regarding factors that may trigger a call to his physical therapist for a reexamination and new episode of physical therapy care.

PSYCHOLOGICAL ASPECTS

Mood and affect may be affected in those with PD.[114] Depression, anxiety, and apathy are recognized to be part of the symptom profile. These psychological aspects are important to recognize and consider when one attempts to motivate patients to comply with a long-range intervention program of compensation strategies, consistent use of assistive devices, and follow through with the home exercise program.

Case Study #1D: Stage 5 Parkinson's Disease

Mr. Barris is now a 79-year-old male who was diagnosed with PD 16 years ago. He is currently seeking physical therapy services due to immobility and complaints of being uncomfortable in his current wheelchair.

PHYSICAL THERAPIST EXAMINATION

Note: Only changes from his previous episodes are included in this case.

HISTORY

♦ General demographics: Mr. Barris is now a 79-year-old male.

♦ Social history: Mr. Barris and his wife moved 2 years ago from Chicago to Minneapolis to be near their daughter.

♦ Living environment: He and his wife live in an assisted living apartment in suburban Minneapolis. They receive daily in-home assistance from the assisted living staff for morning and evening care, bathing, and medication administration. Mrs. Barris provides supervision and assistance at other times of day. Congregate dining is available three times per day. Mrs. Barris assists with meal set up and feeding as needed.

♦ General health status
  • General health perception: Mr. Barris reports continual overall decline in his health and quality of life, noting loss of ability to participate in past leisure interests like travel, difficulty communicating with others, weight loss, and problems swallowing.
  • Physical function: Mr. Barris requires assistance for transfers. He currently ambulates only short distances from his wheelchair to the bathroom with a U-step walker and the assistance of one person twice a day. He experiences episodes of urinary incontinence.
  • Psychological function: He has continued decline in short-term memory and significant bradyphrenia. He is now also experiencing episodes of confusion, and his wife reports that he has visual hallucinations, usually occurring at night.
  • Role function: Husband and father, but wife and daughter have assumed roles of making decisions, handling finances, and managing other household decisions.
  • Social function: He is becoming more isolated with few social contacts and difficulty communicating with others. He rarely attends activities and events within the assisted living community with his wife. While he and his wife were very active in church activities prior to moving 2 years ago to this area, they have not connected with a faith community since then.

♦ Medical/surgical history: His PD was diagnosed 16 years ago. He sustained a right hip fracture 5 years ago that was treated with open reduction internal fixation (ORIF) surgery. He has also experienced weight loss of 12 pounds over the past 4 months.

♦ Prior hospitalizations: He had an appendectomy at age 36, bowel obstruction surgery at age 67, left TKR surgery at age 68, and a right hip fracture with ORIF at age 74.

♦ Preexisting medical and other health-related conditions:

He has depression, OH controlled by medications, occasional complaints of dizziness during transfers and assisted ambulation, confusion, and hallucinations. His cognitive changes have been improved somewhat over the past 6 weeks with the introduction of Seroquel into his medication schedule.

♦ Current condition(s)/chief complaint(s): Mr. Barris is increasingly immobile with inability to perform independent position change. He has a reddened area on his coccyx that was noted by the assisted living staff while providing care assistance. He complains of being uncomfortable when seated in his current wheelchair.

♦ Functional status and activity level: He requires the assistance of the assisted living staff to perform bed, chair, and toilet transfers. He ambulates only 10 to 20 feet with the U-step walker and the assist of one during transfers between bed, wheelchair, and toilet. Mr. Barris sits in the wheelchair for most of the day and uses his wheelchair as his primary mode of transport, transferring to a recliner for a brief rest period each afternoon. He frequently complains of back and knee pain after 1 to 2 hours in the chair. He requires assistance for wheelchair propulsion. Mrs. Barris is with her husband at all times due to episodic confusion and hallucinations, and she appears stressed by her role as caregiver, complaining of fatigue. His sedentary lifestyle includes watching TV and enjoying classical music.

♦ Medications: Carbidopa/levodopa, Proamatine, Seroquel.

SYSTEMS REVIEW

♦ Cardiovascular/pulmonary
  ● BP
    ■ Sitting: 110/62 mmHg
    ■ Standing: 100/54 mmHg
  ● HR: 60 bpm and regular
  ● RR: 18 bpm

♦ Integumentary
  ● Presence of scar formation: Well-healed incisional scars on abdomen, left knee, and right hip from previous surgeries
  ● Skin color: Reddened pressure area noted on coccyx and reddened area also noted in the perineal area due to episodic urinary incontinence
  ● Skin integrity: Skin intact at reddened pressure area on coccyx

♦ Musculoskeletal
  ● Gross range of motion
    ■ Decreased neck and spinal flexibility
    ■ Limitations noted in all four extremities due to muscle rigidity

  ● Gross strength: General weakness and immobility due to moderate to severe rigidity
  ● Gross symmetry
    ■ Significantly increased forward head, thoracic kyphosis, right and forward trunk lean, and hip and knee flexion
    ■ Unable to make good eye contact when sitting in wheelchair
  ● Height: 5'9" (1.75 m)
  ● Weight: 154 lbs (69.85 kg)

♦ Neuromuscular
  ● Balance: Unable to stand unsupported and has history of multiple falls
  ● Locomotion, transfers, and transitions
    ■ He ambulates only short distances using his U-step stabilizer
    ■ He has frequent freezing episodes and has difficulty using cues effectively due to reduced memory and other cognitive changes
    ■ He requires the assistance of a transfer belt and one person when ambulating due to frequent balance loss
    ■ He uses his wheelchair as primary mode of transport

♦ Communication, affect, cognition, language, and learning style
  ● He has decreased voice volume with absent facial expression
  ● His speech is now frequently unintelligible
  ● His cognitive decline has continued to include severe short-term memory deficits, profound bradyphrenia, episodic confusion, and visual hallucinations
  ● Learning style
    ■ He requires frequent repetition and cueing due to memory deficits and confusion, responding best to simple, one-step instructions
    ■ Mrs. Barris prefers written programs

TESTS AND MEASURES

♦ Arousal, attention, and cognition
  ● Poor short-term memory
  ● Profound bradyphrenia
  ● Episodes of confusion and hallucinations reported
  ● MMSE[115,116] is a screening tool to assess cognitive impairment in older adults that can be administered in a brief period of time and is practical for repeated or routine use
    ■ It is an 11-question measure that tests five areas of cognitive function: orientation, registration, attention and calculation, recall, and language (see www.minimental.com/MSRS)

- Maximum score is 30, and a score of 23 or lower is indicative of cognitive impairment
- Patient scores
  - Orientation: 6/10
  - Registration: 2/3
  - Attention and calculation: 2/5
  - Recall: 1/3
  - Language: 5/9
  - Total score: 15/30

◆ Assistive and adaptive devices
- U-step stabilizer with reverse brake mechanism
- Manual folding wheelchair with fixed upright back rest, standard fixed arm rests, and standard removable leg and foot rests
- Currently sits on standard 3-inch vinyl covered foam cushion when up in wheelchair

◆ Ergonomics and body mechanics
- Observations of transfers and care provided to patient by his wife, daughter, and assisted living staff revealed patient to have poor postural alignment and positioning in bed at night and an inadequate repositioning schedule while up in the wheelchair during the day

◆ Gait, locomotion, and balance
- He ambulates only short distances (10 to 20 feet) using his U-step stabilizer with reverse brake mechanism and freezing laser light compensation device
- He ambulates with a narrow base of support with flexed hips and knees and numerous short shuffling steps and with a tendency to walk on tiptoes
- He has frequent freezing episodes when walking and has extreme difficulty turning to sit down on the bed or toilet
- He requires moderate assistance of one person when ambulating due to frequent balance loss
- He uses his manual wheelchair as his primary mode of transport

◆ Integumentary integrity
- Assessment of skin characteristics revealed redness on his coccyx after sitting in his current wheelchair for less than 1 hour
- No skin breakdown or blistering observed at this time
- Skin redness is also evident in perineal area due to episodes of urinary incontinence

◆ Motor function
- UPDRS[21] motor section scores
  - Speech: Grade 3=marked impairment, difficult to understand
  - Facial expression: Grade 4=masked or fixed faces with severe or complete loss of facial expression, lips parted a quarter inch or more

- Tremor at rest
  - RUE: Grade 1=slight and infrequently present
  - RLE: Grade 0=absent
  - LUE: Grade 3=moderate in amplitude and present most of the time
  - LLE: Grade 2=mild in amplitude and persistent or moderate in amplitude but only intermittently present
- Action or postural tremor of hands: Grade 2=moderate in amplitude and present with action
- Rigidity
  - RUE: Grade 4=severe and ROM achieved with difficulty
  - RLE: Grade 4=severe and ROM achieved with difficulty
  - LUE: Grade 4=severe and ROM achieved with difficulty
  - LLE: Grade 4=severe and ROM achieved with difficulty
- Finger taps: Grade 4=can barely perform the task
- Hand movements: Grade 3=severely impaired and frequent hesitation in initiating movements or arrest of ongoing movement
- Rapid alternating movements of hands: Grade 4=can barely perform the task
- Leg agility
  - RLE: Grade 4=can barely perform the task
  - LLE: Grade 4=can barely perform the task
- Arising from chair: Grade 4=unable to arise without help
- Posture: Grade 4=marked flexion with extreme abnormality of posture
- Gait: Grade 3=severe disturbance of gait, requiring assistance
- Postural stability: Grade 4=unable to stand without assistance
- Body bradykinesia and hypokinesia: Grade 4=marked slowness and poverty or small amplitude of movement

◆ Muscle performance
- Unable to demonstrate independent weight shift or position change in bed or wheelchair due to akinesia, severe muscle rigidity, and generalized weakness
- Requires moderate assistance of one person to rise from wheelchair
- Unable to stand without physical support
- Able to assist in transfers and supported standing position by holding on to grab bar in bathroom

◆ Pain
- Pain in neck, low back, and knees when seated in the wheelchair

- Cognition prevents using subjective 0 to 10 NPS for rating pain
- Wife states patient reports pain several times per day, most often during and after meals when seated in wheelchair
- Generalized hip and knee pain with all standing or weightbearing activities that appears to increase as patient attempts to turn during pivot transfers

◆ Posture
  - Photographic assessment and observation of sitting posture in current wheelchair shows significant forward head, thoracic kyphosis, and trunk flexion, with significant lean to right side
  - Poor eye contact while sitting, impacting communication and interaction with external environment
  - Occasionally drowsy during day and dozes in wheelchair with head flexed forward, which contributes to poor posture
  - Poor sitting posture exacerbates swallowing difficulties
  - Standing posture exhibits all of the changes noted in sitting and hip and knee flexion

◆ Range of motion
  - Hip and knee flexion contractures so that he is unable to fully extend hips or knees when in assisted standing position
    - Bilateral hip flexor tightness (20 degree flexion contracture bilaterally)
    - Bilateral hamstring tightness (30 degree flexion contractures bilaterally)
  - Severe muscle rigidity noted in all four extremities

◆ Self-care and home management
  - A general lack of protocol exists for patient care with each aide performing transfers and assistance cues differently, thus contributing to the patient's inability to consistently assist in his care
  - Family members and staff note difficulty performing transfers with the patient, as he has extreme difficulty turning and frequently complains of knee pain during attempts to perform pivot transfers
  - He occasionally reclines in electric lift chair during day
  - Wife or assisted living staff assists with position changes, bed mobility, and toileting
  - Care assistance is becoming increasingly difficult for wife to perform due to her advancing age and own health concerns, which include osteoporosis and history of coronary artery disease with myocardial infarction

EVALUATION

Mr. Barris' history and risk factors previously outlined indicate that he is a 79-year-old male with a diagnosis of Stage 5 PD based on the Hoehn and Yahr rating scale.[20] He demonstrates risk for secondary impairments and skin breakdown due to severe rigidity with resulting inability to perform independent position change, transfers, or ambulation. OH, pain, and cognitive dysfunction are also noted.

DIAGNOSIS

Mr. Barris is a patient with a diagnosis of Stage 5 PD and has pain in his neck, low back, hips, and knees. He has impaired: arousal, attention, and cognition; ergonomics and body mechanics; gait, locomotion, and balance; integumentary integrity; motor function; muscle performance; posture; and range of motion. He is functionally limited in self-care and home management actions, tasks, and activities. He is in need of devices and equipment. These findings are consistent with placement in Pattern E: Impaired Motor Function and Sensory Integrity Associated With Progressive Disorders of the Central Nervous System and in Integumentary Pattern A: Primary Prevention/Risk Reduction for Integumentary Disorders in the APTA's *Guide to Physical Therapist Practice*.[78] The identified impairments, functional limitations, and device and equipment needs will be addressed in determining the prognosis and the plan of care.

In this aspect of Mr. Barris' case, it is his risk of integumentary disorders due to severe rigidity, dependent mobility, and inability to perform independent position change that will drive the primary interventions for this episode of care along with all of the other needs identified during the examination.

PROGNOSIS AND PLAN OF CARE

Over the course of the visits, the following mutually established outcomes have been determined:
◆ Integumentary integrity is improved
◆ New seating system is obtained
◆ Patient, family, and assisted living staff are trained in positioning, body mechanics, and transfer techniques
◆ Risk of integumentary disorders is decreased
◆ Tolerance of sitting position is increased

To achieve these outcomes, the appropriate interventions for this patient are determined. These will include: coordination, communication, and documentation; patient/client-related instruction; therapeutic exercise; functional training in self-care and home management; functional training in work, community, and leisure integration or reintegration; and prescription, application, and, as appropriate, fabrication of devices and equipment.

The *Guide*[78] takes into consideration that patients placed in these patterns have progressive conditions that may have ongoing impairments, functional limitations, and disabilities. Mr. Barris is expected to need four visits over 30 days. He continues to have good social support that will follow through with his home program. He is now significantly impaired and is becoming increasingly at risk for health complications due to impaired cognitive function, dysphagia, and increasing immobility. The health care team is currently using a palliative care model to guide decisions concerning his heath care.

INTERVENTIONS

RATIONALE FOR SELECTED INTERVENTIONS

As PD advances, significant deficits in both physical function and cognitive status may occur.[117,118] A palliative care model has been suggested to manage the complex symptom profile often seen in patients with PD.[119] This model of care helps to ensure that needs are addressed through both pharmacological and nonpharmacological interventions to give patients and family caregivers the best possible quality of life. The focus of physical therapy within the palliative care model will be directed toward patient safety, comfort, and caregiver support.

Increasing immobility puts patients with advanced stage PD at risk for changes in skin integrity. Margolis and associates[120] found that the presence of certain medical conditions, like PD, is associated with the risk of developing pressure ulcers. Deaths associated with pressure ulcers have also been shown to occur more frequently in PD than in age-matched controls.[121] Development of an appropriate seating system and positioning schedule can significantly reduce these risks.

Caregiver instruction in a simple assisted exercise program can also aid in maximizing flexibility and improving patient comfort. These exercises should be designed to be easily incorporated into the daily routine in an effort to maximize likelihood of follow through and reduced caregiver stress. Examples of these exercises may include adding a few extra arm and leg motions during assisted dressing and bathing or performing assisted standing at a grab bar or counter to increase LE weightbearing and ability to retain transfer skills. Involvement in adapted recreational tasks (throwing and catching activities, therapeutic horticulture,[122] or movement to music[123]) also may be successfully used as part of a movement and exercise program.

Injuries may be seen more frequently in family members caring for an elderly or chronically ill person at home.[124] Physical therapy assessment and instruction in proper body mechanics, transfer training, and use of adaptive equipment may reduce caregiver injury risk. Assessment and education relating to caregiver health, stress management, and referral to support services may also be appropriate.[125]

COORDINATION, COMMUNICATION, AND DOCUMENTATION

Communication will occur with the patient, his wife, and his physician during the course of treatment. Mr. Barris and his wife will receive information about the benefits of a comprehensive interdisciplinary team approach to management of PD and will be provided with resources on how to access appropriate team members as needs are identified. Appropriate referrals will be made, including referral to a speech pathologist due to reported swallowing difficulties, a social worker to assist his wife with resources for caregiver respite, and a chaplain to provide spiritual assessment and intervention for both the patient and his wife. Interdisciplinary teamwork will occur through information exchange at team rounds, including discussion about the patient's depression and its impact on his quality of life. All elements of the patient's management will be documented.

PATIENT/CLIENT-RELATED INSTRUCTION

Education will continue regarding his current condition (increasing disability and risk of integumentary disorders). In addition, he and his wife will receive instruction regarding the plan of care including:

♦ Enhancement of performance through development of a schedule for assisted patient position change

♦ Instruction, education, and training of his wife, daughter, and assisted living staff regarding plans for intervention and risk factors related to current and new positioning and seating system

♦ Instruction, education, and training of patient, wife, daughter, and assisted living staff regarding proper body mechanics when assisting patient with position change, ambulation, and transfers

THERAPEUTIC EXERCISE

♦ Body mechanics and postural stabilization
  • Body mechanics training for wife, daughter, and assisted living staff when providing patient assistance during position changes, transfers, and ambulation
♦ Flexibility exercises
  • Assisted ROM exercises with patient twice daily
  • Instruct caregivers in use of music or recreational activities (such as simple games) to achieve increased ROM
♦ Gait and locomotion training
  • Assisted ambulation several times per day with development of short verbal cues to be used consistently by wife, daughter, and assisted living staff
  • Use of transfer belt during ambulation
♦ Strength, power, and endurance training

- LE strengthening, including assisted supported standing at grab bar and allowing LE weightbearing

FUNCTIONAL TRAINING IN SELF-CARE AND HOME MANAGEMENT

- ◆ Self-care
  - Injury prevention or reduction during assisted position change, transfers, and ambulation with use of devices or equipment
  - Safety awareness training during common ADL tasks
  - Use of pivot disc to assist during transfers and reduce torque on patient's painful knee joints during attempts to pivot
  - Instruction in appropriate body mechanics of care assistants

FUNCTIONAL TRAINING IN WORK, COMMUNITY, AND LEISURE INTEGRATION OR REINTEGRATION

- ◆ Community
  - Increased sitting tolerance and comfort to allow patient to attend activities within the assisted living community

PRESCRIPTION, APPLICATION, AND, AS APPROPRIATE, FABRICATION OF DEVICES AND EQUIPMENT

- ◆ Develop seating system, including seat cushion, for improved posture and positioning in wheelchair with decreased integumentary risk
- ◆ Modify current wheelchair to include a reclining back rest, desk style arm rests, and elevating leg rests
- ◆ Instruct family and assisted living staff in use of pivot disc to assist transfer safety and comfort

ANTICIPATED GOALS AND EXPECTED OUTCOMES

- ◆ Impact on impairments
  - Optimal joint alignment and positioning is achieved though wheelchair modification.
  - Pressure on body tissues is reduced through use of new gel-filled wheelchair cushion and with follow through with repositioning schedule.
  - Skin redness is no longer present after sitting in wheelchair 3 to 4 hours.
- ◆ Impact on functional limitations
  - Eye contact and interaction with external environment are improved through modification of current seating system.
  - Participation in care is enhanced through use of consistent care routine and cueing strategies used by family members and assisted living staff.
  - Positioning for eating and swallowing through wheelchair modification is improved.
  - Safety and joint comfort are improved through use of pivot disc during transfers.
- ◆ Impact on disabilities
  - Sitting in wheelchair is tolerated for 3 to 4 hours, allowing attendance at selected activities in the assisted living community.
- ◆ Risk reduction/prevention
  - Risk factors for skin breakdown are reduced through improved seating system and repositioning schedule.
  - Safety and body mechanics during positioning, transfers, and ambulation are improved for patient, family, and assisted living staff through use of consistent care plan and cueing.
- ◆ Impact on societal resources
  - Communication with interdisciplinary health care team and assisted living staff enhances risk reduction and prevention.
  - Decision making for palliative care is enhanced through the use of health care resources by patient, family, significant others, and caregivers.
  - Documentation occurs throughout patient management and follows APTA's *Guidelines for Physical Therapy Documentation*.[78]
- ◆ Patient/client satisfaction
  - Access, availability, and services provided are acceptable to patient and family.
  - Care is coordinated with patient, family, and other health care professionals.
  - Patient and family knowledge and awareness of the diagnosis, prognosis, interventions, and anticipated goals and expected outcomes are increased.
  - Referrals are made to other professionals or resources whenever necessary and appropriate.
  - Sense of well-being is improved.

REEXAMINATION

Reexamination is performed throughout the episode of care.

DISCHARGE

Mr. Barris is discharged from physical therapy after a total of four physical therapy visits over 30 days and attainment of his goals. Mr. Barris and his wife received education regarding factors that may trigger a call to his physical therapist for a reexamination and new episode of physical therapy care.

PSYCHOLOGICAL ASPECTS

Many patients and their family care partners must leave their long-time living environment to move closer to family members or enter residential facilities where more care assistance is available. These transitions can be disruptive to existing social activities and support systems, leaving both patient and care partner more isolated. Numerous caregiving responsibilities frequently overwhelm family caregivers. Adequate caregiver respite and support is needed to reduce caregiver stress. Input into the intervention plan is important as patients and families strive to retain an element of control over their situation, and appropriate referrals to additional services should always be considered.

Case Study #2: Multiple Sclerosis

Mrs. Linda Bernard is a 53-year-old female who was diagnosed with multiple sclerosis 12 years ago and is currently experiencing increasing weakness, balance loss, and dizziness.

PHYSICAL THERAPIST EXAMINATION

HISTORY

♦ General demographics: Linda Bernard is a 53-year-old white female, who is right handed.

♦ Social history: Ms. Bernard lives with her friend and daughter. She has three children (two adult daughters not living at home, who are 28 and 23 years of age, and her daughter living at home, who is 10 years of age). She is divorced, and her ex-husband is not active in her family situation.

♦ Employment/work: Ms. Bernard is a licensed practical nurse who works 4 hours a day, four times a week as a medical nurse. She collects disability for the remaining hours.

♦ Living environment: Ms. Bernard lives in a raised ranch-style house. There are railings on the two stairs to get in the house and on the two sets of six stairs inside the home.

♦ General health status
  • General health perception: Considering her diagnosis of MS, Ms. Bernard perceives her health to be fair to good at this time.

• Physical function: Ms. Bernard reports that she has become progressively less active, feeling increased weakness and fatigue. She is not using any assistive devices, but is experiencing falls more frequently. She attributes this to the "heaviness and sometimes dragging" of her left foot. When she goes to the grocery store, she relies on the use of a grocery cart for support. She is still able to do things around the house without difficulty, such as dusting, washing dishes, and doing the laundry. However, she is having more difficulty with heavy work. She wishes to get stronger, be able to walk and not fall, and to improve her endurance. She wants to continue to be an active parent for her child.

• Psychological function: Ms. Bernard admits to feeling very depressed and says that she cries often. She denies having suicidal ideation.

• Role function: Mother, friend, homemaker, employee, community member.

• Social function: Ms. Bernard lives with her friend and her youngest daughter. She states that many of her social activities revolve around driving and participating in her daughter's activities, such as school, dance, and soccer. Ms. Bernard has been active in the PTA of her daughter's school. She particularly enjoys the theater, music, and movies.

♦ Social/health habits: Ms. Bernard smoked for 20 years, but has not done so in the past 2 years. She is a social drinker. She does not have a history of drug abuse.

♦ Family history: Ms. Bernard has three daughters ages 28, 23 and 10. They all have health issues, including high BP, tuberculosis exposure, and asthma, respectively. She gives evidence of a "difficult" family situation with her mother and father, who are both in their 70s. They live nearby, but they are not available for assistance. Ms. Bernard's mother also has MS and was diagnosed 30 years ago and is now confined to a wheelchair.

♦ Medical/surgical history: Ms. Bernard was diagnosed with MS 12 years ago.

♦ Current condition(s)/chief complaint(s): She currently reports many symptoms related to her MS, including memory loss, depression, dizziness, weakness on one side of her body, balance difficulties, difficulty walking, asthma, shortness of breath, and indigestion.

♦ Functional status and activity level: Ms. Bernard states that over the past few months she has been falling more frequently, usually once a week, she feels unsteady, and is having difficulty on stairs. "I feel like I am going downhill very quickly." She also has been experiencing fatigue when climbing the stairs at her daughter's school, having to stop and rest one or two times. There is a railing on the right when ascending and descending.

◆ Medications: Copaxone 20 mg sub qd, Lexapro 10 mg qd, Xanax 0.25 mg qd, Proventil inhaler, albuterol inhaler.

◆ Other clinical tests
  • MRI spectroscopy
    ▪ Showed two areas of increased T2 signal intensity in the left subependymal white matter adjacent to the precentral sulcus and in the right medullary pyramid
    ▪ Felt to represent demyelinating disease
    ▪ Normal spectroscopy in the left frontal lobe lesion
  • CSF IgG index: Elevated
  • Evoked potential showed delayed but well-preserved wave form

SYSTEMS REVIEW

◆ Cardiovascular/pulmonary
  • BP: 130/80 mmHg
  • Edema: Mild swelling at Copaxone injection sites
  • HR: 80 bpm
  • RR: 12 bpm

◆ Integumentary
  • Presence of scar formation: None noted
  • Skin color: Redness at injection sites, which she states lasts about 1 week after injection
  • Skin integrity: Lipodystrophy secondary to Copaxone in the thighs and abdomen

◆ Musculoskeletal
  • Gross range of motion: WNL throughout all extremities
  • Gross strength
    ▪ Both UEs and RLE: WNL
    ▪ LLE: Decreased strength
  • Gross symmetry: Not impaired
  • Height: 5'4" (1.62 m)
  • Weight: 150 lbs (68.04 kg)

◆ Neuromuscular
  • Balance: Reports increasing balance problems
  • Locomotion, transfers, and transitions
    ▪ Ambulates without assistive devices, but feels unsteady and complains of fatigue
    ▪ No difficulty with transfers or transitions at this time
    ▪ Fatigue with elevation activities

◆ Communication, affect, cognition, language, and learning style
  • Communication, affect, and cognition
    ▪ Able to follow directions and communicate well verbally

▪ Oriented x3 (person, place, and time)
    ▪ Ms. Bernard was teary at times and appeared to be anxious when the task was difficult
  • Learning style and barriers
    ▪ She states that she is a visual learner
    ▪ Barriers to learning include decreased memory (reported by the patient)

TESTS AND MEASURES

◆ Aerobic capacity/endurance
  • Endurance: 150 feet (without assistive device) before fatigue on level surfaces

◆ Arousal, attention, and cognition
  • Oriented x3
  • Memory
    ▪ Difficulties with short-term memory, recalling names and phone numbers
    ▪ Scored 8/10 on the Short Portable Mental Status Questionnaire (SPMSQ), which when adjusted for age and race indicates a mild cognitive impairment[126]
  • Sleep habits: Wakes frequently and has difficulty falling asleep
  • Communicates well
  • Cooperative and motivated

◆ Anthropometric characteristics
  • BMI=705 x (body weight [in pounds] divided by height [in inches])[127]
  • Ms. Bernard's BMI=25.8
  • BMI values between 25 and 29.9 are considered overweight[128]

◆ Assistive and adaptive devices
  • Bracing will be needed to decrease foot drop and to improve balance and endurance during ambulation
  • Assistive devices will be needed for ambulation
  • Assistive devices for the home will be needed to ensure an optimal level of safe function
  • Wheelchair will be considered for transport and use in the community and/or home

◆ Cranial and peripheral nerve integrity
  • Extraocular movements intact without nystagmus, left pupil 4 mm, right 3 mm, both reactive
  • Visual fields full
  • Cranial nerve V: Intact
  • Face moves symmetrically with intact sensation and tongue is midline

◆ Environmental, home, and work barriers
  • Home
    ▪ Raised ranch with two stairs to get in with railings on both sides

- In the home there are two sets of six stairs (going up and down to each level) with railings on both sides
- Bathroom has shower chair
- Additional modifications will be needed
- Work
  - Patient works in a nursing home that is accessible
  - No further examination was indicated
- Gait, locomotion, and balance
  - Sitting balance: No problems demonstrated
  - Standing balance
    - Limited excursion of reach without moving feet
    - Loss of balance with one leg stance and with change in bases of support that increase the demands on trunk performance (ie, a narrow base of support with feet placed together or while on unstable surface)
  - Ambulates without assistive devices
    - Narrow base of support
    - Foot drop on left with mild dragging of the left foot after prolonged walking
    - Difficulty with tandem walking on a flat surface
  - Elevation activities
    - Fatigues easily with stair climbing, even with use of the railing
    - Unable to ascend more than three stairs without a rail
  - Score on Tinetti Assessment Tool for Balance and Gait: 20/28
    - Patients who score below 19 are at high risk for fall
    - Patients who score in the range of 19 to 24 are considered at risk for fall[129-131]
  - Kurtzke Expanded Disability Status Scale (EDSS)
    - Score: 5.0
    - Able to ambulate for about 150 feet when fatigue sets in, indicating that the disability is severe enough to impair full daily activities (eg, to work a full day without special provisions)[132-135]
    - The ordinal EDSS is a reliable and valid measure of impairment and disability
    - It assesses disease severity and the ability to ambulate, to use the upper limbs, and to communicate and swallow on a scale from 0 (normal status) to 10 (death due to MS)[27,134,135]
- Motor function
  - Fine motor skills: WNL
  - Muscle tone or spasticity
    - Minimal increase in tone in LLE distally
    - Patient reports some "stiffness" and occasional night spasms in both LEs

- Modified Ashworth Scale: 1[133,136]
- Trunk: Exhibits stiffening of the trunk with attempts to perform difficult activities with LEs and also when the base of support is decreased or unstable
- Muscle performance
  - MMT
    - Both UEs: 5/5
    - Iliopsoas: R=5/5, L=4+/5
    - Quadriceps: R= 5/5, L=5/5
    - Hamstrings: R=5/5, L=4+/5
    - Tibialis anterior: R=5/5, L=3/5
    - Medial gastrocnemius: R=5/5, L=4+/5
- Neuromotor development and sensory integration
  - No problems with coordination or sensory integration noted in the UEs
  - No finger to nose dysmetria
  - Mild coordination impairments in the LEs with heel to shin and rapid alternating movements
  - Mild swaying on Romberg test
  - No apparent abnormalities of visual-spatial perception
- Posture: Slight elevation of shoulders in standing
- Range of motion: PROM WNL
- Reflex integrity
  - UEs: 2+ bilaterally
  - LEs deep tendon reflexes
    - 3+ knees
    - 4+ ankles with three beats of clonus on the left and two on the right
  - Positive Babinski bilaterally
- Self-care and home management
  - Transfers/transitions
    - Supine to sit and sit to supine: No difficulty, however she does use one arm to push herself to sit
    - Sit to stand
      - Uses one or two arms to assist
      - Able to perform without use of arms but activity is somewhat labored
  - Self-care
    - Uses a shower chair in the tub for bathing
    - Does not have grab bars
    - Sits on the bed or chair when performing LE dressing
  - Home management
    - Able to do light homemaking activities without difficulty, such as dusting, washing dishes, folding laundry, cooking, and light cleaning
    - More difficulty with heavy work, work that requires her to get down to the floor, squat, or climb stairs while carrying things (groceries, laundry basket)

- Sensory integrity
  - Proprioception intact
  - Mild decreased vibratory sense distally in the LEs
- Work, community, and leisure integration or reintegration
  - Gradually cutting back at work and now working only 16 hours a week over the course of 4 days
  - She passes medications in a nursing home and states that all of the information is written and that the job is very structured so she has not had problems with the task itself
  - Primary concern at work is with fatigue, and she has discussed her problems specifically with the nursing supervisor, who is tracking her performance
  - At this time, she continues to drive and has not had difficulty because she has not been experiencing UE or visual-spatial problems and does not have spasms in her legs
  - Community access, especially as it relates to her daughter's soccer activities, has become more difficult secondary to the uneven terrains and her endurance, which worries her
  - She has self-modifying activities (using the grocery cart for support when shopping) and has obtained some devices to help with cleaning and things around the house

EVALUATION

The patient is a 53-year-old female with a 12-year history of MS. At the time of the examination, she demonstrated primary impairments of balance, fatigue, strength, coordination in the LEs, endurance, and cognition, all of which contribute to her decreased functional independence and safety in her home and community environments. Given her diagnosis of MS, a chronic and progressive condition, it was unclear as to what degree of improvement could be expected. She has continued to work, although she has had to cut back. She has a friend who lives with her and who is very supportive of her. These factors were thought to be positive prognostic indicators. It is believed that she will demonstrate good compliance with her home exercise program and therapeutic regimen and this would help to maximize her outcome in therapy.

DIAGNOSIS

Ms. Bernard has had a 12-year diagnosis of MS. She has impaired: aerobic capacity/endurance; anthropometric characteristics; arousal, attention, and cognition; gait, locomotion, and balance; motor function; muscle performance; neuromotor development and sensory integration; posture; reflex integrity; and sensory integrity. She is functionally limited in self-care and home management and in work,

community, and leisure actions, tasks, and activities. She has environmental, work, and community barriers and is in need of assistive devices and equipment. These findings are consistent with placement in Pattern E: Impaired Motor Function and Sensory Integrity Associated With Progressive Disorders of the Central Nervous System. The identified impairments, functional limitations, barriers, and device and equipment needs will be addressed in determining the prognosis and the plan of care.

PROGNOSIS AND PLAN OF CARE

Over the course of the visits, the following mutually established outcomes have been determined:
- Ambulation distance on level indoor surfaces with the use of an assistive device without loss of balance is improved
- Frequency of falls is reduced
- Independence in home exercise program is achieved
- Motor function is improved
- Muscle performance is improved
- Posture is improved
- Relevant community resources to meet discharge needs are identified
- Safety in gait, locomotion, and balance is improved
- Tinetti Scale total score is increased
- Unsupported standing on a variety of surfaces without loss of balance is improved

To achieve these outcomes, the appropriate interventions for this patient are determined. These will include: coordination, communication, and documentation; patient/client-related instruction; therapeutic exercise; functional training in self-care and home management; functional training in work, community, and leisure integration or reintegration; and prescription, application, and, as appropriate, fabrication of devices and equipment. Barriers will be overcome.

It is anticipated that Ms. Bernard will need 16 visits over 8 weeks (twice a week). Although depressed at times, Ms. Bernard is motivated to function at a higher level, and she is in good health.

INTERVENTIONS

RATIONALE FOR SELECTED INTERVENTIONS

MS is a chronic and progressive disorder of the CNS. Because of the chronicity of the disease, often the role of the rehabilitation specialist is to provide education and treatment designed to promote good health and general conditioning and reduce fatigue.[26] With the progression of the disease, the rehabilitation team professionals become more involved with managing symptoms, improving or maintaining function, preserving ADL skills, preventing injury, and augmenting function through assistive devices and environmental modifications.[26] Rehabilitation interventions may be classified as being restorative, improving function, retaining skills, or maintaining function.

Although "MS is characterized by variability and unpredictability,"[26] many symptoms are commonly reported, including fatigue, depression, and cognitive dysfunction. These symptoms, combined with the physical problems associated with MS, contribute to the variability of the disease. The role of the physical therapist is to minimize the impact of existing impairments on the person's ability to function on a day-to-day basis. It is also well-documented that education, medical symptom management, self-care strategies, referrals to other members of the rehab team, and treatment adherence are critical components to effective management of MS.[26,27,78,137-139]

The treatment plan for Ms. Bernard is targeted toward those impairments associated with MS that have been identified in the physical therapist examination, including fatigue, balance, weakness, problems with walking, cognitive changes, and the impact of these on function.

Therapeutic Exercise

Studies on the effect of aerobic exercise in patients with MS has shown that significant improvement in quality of life can be made through changes in physical and psychological well-being and improving functional outcomes.[140-148] Individuals with EDSS scores between 1 and 6 demonstrate the best exercise tolerance.[30] Research has also shown that individuals with MS can achieve the same benefits from exercise programs as people without disabilities if the programs are appropriately modified. Exercise programs need not only to be individually designed, but also modified to accommodate the person's impairments, functional limitations, disability, or activity restriction.[144] In addition to the form of exercise, frequency, intensity, and duration, factors such as fatigue, increased tone, sensory and balance disturbances, and heat intolerance should be considered in the design of a plan of treatment. Vital signs and symptoms of exertion need to be monitored regularly during and after exercise.[27]

Many studies of therapeutic exercise and/or aerobic conditioning have shown improvements in exercise tolerance in subjects with MS with aerobic training and neurological rehabilitation programs when compared with baseline conditions.[140-144,146-148] However, several studies found limited effect on the health-related quality of life.[143,144,149] One study[143] compared aerobic training with a neurological rehabilitation program and found a significant increase in maximum aerobic capacity and work rate in the aerobic training program. The authors suggested that aerobic training may be more effective in improving fitness in patients with MS.

An increase in VO_2 max, lower triglyceride level, low density lipoproteins, increased physical work capacity, and lower skinfold measurements have been experienced by individuals with mild to moderate disability who participated in a 15-week aerobic exercise program for three 40-minute sessions a week.[142] Swimming, treadmill, walking, stationary bikes, rowers, and arm and leg ergometry offer a variety of options for modes of exercise. Recommended exercise parameters to improve aerobic conditioning include[30,150]:

- Frequency of three times per week, alternating days
- Duration 30 minutes per session
- Intensity of 60% to 75% peak HR
- Circuit training may be optimal

An optimal program of increasing the level of physical activity for people with disabilities related to MS would be to integrate "exercise" with "functional training." To accomplish this, Petajan and White[151] created a "physical activity pyramid" model for individuals with MS. This pyramid incorporates at the bottom ADL and IADL, and then goes to modified activities to maximize the level of activity, with active recreation activities increasing the intensity as the individual moves up the pyramid. In the pyramid structure, the most basic physical activities form the base and the most integrated functions are on the top forming a structured exercise program. The overall physical activity at all functional levels may be increased by incorporating appropriate "inefficiencies" into daily activities (ie, parking further away from office and walking). It was reported that individuals with MS with minimum impairment who were 30 to 40 years old were able to engage in aerobic activity at an exercise intensity of 60% to 85% of their peak HR or 50% to 70% of their peak VO_2 for 20- to 30-minute sessions at least three times a week.[151-154]

The use of aerobic exercise in individuals with mild to moderate MS was also supported in a study using a fairly intense program of a 15-week arm and leg ergometry exercise protocol. Participation in the program resulted in improvement in aerobic capacity, strength, depression, anger, and fatigue. Modification of the intensity and duration may be needed for people with more severe disease symptoms.[142]

The need for muscle training in individuals with MS has been underscored in muscle disuse findings. The primary objectives for training programs are to improve decreased oxidative capacity, increased fatigue, and impaired metabolic response to exercise.[155] Petajan and White developed another pyramid exercise model for individuals with MS. This model, a "muscular fitness pyramid," consists of PROM, flexibility exercises combined with resistance, specific muscle strengthening, and moving up to an intensive strength training regime. Different types of programs with modifications for different disabilities are included throughout the program including Tai Chi, yoga, and therapeutic ball exercises; theraband, free weights, and aquatic exercises; and weight training. The weight training protocol recommended consists of three sets of 10 to 12 repetitions though the full ROM, three times a week.[151]

A multitude of factors influence the response to exercise in individuals with MS. Planning an exercise program requires careful attention to these factors.[30] Exacerbations, depending upon the severity, may require modification or suspension of more rigorous portions of the program. Some activities, such as stretching and walking, may still be performed.[156,157] Modifications for muscle weakness or spasticity may be necessary. Equipment or assistive devices may be indicated for successful performance.[153]

Although the typical physiological reaction to submaximal aerobic exercise is expected, HR and BP responses may be dulled because of cardiovascular dysautonomia. In MS, there is a direct relationship between the duration and the extent of the disease and the likelihood of cardiovascular dysautonomia. It is necessary to monitor HR, BP, and RPE during exercise and make appropriate adjustments in intensity.[153,158]

Regulation of body temperature is often a problem with individuals with MS. Uthoff's phenomenon, an increase in body temperature or unfavorable reaction to external heat, which causes fatigue or deterioration of symptoms, often occurs with exercise.[32] Performing exercises in cool environments will assist in meeting the problems of overheating.[153] Quantifiable improvements in motor function, as well as visual function, have been demonstrated through the use of high and low cooling agents.[159] Aquatic exercises and swimming in a cool pool (water temperature at or below 82°F), the use of a cooling vest, ice packs, drinking increased amounts of water, and air conditioning have all been recommended.[146,153,159] Some cooling methods, such as wearing a cooling vest, can be used when a person has to perform an activity outside on a warm day like mowing the lawn. A Schwinn Airdyne bicycle also provides cooling while cycling.[153]

Fatigue is the most common complaint from people with MS. Keeping an activity diary is useful to monitor sleep patterns and the energy expended in certain activities that can also be rated to determine the value of the activity. The type of fatigue (normal muscle, cardiovascular, substitution) can also be differentiated. Schedules can be modified to take into account strenuous activities and to utilize morning times when the body temperature is lower. Adaptive equipment and devices may be used. Rest periods can be scheduled. In addition, education in energy conservation strategies is key to any intervention plan to reduce fatigue.[24,30,160]

Interventions for problems with balance and coordination should be aimed at postural control. Activities such as progression from static holding through activities that increase the postural demands to dynamic postural control may be incorporated into a variety of functional activities. Aquatic exercises, therapeutic ball exercises, and Tai Chi activities may be best used to promote safe and functional balance.[30,146,153]

COORDINATION, COMMUNICATION, AND DOCUMENTATION

Communication will occur with Ms. Bernard's youngest daughter, her friend (housemate), two older daughters, and other members of the multidisciplinary rehabilitation team (medical director, occupational therapist, and speech therapist as appropriate).[26,161] A referral to a neuropsychologist will be discussed with the team because of the presence of depression and memory deficits[26,162] All elements of the patient's management will be documented. Discharge needs will be determined, and discharge planning will be coordinated with all concerned. Follow-up visits will be scheduled at 3-month intervals.

PATIENT/CLIENT-RELATED INSTRUCTION

Education must be a major focus of intervention when working with patients with chronic or progressive disorders. The patient and family will be instructed in the current condition and reasons for the patient's current impairments and functional limitations. Information will also be provided to them regarding community resources for additional support. Ms. Bernard and her family and friend will be involved in the development of the plan of care. They will be taught techniques for energy conservation and fall prevention and techniques to assist Ms. Bernard with safe mobility. Use of a written and pictorial home program will be used to maximize compliance and help to circumvent barriers because of cognitive problems.

Information will be provided regarding the effect of MS on physical and cognitive functioning, ways to improve functional independence at home, and fall risk reduction (eg, use of assistive devices). Factors that would indicate a need for re-referral to physical therapy will also be provided. Risk factors, such as further motor weakness, spasticity, functional decline, bowel and bladder dysfunction, visual disturbances, and cognitive decline, will also be discussed.

THERAPEUTIC EXERCISE

♦ Aerobic capacity/endurance conditioning: For an individual with MS, the optimal recommended aerobic program consists of 30 to 60 minutes of activity with 5 to 15 minutes of warm-up, 20 to 30 minutes of aerobic conditioning at the THR, followed by 5 to 15 minutes of cool down[27,30,150,163-165]
  - Mode
    - LE and arm ergonometry
    - Treadmill training progressing to side stepping and walking backward on the treadmill
    - Aquatic therapy program[145] in a pool with cool

water, starting at chest level with a walking program (contact local MS society to determine if there is a local aquatic program targeted for people with MS or for people with disabilities)

- Duration
  - All activities will be time based, so that if Ms. Bernard tolerates 10 minutes, she will start at 8 minutes and progress each session by 5% to 10% as tolerated[166] up to 30 minutes
- Intensity
  - 60% to 75% of THR
  - Use Borg RPE[167,168]
    - 0=Nothing at all
    - 0.5=Very, very light weak (just noticeable)
    - 1=Very light weak
    - 2=Light weak
    - 3=Moderate
    - 4=Somewhat heavy/strong
    - 5=Heavy/strong
    - 6
    - 7=Very heavy/strong
    - 8
    - 9
    - 10 Extremely heavy/strong (almost maximal)
- Frequency: Three times per week, alternating days
- Eventually join a gym for treadmill, bike, or stepper as able

◆ Balance, coordination, and agility training
- Sitting balance
  - On exercise ball, bounce gently and maintain balance
  - Progress to inclusion of UE and hand activities, such as clapping, catching a ball, jumping jacks while seated on exercise ball
- Standing balance to include tasks that require trunk stability while moving the LEs[169,170]
  - Moving in standing with a variety of foot positions, changing the surface
  - Stepping one foot up to a stool alternating feet
  - Standing with one foot on a stool playing catch
  - Standing with one foot on a mobile surface (playground size ball), rolling the ball in a variety of positions, kicking the ball, and holding the ball while the physical therapist attempts to move it
  - Standing weight shifting, stepping to the side, stepping across, braiding
  - Stepping over objects
  - Jumping with feet landing on different colors (use a Twister mat)
  - Line dancing and dancing on a floor mat
  - Balance boards

- Mini trampoline
◆ Body mechanics and postural stabilization
- Focus on maintaining trunk stability while moving limbs (arm and legs) while providing manual resistance
- Vary demands on trunk by changing the height and size of the base of support (eg, quadruped, kneeling, half kneeling)
- Sit on exercise ball maintaining stability while the physical therapist attempts to move the ball
- Sit on exercise ball and move with lower trunk initiated movements in all directions
◆ Gait and locomotion training
- Walk indoors and outdoors on a variety of surfaces
- Walk and manage doorways and other environmental barriers
- Gradually increase number of tasks performed at one time while walking (talking and walking, carrying items that require attention and walking, looking for objects while walking, crossing the street in traffic)
- Changing the temporal-distance requirements of gait
◆ Strength, power, and endurance training
- T, X, and Y exercises for UE strengthening
  - Begin with strongest elastic band that patient can use with arms extended at sides
  - T: Bring both arms out to the side to shoulder level (abduction) and back down
  - X: Bring both arms up and out to the side and then cross down and in
  - Y: Bring both arms up and out
- Isokinetic strengthening of the LEs with focus on the right iliopsoas, hamstrings, tibialis anterior, and medial gastrocnemius
- Functional strengthening
  - Repeated sit to/from stand
  - Marching in place
  - Toe and heel walking
- Endurance training can be enhanced by decreasing rest time during therapy sessions

FUNCTIONAL TRAINING IN SELF-CARE AND HOME MANAGEMENT

◆ Self-care and home management
- Reinforce self-care and home management actions, tasks, and activities to include ADL training and use of assistive and adaptive devices and equipment during ADL[161]
- A home evaluation would be ideal, providing the most task-specific assessment of readiness of the patient and family to manage at home and predict areas of difficulty

◆ Injury prevention or reduction
  ● Instruction in energy conservation and fatigue management at home
  ● Instruction in safe techniques to assist with ambulation and stair climbing
  ● Instruction in functional activities in the clinic that should mimic those at home as closely as possible, such as the number of stairs and set up of railings

◆ Task-specific activities
  ● Review activities at home and modify them to be more therapeutic
  ● Stand from sit without use of arms, repeat twice each time stands up
  ● Step up and down the stairs backward
  ● "Twister moves"
    ■ A game where the patient has to place feet and/or hands onto colored circles that are on the floor and then change again as requested by the therapist; this challenges balance skills, places demands on ROM, and requires motor control through sequencing and changing the direction of movements
    ■ Can be played with or without musical "instructions," which increase the rate of movement and can add an aerobic component depending on the speed at which it is played
    ■ Activities can be modified to meet the individual's needs

FUNCTIONAL TRAINING IN WORK, COMMUNITY, AND LEISURE INTEGRATION OR REINTEGRATION

◆ Functional training programs
  ● Instruct in strategies for safe and efficient travel to work and in community using appropriate assistive devices
  ● Review work-required activities and attempt to train in task-focused practice

◆ Recommendations for support systems
  ● National Multiple Sclerosis Society[57]
  ● Local Chapter of the National Multiple Sclerosis Society

PRESCRIPTION, APPLICATION, AND, AS APPROPRIATE, FABRICATION OF DEVICES AND EQUIPMENT

◆ Adaptive devices
  ● Adaptive devices for the bathroom (eg, grab bars for the shower, nonskid strips in shower, hand-held shower head, shower/tub bench, toilet versa frame, raised toilet seat)
  ● Adaptive devices for the kitchen (eg, nonskid pads for mixing and cutting and for opening jars, bottles, and cans)
  ● Reacher
  ● Additional rails at the stairs
  ● Night lights
  ● Marking stairs to distinguish one from the other

◆ Assistive devices
  ● Determine need for a wheelchair for long-distance activities in discussion with Ms. Bernard and her family
    ■ If needed, coordinate the wheelchair assessment, documentation, fitting, and ordering of the chair with an appropriate vendor
    ■ To increase Ms. Bernard's mobility performance, stability, and independence in ADL and IADL and to reduce the risk of falls (eg, cane, long-handled reachers, etc)
    ■ Instruct in use and care of the assistive device

◆ Orthotic devices
  ● To increase mobility and stability and reduce risk of falls
  ● Assess need for an AFO to provide ankle and knee stability for standing activities[171]
    ■ Coordinate care with the orthotist to fabricate an AFO based on the physical therapist's recommendations
    ■ If an AFO is needed, Ms. Bernard and her family will be instructed in how to don and doff it, when to wear it, and how to monitor it

ANTICIPATED GOALS AND EXPECTED OUTCOMES

Given the progressive nature of MS and the variability among individuals with the disease, it is often difficult to determine either short- or long-term prognoses for individuals with MS.[172] The following outcomes are based on the examination completed and information provided by the patient. The goals and outcomes will be modified as necessary if Ms. Bernard's status changes significantly during the course of treatment.

◆ Impact on impairments
  ● Ambulation with appropriate assistive device for 800 feet on firm and carpeted surfaces is achieved.
  ● Left foot clears during swing phase of LLE with use of an orthotic gait assistive device during ambulation on all surfaces.
  ● Normal base of support at stance phase during ambulation with an assistive device is demonstrated.
  ● Standing without loss of balance and without UE

support for 5 minutes is achieved.

♦ Impact on functional limitations
   ● Climbing up or down both short flights of stairs in her house using the hand rail without assistance and without the need to stop and rest is achieved.
   ● Standing without loss of balance and without UE support for 5 minutes independently to perform daily grooming tasks is achieved.

♦ Impact on disabilities
   ● Entering the school and ascending and descending six stairs without having to stop and rest and without assistance except for the use of one railing are achieved.
   ● Participation in her daughter's activities as needed is achieved.
   ● Safe ambulation across unlevel terrain for approximately 800 feet with the use of an AFO and assistive device without loss of balance is achieved.

♦ Risk reduction/prevention
   ● Ms. Bernard and her family are able to demonstrate appropriate techniques for energy conservation.
   ● Safety of Ms. Bernard and her family is improved through demonstration by patient of safe techniques during ambulation and stair climbing.

♦ Impact on health, wellness, and fitness
   ● Behaviors that foster healthy habits, wellness, and prevention are acquired.
   ● Fitness is improved.
   ● Physical function is improved.

♦ Impact on societal resources
   ● Available resources are maximally utilized.
   ● Care is coordinated with patient, family, and other professionals.
   ● Documentation occurs throughout patient management in all settings and follows APTA's *Guidelines for Physical Therapy Documentation*.[78]
   ● Interdisciplinary collaboration occurs through patient care rounds and patient family meetings.
   ● Patient will be able to identify relevant community resources to meet her discharge needs.
   ● Referrals are made to other professionals or resources whenever necessary and appropriate.

♦ Patient/client satisfaction
   ● Admission data and discharge planning are completed.
   ● Care is coordinated with patient, family, payor, and other professionals.
   ● Discharge needs are determined.
   ● Patient and family understanding of anticipated goals and expected outcomes is increased.
   ● Patient and family will verbalize an awareness of the

diagnosis, prognosis, interventions, and anticipated goals/expected outcomes.
   ● Results of Physical Therapy Outpatient Satisfaction Survey developed by Roush and Sonstroem[173] indicate patient satisfaction.

REEXAMINATION

Reexamination is performed throughout the episode of care with adjustments to the plan of care as needed.

DISCHARGE

Ms. Bernard is discharged from physical therapy after a total of 16 visits over 8 weeks of outpatient care and attainment of her goals and expectations. These sessions have covered her entire episode of care. It is anticipated that she will require three to four visits over the next year after discharge to home for follow-up and reassessment.

REFERENCES

1. Waters CH. *Diagnosis and Management of Parkinson's Disease.* 3rd ed. Caddo, OK: Professional Communications; 2006.
2. Bear MF, Connors BW, Paradiso MA. *Neuroscience: Exploring the Brain.* 2nd ed. Philadelphia, PA: Lippincott Williams & Wilkins; 2001.
3. Cohen H. *Neuroscience for Rehabilitation.* Philadelphia, PA: Lippincott; 1993.
4. Holland NJ. Overview of multiple sclerosis. *Clinical Bulletin for Health Professionals.* New York, NY: National Multiple Sclerosis Society; 2006. Available at: http://www.nationalmssociety.org/site/PageServer?pagename=hom_gen_homepage. Accessed September 18, 2007.
5. *The Myelin Project: An Overview.* The Myelin Project Headquarters; 2002. Available at: http://www.myelin.org/overview.htm. Accessed September 19, 2007.
6. Gutman SA. *Quick Reference Neuroscience for Rehabilitation Professionals: The Essential Neurologic Principles Underlying Rehabilitation Practice.* Thorofare, NJ: SLACK Incorporated; 2001.
7. Young PA, Young PH. *Basic Clinical Neuroanatomy.* Baltimore, MD: Williams & Wilkins; 1997.
8. Purves D, Augustine GJ, Fitzpatrick D, et al. *Neuroscience.* 2nd ed. Sunderland, MA: Sinauer Associates; 2001.
9. Bear MF, Connors BW, Paradiso MA. *Neuroscience: Exploring the Brain.* 3rd ed. New York, NY: Lippincott Williams & Wilkins; 2007.
10. Fredericks CM, Saladin LK. *Pathophysiology of the Motor Systems: Principles and Clinical Presentations.* Philadelphia, PA: FA Davis; 1996.
11. Schwerin M. The anatomy of movement. Scientific Learning Corporation: Brain Connection; 1997. Available at: http://www.brainconnection.com/topics/?main=anat/motor-anat. Accessed September 26, 2007.
12. Gondim FAA, Thomas FP. Spinal cord, topographical and functional anatomy. eMedicine Specialties: Neurology. Last

Updated: January 11, 2007. Available at: http://www.emedicine.com/neuro/topic657.htm. Accessed September 27, 2007.

13. Shumway-Cook A, Woolacott MH. *Motor Control: Theory and Practical Applications*. 2nd ed. New York, NY: Lippincott Willliams & Wilkins; 2001.

14. Hamani C, Lozano A. Physiology and pathophysiology of Parkinson's disease. *Ann N Y Acad Sci*. 2003;991:15-21.

15. http://en.wikipedia.org/wiki/Saltatory_conduction. Accessed September 29, 2007.

16. Kang PS, Munter FM. *Optic neuritis*. eMedicine from WebMD last updated 2/8/06. Available at: http://www.emedicine.com/radio/topic488.html. Accessed September 27, 2007.

17. Robinson C, Rajput A. The neuropathology of Parkinson's disease and other Parkinsonian disorders. In: Ebadi M, Pfeiffer R, eds. *Parkinson's Disease*. Boca Raton, FL: CRC Press; 2005.

18. Meara RJ. Review—the pathophysiology of the motor signs in Parkinson's disease. *Age Ageing*. 1994;23(4):342-346.

19. Tillerson JL, Caudle WM, Reverón ME, Miller GW. Exercise induces behavioral recovery and attenuates neurochemical deficits in rodent models of Parkinson's disease. *Neuroscience*. 2003;119(3):899-911.

20. Hoehn M, Yahr M. Parkinsonism: onset, progression and mortality. *Neurology*. 1967;17(5):427-442.

21. Fahn S, Marsden CD, Calne DB, Goldstein M, eds. *Recent Developments in Parkinson's Disease*. Vol 2. Florham Park, NJ: Macmillan Health Care Information; 1987.

22. Goodman CC, Boissonault WG, Fuller KS. *Pathology: Implications for the Physical Therapist*. New York, NY: WB Saunders; 2003.

23. Noseworthy JH, Lucchinetti C, Rodriguez M, Weinshenker BG. Multiple sclerosis. *N Engl J Med*. 2000;343(13):938-952.

24. Culpepper WJ, Ehrmantraut M, Wallin MT, et al. Veterans Health Administration multiple sclerosis surveillance registry: the problem of case-finding from administrative databases. *J Rehabil Res Dev*. 2006:43(1):17-24.

25. Courtney SW. *All About Multiple Sclerosis*. 3rd ed. Cherry Hill, NJ: Multiple Sclerosis Association of America; 2006.

26. Kalb R. *Multiple Sclerosis: A Focus on Rehabilitation*. New York, NY: National Multiple Sclerosis Society; 2004.

27. Umphred D. *Neurological Rehabilitation*. 4th ed. St. Louis, MO: Mosby; 2001.

28. Trapp BD, Peterson J, Ransohoff RM, et al. Axonal transection in the lesions of multiple sclerosis. *N Engl J Med*. 1998; 338:278-285.

29. Sowka JW, Gurwood AS, Kabat AG. Demyelinating optic neuropathy (optic neuritis, retrobulbar optic neuritis). *Handbook of Disease Management*. Available at: http://www.revoptom.com/handbook/SECT51a.HTM. Accessed September 26, 2007.

30. O'Sullivan SB, Schmitz TJ. *Physical Rehabilitation: Assessment and Treatment*. 5th ed. Philadelphia, PA: FA Davis; 2007.

31. Cameron MH, Monroe LG. *Physical Rehabilitation: Evidenced Based Examination, Evaluation and Intervention*. St. Louis, MO: WB Saunders; 2007.

32. Sadovnick AD. Familial recurrency risks and inheritance of multiple sclerosis. *Current Opinion in Neurology and Neurosurgery*. 1993;6(2):189-194.

33. Vukusic S, Hutchinson M, Hours M, et al. Pregnancy and multiple sclerosis (the PRIMS study): clinical predictors of post-partum relapse. *Brain*. 2004;127(6):1353-1360.

34. Cook SD, Troiano R, Bansil S, Dowling PC. Multiple sclerosis and pregnancy. *Adv Neurol*. 1994;64:83-95.

35. Confavreux C, Hutchinson M, Hours MM, et al. Pregnancy in multiple sclerosis group. *N Engl J Med*. 1998;339(5):285-291.

36. Saraste M, Väisänen S, Alanen A, et al. Clinical and immunologic evaluation of women with multiple sclerosis during and after pregnancy. *Gender Medicine*. 2007;4(1):45-55.

37. Multiple sclerosis: hope through research. Compiled by the National Institute of Neurological Disorders and Stroke (NINDS). Available at: http://www.ninds.nih.gov/disorders/multiple_sclerosis/detail_multiple_sclerosis.htm. Accessed September 29, 2007.

38. Lublin FD, Reingold SC. Defining the clinical course of multiple sclerosis: results of an international survey. National Multiple Sclerosis Society (USA) Advisory Committee on Clinical Trials of New Agents in Multiple Sclerosis. *Neurology*. 1996;46:907-911.

39. Confavreux C, Vukusic S, Morea T, Adeleine P. Relapses and progression of disability in multiple sclerosis. *N Engl J Med*. 2000;343:1430-1438.

40. Goodin DS, Frohman EM, Garmany GP, et al. Disease modifying therapies in multiple sclerosis: report of the Therapeutics and Technology Assessment Subcommittee of the American Academy of Neurology and the MS Council for Clinical Practice Guidelines. *Neurology*. 2002;22;58(2):169-178.

41. Samkoff LM. Multiple sclerosis: update on treatment. *Hospital Physician*. 2002;38(3):21-27.

42. Baba Y, Wharen R, Uitti R. Parkinson's disease: surgical treatment—stereotactic procedures. In: Ebadi M, Pfeiffer R, eds. *Parkinson's Disease*. Boca Raton, FL: CRC Press; 2005.

43. National Institute of Neurological Disorders and Stroke. Available at: http://www.ninds.nih.gov/disorders/multiple_sclerosis/multiple_sclerosis.htm. Accessed September 26, 2007.

44. Katz RT. Management of spasticity. *Am J Phys Med Rehabil*. 1988;67(3):108-116.

45. Schapiro RT. Spasticity in multiple sclerosis. *MRSQ online*. 2002;21(1).

46. Smyth MD, Peacock WJ. The surgical treatment of spasticity. *Muscle Nerve*. 2000;23:153-163.

47. Healthlink, University of Wisconsin. Treatment for Specific Multiple Sclerosis (MS) Symptoms. Information provided by the National Institutes of Health. Article created: March 29, 2000.

48. Wood J. MR imaging of parkinsonism. In: Ebadi M, Pfeiffer R, eds. *Parkinson's Disease*. Boca Raton, FL: CRC Press; 2005.

49. Jennings D, Marek K, Seibyl J. Dopamine transporter imaging using SPECT in Parkinson's disease. In: Ebadi M, Pfeiffer R, eds. *Parkinson's Disease*. Boca Raton, FL: CRC Press; 2005.

50. Gujar SK, Maheshwari S, Björkman-Burtscher I, Sundgren PC. Magnetic resonance spectroscopy. *J Neuroophthalmol*. 2005;25(3):217-226.

51. http://en.wikipedia.org/wiki/Magnetic_resonance_imaging. Accessed September 17, 2007.

52. Stokes M. *Neurological Physiotherapy*. St. Louis, MO: Mosby; 1998.

53. Marjama-Lyons J, Hubble J, Berchou R, Kittle G. *Parkinson's Disease: Medications*. 2nd ed. Miami, FL: National Parkinson

Foundation Inc; 2005.

54. Ebadi M, Pfeiffer R, eds. *Parkinson's Disease*. Boca Raton, FL: CRC Press; 2005.

55. Silverstein P, Parashos S. *Comprehensive Pharmacological Therapies for Parkinson's Disease*. CNS News.com. McMahon Publishing Group; 2006.

56. Ebadi M, Sharma S, Shavali S, El Refaey H. Neuroprotective actions of selegiline. *J Neurosci Res*. 2002;67(3):285-289.

57. National Clinical Advisory Board of the Multiple Sclerosis Society, Disease Management Consensus Statement. *Expert Opinion Paper*. New York, NY: National Multiple Sclerosis Society; 2007.

58. US Food and Drug Administration, Center for Drug Evaluation and Research. Available at: http://www.fda.gov/cder. Accessed September 18, 2007.

59. Medline Plus Drug Information. Available at: http://www.nlm.nih.gov/medlineplus/druginfo/medmaster/a684001.html. Accessed September 7, 2007.

60. Rudick RA. Neurotherapeutics: disease-modifying drugs for relapsing-remitting multiple sclerosis and future directions for multiple sclerosis therapeutics. *Arch Neurol*. 1999;56:1079-1084.

61. Teva Neurosciences: drug manuafacturer of Copaxone. Available at: http://www.tevaneurosciences.com. Accessed September 17, 2007.

62. Biogen: drug manuafacturer of Avonex. Available at: http://www.avonex.com. Accessed September 7, 2007.

63. Berlex: drug manuafacturer of Betaseron. Available at: http://www.betaseron.com. Accessed September 7, 2007.

64. Merck Serono International: drug manuafacturer of Rebif. Available at: http://www.rebif.com. Accessed September 17, 2007.

65. EMD Serono: drug manuafacturer of Novantrone. Available at: http:// www.Novantrone.com. Accessed September 17, 2007.

66. Berg K, Wood-Dauphine S, William JI, et al. Measuring balance in the elderly: preliminary development of an instrument. *Physiotherapy Canada*. 1989;41:304-311.

67. Shumway-Cook A. Predicting the probability for falls in community dwelling older adults. *Phys Ther*. 1997;77:812-819.

68. Bohannon RW. Comfortable and maximum walking speed of adults 20-79 years: reference values and determinants. *Age Ageing*. 1997;26:15-19.

69. Posiadlo, D, Richardson S. The timed "Up & Go": a test of basic functional mobility for frail elderly persons. *J Am Geriatr Soc*. 1991;39(2):142-148.

70. Shumway-Cook A, Brauer S, Woolacott M. Predicting the probability for falls in community-dwelling older adults using the timed up and go. *Phys Ther*. 2000;80(9):896-903.

71. Morris S, Morris M, Iansek R. Reliability of measurements obtained with the timed up and go test in people with Parkinson's disease. *Phys Ther*. 2001;81(2):810-818.

72. Bohannon RH. Reference values for the timed up and go test: a descriptive meta-analysis. *Journal of Geriatric Physical Therapy*. 2006;29(2):64-68.

73. Bischoff, H, Stahelin, H, Monsch A, et al. Identifying a cut-off point for normal mobility: a comparison of the timed 'up and go' test in community-dwelling and institutionalized elderly women. *Age Ageing*. 2003;32:315-320.

74. Csuka M, McCarty DJ. Simple method for measurement of lower extremity muscle strength. *Am J Med*. 1985;78(1):77-81.

75. Whitney SL, Wrisley DM, Marchetti GF, et al. Clinical performance of sit-to-stand performance in people with balance disorders: validity of data for the fives-times-sit-to-stand test. *Phys Ther*. 2005;85(10):1034-1035.

76. Downie W, Leatham PA, Rhind VM, et al. Studies with pain rating scales. *Ann Rheum Dis*. 1978;37:378-381.

77. Jensen MP, Karoly P, Braver S. The measurement of clinical pain intensity: a comparison of six methods. *Pain*. 1986;27(1):117-126.

78. American Physical Therapy Association. Guide to physical therapist practice. 2nd ed. *Phys Ther*. 2001;81:9-744.

79. deGoede C, Keus S, Kwakkel G, Wagenaar R. The effects of physical therapy in Parkinson's disease: a research synthesis. *Arch Phys Med Rehabil*. 2001;82(4):509-515.

80. Samyra HJ, Keus PT, Bloem BH, et al. Evidence-based analysis of physical therapy in Parkinson's disease with recommendations for practice and research. *Mov Disord*. 2007;22(4):451-460.

81. Shumway-Cook A, Gruber W, Baldwin M, Liao S. The effect of multidimensional exercises on balance, mobility, and fall risk in community dwelling older adults. *Phys Ther*. 1997;77:46-57.

82. Schenkman M, Clark K, Xie T, et al. Spinal movement and performance of a standing reach test in participants with and without Parkinson's disease. *Phys Ther*. 2001;81(8):1400-1411.

83. Morris ME. Impairments, activity limitations and participation restrictions in Parkinson's disease. In: Refshauge K, Ada L, Ellis E, eds. *Science-based Rehabilitation: Theories into Practice*. London, England: Butterworth Heinemann; 2005.

84. Farley BG, Koshland GF. Training BIG to move faster; the application of the speed-amplitude relation as a rehabilitation strategy for people with Parkinson's disease. *Exp Brain Res*. 2005;167(3):462-467. Epub November 11, 2005.

85. Scandalis TA, Bosak A, Berliner JC, et al. Resistance training and gait function in patients with Parkinson's disease. *Am J Phys Med Rehabil*. 2001;80:38-43.

86. Bergen JL, Toole T, Elliott RG, et al. Aerobic exercise intervention improves aerobic capacity and movement initiation in Parkinson's disease patients. *NeuroRehabilitation*. 2002;17:161-168.

87. Miyai I, Fujimoto Y, Ueda Y, et al. Treadmill training with body weight support: its effect on Parkinson's disease. *Arch Phys Med Rehabil*. 2000;81:849-852.

88. Miyai I, Fujimoto Y, Yamamoto H, et al. Long-term effect of body weight-supported treadmill training in Parkinson's disease: a randomized controlled trial. *Arch Phys Med Rehabil*. 2002;83:1370-1373.

89. Baatile J, Langbein WE, Weaver F, et al. Effect of exercise on perceived quality of life of individuals with Parkinson's disease. *J Rehabil Res Dev*. 2000;37:529-534.

90. Morris M. Movement disorders in people with Parkinson's disease: a model for physical therapy. *Phys Ther*. 2000;80:578-597.

91. Schenkman M, Keysor J, Chandler J, et al. *Axial Mobility Exercise Program: An Exercise Program to Improve Functional Ability*. University of Colorado Health Sciences Center, Denver, CO: Physical Therapy Program; 2004.

92. Cianci, H, Walde DM, Wichmann R. *Fitness Counts*. Miami, FL: National Parkinson Foundation; 2005.

93. Morris ME, Iansek R, Matyas T, Summers JJ. Stride length regulation in Parkinson's disease. Normalization strategies and underlying mechanisms. *Brain*. 1996;119(pt2):551-568.

94. Nieuwboer A, Kwakkel G, Rochester L, et al. Cueing training in the home improves gait-related mobility in Parkinson's disease: the RESCUE trial. *J Neurol Neurosurg Psychiatry*. 2007; 78(2):134-140.

95. Li F, Harmer P, Fisher KJ, et al. Tai Chi-based exercise for older adults with Parkinson's disease: a pilot-program evaluation. *Journal of Aging and Physical Activity*. 2007;15(2):139-151.

96. American Thoracic Society. ATS statement guidelines for the six minute walk test. *Am J Respir Crit Care Med*. 2002; 166:111-117.

97. Bean JF, Kiely DK, Leveille SG, et al. The 6-minute walk test in mobility-limited elders: what is being measured? *J Gerontol A Biol Sci Med Sci*. 2002;57(11):M751-M756.

98. Lusardi MM, Pellecchia GL, Schulman M. Functional performance in community living older adults. *Journal of Geriatric Physical Therapy*. 2006;26;(3):14-22.

99. Reuben DB, Siu A. An objective measure of physical dysfunction of elderly outpatients. The Physical Performance Test. *J Am Geriatr Soc*. 1990;38:1105-1112.

100. Paschal K, Oswald A, Oswald R, et al. Test-retest reliability of the Physical Performance Test for persons with Parkinson disease. *Journal of Geriatric Physical Therapy*. 2006;29(3):82-86.

101. Frazier LD. Coping with disease-related stressors in Parkinson's disease. *Gerontology*. 2000;40:53-63.

102. Gill T, Allore H, Guo Z. The deleterious effects of bed rest among community-living older persons. *J Gerontol A Biol Sci Med Sci*. 2004;59:M755-M761.

103. Pepper PV, Golstein MK. Postoperative complications in Parkinson's disease. *J Am Geriatr Soc*. 1999;47(8):967-972.

104. DiMonaco M, Fulvia V, DiMonaco R, et al. Functional recovery and length of stay after hip fracture in patients with neurologic impairment. *Am J Phys Med Rehabil*. 2003;82(2):143-148.

105. Senard JM, Brefel-Courbon C, Rascol O, Montastruc JL. Orthostatic hypotension in patients with Parkinson's disease: pathophysiology and management. *Drugs Aging*. 2001; 18(7):495-505.

106. Wichmann R. *Be Active: An Exericse Program for People with Parkinson's*. New York, NY: American Parkinson's Disease Association; 1988.

107. Suteerawattananon M, Morris GS, Etnyre BR, et al. Effects of visual and auditory cues on gait in individuals with Parkinson's disease. *J Neurol Sci*. 2004;15:63-69.

108. Nieuwboer A, De Weerdt W, Dom R, et al. Development of an activity scale for individuals with advanced Parkinson disease: reliability and "on-off" variability. *Phys Ther*. 2000;80(11): 1087-1096.

109. Koller WC, Tse W. Unmet medical needs in Parkinson's disease. *J Neurol*. 2004;62(Suppl 1):S1-S8.

110. O'Shea S, Morris ME, Iansek R. Dual task interference during gait in people with Parkinson disease: effects of motor versus cognitive secondary tasks. *Phys Ther*. 2002;82(9):888-897.

111. Rochester L, Hetherington V, Jones D, et al. Attending to the task: interference effects of functional tasks on walking in Parkinson's disease and the roles of cognition, depression,

fatigue, and balance. *Arch Phys Med Rehabil*. 2004;85(10):1578-1585.

112. Thaut MH, McIntosh GC, Rice RR, et al. Rhythmic auditory stimulation in gait training for Parkinson's disease patients. *Mov Disord*. 1996;11:193-200.

113. McIntosh GC, Rice RR, Thaut MH. Rhythmic–auditory facilitation of gait patterns in patients with Parkinson's disease. *J Neurol Neurosurg Psychiatry*. 1997;62:22-26.

114. Richard IH. Depression and apathy in Parkinson's disease. *Curr Neurol Neurosci Rep*. 2007;7(4):295-301.

115. Folstein MF, Folstein SE, McHugh PR. Mini-mental state: a practical method for grading the state of patients for the clinician, *J Psychiatr Res*. 1975;12:189-198.

116. Crum RM, Anthony JC, Bassett SS, Folstein MF. Population-based norms for the mini-mental state examination by age and educational level. *JAMA*. 1993;18:2386-2391.

117. Barba A, Molho E, Higgins D, et al. Dementia in Parkinson's disease. In: Ebadi M, Pfeiffer R, eds. *Parkinson's Disease*. Boca Raton, FL: CRC Press; 2005.

118. Dubois B, Pillon B. Cognitive deficits in Parkinson's disease. *J Neurol*. 1997;244:2-8.

119. Bunting-Perry LK. Palliative care in Parkinson's disease: implications for neuroscience nursing. *J Neurosci Nurs*. 2006; 38(2):106-113.

120. Margolis DJ, Knauss J, Bilker W, Baumgarten M. Medical conditions as risk factors for pressure ulcers in an outpatient setting. *Age Ageing*. 2003;32(3):259-264.

121. Redelings MD, Lee NE, Sorvillo F. Pressure ulcers: more lethal than we thought? *Advances in Skin and Wound Care*. 2005;18(7):367-372.

122. Hewson ML. *Horticulture as Therapy*. Guelph, Ontario, Canada: Greenmor Printing Company Limited; 1994.

123. Kravitz L. The effects of music on exercise. *IDEA Today*. 1994; 12(9):56-61.

124. Brown AR, Mulley GP. Injuries sustained by caregivers of disabled elderly people. *Age Ageing*. 1997;26(1):21-23.

125. Caap-Ahlgren M, Dehlin O. Factors of importance to the caregiver burden experienced by family caregivers of Parkinson's disease patients. *Aging Clin Exp Res*. 2002;14(5):371-377.

126. Pfeiffer E. A short portable mental status questionnaire for the assessment of organic brain deficit in elderly patients. *J Am Geriatr Soc*. 1975;23(10):433-441.

127. Oatis C. *Kinesiology: The Mechanics and Pathomechanics of Human Movement*. Philadelphia, PA: Lippincott Williams & Wilkins; 2004.

128. USDA Center for Nutrition Policy and Promotion. Body mass index and health. *Nutritional Insight*. 2000.

129. Tinetti ME, Richman D, Powell L. Falls efficacy as a measure of fear of falling. *J Gerontol B Psychol Sci Soc Sci*. 1990;45(6):239-243.

130. Lewis C. Balance, gait test proves simple yet useful. *PT Bulletin*. 1993;2(10):9,40.

131. Lewis C, McNerney PT. *The Functional Toolbox*. Washington, DC: Learn Publications; 1994.

132. Kurtzke JF. Rating neurological impairment in multiple sclerosis: an extended disability status scale (EDSS). *Neurology*. 1983; 33:1444-1452.

133. Herndon RM. *Handbook of Neurologic Rating Scales. 2nd ed.* New York, NY: Demos Med Publisher; 2006.

134. United States Food & Drug Administration. P&CNS advisory

committee briefing document. Available at: http://www.fda.gov/ohrms/dockets/ac/00/backgrd/3582b1px.pdf. Accessed September 4, 2007.

135. Quirk DC, Schapiro RT. Population dynamics of the disability status scales for multiple sclerosis. *Neurorehabil Neural Repair.* 1996;10(2):127-134.

136. Blackburn M, vanVliet P, Mockett SP. Reliability of measurements obtained with the modified Ashworth Scale in the lower extremities of people with stroke. *Phys Ther.* 2002;182:25-34.

137. Thomas PW, Thomas S, Hillier C, et al. Psychological interventions for multiple sclerosis. *Cochrane Database Syst Rev.* 2006;(1):CD004431. DOI: 10.1002/14651858.CD004431. pub2.

138. Ko Ko C. Effectiveness of rehabilitation for multiple sclerosis. *Clin Rehabil.* 1999;13(Suppl):S33-S41.

139. Patti F, Ciancio MR, Reggio E, et al. The impact of outpatient rehabilitation on quality of life in multiple sclerosis. *J Neurol.* 2002;249(8):1027-1033.

140. Mostert S, Kesselring J. Effects of a short-term exercise training program on aerobic fitness, fatigue, health perception and activity level of subjects with multiple sclerosis. *Mult Scler.* 2002;8:161-168.

141. Newman MA, Dawes H, van den Berg M, et al. Can aerobic treadmill training reduce the effort of walking and fatigue in people with multiple sclerosis: a pilot study. *Mult Scler.* 2007; 13(1):113-119.

142. Petajan JH, Gappmaier E, White AT, et al. Impact of aerobic training on fitness and quality of life in multiple sclerosis. *Ann Neurol.* 1996;39:432-441.

143. Rampello A, Franceschini M, Piepoli M, et al. Effect of aerobic training on walking capacity and maximal exercise tolerance in patients with multiple sclerosis: a randomized crossover controlled study. *Phys Ther.* 2007;87(5):545-555.

144. Rietberg MB, Brooks D, Uitdehaag BMJ, Kwakkel G. Exercise therapy for multiple sclerosis. *Cochrane Database Syst Rev.* 2005;(1):CD003980.

145. Roehrs T, Karst G. Effects of an aquatics exercise program on quality of life measures for individuals with progressive multiple sclerosis. *Journal of Neurologic Physical Therapy.* 2004;28(2):63.

146. Surakka J, Romberg A, Ruutiainen J, et al. Effects of aerobic and strength exercise on motor fatigue in men and women with multiple sclerosis: a randomized controlled trial. *Clin Rehabil.* 2004;18:737-746.

147. Svensson B, Gerdle B, Elert J. Endurance training in patients with multiple sclerosis: five case studies. *Phys Ther.* 1994; 74:1017-1026.

148. White LJ, Dressendorfer RH. Exercise and multiple sclerosis. *Sports Med.* 2004;34:1077-1100.

149. Romberg A, Virtanen A, Ruutiainen J. Long-term exercise improves functional impairment but not quality of life in multiple sclerosis. *J Neurol.* 2005;252(7):839-845.

150. Pariser G, Madras D, Weiss E. Case report: outcomes of an aquatic exercise program including aerobic capacity, lactate threshold, and fatigue in two individuals with multiple sclerosis. *Journal of Neurologic Physical Therapy.* 2006;30(2):82-90.

151. Petajan, JH, White AT. Recommendations for physical activity in patients with MS. *Sports Med.* 1999;27(3):179-191.

152. Winnick JP. *Adapted Physical Education and Sport.* Champaign, IL: Human Kinetics; 1995.

153. Ponichtera-Mulcare JA, Mathews T, Barrett PJ, et al. Change in aerobic fitness of patients with multiple sclerosis during a 6-month training program. *Sports Medicine, Training, and Rehabilitation.* 1997;7:265-272.

154. Peterson JL, Bell GW. Aquatic exercise for individuals with multiple sclerosis. *Clinical Kinesiology.* 1995;49(3):69-71.

155. Ng AV, Kent-Braun JA. Quantitation of lower physical activity in persons with multiple sclerosis. *Med Sci Sports Exerc.* 1997; 29(4):517-523.

156. Sherrill C. *Adapted Physical Activity, Recreation and Sport: Crossdisciplinary and Lifespan.* Boston, MA: McGraw-Hill Higher Education; 1998.

157. Benyas P. Don't be afraid to ask: yoga and multiple sclerosis. *Real Living with Multiple Sclerosis.* 1999;6(6):6.

158. Pepin EB, Hicks RW, Spenser MK, et al. Pressor response to isometric exercise in patients with multiple sclerosis. *Med Sci Sports Exerc.* 1996;28:656-660.

159. Schwid SR, Petrie MD, Murray R, et al. NASA/MS Cooling Study Group. A randomized controlled study of the acute and chronic effects of cooling therapy for MS. *Neurology.* 2003; 60(12):1955-1960.

160. Harmon M. Redefining exercise: no fun, no gain. *Inside Multiple Sclerosis.* 1998;16(1):14-20.

161. Chard SE. Community neurorehabilitation: a synthesis of current evidence and future research directions. *Neuro Rx.* 2006; 3(4):525-534.

162. Goldstein MS, Elliot SD, Guccione AA. The development of an instrument to measure satisfaction with physical therapy. *Phys Ther.* 2000;80(9):853-863.

163. Costello E, Curtis C, Sandel I, Bassile C. Exercise prescription for individuals with multiple sclerosis. *Neurology Report.* 1996; 20:24-29.

164. Mulcare J. Multiple sclerosis. In: American College of Sports Medicine. *ACSM's Exercise Management for Person's with Chronic Disease and Disabilities.* Champaign, IL: Human Kinetics; 1997.

165. Basmajian JV, Wolf SL, eds. *Therapeutic Exercise.* 3rd ed. Baltimore, MD: Williams & Wilkins; 1990.

166. Moffat M, Rosen E, Rusnak-Smith E, ed. *Musculoskeletal Essentials: Applying the Preferred Physical Therapist Practice Patterns^SM.* Thorofare, NJ: SLACK Incorporated; 2006.

167. Borg G. *Borg's Perceived Exertion and Pain Scales.* Champaign, IL: Human Kinetics; 1998.

168. Lewis C, McNerney PT. *The Functional Toolbox II.* McLean, VA: Learn Publications; 1997.

169. Smedal T, Lygren H, Myhr KM, et al. Balance and gait improved in patients with MS after physiotherapy based on the Bobath concept. *Physiother Res Int.* 2006;11(2):104-116.

170. Frzovic D, Morris M, Vowels L. Clinical tests of standing balance: performance of persons with multiple sclerosis. *Arch Phys Med Rehabil.* 2000;81:215-221.

171. Mount J, Dacko S. Effects of dorsiflexor endurance exercises on foot drop secondary to multiple sclerosis: a pilot study. *NeuroRehabilitation.* 2006;21(1):43-50.

172. Grasso MG, Troisi E, Rizzi F, et al. Prognostic factors in multidisciplinary rehabilitation treatment in multiple sclerosis: an outcome study. *Mult Scler.* 2005;11:719-724.

173. Roush SE, Sonstroem RJ. Development of the physical therapy outpatient satisfaction survey (PTOPS). *Phys Ther.* 1999; 79(2):159-170.

ADDITIONAL RESOURCES

Ashburn A, Stack E, Picketing RM, Ward CD. A community-dwelling sample of people with Parkinson's disease: characteristics of fallers and non-fallers. *Age Ageing.* 2001;30:47-52.

Balogun JA, Olokungbemi AA, Kuforiji AR. Spinal mobility and muscular strength: effects of supine- and prone-lying back extension exercise training. *Arch Phys Med Rehabil.* 1992; 73:745-751.

Bridgewater KJ, Sharpe MH. Trunk muscle performance in early Parkinson's disease. *Phys Ther.* 1998;78:566-576.

Hafler DA. Multiple sclerosis. *J Clin Invest.* 2004;113(6):788-794.

Hausdorff JM, Balash J, Giladi N. Effects of cognitive challenge on gait variability in patients with Parkinson's disease. *J Geriatr Psychiatr Neurol.* 2003;16:53-58.

Jacobs JV, Horak FB, Tran VK, Nutt JG. Multiple balance tests improve the assessment of postural stability in subjects with Parkinson's disease. *J Neurol Neurosurg Psychiatry.* 2006; 77(3):322-326.

Johnson AM, Almeida QJ. The impact of exercise rehabilitation and physical activity on the management of Parkinson's disease. *Geriatr Aging.* 2007;10(5):318-321.

Light KE, Behrman AL. The 2-minute walk test: a tool for evaluating walking endurance in clients with Parkinson's disease. *Neuroreport.* 1997;21(4):136-139.

Morris ME, Huxham F, McGinley J, et al. Three-dimensional gait biomechanics in Parkinson's disease: evidence for a centrally mediated amplitude regulation disorder. *Mov Disord.* 2005;20(1):40-50.

Morris ME, Iansek R, Matyas TA, et al. The pathogenesis of gait hypokinesia in Parkinson's disease. *Brain.* 1994;117:1169-1181.

Morris ME, Iansek R, Matyas T, Summers JJ. Abnormalities in the stride-length-cadence relation in Parkinsonian gait. *Mov Disord.* 1998;13:61-69.

Nieuwboer A, DeWeerdt W, Dom R, et al. The effects of a home physiotherapy program for persons with Parkinson's disease. *J Rehabil Med.* 2001;33:266-272.

Reuter I, Engelhardt M, Stecker K, et al. Therapeutic value of exercise training in Parkinson's disease. *Med Sci Sports Exerc.* 1999;31:1544-1549.

Rochester L, Hetherington V, Jones D, et al. Attending to the task: interference effects of functional tasks on walking in Parkinson's disease and the roles of cognition, depression, fatigue, and balance. *Arch Phys Med Rehabil.* 2004;85:1578-1585.

Schenkman M, Morey M, Kuchibhaita M. Spinal flexibility and balance control among community dwelling adults with and without Parkinson's disease. *J Gerontol A Biol Sci Med Sci.* 2000;55:M441-M445.

Temlett JA, Thompson PD, Reasons for admission to hospital for Parkinson's disease. *Intern Med J.* 2006;36(8):524-526.

Impaired Peripheral Nerve Integrity and Muscle Performance Associated With Peripheral Nerve Injury (Pattern F)

Tsega Andemicael Mehreteab, PT, MS, DPT
Gary Krasilovsky, PT, PhD
Sue Sandvik, PT
Lisa Kuehn, PT
Anne Gallentine, PT

ANATOMY

CARPAL TUNNEL

Bony Anatomy

The skeleton of the wrist or carpus is made up of eight carpal bones, known as carpals. The carpals are arranged in two rows of four bones each. The carpus is markedly concave anteriorly and convex posteriorly. The carpal tunnel is formed dorsally by the concave arch of the carpal bones and ventrally by the overlying transverse ligament. The median nerve lies immediately ventral to the flexor digitorum superficialis and flexor digitorum profundus tendons of the index finger. Synovial tendon sheaths surround the flexor tendons in the carpal tunnel.[1]

Median Nerve

The median nerve arises from the brachial plexus, lateral cord (C5 to C7), and medial cord (C8 to T1). The median nerve supplies motor innervation primarily to the flexor muscles in the anterior compartment of the five forearm muscles of the hand and supplies cutaneous innervations to only the palmar skin over the lateral three-and-one-half fingers. It has no branches in the upper arm. The median nerve courses down the medial side of the arm to the antecubital fossa and the forearm, providing motor innervations to the pronator teres, flexor carpi radialis, palmaris longus, the flexor digitorum superficialis, and the anterior interosseous nerve. Further distally, the anterior interosseous nerve supplies motor innervation to the flexor pollicis longus, flexor digitorum profundus of the index and long fingers, and the pronator quadratus. The median nerve supplies all the flexor muscles in the forearm and hand except the flexor carpi ulnaris and the medial half (digits four and five) of the flexor digitorum profundus, which are supplied by the ulnar nerve. Motor fibers from C7 to C8 innervate the abductor pollicis brevis, flexor pollicis brevis, opponens pollicis, and first and second lumbrical muscles in the hand.[1]

Sensory median nerve fibers arise from C6 and C7. Proximal to the transverse carpal ligament and before the median nerve enters the carpal tunnel, the palmar sensory cutaneous nerve branches off the median nerve, runs deep to the antebrachial fascia, and enters its own tunnel. The nerve passes over the flexor retinaculum and supplies the lateral

	Table 6-1	
MUSCLES INNERVATED BY THE FACIAL NERVE AND THEIR FUNCTIONAL MOVEMENTS		
Muscle	*Functional Movement*	
Frontalis	Raise eyebrows	
Corrugator	Frown	
Orbicularis oculi	Close eyelid	
Procerus	Wrinkle bridge of nose	
Zygomaticus major	Raise corner of mouth, smile	
Zygomaticus minor	Sad expression	
Levator labii superioris	Raise upper lip	
Nasalis, alar	Widen nostrils	
Buccinator	Mouth closure, blow a horn, pull angle of mouth posteriorly	
Orbicularis oris	Close and protrude lips	
Levator anguli oris	Elevate the angle of the mouth, sneer	
Risorius	Transverse smile	
Depressor anguli oris	Pull down angle of the mouth, frown	
Depressor labii inferioris	Pull lower lip and angle of mouth down and laterally	
Mentalis	Pout, close and protrude lips	
Platysma	Pull down fascia of neck	

part of the palm, the thenar eminence, index finger, middle finger, and the radial half of the ring finger. In carpal tunnel syndrome (CTS), the palmar cutaneous branch is spared and is a useful guide in differentiating CTS from proximal median nerve compression. The median nerve is supplied by the radial and ulnar arteries. Inflammation may lead to local swelling especially in patients with vascular impairments and in women who are pregnant.[1]

FACIAL NERVE

The seventh cranial nerve, commonly known as the facial nerve, provides the primary innervation to the muscles of the face. The fibers that control facial expression originate in the motor area of the primary motor cortex of each hemisphere and synapse at the motor nucleus for the seventh cranial nerve. The innervation of the muscles on each side of the face comes from the opposite hemisphere, with the exception of the muscles of the forehead, which are innervated by dual (bilateral) innervation via the temporal branch. The implications of this pattern of innervation enable differential diagnosis of facial nerve paralysis from paralysis that occurs as a result of CNS involvement and that spares the frontalis muscle and typically results in less severe involvement.[1]

The facial nerve has primary motor functions and minor sensory functions. The motor nucleus of the facial nerve is located in the pons, and the fibers travel to the internal auditory canal. The fibers then pass through the facial canal.

Of note is the fact that the proximal segment of the facial canal is the narrowest segment, and this is the most common site of involvement of the nerve from edema secondary to inflammation or infection.[2] The geniculate ganglion of the facial nerve is also located in this segment of the facial canal and is the most common site of injury in temporal bone fractures.[3] Traveling with the labyrinthine artery, the nerve then bends (genu segment) posteriorly in the direction of the internal auditory meatus. The facial nerve is in close proximity to the middle ear and tympanic membrane before it exits the skull via the stylomastoid foramen,[4] which is located between the mastoid process and styloid process. Prior to or just after exiting the skull, the nerve is in close proximity with the acoustic nerve, the parotid gland, and the temporomandibular joint. Surgical procedures related to these structures require careful identification of the facial nerve, and tumors or other pathological processes in any of these structures may result in facial nerve damage.[5]

After the facial nerve exits the skull, it ultimately divides into four branches and one ramus. From superior to inferior, they are the temporal, zygomatic, buccal, and mandibular branches and the cervical ramus. The muscles innervated by the facial nerve include all muscles of facial expression, oral closure (mentalis, orbicularis oris inferior and superior), eyelid closure (orbicularis oculi inferior and superior), forehead wrinkling (frontalis), and neck wrinkling with depression of the corner of the mouth (platysma) (Table 6-1). The anatomical

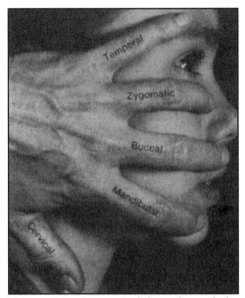

Figure 6-1. Anatomical branches of the facial nerve. Reprinted with permission from *Clinically Oriented Anatomy*, 4th ed, Moore KL, Dalley AF, eds, Lippincott Williams & Wilkins, 1999, 863.

distribution and pathways of the facial nerve and its branches and ramus are seen in Figures 6-1 and 6-2. The facial nerve also provides sensory innervation to the anterior two thirds of the tongue and a localized area around the external acoustic meatus.[1] Fibers anatomically associated with the facial nerve in the facial canal are often affected in a patient with Bell's palsy. These include the nervus intermedius, which controls the lachrymal gland (tear production), and the salivary glands.[2,4]

VESTIBULAR SYSTEM

The body receives sensory input for movement and postural stability from three systems: the visual, proprioceptive, and vestibular. Information from these systems is used by the CNS to maintain equilibrium. The CNS requires at least two of the systems for postural stability. A person's experience with the environment or situation also contributes to how the sensory information from the three systems is interpreted and relied upon by the CNS.[6]

The vestibular system is composed of both peripheral and central components. The peripheral system (Figure 6-3) is found in the inner ear and includes three semicircular canals (anterior, posterior, and horizontal/lateral) and the otoliths (utricle and saccule).[6] The peripheral vestibular system is comprised of a membranous labyrinth suspended within a bony labyrinth by endolymphatic fluid and supportive tissues. One end of each semicircular canal is widened where it connects to the utricle to form the ampulla.[6-10] Within the ampulla of each semicircular canal are hair cells that protrude into a gelatinous matrix called the cupula. Each hair cell is

innervated by an afferent neuron. Angular head acceleration (rotation) imposes forces on the endolymph fluid within the canal, which causes it to flow around the canal in the direction opposite to that of the head acceleration. This flow deflects the cupula and bends the hair cells. Normal neuronal firing rate is increased for the same side angular head movement and decreased for the opposite side angular head movement (Figure 6-4).[7] The input from the semicircular canals is transmitted via cranial nerve VIII and used primarily to generate compensatory eye movement that occurs with head movement, which is known as the VOR, or vestibulo-ocular reflex. This input is also used to generate postural responses via the vestibulospinal reflex (VSR).[7-9]

The utricle and saccule are at right angles to each other and also contain hair cells. The hair cells protrude into another gelatinous matrix called the maculae, which is covered by calcium carbonate crystals called otoconia (Figure 6-5). The otoconia cause the maculae to be gravity sensitive. Each hair cell innervated by an afferent neuron allows displacement due to linear acceleration and sustained head tilt to be converted into neuronal firing. The firing rate is increased for the same side linear head movements or tilt and is decreased for the opposite side linear head movement or tilt just as in angular movements.[7] Input from the utricle and the saccule contributes primarily to postural responses.[7-10] Table 6-2 provides

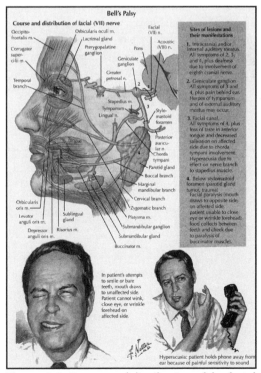

Figure 6-2. Course and distribution of the facial nerve. Reprinted with permission from Misulis KE, Head TC. *Netter's Concise Neurology.* Philadelphia, PA: Elsevier; 2007:481. All rights owned by Elsevier Inc.

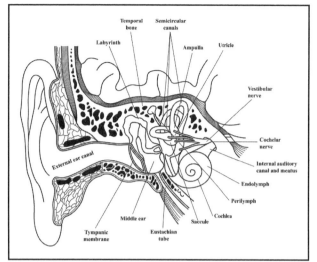

Figure 6-3. Peripheral vestibular system.

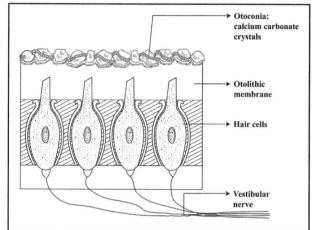

Figure 6-5. Otoconia cause the maculae to be gravity sensitive. Adapted from Baloh RW, Honrubia V. *Clinical Neurophysiology of the Vestibular System*. 2nd ed. Philadelphia, PA: FA Davis Co, 1990:4.

examples of movements that stimulate vestibular sensory organs.

The central vestibular system includes cranial nerve VIII, vestibular nucleus complex, and the cerebellum.[10] The vestibular nuclei are primarily located in the pons but are also found in the medulla. They receive information from the peripheral vestibular system via the vestibular portion of cranial nerve VIII. The vestibular nucleus complex is the primary processor of vestibular input. The complex makes fast direct connections between the afferent information and the motor output. The vestibular nuclei communicate with each other via a system of commissures. These commissures allow information to be shared between the two sides of the brainstem.

The cerebellum is the adaptive regulator receiving information from the vestibular nuclei and from the vestibular nerve and readjusts as needed. The CNS processes these signals and combines them with other sensory, proprioceptive, and visual information to estimate head orientation.[7-12]

The motor output of the CNS produces the VOR and VSR. The VOR stabilizes the eyes during movements of the head, keeping the vision clear. It involves ascending tracks receiving information from the vestibular nuclei and sending information to the extraocular musculature. The VSR generates compensatory body movement to maintain head and postural stability. It involves descending tracts that receive information from the vestibular nuclei and send information to the musculature of the body.[7-9,11,12]

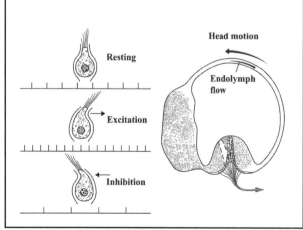

Figure 6-4. Cupula deflection with angular head acceleration. Adapted from Bach-Y-Rita P, Collins CC, Hyde JE, eds. *The Control of Eye Movements*. New York, NY: Academic Press; 1971.

Table 6-2	
EXAMPLES OF MOVEMENTS THAT STIMULATE VESTIBULAR SENSORY ORGANS[6,32]	
Movement	*Vestibular Sensory Organ Stimulated*
Moving head up and down: "Yes"	Anterior and posterior semicircular canal
Turning head horizontally: "No"	Horizontal semicircular canal
Linear movement up and down: Riding in an elevator	Saccule
Linear movement horizontally: Riding in a train	Utricle

PATHOPHYSIOLOGY

CARPAL TUNNEL SYNDROME

As the median nerve passes distally through the carpal tunnel, it is susceptible to compression. Pressure interferes with median nerve perfusion and eventually leads to sensory and motor impairment. The increased tunnel pressure on the median nerve and tendons is usually the main cause of the symptoms and subsequent impairment of the median nerve, known as CTS. Other common causes of CTS include congenital narrowing of the carpal tunnel; acute injury, such as sprains or strains; chronic trauma; and chronic stresses related to use of vibrating hand tools, work, or sports-repetitive movements. Swelling and microtrauma at the wrist causes compression and irritation of the median nerve and tendons leading to bursitis, tendonitis, and fibrosis. Chronic soft tissue inflammatory processes may lead to thick restrictive tendon sheaths and eventual fibrosis. These changes may limit gliding of the median nerve in the carpal tunnel during wrist flexion and extension, further aggravating the symptoms. Progressive worsening of CTS may involve three stages: muscle fatigue that is relieved with rest; discomfort that may continue to the next day; and chronic aching, fatigue, and weakness that persist at rest. Compared to individuals without impairment, those with CTS have a higher baseline pressure and a more marked increase in pressure when the wrist is flexed or extended.[13]

The following are major risk factors that may lead to median nerve entrapment or chronic injury at the wrist[14-16]:

♦ Systemic conditions, such as diabetes, chronic renal insufficiency, alcoholism, circulatory disorders, overactivity of the endocrine system, hypothyroidism, rheumatoid arthritis, or fluid retention during pregnancy or menopause

♦ Ischemia or traumatic injuries (fractures, traction, and soft tissue injuries)

♦ Progressive mechanical compression pressures ranging from mild compression (~20 to 30 mmHg) that results in reduced blood flow, moderate compression (~30 to 40 mmHg) that results in paresthesia, and more severe compression (>40 mmHg) that results in ischemia and complete loss of sensory and motor functions

♦ Proximal nerve impairments, such as cervical root compression, leading to proximal compression syndromes

♦ Overuse syndromes from compression, repetitive, or forced hand and finger movements (keyboard operators, musicians, carpenters, and athletes) that may lead to microtrauma of the median nerve resulting in intermittent paresthesia, tingling, and numbness, and if severe, complete loss of sensory and motor functions of the median nerve

CTS is three times more prevalent in women than it is in men. The dominant hand is usually affected first, and symptoms in that hand may be more severe than in the nondominant hand. Bilateral involvement is also common.[16]

According to MacKinnon[17] peripheral nerve compression can be classified based on the extent of the structural damage. Grade I or neuropraxia involves transient conduction block with possible demyelination, but the integrity of the nerve axon is preserved. Provocative tests in this type of injury may aggravate the symptoms of paresthesia. Changes in large sensory nerve fibers may be indicated by changes in touch and vibration thresholds. Grade II or axonotmesis represents axonal damage resulting in wallerian degeneration of nerve axons. In addition to the findings of EMG fibrillation potentials, a positive Tinel's test (ie, paresthesias in the distribution of the median nerve when the clinician taps on the distal crease over the median nerve), and a loss of motor function, symptoms may include changes in two-point discrimination, and numbness. Grade III or neurotmesis is more severe than axonotmesis and occurs as a result of severe contusion, stretch, or laceration. Depending on the severity of the injury, neurotmesis may be classified as Grade III, IV, or V. In CTS, damage to the median nerve may progress through Grade III. Grades IV and V apply to complete severance of the nerve and not to CTS. Grade III involves disruption of the endoneurium, but the epineurium and perineurium are intact. Symptoms include constant numbness and loss of motor function and muscle atrophy. Grade IV represents interruption of all neural and supporting elements, but the epineurium is intact. Grade V represents more severe injury with complete nerve transaction, loss of continuity, and scarring of the nerve.[17]

Other proximal compression injuries of the median nerve may mimic the symptoms of CTS and need to be differentiated. Intact sensation over the thenar eminence and normal muscle tests of the flexor pollicis longus, pronator quadratus, and flexor carpi radialis are used to rule out proximal median neuropathy. Proximal compressive neuropathies include cervical radiculopathy (usually at level C6), thoracic outlet syndrome, pronator syndrome, and anterior interosseous nerve syndrome. Neck and shoulder pain with weakness of C6 innervated muscles, reflex changes, sensory loss restricted to the thumb, absence of nocturnal paresthesia, and inability to reproduce symptoms with root compression maneuvers are indicative of cervical radiculopathy.[14]

Pronator syndrome results from entrapment of the median nerve in the forearm as it passes through the two heads of the pronator teres or compression by thickening of the flexor digitorum superficialis. Such compression causes pain in the proximal anterior aspects of the forearm, which is aggravated by repetitive pronation and supination of the forearm. Paresthesia or numbness of the medial three-and-one-half digits and the palm are common findings. The clinical presentation of pronator syndrome that includes localized proximal forearm pain, sensory deficits of the palm, weakness of the median and anterior interosseous innervated muscles distal to the entrapment, and the absence of nocturnal symptoms help differentiate this syndrome from impairments produced by CTS.[18-21]

IDIOPATHIC FACIAL NERVE BELL'S PARALYSIS

Facial nerve paralysis (Figure 6-6) may result from either CNS involvement or peripheral involvement distal to the motor nucleus. The most common etiology of facial paralysis from CNS involvement is a CVA, which may result in moderate weakness on one side of the face with sparing of the frontalis muscle because of its dual innervation. This chapter will focus on peripheral involvement of the facial nerve commonly referred to as idiopathic facial nerve paralysis or Bell's palsy.

Bell's palsy is typically a unilateral, acute, idiopathic weakness or total paralysis of the facial nerve. It is strictly a mononeuropathy, and associated neurological symptoms should immediately rule out idiopathic Bell's palsy. The presentation is usually within a 24- to 48-hour period,[2] and the severity progresses over a period of 7 to 10 days. The progression includes inability to close one eyelid due to involvement of the orbicularis oculi, loss of the blinking reflex, drooling and difficulty drinking due to loss of control of the orbicularis oris, loss of voluntary facial gesturing, and overall drooping on one side of the face. It may be accompanied by a dry eye and impairment of taste. The severity can vary from total paralysis as described above to partial involvement of one or more branches of the facial nerve. Paralysis develops as nerve function deterioration occurs as a result of the pathological process.[2]

More than 70% of individuals with a diagnosis of Bell's palsy recover within 1 year without treatment, and the majority of these patients have a full recovery within 3 weeks of onset.[22] Patients with incomplete paralysis do very well without treatment. Age is a factor in ultimate recovery, and only 33% of patients over the age of 60 have a full recovery. Other factors that inhibit optimal recovery are complete paralysis of all facial muscles, presence of Herpes zoster infection (Ramsey-Hunt syndrome), minimal recovery by 3 weeks, pregnancy, axonal degeneration of the facial nerve (as demonstrated by testing), diabetes, and HTN.[22]

Etiologies for Bell's palsy include: idiopathic (50%); infectious processes, such as Lyme disease or otitis media (15%); neurogenic, such as MS or Guillain-Barré syndrome (14%)[23]; neoplasms, such as acoustic neuroma, parotid tumors, or facial nerve schwannomas (14%)[24]; and trauma, such as temporal bone fractures[25] and trauma during tumor surgical resections (7%). Eighty-five percent of infectious cases in pediatric patients are due to acute otitis media with effusion.[26] The literature has more recently supported

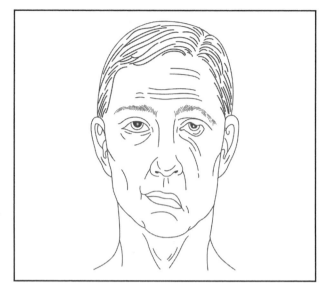

Figure 6-6. Facial nerve paralysis.

Herpes zoster virus[2,27,28] infection as the possible etiology of the majority of idiopathic facial nerve paralysis. Patients who are also at high risk for facial nerve paralysis include those with diabetes,[28] pregnancy, and HTN.[29]

The typical mechanism of damage of the facial nerve is secondary to an inflammatory response or infection in the region of the facial canal or the stylomastoid foramen. Similar to any nerve compression syndrome, swelling and edema in a confined space compromises the conduction capabilities of the nerve. If the resultant edema is mild, a neuropraxia may result, which often results in a temporary conduction block. Recovery can occur within minutes if no localized anatomical changes occur to the myelin sheath. If the compression progresses, localized ischemia can lead to demyelination. Although recovery will be excellent, it may take a few weeks. If the compression continues to progress, more severe anoxia will occur to the nerve, and the nerve will undergo demyelination and axonal degeneration or axonotmesis.[30] The greater the number of axons that degenerate, the more severe the involvement and the greater the chance of incomplete recovery. Recovery can only begin after the cause of nerve damage is removed, allowing the nerve axons to begin their slow (approximately 1 mm/day average) regeneration and eventual reinnervation. The key to optimal recovery is reducing the severity and duration of the infection and/or inflammatory response, so the edema can resolve quickly and the internal architecture of the nerve sheaths is preserved. This progression of nerve damage associated with fluid retention is one reason why women who are pregnant and develop Bell's palsy have a poor prognosis.[29]

The most severe form of nerve damage is neurotmesis, which has been classified by Sunderland.[31] His subclassifications (I, II, and III) relate to the destruction of the different sheaths (endoneurium, perineurium, and epineurium) that surround and compartmentalize a peripheral nerve (Figure 6-7). The classifications of neurotmesis are:

I. Damage to the axon and endoneurium but with preservation of perineurium and fascicular arrangement; regeneration is less complete than axonotmesis, but relatively functional.

II. Damage to the axon, endoneurium, and perineurium, although the nerve remains visually intact (due to the external sheath being intact); regeneration is poorly oriented and less functional.

III. Complete anatomical transection of the nerve; regeneration is poor.

Whether the internal architecture of the peripheral nerve is intact has a significant impact on overall recovery. Axonal regeneration is the key to recovery in any of these classifications. For axonal regeneration to proceed to the original muscle fibers that became denervated, it is extremely important that hollow tubes are left by the intact sheaths. Destruction of these internal nerve sheaths results in regeneration of motor axons down random nerve sheaths and will greatly reduce the percentage of motor fibers that eventually reinnervate a facial muscle. The random reinnervation that does occur after more severe nerve damage is what results in synkinesis and the relative poor prognosis in any nerve lesion classified as a neurotmesis.

BILATERAL AND UNILATERAL HYPOFUNCTION

Symptoms of vertigo, imbalance, and even nausea occur after damage or impairment of the function of the peripheral vestibular system. In unilateral hypofunction, the damage can be due to trauma, infection, inflammation, or tumor growth. In bilateral hypofunction, the damage is most commonly attributed to idiopathic or hereditary, sequential vestibular neuritis, or ototoxicity causes. Decreased afferent information is sent to the CNS from the damaged ear(s) during head rotation. The decrease of information resulting from the damaged ear(s) results in an impaired VOR and feelings of dizziness.[6,7] The VOR is impaired causing retinal slip during attempted gaze stabilization. This causes decreased visual acuity, oscillopsia (the false illusion of movement of objects in the environment), and the sensation of dizziness. With bilateral involvement, oscillopsia is a hallmark symptom that leads to decreased balance, especially in situations where visual or somatosensory input is altered.[32]

An individual with unilateral hypofunction of the vestibular system may initially exhibit nystagmus, the repeated rhythmical movement of the eyes.[33-35] Nystagmus is characterized by a slow phase ("slow" movement in one direction) followed by a fast phase (rapid return to the original position). The type of nystagmus is named after the direction of the fast phase. It can be horizontal, vertical, rotatory, or any combination of these.[33,35] Nystagmus that is the result of an infection should spontaneously resolve.

The CNS compensates for vestibular disorders by adapting the VOR and VSR directly or by substituting other reflexes and strategies[36,37] that occur in the cerebellum, vestibular commissure, reticular formation, cerebral cortex, and cerebral hemispheres. A lesion in any of these areas may prevent, reduce, or slow down the process of compensation.[38] Compensation occurs through three possible mechanisms: adaptation, substitution, and habituation.[7,11,36,39,40] Adaptation is the capability of the vestibular system to make long-term plastic changes in neuronal responses to head movement. Adaptation (see Case Study #3D, Unilateral Peripheral Hypofunction) can be used as a treatment strategy for patients with incomplete vestibular deficits. An effective stimulus for inducing adaptation of the vestibular system is movement of an image across the retina at the same time there is head movement. Substitution (see Case Study #3E, Bilateral Vestibular Hypofunction) is the use of alternative strategies to replace lost or compromised function (eg, bilateral vestibular loss). Effective stimuli for inducing substitution of the vestibular system are exercises that decrease the use of somatosensory and visual systems. Habituation (see Case Study #3D, Unilateral Peripheral Hypofunction) is the long-term reduction of a response to a noxious stimulus by repeated exposure to the stimulus.[38,41]

MENIERE'S DISEASE

Meniere's disease is an idiopathic disease characterized by episodic spells of vertigo associated with fluctuating, unilateral ear fullness, tinnitus (ringing in the ear), and a hearing loss.[7,42] Over time the hearing loss and tinnitus may become permanent. Hearing typically diminishes in lower frequencies first, and the higher frequencies are affected later in the course of the disease.[42] Vertigo is a spontaneously occurring sensation of movement accompanied by unsteadiness. Vertigo in Meniere's disease often decreases in frequency and

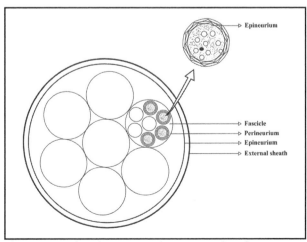

Figure 6-7. Sheaths surrounding a peripheral nerve.

severity and eventually stops all together many years after the onset of symptoms. This is known as "burnt-out" Meniere's disease.[42] Over time disequilibrium and constant ear fullness occur as a result of unilateral vestibular weakness.

A Meniere's episode generally involves severe vertigo, imbalance, nausea, and vomiting. The average attack lasts 2 to 4 hours.[7] After a severe attack, most people are extremely tired and sleep for several hours. In some cases Meniere's episodes may occur in clusters (several attacks within a short time), while in other cases weeks, months, or even years may pass between episodes. Most people are symptom free or note a mild imbalance and tinnitus between the attacks.[36]

The most common etiological theory is that Meniere's disease is caused by overdistension of the membranous labyrinth due to excessive endolymphatic fluid. Ears affected by Meniere's disease typically have a narrow vestibular aqueduct that may diminish the flow of endolymph into the endolymphatic sac. It is thought that the cochlea produces some metabolic debris that silts up the lumen of the duct. The endolymphatic sac senses the lack of endolymph and responds by both secreting a hormone, saccin, to increase the amount of endolymph and by secreting glycoproteins to attract endolymph. This combination clears the duct from obstruction. A sudden restoration of movement of endolymph toward the endolymphatic sac results in the sensation of vertigo.[43]

Meniere's disease has been classically managed by low salt dietary modifications, vestibular rehabilitation at the end stages of the disease or post surgically, psychological support, and pharmacologic intervention. A lack of understanding of the pathophysiology of Meniere's disease exists, and thus, most medical therapy is based on clinical experience.[44] When the treatment of Meniere's disease becomes refractory to medical management a variety of surgical options are available.[45,46] A vestibular nerve section can relieve the disabling vertigo while preserving hearing. When hearing on the involved side is not present, a labyrinthectomy is a possibility. An eighth nerve section, or translabyrinthine cochleovestibular neurectomy, may be performed when the patient is suffering from severe tinnitus.[45]

BENIGN PAROXYSMAL POSITIONAL VERTIGO

Benign paroxysmal positional vertigo (BPPV) is characterized by nystagmus with position change. The otoconia from the utricle become displaced into one of the semicircular canals.[7] In the canal they may either be free floating in the endolymph or adhere to the cupula, making them gravity sensitive. A change in head position results in a deflection of the cupula, which sends an afferent message to the vestibular nuclei that in turn sends a message to the extraocular musculature resulting in nystagmus. Nystagmus caused by the peripheral vestibular system can be suppressed with visual fixation.[32]

A 5- to 10-second delay of onset of symptoms once the specific position change has occurred is a characteristic finding with BPPV. The symptoms last less than 1 minute, the response decreases upon repetition, and upbeating, rotary nystagmus toward the undermost ear is seen with the Dix-Hallpike test (see page 176 for description of test).[7,33-35]

Advanced age (most commonly between the fifth and seventh decade), head trauma, labyrinthitis, or ischemia of the labyrinth predispose one to BPPV.[47-49] Approximately 50% to 70% of the cases of BPPV are "idiopathic."[47] BPPV is more common with advanced age due to degeneration of the otoconia and the maculae in which they rest. It has an incidence of up to 64 per 100,000.[48] Head trauma is the most common cause of simultaneous bilateral posterior canal BPPV.[35]

The vast majority of all BPPV cases are the posterior canal variant. Less than 30% of BPPV may be of the horizontal (lateral) canal type,[35,50] which resolves much more quickly than the posterior canal BPPV. This is in part due to the posterior canal, which hangs inferiorly and has its cupular barrier at its more dependent end, thus more likely trapping debris entering the canal.[35] In contrast, the horizontal canal slopes upward and has its cupular barrier at the upper end allowing free-floating debris to more likely float back into the utricle with normal head movement.

BPPV most often involves a single semicircular canal but may involve both posterior and horizontal semicircular canals in the same inner ear. Following the canalith repositioning maneuvers, posterior semicircular canal BPPV may convert to horizontal canal BPPV.[35]

PHYSICAL THERAPIST DIFFERENTIAL DIAGNOSES OF VESTIBULAR DYSFUNCTION

The physical therapist must make a differential diagnosis to determine the basis of the dizziness. It is important to keep in mind that a patient may have more than one diagnosis. For example, the patient may have a positional vertigo and a concurrent nonvestibular diagnosis. The following are examples of medical diagnoses or conditions that may be referred to physical therapists for vestibular rehabilitation.

♦ Unclear cervicogenic dizziness[51]: Controversy exists over whether this is a true diagnosis, and no definitive test for the diagnosis exists. It is a diagnosis of exclusion. Initially the physical therapist must rule out central or peripheral causes. The patient may have a history of cervical trauma. Complaints may include dizziness, lightheadedness, nausea and vomiting, neck pain, and/or frequent headaches. To test for cervicogenic dizziness, begin with the patient sitting in a chair and rotate the patient with the head and body moving together and evaluate for symptoms. Next keep the patient's head still and rotate the body only. If the first test does not cause symptoms but the second does, the patient may have cervicogenic dizziness. Treatment may include manual intervention to the cervical spine, exercises (described in the vestibular case studies in this chapter), balance training, and postural training.

♦ Mal de debarquement[52]: This patient would have an onset of dizziness immediately or within hours of finishing a cruise or boat ride, a long train ride, or possibly an airplane trip. The symptoms include rocking or swaying, nausea, and general dizziness that occur throughout most of the day. The symptoms may worsen with movement, but do not go away with lying still. The patient usually feels better when riding in a car. Current research[52] is controversial regarding whether physical therapy is helpful for this diagnosis. Controversy also exists within the medical profession whether this is a true diagnosis. It may be appropriate to alleviate symptoms by treating the balance problems, advising on available support groups and sources of information, such as the Vestibular Disorders Association Web site, and beginning an aerobic exercise program, since these patients become deconditioned as they increasingly avoid activity that triggers symptoms.

♦ Migraine[53,54]: This patient has episodes of dizziness that last minutes to hours and symptoms of vertigo, dizziness, or motion sickness. Symptoms may precede a headache. The vestibular evaluation may show an intolerance of motion, in which case the patient should be referred back to the physician regardless of whether he or she has been formally diagnosed with migraines.

♦ Orthostatic hypotension (OH): This patient typically describes the symptoms as lightheadedness, dizziness, headache, or blurred vision which occur when coming to sitting or standing from supine or are more ongoing in the case of orthostatic intolerance. OH is a decrease in systolic pressure of at least 20 mmHg or a decrease in diastolic pressure of at least 10 mmHg that occurs 3 minutes after rising from supine to standing. If orthostatic intolerance is suspected as the patient's only problem, it would be appropriate to refer the patient back to the physician.

♦ Panic attacks[55-57]: This patient typically describes the symptoms as dizziness, nausea, diaphoresis, fear, palpitations, or paresthesias. The occurrence may last for minutes or longer. The circumstances may be spontaneous or situational, but will not be provoked by position change or movements. The examination may otherwise be normal or may show an intolerance to motion. The score on the Positive and Negative Affective Scale (PANAS) may be positive for depression or anxiety.[58] This patient should be referred back to his or her physician and may need to see a psychiatrist.

♦ TIA[59]: This patient typically describes the symptoms as

vertigo, lightheadedness, disequilibrium, parasthesias, and decreased visual field. The symptoms may last minutes to hours. The vestibular examination tests should not provoke the symptoms. If a TIA is suspected, the patient should be immediately referred back to the physician.

♦ Aging[60]: With age, the peripheral vestibular system deteriorates in many ways. There is a decrease in number of hair cells and neurons to the ears. The otoconia of the utricle and saccule and the matrix upon which they rest degenerate. The CNS also demonstrates a decreased adaptive ability and less ability to augment the VOR with vision.

♦ Other factors associated with aging[61-64]: Many other changes in the body, all of which may have an effect on mobility and balance, are well documented. The visual system shows decreased acuity, contrast sensitivity, depth perception, color discrimination, and ability to focus. The somatosensory system demonstrates less kinesthesia, vibration sensation, and light touch. The musculoskeletal system deteriorates resulting in fewer muscle fibers and decreases in recruitment, reaction time, conduction velocity, and muscle contraction speed. Along with these changes, age-related changes in the cardiovascular and pulmonary systems also occur, which may result in symptoms of dizziness.

IMAGING

CARPAL TUNNEL SYNDROME

♦ Routine x-ray of the wrist and hand may reveal wrist fractures

IDIOPATHIC FACIAL NERVE BELL'S PARALYSIS

♦ CAT or CT scans and MRI scans have been advocated for specific cases of peripheral facial nerve paralysis[65]
  • These tests are most important when an acoustic neuroma, parotid tumor, facial nerve schwannoma,[24] or other surgically treatable etiology is suspected
  • Imaging should also be performed with direct trauma or when multiple system involvement is apparent

VESTIBULAR DYSFUNCTION

♦ CAT scans evaluate central and peripheral causes of vestibular dysfunction[66]

♦ MRI evaluates central and peripheral causes of vestibular dysfunction[66]

OTHER CLINICAL TESTS

CARPAL TUNNEL SYNDROME

♦ Ultrasonography
  • A promising technique for evaluation of morphologic changes of the median nerve in patients with CTS
  • Is non-invasive and is a relatively well-tolerated technique
  • An enlarged cross-sectional area at the middle of the carpal tunnel is seen with CTS
  • Preliminary results of ultrasonography research indicate that it has potential as a diagnostic tool for CTS[67]

♦ Electrodiagnostic tests, including needle EMG and nerve conduction velocity (NCV) tests
  • The first change that tends to occur when testing nerve function and integrity is a decrease in the amplitude of the sensory nerve action potential (SNAP)
  • In more severe conditions, positive NCV findings may include loss or prolongation/distal latency of the motor nerve action potential
  • Positive EMG findings may indicate denervation of thenar muscles
  • In a systemic review of the utility of electrodiagnositic tests in CTS, Jordan and associates concluded that "in cases of clear-cut clinical CTS, electrodiagnosis is not warranted either as a diagnostic test, where clinical symptoms are well defined, or as a predictive indicator of surgical outcome"[68]

IDIOPATHIC FACIAL NERVE BELL'S PARALYSIS

♦ Audiogram: Rules out a unilateral hearing impairment
♦ Physiological nerve testing
  • First week post onset: Nerve degeneration has not occurred, and therefore physiological nerve testing results may be normal even with severe pathology
  • After 1 week post onset: Other tests may be appropriate 1 week post depending upon the level and duration of the facial nerve involvement
    ■ Maximal stimulation test (MST)[69]
      ► Utilizes a nerve stimulator to evaluate the response to maximal nerve stimulation
      ► Although MST is a subjective evaluation of the neuromuscular function evoked by voluntary contractions, it is still considered useful to determine a prognosis[4,69]
      ► Eighty-five percent of patients who did not have a response to the MST after 10 days did

not have a full recovery[69]
      ► With strong stimulation, overflow of the stimulation pulse may result in activation of the masseter muscle and may lead to an erroneous more positive prognosis[70]
    ■ Nerve excitability test (NET)
      ► Utilizes a nerve stimulator to determine the threshold for a motor response
      ► Normal threshold ranges from 3.0 to 8.0 mA and should not vary by more than 2.0 mA between the involved and uninvolved sides[70]
      ► A 3.5 mA difference between the involved and uninvolved facial nerves on the NET indicates over 90% degeneration of the facial nerve[71]
    ■ Electroneuronography (ENog)
      ► Compares the amplitude of the compound motor unit action potential on both sides
      ► When there is a reduction of more than 90% on the involved side vs the unaffected side, the prognosis is poor[72]

♦ EMG
  • Has definite role in the diagnosis and prognosis of patients with facial nerve paralysis[70,73,74]
  • Needle EMG of specific facial muscles representing the different branches of the facial nerve confirms or rules out involvement of each branch of this cranial nerve
  • Pathological discharges at rest, such as fibrillation potentials and/or positive sharp waves, support a diagnosis of denervation of each particular muscle and reveal degeneration of the associated branch of the facial nerve
  • Absence of pathological discharges at rest indicates that the branch being tested may be intact
  • Types of motor units and the interference pattern found during voluntary contraction help reveal the state of the facial nerve
  • Normal motor units with a complete interference pattern would be expected in fully innervated muscles
  • Long duration polyphasic motor units would indicate a neuropathic process, and the interference pattern would reflect the ability of the patient to recruit motor units and/or degree of nerve damage
  • Absence of any motor units would indicate complete denervation or a complete nerve block
  • Electrical stimulation anterior to the external auditory meatus, where the facial nerve exits the skull, can be used to artificially test whether each branch of the facial nerve is intact
    ■ Recording over a muscle representative of each branch of the facial nerve allows determination of

a motor latency from this point of stimulation to the target muscle

- Prolonged latencies or absent responses indicate either demyelination or complete axonal degeneration of each branch
- If conduction study results are borderline or questionable, the results may be compared with testing on the intact side of the face
- Muscles most often selected for this testing include the orbicularis oculi, the orbicularis oris, and/or the frontalis

VESTIBULAR DYSFUNCTION

- Electronystagmography (ENG)[75]
  - Is a battery of tests that evaluates eye movement
  - Electrodes are placed around the eye or infrared goggles are used to record movement of the eye during different tasks
  - The tests may include any of the following
    - Saccade test
      - Tests movement of the eyes between specific visual points
      - An abnormal result may indicate CNS injury
    - Spontaneous nystagmus and gaze test
      - Observation of the eyes in a dark environment that prevents visual fixation followed by visual fixation on targets in various locations
      - An abnormal result may suggest CNS injury, if unable to suppress nystagmus with visual fixation
      - If able to suppress with visual fixation, it may more likely indicate a peripheral injury
    - Pursuit test
      - Tests movement of the eyes as they follow a visual target back and forth
      - An abnormal result may be a sign of CNS injury
    - Optokinetic test
      - Tests the development of nystagmus when a series of vertical lines are moving across the field of vision
      - The nystagmus has a slow phase in the direction that the vertical lines are moving
      - An abnormal response may indicate that the person has some type of damage in the CNS
    - Dix-Hallpike maneuver: Refer to Physical Therapist Clinical Tests for description
    - Positional test
      - Monitors for nystagmus provoked by various positions with the ability to visually fixate removed

- Bithermal caloric test
  - Warm/cold air or water is placed in the ear canal and should induce nystagmus
  - The nystagmus is measured
  - If the response does not match what is considered a normal response, the patient has a peripheral weakness (see Case Study #3D, Unilateral Peripheral Hypofunction)
- Hearing test: Hearing loss may help define a vestibular diagnosis
- Rotational chair test[75]
  - Tests a person's response to rotational movement
  - The person is placed in a rotating chair in a dark room
  - The chair is rotated at various speeds, and the eye movements of the person are observed with the use of infrared goggles or electrodes
  - The test compares velocity of the eyes with the velocity of the head at different chair speeds
  - An abnormal result may indicate central or peripheral damage, and at times the results may need to be compared with other test results
- Computerized dynamic posturography tests[75,76]
  - Test a person's visual, proprioceptive, and vestibular abilities while maintaining balance
  - During the tests the person stands on force plates, which can detect changes in force caused by postural sway
  - There are six tests
    1. Stable surface with vision present
    2. Stable surface with vision absent
    3. Stable surface with visual reference moving
    4. Sway reference surface with vision present
    5. Sway reference surface with vision absent
    6. Sway reference surface with visual reference moving
- Physical therapist clinical tests[32]
  - Positional tests (Note: If equipment, such as Frenzel glasses or infrared goggles, to prevent visual fixation are not available, the nystagmus may not be seen or the eyes may be seen to jump for a brief moment.)
  - In each test, observe for nystagmus and subjective symptoms
    - Sit to supine: Patient begins in long sitting and quickly lies flat
    - Supine to sit: Patient begins in supine and then quickly sits up
    - Roll test
      - Patient begins in supine with head in 20 degrees of flexion
      - Patient quickly rolls head to right (left)

- Dix-Hallpike maneuver
  - ▶ Patient begins in long sitting with head rotated 30 to 45 degrees to right (left)
  - ▶ While maintaining this head rotation, the patient is quickly laid flat so head/neck are extended over edge of table approximately 30 degrees below the horizontal (Figure 6-8); the therapist observes for nystagmus and subjective symptoms
- Seated cervical flexion: Patient begins in a sitting position and is asked to flex the neck forward toward the feet
- Seated cervical extension: Patient begins in a sitting position and is asked to extend the neck and look up toward the ceiling
- Visual tests
  - Smooth pursuits
    - ▶ Patient begins in a sitting position with the physical therapist seated directly in front
    - ▶ Patient's head remains still during this test
    - ▶ Patient is asked to follow the physical therapist's finger with his or her eyes, as the finger tracks 30 to 40 degrees for 2 to 3 seconds in each direction up and down and side to side
    - ▶ Observe for patient's ability to maintain focus on finger throughout activity
  - Saccades
    - ▶ Patient begins in a sitting position with physical therapist seated directly in front
    - ▶ Patient's head remains still during this test
    - ▶ Patient eyes start in center focused on the physical therapist's nose
    - ▶ On command patient moves eyes to a target that is 40 degrees from center
    - ▶ The timing of the commands must be varied so that the testing is unpredictable
    - ▶ Observe for overshooting and undershooting of the eyes
  - Head thrust test for VOR[77]
    - ▶ Prior to this test the cervical spine must be cleared, and the patient must be informed that the head will be turned from side to side
    - ▶ Patient is asked to fixate on a stationary target (eg, the physical therapist's nose) while the head is turned side to side by the physical therapist
    - ▶ The head is then turned with a small amplitude rapid head thrust
    - ▶ The physical therapist watches for the patient's ability to keep the eyes stable on the target
    - ▶ If the patient performs a small corrective saccade to bring the eyes back on the target after

the physical therapist completes the head thrust, it is a positive test
  - ▶ If this occurs when the head is turned to the right, the impairment is in the right ear, and vice versa
- VOR cancellation
  - ▶ Patient is instructed to move head, eyes, and target together

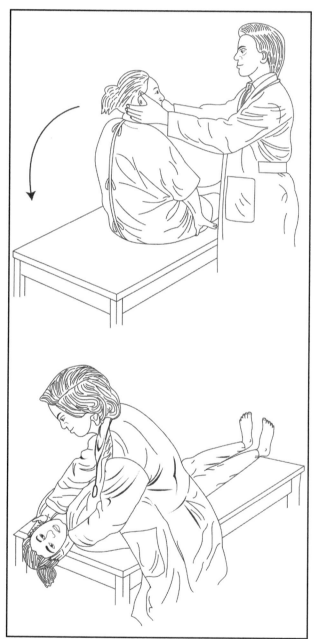

Figure 6-8. Dix-Hallpike maneuver. Adapted from Herdman SJ. Treatment of benign paroxysmal positional vertigo. *Phys Ther.* 1990;70(6):382, with permission of the American Physical Therapy Association. This material is copyrighted, and any further reproduction or distribution is prohibited.

- One way of doing this is having the patient extend both arms in front clasping hands together with thumbs held up
- Patient is instructed to focus on the thumbs and then rotate side to side
- Observe for the patient's ability to maintain focus on the target and for symptoms
- These results should agree with the results from the smooth pursuit test

PHARMACOLOGY

CARPAL TUNNEL SYNDROME

♦ Antihypertensive drugs
  - Example: Ramipril
  - Action: An ace inhibitor, lowers BP by decreasing arterial spasm
  - Side effects: Cough, dizziness, tiredness, diarrhea, runny nose
♦ Corticosteroid drugs
  - Example: Methylprednisone acetate
  - Action: Pain relief
  - Side effects: Upset stomach, vomiting, headache, easy bruising, dizziness, insomnia, depression, anxiety, acne, increased hair growth
♦ Diuretics for controlling fluid retention
  - Loop
    - Example: Furosemide (Lasix)
    - Action: Acts on the ascending loop of Henle in the kidney to decrease fluid volume
    - Side effects: Arrhythmias, dehydration, electrolyte imbalance, impairment of glycemic control
  - Potassium sparing
    - Examples: Amiloride (Midamor), spironolactone (Aldactone)
    - Actions: Decrease fluid volume, spare potassium, and decrease risk of arrhythmias
    - Side effects: Dehydration and impaired glycemic control
♦ NSAIDs
  - Examples: Ibuprofen (Advil, Motrin)
  - Actions: Relieves pain, tenderness, swelling
  - Side effects: Dizziness, constipation, diarrhea, ringing in ears

IDIOPATHIC FACIAL NERVE BELL'S PARALYSIS

Pharmacological interventions for the management of this disorder are still being debated, but some are considered appropriate.[4] Pharmacologic intervention is supported by studies demonstrating that the treatment of patients with "idiopathic" facial nerve paralysis with acyclovir (an antiviral medication) and steroids (such as prednisone) have produced significant, earlier recovery compared to no intervention.[78] Acyclovir is a specific drug that inhibits the replication of the herpes simplex virus (HSV) and has been shown to be the most effective drug for the treatment of HSV infection.[79] As stated earlier, more recent literature has supported the belief that a majority of the patients with "idiopathic" Bell's palsy may be due to the HSV, and therefore, treatment with a medication that inhibits HSV replication is appropriate. Steroids are well established as being extremely effective anti-inflammatory medications. In combination, these two medications have been shown to reduce the severity of HSV-induced facial nerve paralysis.[79,80] The key factor in the effectiveness of this pharmaceutical approach is that both acyclovir (400 mg five times/day) and prednisone (minimum of 30 mg twice/day) must be used in combination and started within 3 days of onset.[78,81]

For eye protection, the cornea and the full eyeball must be completely bathed to prevent drying and permanent damage. Artificial lubrication of the eye is the primary treatment. Preservative-free teardrops should be applied during the day, whereas a longer duration ointment should be applied at night.[4]

♦ Anti-inflammatory medication
  - Examples: Corticosteroid (prednisone)
  - Actions: Replaces steroids normally produced naturally by the body and counteracts inflammation
  - Side effects: Dizziness, mood changes, headache, acne, delayed healing, hair growth, muscle weakness
♦ Antiviral medication
  - Example: Acyclovir
  - Action: A synthetic nucleoside analogue that inhibits replication of HSV
  - Side effects: Vomiting, diarrhea, tiredness, dizziness, joint pain, hair loss
♦ Artificial tears
  - Examples: Carboxymethyl cellulose, hydroxypropyl cellulose
  - Actions
    - Used as a lubricant in nonvolatile eye drops
    - Stabilize and thicken the precorneal tear film and prolong the tear film breakup time
  - Side effects: Eye pain, irritation, continued redness, hyperemia, photophobia, stickiness of eyelashes

VESTIBULAR DYSFUNCTION[82-84]

Pharmacological agents utilized in the management of patients/clients who have a vestibular pathology include vestibular sedatives and anti-emetic agents. Vestibular sedative agents have a suppressant effect on the vestibular system that decreases vertigo symptomatically by suppressing vestibular activity. Medications are included in the class of antihistamines, anticholinergics, and benzodiazepines. Except in the case of chronic diseases, such as Meniere's, neurological conditions, and recurrent vertigo due to migraine, use of these agents should be limited as much as possible due to the risk of limiting recovery. Meniere's disease has been classically managed with diuretics. Anti-emetic agents suppress the central and peripheral components of the nervous system associated with vomiting. Many of the medications listed below have properties that allow them to act as anti-emetic, antihistamines, and anticholinergic agents. Typically medications do not help oscillopsia.

It is important to identify any medications being taken by the patient on examination, as a muted response may occur during vestibular testing with certain medications. It is also important for the physical therapist to know if the patient in rehabilitation is taking any medications, because responsiveness to vestibular rehabilitation activities may be affected by a sedated vestibular system. In addition, dizziness or vestibular dysfunction may be side effects of some medications.

- ◆ Anticholinergic
  - Scopolamine
    - Example: Transderm scop
    - Actions: Blocks receptor sites in parasympathetic nervous system, blocks receptors in smooth muscle resulting in decreases in involuntary movement, believed to block cholinergic transmission from vestibular nuclei to CNS
    - Functional class: Cholinergic blocker
    - Administered: Transdermal patch
    - Side effects: Paralytic ileus, dryness of mouth, constipation, drowsiness, blurring vision, dilation of pupils, disorientation, memory disturbances, dizziness, palpitations, skin rashes
    - Precautions/contraindications: Glaucoma, children, elderly, myasthenia gravis, intestinal obstruction, impaired renal or kidney function, enlarged prostate, HTN, dysrhythmia
- ◆ Anti-emetic
  - Droperidol
    - Example: Inapsine
    - Actions: Acts on CNS to produce sleep, tranquility, and anti-emetic
    - Functional classes: Neuroleptic, anti-emetic
    - Administered: Injected in muscle or administered intravenously
    - Side effects: Laryngospasm, bronchospasm, tachycardia, hypotension, chills, facial sweating, shivering
    - Precautions/contraindications: Elderly, cardiovascular disease, renal disease, liver disease, PD

- Ondansetron
  - Example: Zofran
  - Actions: Blocks serotonin, may be effective in controlling vertigo and nausea due to CNS disease[82,85,86]
  - Functional class: Anti-emetic
  - Administered: Tablet or may be injected in muscle or administered intravenously
  - Side effects: Bronchospasms, diarrhea, constipation, headache, dizziness, drowsiness, fatigue, extrapyramidal syndrome, musculoskeletal pain, wound problems, shivering, fever, hypoxia, urinary retention, rash
  - Precautions/contraindications: Pregnancy, lactation, children, elderly
- Prochlorperazine
  - Example: Compazine
  - Action: Acts centrally to decrease vomiting
  - Functional classes: Anti-emetic, antipsychotic
  - Administered: Tablet, may be injected in muscle, or administered intravenously
  - Side effects: Neuroleptic malignant syndrome, depression, circulatory failure, tachycardia, respiratory depression, extrapyramidal reactions, tardive dyskinesia, euphoria, restlessness, tremor, dizziness, nausea
  - Precautions/contraindications: Coma, seizure, encephalopathy, bone marrow depression, elderly, pregnancy
- Trimethobenzamine
  - Examples: Tigan, Arestin, Benzacot, Ticon
  - Action: Act centrally to decrease vomiting
  - Functional classes: Anti-emetic, anticholigenic
  - Administered: Tablet, may be injected in muscle, or administered intravenously
  - Side effects: Drowsiness, vertigo, restlessness, headache, dizziness, nausea, anorexia, HTN, hypotension, palpitation, rash, dry mouth, blurred vision
  - Precautions/contraindications: Children, cardiac dysrhythmias, elderly, asthma, pregnancy, enlarged prostate, glaucoma
- ◆ Antihistamines
  - Cyclizine
    - Example: Marezine
    - Actions: Relieves motion sickness, prevents postoperative vomiting, is an antihistamine
    - Administered: Tablet or may be injected in muscle
    - Precautions/contraindications: Hypersensitivity to cyclizines, shock
  - Dimenhydrinate

- Examples: Dramamine, Children's Dramamine
- Action: Decrease vestibular stimulation
- Functional classes: Anti-emetic, antihistamine, anticholinergic
- Administered: Tablet may be swallowed, chewed, dissolved, may be injected in muscle, or administered intravenously
- Side effects: Drowsiness, constipation, hypotension, dry mouth, anaphylaxis, headache, dizziness, confusion, nervousness, tingling, vertigo, HTN, palpitation, rash, blurred vision
- Precautions/contraindications: Children, cardiac dysrhythmias, elderly, asthma, pregnancy, prostate enlargement, glaucoma

- Diphenhydramine
  - Example: Benadryl
  - Actions
    - Blocks histamine action in blood vessels, gastrointestinal system, and respiratory system
    - Is a sedative at CNS level
  - Administered: Tablet or liquid
  - Side effects: Dizziness, drowsiness, seizures, urinary retention, thrombocytopenia, agranulocytosis, hemolytic anemia, fatigue, anxiety, paresthesia, neuritis, dry mouth, nausea, blurred vision
  - Precautions/contraindications: Glaucoma, cardiac condition, renal condition, prostate enlargement, asthma, seizure disorder, pregnancy

- Meclizine
  - Examples: Antivert, Bonine, Dramamine II, Meni-D, Ru-Vert-M
  - Actions: Act centrally to decrease vomiting and less sedative than some other medications
  - Functional classes: Anti-emetic, antihistamine, anticholinergic
  - Administered: Tablet may be swallowed, chewed, or dissolved
  - Side effects: Drowsiness, fatigue, restlessness, headache, insomnia, hypotension, urinary retention, nausea, anorexia
  - Precautions/contraindications: Children, glaucoma, urinary retention, prostate enlargement, asthma

- Promethazine
  - Example: Anergan 50[34]
  - Actions: Blocks histamine action in blood vessels, gastrointestinal system, and respiratory system and acts as sedative at CNS level
  - Administered: Tablet, liquid, may be injected in muscle, or administered intravenously
  - Side effects: Dizziness; drowsiness; constipation; urinary retention; thrombocytopenia; agranulocytosis; hemolytic anemia; poor coordination;

fatigue; hypotension; palpitations; tachycardia; dry mouth; nausea; anorexia; apnea in neonates, infants, and young children
  - Precautions/contraindications: Glaucoma, cardiac condition, renal condition, prostate enlargement, bronchial asthma, seizure disorder, pregnancy

- Benzodiazepines
  - Diazepam
    - Examples: Valium, Diazepam Intensol, Valrelease, Zetran
    - Actions: Is a sedative at CNS level, increase presynaptic inhibition, potentiate the actions of GABA
    - Functional class: Anti-anxiety
    - Administered: Tablet, may be injected in muscle, or administered intravenously
    - Side effects: Neutropenia, respiratory depression, ECG changes, tachycardia, dizziness, drowsiness, blurred vision, OH
    - Precautions/contraindications: Glaucoma, elderly, debilitated, hepatic disease, renal disease, pregnancy, potential addiction to drug
  - Hydroxyzine
    - Examples: Vistaril, Vistazine 50[34]
    - Action: Depress CNS
    - Functional classes: Anti-anxiety, antihistamine, sedative, hypnotic
    - Administered: Tablet or may be injected in muscle
    - Side effects: Convulsions, dizziness, drowsiness
    - Precautions/contraindications: Elderly, debilitated, hepatic disease, renal disease, glaucoma, chronic obstructive pulmonary disease
  - Lorazepam
    - Example: Ativan
    - Actions: Is a sedative at CNS level and potentiates the actions of GABA
    - Functional classes: Sedative, hypnotic, anti-anxiety
    - Administered: Tablet, may be injected in muscle, or administered intravenously
    - Side effects: ECG changes, tachycardia, dizziness, drowsiness, blurred vision, OH
    - Precautions/contraindications: Glaucoma, elderly, debilitated, hepatic disease, renal disease, pregnancy, potential addiction to drug

Alternative Remedies

- Ginger root
  - Latin name: Zingiber officinale roscoe
  - Actions: Relieves motion sickness and postoperative nausea, does not have sedative effects of other vestibular sedative drugs

■ Effectiveness not established for vertigo and nausea of vestibular dysfunction[82]
  ● Side effects: Heartburn
  ● Precautions/contraindications: Pregnancy
◆ Vertigoheel
  ● Homeopathic preparation available by prescription
  ● Actions: FDA approved for vertigo, related imbalance disorders, and related symptoms such as nausea[82]

Medications That May Cause Vestibular Dysfunction

◆ Gentamicin
  ● Example: Garamycin IV piggyback
  ● Actions: Interferes with bacteria protein resulting in cell death, used for severe systemic infections
  ● Functional class: Anti-infective
  ● Administered: Injected in muscle or administered intravenously
  ● Side effects: Ototoxicity, convulsions, neurotoxicity, nephrotoxicity, hepatic necrosis
  ● Precautions/contraindications: Neonates, mild renal disease, pregnancy, hearing deficits, myasthenia gravis, elderly, PD
  ● Studies indicate that drug may cause[87,88]
    ■ Idiosyncratic response in <3% of people
    ■ Bilateral vestibular hypofunction due to selective uptake by vestibular hair cells
      ► Occurs in 10% to 20% of those with renal impairment >65 years old, on loop diuretics, or with previous vestibular loss
      ► Occurs in 20% of those on renal dialysis

Case Study #1: Carpal Tunnel Syndrome

Mrs. Joann Carpenter is a 35-year-old female with a diagnosis of carpal tunnel syndrome with complaint of pain and intermittent tingling with occasional numbness of both hands and was referred to outpatient physical therapy.

PHYSICAL THERAPIST EXAMINATION

HISTORY

◆ General demographics: Mrs. Carpenter is a 35-year-old white female whose primary language is English. She is right-hand dominant. She is a high school graduate with on-the-job computer training.

◆ Social history: Mrs. Carpenter is married and has two young sons, ages 7 and 9.

◆ Employment/work: She is a data entry keyboard operator for a major Internet mail order company and is currently on medical leave from her employment.

◆ Living environment: She lives in a single-family home with her husband and her children.

◆ General health status
  ● General health perception: Mrs. Carpenter reports that her health has been fairly good prior to this episode.
  ● Physical function: Normal for her age prior to current episode.
  ● Psychological function: She states that she feels depressed and concerned about her job and her family's welfare.
  ● Role function: Wife, mother, keyboard operator.
  ● Social function: Mrs. Carpenter actively participates in her children's school activities. She often volunteers in making arts and crafts for fundraising projects for her church.

◆ Social/health habits: Mrs. Carpenter does not smoke and considers herself a social drinker (one or two drinks per week).

◆ Family history: Her mother had diabetes that resulted in an above knee amputation and died of natural causes at age 75, and her father died of congestive heart failure at age 69.

◆ Medical/surgical history: She had a C-section with the birth of her second child, and she currently has HTN.

◆ Current condition(s)/chief complaint(s): She complains of intermittent tingling, swelling, and pain in her hands. Her hands fall asleep. She is often awakened in the night by pain in one or both hands and fingers. Gentle rubbing, wringing, or shaking of her hands "make them feel better." She states that her symptoms are worse at the end of the work day or when she knits. At present she is unable to work due to worsening of her symptoms and is on a medical leave from her job. She complains that her symptoms have progressively increased, and her condition has worsened over the past 4 months. She has recently noticed that she occasionally drops objects and is finding it increasingly difficult to use her hands and fingers for opening jars and for fine hand activities, such as knitting, buttoning, threading needles, and playing the piano.

◆ Functional status and activity level: Prior to the onset of symptoms, Mrs. Carpenter was independent in all basic ADL and IADL.

- Medications: She is currently taking diuretics for control of her fluid retention, ramipril for her HTN, and oral NSAIDs as needed for pain control. She reported that she had two (40 mg and 80 mg) local injections of methylprednisone acetate to the wrist for transient relief 4 months ago.
- Other clinical tests
  - EMG: Normal
  - NCV
    - Motor NCV: Positive and revealed a decreased motor nerve action potential amplitude and prolonged distal latency (amplitude decreases before latency changes).
    - Sensory NCV: Positive with prolonged distal latency and decreased amplitude.
    - Motor and sensory NCV confirmed the clinical diagnosis of CTS.

SYSTEMS REVIEW

- Cardiovascular/pulmonary
  - BP: 140/84 mmHg (with antihypertensive medication)
  - Edema
    - Tends to retain fluids
    - Edema (2+) over wrist joint and volar and dorsal aspects of both hands
    - Edema (2+) over the dorsum of both feet and around the medial malleolus bilaterally
  - HR: 78 bpm
  - RR: 18 bpm
- Integumentary
  - Presence of scar formation: C-section surgical scar
  - Skin color: WNL
  - Skin integrity: WNL
- Musculoskeletal
  - Gross range of motion:
    - Bilateral UEs and LEs WNL
    - Minimal limitations in wrist flexion and extension and thumb abduction bilaterally
  - Gross strength: Minor limitations demonstrated in wrist flexion, wrist extension, and hand function requiring prehension
  - Gross symmetry: WNL
  - Height: 5'3" (1.6 m)
  - Weight: 152 lbs (69 kg)
- Neuromuscular
  - Balance: WNL
  - Locomotion, transfers, and transitions: WNL
- Communication, affect, cognition, language, and learning style

- Communication, affect, and cognition: WNL
- Learning style: Visual learner

TESTS AND MEASURES

- Aerobic capacity/endurance: WNL
- Anthropometric characteristics
  - Body mass index=weight divided by height^2=69/2.56=26.95
  - Mrs. Carpenter is overweight (normal=18.5 to 24.9; overweight=25 to 29.9; obese=30 to <40)
- Assistive and adaptive devices: None
- Cranial and peripheral nerve integrity
  - Two-point discrimination
    - Poor threshold (using the Disk Criminator)
    - Patient averaged 12 mm discrimination over digits one through three (normal less than 6 mm)
    - Test results indicated difficulty in handling precision tools[89]
  - Decreased sensation with paresthesia and tingling in wrist, index, middle, and radial half of ring fingers in both hands
  - Ten Test[90]
    - Quick test for clinical sensibility
    - Lightly stroke normal body part, which is assigned a 10, and then simultaneously and with equal pressure stroke abnormal area and ask patient to compare on scale of 1 to 10 (10=best sensibility)
    - Decreased touch sensibility over digits one through three (as compared to that over the fifth digit)
    - Digits one through three=6
  - Vibration threshold: WNL in palm and dorsum of each hand as measured by response to tuning forks
- Ergonomics and body mechanics
  - Analysis of sitting and standing postures revealed slight kyphotic posture with rounded shoulders and forward head
- Muscle performance
  - MMT of RUE and LUE revealed the following deviations from normal in her wrist and hand
    - Right wrist flexion=4-/5
    - Left wrist flexion=4-/5
    - Right wrist extension=3-/5
    - Left wrist extension=4-/5
    - Right thumb abduction=4/5
    - Left thumb abduction=4/5
    - Right thumb opposition=3-/5
    - Left thumb opposition=3-/5
    - Right thumb flexion=3/5
    - Left thumb flexion=4-5
    - Right finger flexion—first and second digits (lum-

bricals 1-2)=3-/5
- Left finger flexion—first and second digits (lumbricals 1-2)=3-/5
● No significant muscle atrophy of thenar muscles noted
◆ Orthotic, protective, and supportive devices
● Mrs. Carpenter wears bilateral over-the-counter wrist splints when sleeping at night
◆ Pain
● Symptoms Severity Scale (SSS) of the Boston Carpal Tunnel Scales Questionnaire[91]
  - The 11-item Boston SSS questionnaire relates to the severity of nocturnal pain and paresthesia, frequency of wakening at night, pain in the hand and wrist during the day, presence of numbness or weakness in the hand, and difficulty manipulating small objects
  - Each area is scored 1 through 5, with 5 being the most severe
  - All scores are added and divided by 11 and the reported score is out of a total of 5
  - Patient's baseline score was 3/5
● Provocative CTS tests[92]
  - Phalen's test
    ▶ Procedures: Back of the hands are held together, fingers pointing down for gravity-assisted maximum flexion of wrists, held for approximately 1 minute
    ▶ Results: Positive test with increased symptoms of paresthesia in wrist and digits one through three
  - Reversed Phalen's test
    ▶ Procedures: Active extension of wrist and fingers held for approximately 2 minutes
    ▶ Results: Positive test resulted in increased symptoms of paresthesia in wrist and digits one through three bilaterally
  - Carpal compression test
    ▶ Procedures: Examiner presses over carpal tunnel (proximal crease) with thumbs for approximately 30 seconds
    ▶ Results: Positive test resulted in increased symptoms of paresthesia
  - Tinel's test
    ▶ Procedures: Examiner taps over the median nerve as is runs under the carpal tunnel
    ▶ Results: Positive test resulted in tingling and numbness along the median nerve distribution to digits one through three
  - Tethered median nerve stress test
    ▶ Procedures: Examiner hyperextends the index finger and wrist with the forearm in supination

▶ Results: Positive test resulted in increased pain radiating to the forearm
  - Flick sign
    ▶ Procedures: Patient shakes the hand
    ▶ Results: Positive test resulted in relief of symptoms
  - Tests to rule out more proximal median nerve entrapment[92]
    ▶ Resisted full elbow flexion or resisted supination: Negative for entrapment at the ligament of Struthers and lacertus fibrosus
    ▶ Resisted forearm pronation: Negative for pronator teres compression
    ▶ Resisted middle finger flexion: Negative for flexor digitorum superficialis
● Patient reported pain of 3-4/10 on the NPS (where 0=no pain and 10=worst possible pain)[93]
◆ Posture
● Observation of postural alignment and position (static and dynamic)
  - Slightly increased thoracic kyphosis
  - Rounded shoulders
  - Forward head
◆ Range of motion
● Goniometry: All ROM reported in degrees limited secondary to complaint of pain/poor tolerance[94]
  - Forearm pronation/supination: WNL (~85 to 90)
  - Wrist flexion: R=0 to 60, L=0 to 65, normal=80 to 90
  - Wrist extension: R=0 to 50, L=0 to 55, normal=70 to 90
  - Wrist abduction/radial deviation: R=0 to 10, L=0 to 10, normal=~15
  - Wrist adduction/ulnar deviation: R=0 to 25, L=0 to 25, normal=~30 to 45
  - Digits one and two finger MCP flexion: R=0 to 70, L=0 to 75, normal=85 to 90
  - Digits three and four: Right and left WNL
  - Thumb CMC flexion: R=0 to 40, L=0 to 40, normal=~45 to 50
  - Thumb MCP flexion: R=0 to 45, L=0 to 45, normal=~50 to 55
  - Thumb abduction: R=0 to 50, L=0 to 55, normal=~60 to 70
  - Thumb adduction: Right and left WNL (~30)
◆ Self-care and home management
● The eight-item Functional Status Scale (FSS) portion of the Boston Carpal Tunnel questionnaire assessed functional activities, such as writing, buttoning, holding a telephone, carrying groceries, holding a

book to read, opening jars, household chores, and bathing and dressing[91]

- Indicated moderate functional difficulties (3/5) with writing, opening jars, bathing and dressing especially buttoning or zipping clothes, lacing shoes, and grooming
- In addition, Mrs. Carpenter has difficulty in typing, knitting, and performing household chores, such as cooking, cutting, and preparing food, opening jars, taking things in and out of the oven, turning on twist light switches, cleaning windows, scrubbing the tub/shower, doing the laundry, holding a telephone, writing, sewing, carrying groceries, and picking up small, large, or heavy objects

- Jebsen-Taylor hand function test, which is a timed test of common hand functions such as writing, card turning, simulated feeding, and picking up small, large, or heavy objects[95]

- Similar functional difficulties observed as above

- Difficulty with self-care and home management especially those activities that require dexterity and fine hand movements including grooming, buttoning, completing dressing, cutting, and preparing food

♦ Work, community, and leisure integration or reintegration

- Mrs. Carpenter has been unable to work as a keyboard data entry operator and is currently on medical leave
- She is unable to keep up with her church arts and crafts fundraising activities
- Her leisure activities have also been decreased

EVALUATION

Mrs. Carpenter's risk factors previously outlined indicated that she is a 35-year-old white female with complaints of intermittent pain, tingling with occasional numbness of both hands, and weakness of both hands. She complains of nocturnal symptoms that are relieved by shaking or massaging her hands and is using a wrist/hand splint during sleep to relieve her discomfort. She is a keyboard operator and currently on medical leave due to her CTS. Mrs. Carpenter has muscle weakness, decreased ROM, and altered sensation. She is limited in ADL and IADL. She has difficulty in performing and sustaining tasks that require repetitive hand movements and dexterity. She is currently unable to continue with her community responsibilities due to her inability to make arts and crafts items for fundraising for her church and school.

DIAGNOSIS

Mrs. Carpenter is a patient with CTS with pain involving both hands. She has impaired: anthropometric characteris-

tics; cranial and peripheral nerve integrity; ergonomics and body mechanics; muscle performance; posture; and range of motion. She is functionally limited in self-care and home management and in work, community, and leisure actions, tasks, and activities. She is in need of devices and equipment. These findings are consistent with placement in Pattern F: Impaired Peripheral Nerve Integrity and Muscle Performance Associated With Peripheral Nerve Injury. The identified impairments, functional limitations, and device and equipment needs will be addressed in determining the prognosis and the plan of care.

PROGNOSIS AND PLAN OF CARE

Over the course of the visits, the following mutually established outcomes have been determined:

♦ Ability to perform home management activities is improved
♦ Ability to perform physical activities including ADL is improved
♦ Edema is reduced
♦ Functional independence in ADL and IADL is increased
♦ Muscle performance is increased
♦ Pain is decreased
♦ Peripheral nerve integrity is increased
♦ Physical function is improved
♦ Postural control is improved
♦ ROM is improved
♦ Self-management of symptoms is improved

To achieve these outcomes, the appropriate interventions for this patient are determined. These will include: coordination, communication, and documentation; patient/client-related instruction; therapeutic exercise; functional training in self-care and home management; functional training in work, community, and leisure integration or reintegration; prescription, application, and, as appropriate, fabrication of devices and equipment; electrotherapeutic modalities; and physical agents and mechanical modalities.

Based on the diagnosis and prognosis, Mrs. Carpenter is expected to require between 20 and 25 visits over an 8-week period of time. Mrs. Carpenter has good family and social support, is motivated, and will follow through with her home exercise program. She is only moderately impaired and is generally in good health.

INTERVENTIONS

RATIONALE FOR SELECTED INTERVENTIONS

Therapeutic Exercise

Inflammation and tissue structural changes limit the nerve and tendon excursion within the carpal tunnel. This leads to tethering of the nerve, which reduces nerve perfusion and compromises function.[96] The benefits of therapeutic exercise in the management of CTS are well established and supported by numerous studies. By measuring carpal tunnel pressure, Seradge and colleagues[97] showed that 1-minute intermittent active wrist and finger exercise can lower pressure in the carpal tunnel. Tendon and nerve gliding exercises have been reported to be effective in the conservative intervention of CTS.[98,99] The beneficial effects are thought to be due to stretching of the tendon and nerve tissues directly and due to enhancing venous return and edema reduction.[100] Seradge and associates[101] found reduced post-intervention scores on the SSS and FSS of the Boston Carpal Tunnel Scales questionnaires in patients treated with carpal tunnel decompression wrist and hand exercises involving gliding of the tendon and nerve tissues. Exercise techniques, such as grip-strengthening exercises with either putty or hand grippers, tend to increase pressure within the carpal tunnel and are not appropriate interventions for CTS.[102]

Prescription, Application, and, as Appropriate, Fabrication of Devices and Equipment

Application of a custom-fitted hand splint during the day and night or only during the night (nocturnal splinting) has been recommended for reducing wrist, hand, and finger discomfort. The rationale for using splinting is based on the reduced pressure in the carpal tunnel when the wrist is in neutral (0 degrees) anatomical position with respect to extension, flexion, and ulnar and radial deviation and when the forearm is in neutral rotation.[103] Mrs. Carpenter has been wearing an over-the-counter splint, which does not provide a proper fit. The literature indicates that a custom fabricated thermoplastic splint or a properly fitting prefabricated splint with adjustable angle bar or insert has been recommended as the first line of intervention in the conservative management of the symptoms associated with CTS.[102] The benefits of splinting are supported by numerous studies.[14,104] Seradge and colleagues[100,101] and Akalin and associates[98] also reported the beneficial effects of a combined program of splinting and tendon/nerve gliding exercises. In a randomized controlled trial, Manente and coworkers[105] used the SSS and FSS scales of the Boston Carpal Tunnel questionnaire to compare outcome scores of night splinting with control

subjects who did not use splinting. Their study showed that the splinting group had a significant reduction in SSS and FSS scores indicating improvement of both symptoms and function. Splinting for 6 weeks is supported by a study by Walker and colleagues,[106] who compared the results of 6 weeks of night-only use to the results of full-time, night-and-day use of splinting in patients with CTS. The study showed improvement in symptoms, function, and electroneuromyographic test results. For optimal physiologic response, they recommended full-time, night and day, splinting.[106]

Device and equipment needs or modification are also important in the workplace. The normal pressure in the carpal tunnel is reported to be least when the wrist is in a neutral position. Pressure markedly increases when the wrist is moved into flexion or extension.[98]

Electrotherapeutic Modalities

Iontophoresis is effective in disseminating local concentrations of drugs to the carpal tunnel with little systemic effects. Dexamethasone sodium phosphate is an effective anti-inflammatory agent, and iontophoresis deposits the drug in the area of the epidermis with deeper penetration apparently occurring with passive diffusion. Iontophoresis of dexamethasone sodium phosphate was reported to be an effective analgesic and anti-inflammatory agent in the management of CTS. Gokoglu and associates[107] compared the effects of corticosteroid injection and dexamethasone sodium phosphate iontophoresis on relieving CTS symptoms. They reported that iontophoresis of 0.4% dexamethasone sodium phosphate with 40 to 45 mA continuous direct current applied for 20 minutes was effective in relieving CTS symptoms. Treatment was given every other day for 1 week. Compared to injection, iontophoresis provided a less invasive means of delivering corticosteroids to the tissues. Although symptom relief was greater with corticosteroid injection, the noninvasive application of iontophoresis does seem to have an advantage over invasive techniques.

Physical Agents and Mechanical Modalities

Ebenbichler and colleagues[108] compared the use of pulsed ultrasound treatment to sham (no ultrasound) treatment in CTS. They used pulsed ultrasound with 1 MHz frequency at 1.0 W/cm^2 in the pulsed mode of 1:4 (20% duty cycle) for 15 minutes a session. Pulsed ultrasound was applied daily for 2 weeks followed by twice a week for 5 weeks for a total of 20 sessions. Compared to the sham treatments, pulsed ultrasound was found to significantly reduce symptoms and complaints of pain and to significantly improve handgrip and finger pinch strength. Positive effects of ultrasound were shown in both short- and long-term effects, at 2 to 7 weeks and at 8 months, respectively. Increased circulation to the treated area was thought to be the basis for the observed improvements. Other studies have indicated conflicting evidence for ultrasound effectiveness in CTS. In contrast to the use of pulsed ultrasound, Oztas and coworkers[109] found no support for the use of continuous ultrasound and stated that continuous ultrasound is not recommended due to the potential of tissue overheating and subsequent adverse effects on the median nerve.

COORDINATION, COMMUNICATION, AND DOCUMENTATION

Communication will occur with Mrs. Carpenter regarding all components of her care to engender support for her program. Management will start in the outpatient environment and will continue at home through her return to work, community, and leisure activities. Assessment and modification of her work environment and recommendations regarding transition back to work will be communicated to the appropriate individuals managing her case. All elements of the patient's management, including examination, evaluation, diagnosis, prognosis, and interventions, will be documented.

PATIENT/CLIENT-RELATED INSTRUCTION

The patient will be fully instructed about her current condition, impairments, and functional limitations. The patient will be instructed in a home exercise program and will understand the importance of her home exercise program and the outcomes that can be expected. Mrs. Carpenter will be instructed in strategies to prevent further exacerbation of her condition. She will be instructed to modify her work environment both at home and at the workplace. Mrs. Carpenter will be instructed to raise her chair and adjust her desk and arm rest/support both at home and at work. She will be instructed to place her wrist at an optimum neutral position. She will also be instructed in correct shoulder mechanics so that she does not elevate her scapula and internally rotate her shoulders to compensate for decreased mobility of her wrists. Altered posture of her shoulders could potentially lead to a secondary problem of shoulder tendonitis. In addition, she will be instructed to incorporate frequent breaks during her workday and practice her stretching exercises.

She will use correct posture, body mechanics, and wrist position; perform stretching exercises; take rest breaks as frequently as may be allowed at work; and wear splints to keep wrists in neutral position. She will receive ongoing instruction/modification and progression of her therapeutic exercise and home exercise program. She will be instructed in enhancement of performance, health, wellness, and fitness programs. She will also be informed of the plan of care that will include transitioning back into her work, community, and leisure activities.

Her leisure craft activities will be reviewed to identify exactly what types of crafts she does and then determine what she should/should not be doing and/or implement modifications or alternative crafts. Mrs. Carpenter will be referred to a clinical psychologist and a social worker for career counseling and to explore alternative positions at her job. She will also be referred to a nutritionist for improving her diet and weight loss.

THERAPEUTIC EXERCISE

◆ Balance, coordination, and agility training
  ● Practice of hand movements requiring dexterity and fine movements, such as picking up coins, writing, shuffling and dealing cards
◆ Body mechanics and postural stabilization
  ● Postural control training
    ■ Proper alignment of head, cervical and thoracic spines, and shoulders
    ■ Axial extension
    ■ Scapula retraction and depression
  ● Postural stabilization activities
    ■ Maintenance of axial extension position with hand activities
    ■ Core stabilization while sitting on ball
  ● Postural awareness training
    ■ Postural corrections in sitting to achieve upright head, neck, and trunk
◆ Flexibility exercises
  ● Stretching exercises should be done after warming up, using a slow and steady stretch accompanied by deep breathing, and building hold up to 30 to 60 seconds
    ■ Stretch soft tissues and muscles of the shoulder, neck, and arms including the trapezius, rhomboids, levator scapulae, deltoids, infraspinatus, teres major, and teres minor
    ■ ROM for elbow flexion/extension, wrist flexion/extension, and pronation/supination
  ● Tendon gliding exercises
    ■ Hold each hand/finger position for approximately 5 seconds
    ■ Repeat each exercise 10 times
    ■ Performed twice a day for 4 weeks
    ■ Hand and fingers are placed in five positions (Figure 6-9)
      ▶ Straight
      ▶ Hook
      ▶ Fist
      ▶ Tabletop
      ▶ Straight fist
  ● Median nerve gliding exercises
    ■ Exercises start with patient in a sitting position with head, neck, and shoulders well aligned in neutral position, elbows in 90 degrees flexion, and wrist in supination

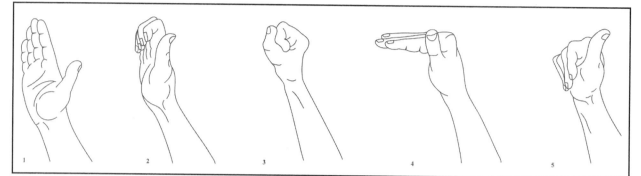

Figure 6-9. Tendon gliding exercises

- Hold each hand/finger position for approximately 5 seconds
- Repeat each exercise 10 times
- Perform twice a day for 4 weeks
- With the elbow flexed and on the table, the wrist, thumb, and fingers are placed in the following six positions (see Figure 6-10 for some examples)
  ▶ Wrist in neutral position, fingers and thumb in flexion (fist)
  ▶ Wrist in neutral position, fingers and thumb extended
  ▶ Wrist and fingers extended, thumb in neutral position
  ▶ Wrist, fingers, and thumb extended
  ▶ Wrist, fingers, and thumb extended with forearm in supination
  ▶ Wrist, fingers, and thumb extended and the opposite hand applies gentle stretch to the thumb

◆ Strength, power, and endurance training
  • Progressive resistive exercise using weights or elastic bands for UEs as tolerated, including shoulder flexion/extension, abduction/adduction, external/internal rotation, and elbow flexion/extension
  • Active exercises of the fingers and hands using pegs of various shapes and sizes and rubber bands of various resistance
  • Timed hand functional exercises using blocks, playing cards, pegs, or paper clips

FUNCTIONAL TRAINING IN SELF-CARE AND HOME MANAGEMENT

◆ Self-care
  • Review of correct positions and appropriate training in self-care activities, including bathing, grooming, feeding, and dressing, especially buttoning or zipping clothes and lacing shoes
  • Timed functional training in all activities above

◆ Home management
  • Using adapted equipment as needed, review of correct positions and appropriate training in home management activities, including household chores; cooking, cutting, and preparing food; writing; holding a telephone; carrying groceries; picking up small or large or heavy objects; opening jars; taking things in and out of the oven; scrubbing a pot; turning on twist lights; cleaning windows; scrubbing the tub/shower; and doing laundry
  • Timed functional training in all activities above
  • Ensure wrists and shoulders are in neutral position with arms resting on a support

FUNCTIONAL TRAINING IN WORK, COMMUNITY, AND LEISURE INTEGRATION OR REINTEGRATION

◆ Work
  • Review of correct positions and appropriate training in work actions, tasks, and activities, including keyboard use, filing, and using scissors
  • Timed functional training in all activities above
  • Workplace modifications
    ■ Instruction and practice of proper body alignment in sitting, including head, neck, and upper back alignment
    ■ Adjustment of chair height so work desk allows for correct arm and hand positioning (shoulder in anatomical position, elbow and forearm supported)
    ■ Determine appropriate position of materials being typed while on computer (so that eye level allows for good body alignment and optimum sitting posture is maintained)
    ■ Determine need for ergonomic computer mouse
    ■ Ensure wrists are in optimum neutral position and forearms are supported on arm rest
    ■ Use a back support and a small footstool when

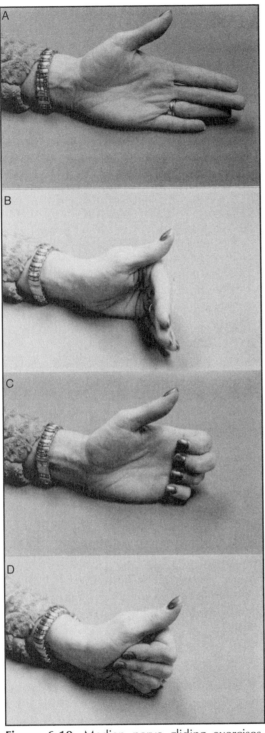

Figure 6-10. Median nerve gliding exercises. Reprinted from Michlovitz SL. Conservative interventions for carpal tunnel syndrome. *J Orthop Sports Phys Ther.* 2004;34(10):589-600. doi:10.2519/jospt.2004.1562, with permission of the Orthopaedic Section and the Sports Physical Therapy Section of the American Physical Therapy Association.

sitting to ensure correct alignment
- Breaks should be frequent during the work day with maximum time period allowed by employer
- Perform stretching exercises throughout the day

◆ Community
  - Review of correct positions and appropriate training in community actions, tasks, and activities, including arts and crafts

◆ Leisure
  - Review of correct positions and appropriate training in leisure actions, tasks, and activities, including knitting, card shuffling and playing, and holding a book to read

PRESCRIPTION, APPLICATION, AND, AS APPROPRIATE, FABRICATION OF DEVICES AND EQUIPMENT

◆ Custom fabricated and well-fitted hand splint
  - Wrists are supported by the splint to the level of the MCP joints
  - Worn initially during the day and night and later when symptoms resolve worn at night only for a total of 6 weeks

ELECTROTHERAPEUTIC MODALITIES

◆ Iontophoresis of 0.4% dexamethasone sodium phosphate
  - Electrode placement
    - Active electrode with dexamethasone applied longitudinally over the median nerve of each wrist
    - Dispersive electrode is placed over the dorsum of the hand
  - Intensity: 40 to 45 mA continuous direct current
  - Duration: 20-minute sessions
  - Frequency: Three times a week for 2 weeks

PHYSICAL AGENTS AND MECHANICAL MODALITIES

◆ Pulsed ultrasound
  - Dosage: 1.0 W/cm^2 1 MHz frequency
  - Mode: Pulsed mode with 1:4 (20%) duty cycle
  - Duration: 15 minutes a session, applied three times a week, for 2 weeks and two times a week for up to 5 weeks up to a total of 20 sessions

ANTICIPATED GOALS AND EXPECTED OUTCOMES

◆ Impact on pathology/pathophysiology
  - Compression on nerve is reduced.

- Nerve and soft tissue swelling and inflammation are reduced.
- Pain is decreased.
- Self-management of symptoms is improved.

◆ Impact on impairments
- Motor and sensory function, muscle performance, and postural control are improved.
- Pain-free ROM of both wrists and finger extension and flexion is achieved.

◆ Impact on functional limitations
- Ability to independently perform physical activities and tasks related to ADL/IADL in self-care, such as grooming and dressing, and in home management activities, such a food preparation, return to normal.
- Ability to independently perform physical activities and tasks in work-related activities, such as typing and filing, and in community activities, such as arts and crafts and knitting, return to normal.
- Ability to use both hands functionally is improved.
- Level of assistance required for hand function and task performance is normal.
- Safety during self-care, home management, work, community, and leisure is improved.

◆ Risk reduction/prevention
- Ergonomics and workplace are modified.
- Risk factors and the risk of secondary impairments are reduced.

◆ Impact on health, wellness, and fitness
- Behaviors that foster healthy habits, wellness, and fitness are acquired.
- Behaviors that incorporate prevention are acquired.
- Decision making is enhanced regarding health, wellness, and fitness needs.
- Fitness, health status, physical capacity, and physical function are improved.

◆ Impact on societal resources
- Available resources are maximally utilized.
- Documentation occurs throughout patient management and follows the APTA's *Guidelines for Physical Therapy Documentation.*[110]
- Physical therapy services will be utilized optimally and result in the efficient use of health care dollars.
- Utilization and cost of health care services are decreased.

◆ Patient/client satisfaction
- Care is coordinated with family and other professionals.
- Patient and family are satisfied with the access, availability, and services provided and the clinical proficiency and interpersonal skills of the physical therapist.

- The patient and family knowledge and awareness of the diagnosis, prognosis, interventions, and understanding of anticipated goals and expected outcomes are increased.

REEXAMINATION

Reexamination is performed throughout the episode of care. The SSS and FSS of the Boston Carpal Tunnel questionnaires were used to determine post-intervention outcomes.[91]

DISCHARGE

Mrs. Carpenter is discharged from physical therapy after a total of 25 outpatient physical therapy sessions over 8 weeks and attainment of her goals and expectations. These sessions have covered her entire episode of care. She is discharged because she has achieved the goals and expected outcomes.

Case Study #2: Bell's Palsy

Mrs. Pamela Rivera is a 37-year-old female who had difficulty controlling her mouth while brushing her teeth earlier today and noticed a drooping of the right side of her face and fears she may have had a stroke.

PHYSICAL THERAPIST EXAMINATION

HISTORY

◆ General demographics: Mrs. Rivera is a 37-year-old Hispanic woman whose primary language is Spanish, but she speaks fluent English. She is right-hand dominant.

◆ Social history: She lives with her husband, two teenage children, and her parents. Her children are both in high school.

◆ Employment/work: Mrs. Rivera is an elementary school teacher. Her husband is an investment banker.

◆ Living environment: The family owns their home, which is a ranch-style house with three bedrooms and three full baths. The parents have one of the three bathrooms off of their bedroom.

◆ General health status
- General health perception: Mrs. Rivera has no specific health conditions and has been healthy until today.

- Physical function: She is physically active, on her feet most of the working day. She has been independent in all ADL, drives a car, and does the family shopping.
- Psychological function: She is concerned about her acute symptoms and is anxious about whether she had a stroke. Her husband reports that she is typically somewhat anxious but that their family interactions have all been very supportive and positive.
- Role function: Wife, mother, teacher, housekeeper.
- Social function: She is active socially with her husband. Mrs. Rivera is an active member in her children's high school activities and in her local church activities.

◆ Social/health habits: She does not drink or smoke.

◆ Family history: Both parents are alive and well.

◆ Medical/surgical history: She gave birth to both her children via normal vaginal delivery.

◆ Preexisting medical and other health-related conditions: She has an elevated cholesterol level that is under control with medication.

◆ Current condition(s)/chief complaint(s): Mrs. Rivera reported that she was aware of pain near her right ear that started about 2 days ago. While performing basic dental/facial hygiene this morning, she reported difficulty brushing her teeth and rinsing her mouth, drooping of the right side of her face, inability to close her right eyelid, and difficulty frowning and moving the right side of her face. She was anxious about the cause of this and wondered if she was having a stroke. Her husband has been very supportive and took off the day from work to drive her to her medical appointment today.

◆ Functional status and activity level: Prior to today, she was fully independent and had no limitations in her desired level of physical activity.

◆ Medications: She is presently taking Lipitor for elevated cholesterol levels.

◆ Other clinical tests
  - Complete blood tests have been done every year to check all levels, especially high-density lipoproteins, low-density lipoproteins, and liver function, which are reported to be WNL (on meds for elevated cholesterol) at this time.

SYSTEMS REVIEW

◆ Cardiovascular/pulmonary
  - BP: 125/85 mmHg
  - Edema: WNL
  - HR: 73 bpm
  - RR: 14 bpm

◆ Integumentary
  - Presence of scar formation: None
  - Skin color: WNL
  - Skin integrity: WNL

◆ Musculoskeletal
  - Gross range of motion: WNL
  - Gross strength: Severe weakness of right side of face with minimal to no voluntary movement of facial muscles
  - Gross symmetry: Right side of face presents with severe drooping representing all branches of the facial nerve (cranial nerve VII)
  - Height: 5'2" (1.57m)
  - Weight: 135 lbs (61.2 kg)

◆ Neuromuscular
  - Balance: WNL
  - Locomotion, transfers, and transitions: WNL

◆ Communication, affect, cognition, language, and learning style
  - Communication, affect, cognition
    - Some slurring of speech due to impaired oral motor control
    - Word finding, affect, cognition, and ability to communicate are all WNL
  - She is currently wearing eyeglasses, although she normally wears contact lenses
  - Learning style: Visual learner

TESTS AND MEASURES

◆ Cranial and peripheral nerve integrity
  - All peripheral nerve testing reveals sensory and motor intact and WNL
  - Cranial nerve testing results are found in Table 6-3
    - Based upon the initial assessment and using the House-Brackmann Facial Nerve Grading System,[111] this patient is a Grade V indicating severe dysfunction
    - During assessment of eyelid closure there is inability to close the eyelid on the involved side along with an upward movement of the eye on the same side, which is called Bell's phenomenon[111]
  - Examination of the orbit reveals tear production is decreased, and the eyeball and cornea are at risk of drying
  - Sensation of taste is impaired
  - Sensitive to sound, which she reports as almost painful

◆ Integumentary integrity: WNL
  - No signs of skin eruptions in the ear canal

◆ Muscle performance

Table 6-3
CRANIAL NERVE TESTING RESULTS

CN Number	CN Name	Main Function	Sensory Results	Motor Results
I	Olfactory	Smell	WNL	–
II	Optic	Sight	WNL	–
III	Oculomotor	EOM	–	WNL
IV	Trochlear	EOM	–	WNL
V	Trigeminal	Facial sensation, chewing	WNL	WNL
VI	Abducens	EOM	–	WNL

VII	Facial	Facial expression, taste	Loss of taste on anterior two thirds of tongue	Facial nerve branches:
				Temporal
				  Frontalis:1+
				Zygomatic
				  Orbicularis oculi: 1+
				Buccal
				  Buccinator: 1
				  Orbicularis oris: 1+
				Mandibular
				  Depressor anguli oris: 0
				Cervical
				  Platysma: 0

VIII	Vestibulocochlear	Hearing, equilibrium	WNL	–
IX	Glossopharyngeal	Taste, swallowing	WNL	WNL
X	Vagus	Speech, swallowing, thoracic and abdominal viscera	WNL	WNL
XI	Accessory	Motor—SCM and trapezius	–	WNL
XII	Hypoglossal	Tongue movements	–	WNL

EOM=Extraocular movements.

Adapted from Agur AMR, Dalley AF. *Grant's Atlas of Anatomy.* 11th ed. Philadelphia, PA: Lippincott Williams & Wilkins; 2005 and Nolte J. *The Human Brain.* 3rd ed. St. Louis, MO: Mosby Year Book; 1993. See p 602 of Agur and Dalley for samples of pictures of each muscle testing facial movement.

- All voluntary facial and neck muscles innervated by the facial nerve are within a range of 0 to 1+ (Table 6-4)
- Unable to purse lips, close eyelids, raise eyebrows
- Extraocular muscles: WNL
- All other skeletal muscles: WNL

♦ Orthotic, protective, and supportive devices: None being used at this time
♦ Pain
  - Using the NPS[112] (0=no pain and 10=the worst possible), pain rated as 2/10 in the posterior auricular area

Table 6-4
MANUAL MUSCLE TESTING RESULTS— RIGHT SIDE

Muscle	MMT Grade
Frontalis	1+/5
Corrugator	1/5+
Orbicularis oculi	1/5
Procerus	0/5
Zygomaticus major	1/5
Zygomaticus minor	0/5
Levator labii superioris	0/5
Nasalis, alar	0/5
Buccinator	1/5
Orbicularis oris	1/5
Levator anguli oris	1/5
Risorius	1/5
Depressor anguli oris	0/5
Depressor labii inferioris	0/5
Mentalis	0/5
Platysma	1/5

◆ Posture: WNL

◆ Range of motion: WNL

◆ Reflex integrity: WNL

◆ Self-care and home management

- Patient reports difficulty drinking liquids, drooling of her saliva, and difficulty chewing foods

- She is independent in all tasks preparing meals and performing all self-care

◆ Sensory integrity: WNL except as noted taste is impaired

◆ Work, community, and leisure integration or reintegration

- Patient is concerned about returning to work and community activities

- She is very self-conscious of her facial asymmetry and the drooling from the right corner of her mouth during her work and community activities

EVALUATION

Mrs. Rivera's history and findings are consistent with a diagnosis of Bell's palsy with a rapid onset. The location of involvement is most likely distal to the acoustic nerve, which helps rule out an acoustic neuroma as a possible etiology.

She has severe involvement in all branches of the facial nerve and involvement in tear production. Electrodiagnostic testing, such as nerve conductions and needle EMG, cannot be performed until at least 10 to 14 days post onset. She has significant involvement of all facial muscles and associated findings of involvement of cranial nerve VII in the region of the geniculate ganglion or the facial canal. She has a supportive family who can assist her as needed.

DIAGNOSIS

Mrs. Rivera has what presently appears to be idiopathic facial nerve Bell's paralysis, also known as Bell's palsy, with pain in the right posterior auricular area. She has impaired: cranial and peripheral nerve integrity; muscle performance; and sensory integrity. She is functionally limited in self-care and home management and in work, community, and leisure actions, tasks, and activities. She is at risk for cornea drying and/or abrasion, which can result in blindness if not treated. These findings are consistent with placement in Pattern F: Impaired Peripheral Nerve Integrity and Muscle Performance Associated With Peripheral Nerve Injury. The identified impairments, functional limitations, and risks will be addressed in determining the prognosis and the plan of care.

PROGNOSIS AND PLAN OF CARE

Over the course of the visits, the following mutually established outcomes have been determined:

◆ Ability to perform all self-care, eye care, facial interventions, and self-monitoring of recovery is optimized

◆ Communication between the patient, family, employer, and medical team is optimized

◆ Education is provided to the patient and family members on the risks associated with facial paralysis

◆ Motor performance is increased

◆ Precautions and contraindications to optimize normal neuromuscular recovery and facial symmetry are incorporated into the daily routine of the patient

◆ Sensory integrity is increased

◆ Therapeutic and pharmacological interventions and recovery of function are closely administered and monitored by patient and health care team

To achieve these identified outcomes, the appropriate interventions for this patient are determined. These will include: communication, coordination, and documentation; patient/client-related instruction; therapeutic exercise; functional training in self-care and home management; functional training in work, community, and leisure integration or reintegration; prescription, application, and, as appropriate, fabrication of devices and equipment; and electrotherapeutic modalities.

Based on the diagnosis and prognosis, Mrs. Rivera is expected to require seven visits over the course of the next 4 weeks. If the improvement occurs as expected, recovery of function of the facial nerve will occur within this time period, allowing for follow-up and discharge with instructions on further self-monitoring of any residual effects. Many factors may influence the frequency of visits and the overall duration of physical therapy intervention including the patient's level of initial impairment, the response of nerve function secondary to pharmacological intervention, the ability to correctly perform therapeutic exercises, the compliance with cornea protection, the achieved mobility of muscle/soft tissue on the right side of the face, and the recurrence of any symptoms. Mrs. Rivera is very motivated and the prognosis is good to excellent.

INTERVENTIONS

RATIONALE FOR SELECTED INTERVENTIONS

Protection of the affected areas and close monitoring for recovery of nerve/muscle function are important for the appropriate progression of therapeutic interventions while preventing undesired side effects, such as loss of ROM, loss of isolated control, and synkinesis.[113]

Therapeutic Exercise

A program of progressive physical therapy interventions will be implemented based upon the amount of recovery and the patient's responses to tests and measurements. This patient will undergo an abbreviated version of the treatment-based categories and corresponding treatment approach for facial nerve paralysis as described by Brach and VanSwearingen.[113]

During the initial stage, instruction in PROM or AAROM will lessen the effects of gravity pulling the facial muscles downward. A mirror will be used to show the patient the range and direction of upward movements that are performed using the patient's fingers.[114] Applying other rehabilitation approaches should be beneficial to this population. Bilateral, symmetrical movements performed in front of a mirror for muscles that have some preservation of voluntary control will enhance muscle function and preclude irradiation to other facial muscles.[115] When minimal voluntary movement occurs, surface EMG demonstrates voluntary motor unit recruitment. As voluntary control appears, PROM is replaced with passive positioning of affected facial muscles into shortened ranges, and then isometric contraction further enhances muscle contraction.[116] Muscle fatigue should be avoided during the early stages of peripheral or cranial nerve recovery.[31]

As recovery occurs in more facial muscles, active exer-

cises replace AAROM. Symmetry must be maintained, and irradiation to other muscles must be avoided.[117] If undesired muscles are also being recruited during specific exercises, EMG biofeedback may be used to monitor the target muscles for recruitment and to monitor undesired movements.[114] Strategies for recruiting muscles can also include surface EMG coupled with functional movements.[118] Performing bilateral, functional movements in front of a mirror will provide feedback to the patient on the quality and symmetry of these movements.[118] If recovery is occurring within a few weeks, the probability of synkinesis from aberrant innervation is minimal. To optimize patient compliance with a home exercise program, it is important for Mrs. Rivera to know the rationale for each exercise and for the number of exercises to be kept to a minimum while focusing on the most important muscle impairments.[116]

As recovery continues, the focus of physical therapy exercise interventions would be to achieve fully functional, symmetrical movements within the complete AROM. Goals will include inhibition of excess movement patterns, full control over Bell's phenomena, and symmetry at rest.[113] Residual deficits in complete active movements should be eliminated through targeted strengthening. Appropriate resistance to impaired muscles may be effective in improving motor unit recruitment and AROM.[119] Mental practice of these movements prior to actual training has been proven to be an effective strategy for the extremities and should be effective in this patient population.[120]

Prescription, Application, and, as Appropriate, Fabrication of Devices and Equipment

In patients without full eyelid closure an important consideration is protection of the cornea. Even a patient with full eyelid closure is at risk for corneal drying and damage. An eye patch to protect the cornea is often suggested, but due to the risk of eye abrasion, the literature supports other interventions. These include use of artificial tears and lubricants to protect the cornea and a moisture chamber. For short-term interventions, no other devices are recommended.[4]

Taping the eyelids closed at night is effective and safer than patching the eye, which has been shown to produce abrasive trauma to the cornea.[121] The author of this case would strongly recommend not using artificial closure of the eyelid as a means of protection for any patient with facial nerve palsy who is in a coma. Clinical experience with such a patient, who had her eyes taped shut while in a coma, resulted in a reduction of visual stimuli to the patient that produced an increased stress response (to loss of visual stimuli) that led to internal hemorrhaging that did not resolve until the eyelid tape was removed. For patients with potentially long-term lagophthalmos (incomplete eyelid closure), temporary external eyelid weights, placed on the upper eyelid, have been shown to be an effective intervention. They help to produce full eyelid closure during blinking and thereby prevent corneal damage.[122] At night, due to the supine position, weights would not be effective. A moisture chamber, which is available through prescription, provides a protective shield combined with a controlled environment to prevent eye drying.

Electrotherapeutic Modalities

Neuromuscular electrical stimulation, while advocated by some physical therapists, is not supported by the literature as an intervention for Bell's palsy. Ohtake and associates[123] found few controlled trials using electrical stimulation, and none concluded that electrical stimulation was of benefit. If a patient has idiopathic facial paralysis and recovery is expected through recovery of function of the involved cranial nerve, then electrical stimulation would, at best, reduce the effects of disuse atrophy. However, most reported treatment interventions using electrical stimulation do not clarify pulse duration, number of contractions per muscle, nor any other parameters that would produce true exercise of the involved muscles and therefore reduce atrophy.

When severe nerve damage is present and the facial nerve is not expected to fully regenerate, then recovery is partially due to collateral sprouting and reinnervation by foreign nerves (other than the original nerve). Reinnervation is facilitated by increased Ach sensitivity along the entire surface of the denervated muscle. Electrical stimulation reduces this Ach sensitivity and has been shown to impair reinnervation from an adjacent (foreign) nerve and therefore could ultimately reduce the optimal recovery of the patient.[124,125]

Surface EMG biofeedback assists patient awareness of muscle performance. It can provide external awareness of muscle activation even before movement is visually observed, which may provide strong motivation for the patient.[114,118] If undesired muscles are being recruited during specific exercises, EMG biofeedback can be used to monitor target muscles for recruitment and to monitor undesired movement.[114] Surface EMG coupled with functional movements can also facilitate muscle recruitment.[118]

COORDINATION, COMMUNICATION, AND DOCUMENTATION

Communication will occur with family members to gain their support and encouragement for optimal safety and compliance by the patient. If returning to work is planned, communication with school personnel will be encouraged to gain their support and optimize safety and comfort for the patient. Psychosocial issues related to Mrs. Rivera's self-image and acceptance by her peers will be addressed before her return to the classroom, and referral will be made as needed. All elements of the patient's management will be documented.

PATIENT/CLIENT-RELATED INSTRUCTION

The patient and family members will be instructed in proper protection of her eye and performing the recommended home program. A diagram showing the specific movements performed by each facial muscle will be provided to the patient (see p 602 of *Grant's Atlas of Anatomy, 11th ed*). Use of contact lenses must be discontinued until complete, voluntary eyelid closure is achieved. The etiology of the disorder will be clearly delineated and understood by all those involved. The role of Mrs. Rivera's family in providing emotional and physical support will be reviewed. The entire family must fully understand the importance of each aspect of the home program and protection of the eye. Safety precautions should be issued for any driving, since depth perception may be impaired if the involved eye is covered.

THERAPEUTIC EXERCISE

♦ Initial stage
  ● PROM or AAROM of the involved facial muscles, using fingers to assist the movements
  ● Use mirror so patient can see the range and direction of upward movements of the involved muscles
  ● Bilateral movements in front of a mirror for muscles that have some preservation of voluntary control
  ● As voluntary control appears
    ■ Replace PROM with passive positioning of affected facial muscles into shortened ranges followed by a holding isometric contraction of the muscles
  ● Avoid fatigue during this stage of recovery
♦ As innervation returns to more facial muscles
  ● Replace AAROM with active exercises
  ● Maintain symmetry and avoid irradiation to other muscles
  ● Increase muscle recruitment with functional movement coupled with surface EMG
  ● Perform bilateral, functional movements in front of a mirror
    ■ Raise the corner of the mouth
    ■ Raise the upper lip
    ■ Close the eyelid while looking down at an object
    ■ Close and protrude the lips
    ■ Close the lips, hold, and puff the cheeks
    ■ Raise the eyebrows
  ● Avoid powerful contractions from the uninvolved side
  ● Keep number of specific exercises on any given day to a minimum to optimize compliance
♦ As recovery continues
  ● Achieve fully functional, symmetrical movements within complete AROM (see bilateral functional movements above)
  ● Inhibition of excess movement patterns

- Control Bell's phenomena
- Achieve symmetry at rest
- Targeted strengthening in areas of residual deficits as determined by reevaluation
- Use appropriate resistance exercises to impaired muscles
  - Use fingers to resist the movements listed above
  - Do not prevent the full movement
  - Use movement on the uninvolved side for comparison
- Instruct in techniques of mental practice of movements prior to actual training

FUNCTIONAL TRAINING IN SELF-CARE AND HOME MANAGEMENT AND FUNCTIONAL TRAINING IN WORK, COMMUNITY, AND LEISURE INTEGRATION OR REINTEGRATION

- ADL training for protecting her eye during bathing, upper body dressing, grooming activities, and dental care
- IADL training when going outdoors for proper eyewear to protect her eye due to absent blink reflex
- Instruction in eye protection in windy and/or dusty environments or when performing any outdoor activities
- Caution when around children and/or infants to protect her eye
- Wearing protective eyewear at all times
- Do not wear contact lenses as long as problems exist

PRESCRIPTION, APPLICATION, AND, AS APPROPRIATE, FABRICATION OF DEVICES AND EQUIPMENT

- Instruct in taping technique to keep eyelid closed at night
  - Use only surgical tape, since paper tape will not stay in place all evening
  - Apply the tape vertically over the manually closed eyelid, while standing in front of a mirror
- A moisture chamber, which is a clear cover for the eye, is another device to protect the eye
  - The chamber must be provided by an ophthalmologist
  - It will hold moisture in after using artificial tears
- If needed, provide instruction in use of temporary external eyelid weights,[122] which are applied to the outside of the upper eyelid with double-backed adhesive strips

ELECTROTHERAPEUTIC MODALITIES

- Surface EMG to demonstrate awareness of muscle activation even before movement is visually observed and to demonstrate voluntary motor unit recruitment
  - Use one-channel EMG biofeedback unit with auditory and visual feedback modes
  - Instruct patient in application of electrodes to selected muscles using diagram of facial muscles
  - Instruct patient to raise the signal on the targeted muscles according to selected goals
  - Daily 30-minute sessions recommended supplemented by use of a mirror
  - Repetitions are kept under 10 to avoid fatigue
- Surface EMG biofeedback to reduce any undesired muscle activity
  - Use a two-channel EMG unit if strong activation of facial muscles on the intact side is occurring with no visible activity on the involved side
  - Instruct patient to keep down the signal on the intact side and try to raise the signal from the targeted muscle on the involved side
  - This technique reduces volume conduction, which can result in false positive EMG feedback[114]
- As voluntary control improves, then use of EMG feedback is continued only if synkinesis occurs
  - EMG electrodes are placed over the abnormally active muscle (synkinesis) and the patient attempts to keep down the signal from this muscle, while activating the desired muscle

ANTICIPATED GOALS AND EXPECTED OUTCOMES

- Impact on pathology/pathophysiology
  - Corneal protection is fully achieved.
- Impact on impairments
  - Muscle strength, coordination, and endurance return to normal.
  - ROM and facial symmetry return to normal.
- Impact on functional limitations
  - Facial and oral self-care are independently performed with no limitations.
  - Functional independence is optimized.
- Impact on disabilities
  - Ability to resume all indoor, outdoor, and work activities is achieved.
- Risk reduction/prevention
  - Risk of secondary impairment is decreased.
  - Self-management of corneal protection is improved.
- Impact on health, wellness, and fitness

- Physical well-being is improved.
- Self-esteem is improved.

♦ Impact on societal resources
- Documentation occurs throughout patient management and follows the APTA's *Guidelines for Physical Therapy Documentation.*[110]
- Use of physical therapy services is optimized.

♦ Patient/client satisfaction
- Patient and family demonstrate understanding of the diagnosis and their role in management.
- Patient education and availability of services are deemed acceptable by the patient.
- Sense of well-being is improved.

REEXAMINATION

Reexamination is performed throughout the entire episode of care.

DISCHARGE

Mrs. Rivera is discharged from physical therapy after a total of seven outpatient physical therapy sessions over 4 weeks and the attainment of her goals and expectations. She was discharged because she has achieved the majority of her goals and outcomes and is fully capable of self-monitoring her expected full recovery.

Case Study #3A: Disuse Disequilibrium

Mrs. Fern Peterson is a healthy 79-year-old woman with complaints of dizziness.

PHYSICAL THERAPIST EXAMINATION

HISTORY

♦ General demographics: Mrs. Peterson is a 79-year-old white female whose primary language is English. She is a high school graduate.

♦ Social history: Mrs. Peterson was widowed 10 years ago. She has one son, who is married and has three children, and all are living in the area.

♦ Employment/work: She retired from office work and currently is a volunteer for the Red Cross once a week providing refreshments after people donate blood.

♦ Living environment: She lives alone in a one-level home with three steps to enter without hand rails.

♦ General health status
- General health perception: She perceives herself to be generally healthy, although not as active as she used to be. She has no major health concerns.
- Physical function: While generally good, she feels less sure of herself during movement due to the dizziness. She is afraid of falling.
- Psychological function: Normal.
- Role function: Mother, grandmother, friend, volunteer.
- Social function: Mrs. Peterson plays bridge once a week with friends and attends church regularly.

♦ Social/health habits: She does not smoke and rarely drinks alcohol.

♦ Family history: Noncontributory.

♦ Medical/surgical history: She had an appendectomy at the age of 40 and a unilateral left mastectomy for breast cancer at the age of 55.

♦ Prior hospitalizations: She has been hospitalized for the delivery of her son, the appendectomy, and the mastectomy.

♦ Preexisting medical and other health-related conditions: She has mild allergies that are managed without medication.

♦ Current condition(s)/chief complaint(s): Mrs. Peterson states that getting around has gradually been getting more difficult, mainly because she feels dizzy. She does not use an assistive device, but finds she is beginning to occasionally reach for furniture to steady herself. She has kept up with her regular activities, but she is not sure she will continue to do so if she feels increasingly unsteady. When asked for a more detailed description of her dizziness, she states that she feels fine when she is sitting down; it only occurs when she is up and moving. She reports that it is a feeling in her head. She does not feel like the world is spinning. She offers no other description except to say that she feels dizzy and off balance.

♦ Functional status and activity level: Mrs. Peterson is independent with all ADL. She does not drive and never has. She relies on friends and family for rides or uses public transportation.

♦ Medications: Mrs. Peterson has tried meclizine in the past for the dizziness without any improvement in symptoms. She currently is taking a multivitamin and calcium supplement daily.

♦ Other clinical tests: No specific testing has been performed in the past. A review of the medical record and doctor's notes dated 1 month ago show that her cardiovascular/pulmonary function is normal for her age, she is close to being overweight, and has no other significant findings.

SYSTEMS REVIEW

- Cardiovascular/pulmonary
  - BP: 120/80 mmHg
  - Edema: None noted
  - HR: 78 bpm and regular
  - RR: 15 bpm
- Integumentary
  - Presence of scar formation: Well-healed incisions from previous surgeries
  - Skin color: WNL
  - Skin integrity: WNL
- Musculoskeletal
  - Gross range of motion: WFL
  - Gross strength: Grossly WNL
  - Gross symmetry: Appropriate
  - Height: 5'4" (1.63 m)
  - Weight: 145 lbs (65.77 kg)
- Neuromuscular
  - Transfers and transitions: Independent, but requires some effort to go from sit to stand
  - Balance and locomotion: Able to walk forward without difficulty, but slows down to turn around
- Communication, affect, cognition, language, and learning style
  - Communication, affect, and cognition: Grossly WNL
  - Learning style: Mixed including both verbal and written

TESTS AND MEASURES

- Anthropometric characteristics
  - Body mass index=weight divided by height^2=24.9
  - Mrs. Peterson is at the very upper limit of normal (normal=18.5 to 24.9, overweight=25 to 29.9, obese=30 to <40)
- Circulation
  - OH
    - BP checked after 5 minutes of lying supine and then initially upon standing up and 3 minutes later
    - Supine: 120/80 mmHg
    - Standing: 124/82 mmHg
- Cranial and peripheral nerve integrity (see Other Clinical Tests, Vestibular Dysfunction, pages 175 through 177)
  - Positional tolerance tests[32]
    - Sit to supine: Negative
    - Rolling right and rolling left: Negative
    - Dix-Hallpike[33]: Negative
  - Visual testing
    - Smooth pursuits: Negative
    - Saccades: Negative
    - VOR: Negative
- Gait, locomotion, and balance
  - BBS[126]
    - Tests: Sit to stand, standing unsupported, sitting unsupported, standing to sitting, transfers, standing unsupported with eyes closed, standing unsupported with feet together, reaching forward with outstretched arm, pick up object from floor, turn to look behind/over left and right shoulders, turn 360 degrees, alternating steps on stool, standing unsupported-one foot in front, and stand on one leg
    - She had difficulty with eyes closed, narrow base of support, single leg stance, and forward reach
    - Score: 46/56
    - She has a 26% probability of falling
  - Other gait/balance activities
    - Stepping over obstacles: Slows down, unsteady but self-recovers
    - Gait with head turns: Weaves and occasional loss of balance
    - Steps: Ascends/descends without rails, one at a time
    - Standing on thick foam: Loss of balance when attempting
    - Patient complained of dizziness several times during activities that challenged her balance, specifically when she would stagger or have loss of balance
    - When questioned, she confirmed that she does not feel dizzy in her head, she used the word "dizzy" when she lost her balance
- Muscle performance
  - Dorsiflexors: R=3/5, L=3/5
  - Remainder of LE musculature: 4/5
- Self-care and home management
  - She is independent with all ADL
  - Dizziness Handicap Inventory (DHI)[127]
    - Mrs. Peterson filled out the DHI, which is an objective test of the patient's subjective symptoms and their effect on daily life
    - The higher the number the greater the handicap and impact on functional ability
    - This patient scored 48/100 on the DHI
- Work, community, and leisure integration or reintegration
  - Mrs. Peterson plays bridge once a week with friends and attends church regularly, but she has less confidence walking to and from these activities

EVALUATION

Mrs. Peterson is a healthy elderly woman who has mildly impaired LE strength and balance. She demonstrates no vestibular impairment. Her original complaint of "dizziness" should actually be described as imbalance. Her imbalance is affecting her confidence and ability to perform activities at home and participate in community and places her at risk for falls.

DIAGNOSIS

Mrs. Peterson is a patient with disuse disequilibrium. She has impaired: circulation; gait, locomotion, and balance; and muscle performance. She is somewhat functionally limited in self-care and home management actions, tasks, and activities. As a result of her referring diagnosis, she initially was placed in Pattern F: Impaired Peripheral Nerve Integrity and Muscle Performance Associated With Peripheral Nerve Injury. However, the results of the physical therapist examination indicated that her findings were consistent with placement into Pattern A: Primary Prevention/Risk Reduction for Loss of Balance and Falling. The identified impairments will be addressed in determining the prognosis and the plan of care.

PROGNOSIS AND PLAN OF CARE

Over the course of the visits, the following mutually established outcomes have been determined:

- Balance is improved
- Gait and locomotion are improved
- Muscle performance is increased
- Participation in work, community, and leisure actions, tasks, and activities are enhanced
- Performance of ADL and IADL is improved

To achieve these outcomes, the appropriate interventions for this patient are determined. These will include: coordination, communication, and documentation; patient/client-related instruction; therapeutic exercise; functional training in self-care and home management; and functional training in work, community, and leisure integration or reintegration.

Mrs. Peterson is expected to need 6 to 24 visits over 8 to 12 weeks. She has good social support, is motivated, and will follow through with her home exercise program. While at risk for falls, she is not severely impaired and is healthy.

INTERVENTIONS

For additional rationale and additional interventions for loss of balance and falls, see Pattern A: Primary Prevention/Risk Reduction for Loss of Balance and Falling.

RATIONALE FOR SELECTED INTERVENTIONS

Therapeutic Exercise

As people age, their strength, balance, reflexes, and vestibular systems deteriorate. Research has shown that targeted physical therapy programs for strengthening, balance, and gait training result in improvements in all of these areas.[128-133] Individuals are better able to maintain mobility at the highest possible level of independence, are at lower risk of falls, and have greater confidence in performing ADL and IADL.[134-136]

COORDINATION, COMMUNICATION, AND DOCUMENTATION

Communication will occur with the Mrs. Peterson both in written and verbal format. All elements of the client's management will be documented. Communication will also occur with the physician to inform her of the results of the physical therapist examination, diagnosis, and plan of care.

PATIENT/CLIENT-RELATED INSTRUCTION

Mrs. Peterson will be provided instruction about the factors that contribute to her disequilibrium. She will be instructed in her risk for falls and the measures she can take to help prevent falls. She will have full knowledge of her home exercise program and its importance if progress is to occur.

THERAPEUTIC EXERCISE

- Balance, coordination, and agility training
  - Static balance
    - Standing with progressively narrower base of support with eyes open and closed
    - Standing on varied surfaces
    - Standing with and without head turns
  - Dynamic balance
    - Stepping over obstacles
    - Picking up objects
    - Quick starts and stops
    - Turning
    - Lunges forward/backward/sideways
    - Ball activities sitting
    - Standing with one foot on a phone book progressing to stool and then to ball
    - Line dancing
    - Putting/getting clothes from washer/dryer
    - Hanging clothes on a clothesline
    - Carrying a clothes basket so vision is blocked
- Gait and locomotion training
  - Gait on varied surfaces with and without head turns

- Walking in Figure 8's
- Walk forward/backward/circle sway

♦ Strength, power, and endurance training
  - Bilateral or single leg heel raises
  - Toe raises
  - Step-ups
  - PREs for dorsiflexors
  - Repeated sit to stand

FUNCTIONAL TRAINING IN SELF-CARE AND HOME MANAGEMENT

♦ Home management
  - Remove throw rugs
  - Use nightlights or turn on lights when up at night
  - Add railings to outdoor steps

FUNCTIONAL TRAINING IN WORK, COMMUNITY, AND LEISURE INTEGRATION OR REINTEGRATION

♦ Community and leisure
  - Continue volunteering at the Red Cross
  - Walk to and from church
  - Continue outings with family and friends

ANTICIPATED GOALS AND EXPECTED OUTCOMES

♦ Impact on impairments
  - Balance as measured by the Berg scale will increase to >48/56 to decrease fall risk.
  - Gait is improved, and Mrs. Peterson will be able to walk and turn her head without loss of balance.
  - Mrs. Peterson will increase strength in her ankles.

♦ Impact on functional limitations
  - Ability to perform activities related to self-care, home management, work, community, and leisure is improved.
  - Increased confidence during her community activities is achieved.
  - Increased confidence in mobility is achieved within her home.
  - Mrs. Peterson is capable of continuing to volunteer at the Red Cross.
  - Mrs. Peterson's score (<48/100) on the DHI is decreased.
  - Performance and safety levels in self-care, home management, work, community, and leisure activities are improved.

♦ Risk reduction/prevention

- Behaviors that foster healthy habits, wellness, and prevention are acquired.
- Patient's knowledge of personal and environmental factors associated with the condition is increased.
- Risk of falls or injury is reduced as evidenced by improvement in the BBS.

♦ Impact on health, wellness, and fitness
  - Mrs. Peterson will participate in her home program on a regular basis.

♦ Impact on societal resources
  - Communication enhances risk reduction and prevention.
  - Documentation occurs throughout patient management and follows APTA's *Guidelines for Physical Therapy Documentation*.[110]
  - The physical therapist will understand the patient's goals and concerns.

♦ Patient/client satisfaction
  - Mrs. Peterson's and family's knowledge and awareness of the diagnosis, prognosis, interventions, and anticipated goals and expected outcomes are increased.
  - Sense of well-being is improved.

REEXAMINATION

Reexamination is performed throughout the episode of care.

DISCHARGE

Mrs. Peterson is discharged from physical therapy after a total of 10 physical therapy visits over a 10-week period of time and attainment of her goals.

Case Study #3B: Meniere's Disease

Mrs. Richards is a 60-year-old female with Meniere's disease who has been referred to physical therapy for her dizziness and decreasing balance.

PHYSICAL THERAPIST EXAMINATION

HISTORY

♦ General demographics: Mrs. Richards is a 60-year-old white female whose primary language is English. She is right-hand dominant. She is a college graduate.

♦ Social history: She is married and has no children.

♦ Employment/work: She is a retired medical transcriber.

♦ Living environment: She lives in a one-story home with no stairs to enter.

♦ General health status
  ● General health perception: Mrs. Richards states that she is in generally good health.
  ● Physical function: She reports when she gets these episodes of dizziness she remains in bed for several hours, but she still feels imbalanced for a number of days afterward.
  ● Psychological function: Mrs. Richards' reports that she is feeling a bit overwhelmed with the dizziness. It limits her life for a while after each episode in many ways, particularly going on outings with friends, getting chores done around the home, and dancing.
  ● Role function: Wife, friend, housekeeper, volunteer.
  ● Social function: She is socially active with her husband and friends. She is active in her church, likes recreational dancing, and goes to the movies.

♦ Social/health habits: Mrs. Richards has an occasional drink on the weekend and is a nonsmoker.

♦ Family history: She reports that her aunt had Meniere's disease. Both of her parents are alive and living in a retirement community. Her mother, who is 84 years of age, has osteoarthritis, osteoporosis, and a history of a myocardial infarction that was treated with clot-dissolving drugs. Her father, who is 85 years of age, has peripheral vascular disease and has had a knee replacement.

♦ Medical/surgical history: She reports no significant history other than her Meniere's disease, which was diagnosed 20 years ago. She reports she has a hearing loss in her left ear in the lower frequencies that comes and goes with the dizziness and seems to be getting worse. She reports that she is sensitive to loud noises and has tinnitus (ringing in her ear).

♦ Prior hospitalizations: None.

♦ Preexisting medical and other health-related conditions: Meniere's disease.

♦ Current condition(s)/chief complaint(s): Mrs. Richards reports that 3 weeks ago she had a sudden onset of dizziness (vertigo) she rated as an 8/10 with 10 being the worst dizziness. She was unable to walk without losing her balance and hitting into the walls and felt better lying still with her eyes focused on a spot. When she did need to get up out of bed, the vertigo would increase for a brief time making her want to return to lying down. She reports that the vertigo lasted most of the day before she could sit up without an increase in the symptoms. For the next couple of days after the vertigo attack, she was off balance requiring her to reach out for furniture or just move slowly and cautiously. At this time she feels that her balance is not back to normal, which concerns her. She notes that walking to the bathroom at night is hard, and she now has to put on a light. In the past her balance had returned more quickly.

♦ Functional status and activity level: Mrs. Richards usually walked 1 to 2 miles a day 5 days a week. Currently she is able to walk independently but occasionally reaches out for furniture for reassurance. She is independent with all transitional movements. She is back to her volunteer work at church and socializing with friends. She has not tried dancing yet.

♦ Medications: Multivitamin, hydrochlorothiazide (diuretic), diazepam (Valium).

♦ Other clinical tests: Audiogram and ENG were retested a year ago. The audiogram displayed a unilateral sensorineural hearing loss involving the lower frequencies of the involved ear. Note: Fluctuation in discrimination scores is often seen with a trend toward poor scores as time goes by. The ENG demonstrated a unilateral vestibular weakness on caloric testing involving the left ear.

SYSTEMS REVIEW

♦ Cardiovascular/pulmonary
  ● BP: 118/72 mmHg
  ● Edema: None noted
  ● HR: 68 bpm
  ● RR: 14 bpm

♦ Integumentary
  ● Presence of scar formation: None
  ● Skin color: Normal
  ● Skin integrity: Normal

♦ Musculoskeletal
  ● Gross range of motion: WNL and no dizziness with cervical ROM
  ● Gross strength: WNL
  ● Gross symmetry: Symmetrical
  ● Height: 5'2" (1.575 m)
  ● Weight: 130 lbs (69.68 kg)

♦ Neuromuscular
  ● Gross coordinated movements: Mrs. Richards ambulates independently without any loss of balance but with a wider base of support and at a slow cautious pace
  ● Transfers and transitions: Appear normal

♦ Communication, affect, cognition, language, and learning style
  ● Communication, affect, cognition: WNL
  ● Learning style: Mixed

TESTS AND MEASURES

◆ Aerobic capacity/endurance
  ● Walks 1 to 2 miles 5 days per week
◆ Anthropometric characteristics
  ● Body mass index=weight divided by height^2=26.95
  ● Mrs. Richards is overweight (normal=18.5 to 24.9; overweight=25 to 29.9; obese=30 to <40)
◆ Assistive and adaptive devices
  ● Mrs. Richards has not used any device to assist with walking but will reach out for furniture or walls when feeling dizzy or imbalanced
  ● A device to assist with balance when experiencing extreme dizziness or imbalance will be recommended
◆ Cranial and peripheral nerve integrity
  ● Positional tolerance tests (see Other Clinical Tests, Vestibular Dysfunction, pages 175 through 177)[32]
    ■ Sit to supine: Negative
    ■ Supine to sit: Slight feeling of vertigo rated as 2/10 on a VAS (0 to 10 scale with 0 as none and 10 as the worst vertigo), lasting 15 seconds with no nystagmus noted, but increased symptoms with speed of the maneuver
    ■ Rolling right: Negative
    ■ Rolling left: Slight feeling of vertigo rated as 2/10 lasting 5 seconds with no nystagmus
    ■ Dix-Hallpike (see Figure 6-8) right: Negative
    ■ Dix-Hallpike left: Slight feeling of vertigo rated as 2/10, lasting 10 seconds with no nystagmus and a movement sensation with the return to upright
    ■ Seated flexion/extension: Negative
  ● Visual tests (see Other Clinical Tests, Vestibular Dysfunction, pages 175 through 177)[32]
    ■ Pursuit: Negative
    ■ Saccade: Negative
    ■ VOR cancellation: Negative
    ■ Head thrust test: Positive on the left indicating an abnormal VOR
◆ Gait, locomotion, and balance
  ● Key tests in this area are the Berg[126] (particularly the components of functional reach, single leg stance, and tandem stance), computerized posturography, and the Clinical Test of Sensory Interaction on Balance (CTSIB) for monitoring balance between episodes and overtime[38]
    ■ BBS: 49/56 (low risk of falls, however the probability of falling with her history of no falls in the last 6 months is still 14%)[137,138]
    ■ Computerized dynamic posturography
      ▶ Patient able to weight shift at 68% of limits of stability with appropriate ankle strategies, initiation, and timing

■ CTSIB
  ▶ This test can simulate computerized posturography, when that equipment is not available
  ▶ The CTSIB tests standing balance in four categories: On a firm surface with eyes open, on a firm surface with eyes closed, on a foam surface with eyes open, and on a foam surface with eyes closed
● Ambulation
  ■ With head rotation right and left and with head flexion and extension
    ▶ Positive for vertigo, which she rated as 3/10 in all directions
    ▶ Has slight loss of balance on the left
  ■ At a fast pace with quick stops or turns upon command
    ▶ Slows with turns and slows anticipating the command
    ▶ When asked to walk faster during the test, she exhibits a slight stagger with turns to the left
◆ Self-care and home management
  ● Unable to do self-care or home management when dizzy as she needs to stay in bed for several hours at a time
  ● Unable to get chores done following an episode of dizziness since she feels unbalanced for several days
  ● Needs lights on at night to walk to bathroom
◆ Work, community, and leisure integration or reintegration
  ● Had stopped going out into the community but is now able to do her volunteer work at church and socialize with friends
  ● Has stopped driving as she does not feel safe
  ● Has stopped dancing

EVALUATION

Mrs. Richards is a generally healthy woman other than being diagnosed with Meniere's disease. However, as of late she has been experiencing a decline in balance in between her attacks. She is having more difficulty with her balance in situations that alter her visual and somatosensory information. She has some positional symptoms with Dix–Hallpike, supine to sit, and quick movements. She has balance impairments with functional movements (loss of balance with head turns while walking, loss of balance with quick movements, loss of balance with narrow base of support) especially with increased speed. The patient's left VOR is abnormal upon testing.

DIAGNOSIS

Mrs. Richards has Meniere's disease. She has impaired: cranial and peripheral nerve integrity and gait, locomotion, and balance. She is functionally limited in self-care and home management and in work, community, and leisure actions, tasks, and activities. She is in need of devices and equipment. The results of her physical therapist examination indicate findings consistent with a developing loss of her vestibular function on the left, which can occur in the end stages of Meniere's disease. These findings are consistent with placement in Pattern F: Impaired Peripheral Nerve Integrity and Muscle Performance Associated With Peripheral Nerve Injury. The identified impairments, functional limitations, and device and equipment needs will be addressed in determining the prognosis and the plan of care.

PROGNOSIS AND PLAN OF CARE

Over the course of the episode of care, the following mutually established outcomes have been determined:

♦ Ability to perform physical activities related to self-care, home management, work, community, and leisure is improved

♦ Balance is improved

♦ Fitness is improved

♦ Knowledge of behaviors that foster healthy habits, wellness, and prevention is increased

♦ Physical capacity is improved

♦ Risk factors (decreased physical activity, balance, ROM, muscle performance) are reduced

To achieve these outcomes, the appropriate interventions for this patient are determined. These will include: coordination, communication, and documentation; patient/client-related instruction; therapeutic exercise; functional training in self-care and home management; functional training in work, community, and leisure integration or reintegration; and prescription, application, and, as appropriate, fabrication of devices and equipment.

It is anticipated that Mrs. Richards will require two to eight visits over the course of 4 to 6 weeks to address her increasing imbalance related to her Meniere's disease.

INTERVENTIONS

RATIONALE FOR SELECTED INTERVENTIONS

Therapeutic Exercise

In the past, individuals with Meniere's disease had not been considered candidates for vestibular rehabilitation. They were managed with diuretics, labyrinthine sedatives (eg, meclizine), sometimes benzodiazepines (eg, Valium), and a diet that regulates the sodium and sugar intake.[44,139] If the disease progressed and became uncontrolled for an extended

interval, surgery may have been recommended. Since the late 1990s research has shown that individuals who opt for surgical management and vestibular rehabilitation show improvement with postural stability and have a decreased perception of disequilibrium, whereas individuals who have not been treated with surgery complain of having difficulty with ADL and with work.[42] Cohen and associates found that between attacks, 90% of patients with Meniere's could independently transfer, walk, bathe, and dress. However, during an attack, only 10% could independently transfer, 5% could independently walk, 15% could independently bathe, and 10% could independently dress themselves. Over time, their jobs were either hindered to some degree or they needed to change jobs.[42]

Once the physical therapist determines the specific impairments and functional limitations, a home exercise program may be tailored to the patient's needs in terms of balance, postural stability, and function. Vestibular rehabilitation to promote adaptation to the unilateral vestibular loss may be beneficial once a patient is not experiencing an active episode.[139] Some patients with a progressive unilateral vestibular hypofunction will adapt on their own. Others will require vestibular rehabilitation to aide in adaptation. Whitney and Metzinger recommended that patients recently diagnosed with Meniere's disease should be referred for an examination by a physical therapist during an inactive phase for education on the disease process, support groups, and falls prevention during an attack of Meniere's disease.[139]

COORDINATION, COMMUNICATION, AND DOCUMENTATION

Communication will occur with the patient, both in written and verbal format. Communication will also occur with the physician on an ongoing basis. All elements of the patient's management will be documented.

PATIENT/CLIENT-RELATED INSTRUCTION

The patient and her husband will be provided education about Meniere's disease. They will be instructed to anticipate the possibility of an occasional sudden loss of balance that can occur in this late stage of Meniere's disease and is of vestibular origin. They will also understand that the loss of balance becomes more problematic in conditions of low lighting, fatigue, or when Mrs. Richards is exposed to visually stimulating situations.[140]

Mr. and Mrs. Richards will be informed of support groups due to the psychological impact of the disease.[141] Support groups can be found through the Vestibular Disorders Association's Web site (www.vestibular.org/menieres). She will be referred to her physician or dietician for any questions related to diet or fluid restrictions. The association's Web site is also a valuable resource for information about dietary modifications and other facts related to Meniere's disease.

Mrs. Richards will also be provided with information

about the benefits of an ambulatory assistive device for safety during an episode of dizziness with balance issues.

THERAPEUTIC EXERCISE

A general rule for the patient's home exercise program is that the exercises should not increase her symptoms for more than 1 hour after she performs the exercises.

♦ Aerobic capacity/endurance conditioning
  ● Continue her walking program to help prevent deconditioning from inactivity, to encourage postural control, and to help her get back to an activity she enjoys[139]

♦ Balance, coordination, and agility training
  ● Static balance activities
    ▪ Single leg stance with UE support progressing toward no UE support
      ▸ Variations of single leg stance: Eyes open, eyes closed, head position with a tilt of 30 degrees forward then back, head turned right/left, head tilted sideways right/left
      ▸ Then change the surface (eg, foam pads) upon which she is standing with variations of eye and head positions to make it more challenging
    ▪ Tandem stance/sharpened Romberg
      ▸ Variations of environments, visual input, somatosensory input, and vestibular information with head position changes
  ● Dynamic balance activities
    ▪ Ambulation with head turns
      ▸ Start with shifting the gaze side to side and progress to small slow head turns while walking
      ▸ As she improves, change the speed of head or eye movements, change base of support, or change direction of eye or head movement
    ▪ Ambulation with head tilts forward, backward, and sideward
    ▪ Ambulation with 180-degree and 360-degree turns
      ▸ Progress to making tighter turns with eyes open and with eyes closed
    ▪ Practice easy dance steps
      ▸ Start without turns and progress to turns
      ▸ Start with lights on and progress to dim light
      ▸ Start slow and then increase the pace
  ● Vestibular training
    ▪ Exercises to enhance the VOR for adaptation
      ▸ Vestibular stimulation exercises[32]
        ○ Patient begins sitting facing a wall with a plain background and focuses on a target taped on the wall that can be clearly seen or read

        ○ Patient turns head from side to side for 30 seconds and gradually progresses the duration to 2 minutes of head turns still focusing on the target
        ○ As she progresses, advance the exercise by increasing the speed of head turns, putting the target on a busy background, or having her stand or march in place while turning the head
        ○ Exercise may also be done with head moving up and down
      ▸ Visuovestibular interactions[32]
        ○ Patient begins sitting facing a wall with a plain background and holds the target (ie, business card) so she can read it
        ○ She moves the target and her head back and forth horizontally in opposite directions keeping the target in focus for 30 seconds and gradually progresses the duration to 2 minutes
        ○ Further progression would be the same as in vestibular stimulation exercises
    ▪ Three habituation exercises[7]
      ▸ Rolling, supine to sit, and sit to stand
      ▸ Performed three or four times per day
      ▸ Three to five repetitions each
    ▪ Encourage postural control during all vestibular exercises

♦ Gait and locomotion training
  ● See Dynamic Balance Activities

FUNCTIONAL TRAINING IN SELF-CARE AND HOME MANAGEMENT

♦ Home management
  ● Use nightlights or turn on lights when up at night
  ● Emergency lighting in case of a power failure
  ● Make sure the pathway to the bathroom is free of throw rugs, furniture, or other obstacles

FUNCTIONAL TRAINING IN WORK, COMMUNITY, AND LEISURE INTEGRATION OR REINTEGRATION

♦ Leisure
  ● Use a flashlight when walking outside at night
  ● Choose a level path when walking in dim light
  ● Practice easy dance moves in community setting

PRESCRIPTION, APPLICATION, AND, AS APPROPRIATE, FABRICATION OF DEVICES AND EQUIPMENT

◆ Assistive devices
  ● Mrs. Richards will be given a cane to use when experiencing extreme dizziness or imbalance

ANTICIPATED GOALS AND EXPECTED OUTCOMES

◆ Impact on pathology/pathophysiology
  ● Vertigo is decreased to 0-1/10.
◆ Impact on impairments
  ● A target is kept in focus while shaking her head yes and no without symptoms in 3 to 6 weeks.
  ● Balance is maintained with altered somatosensory or altered visual information.
  ● Gaze stability during head movements is improved.
  ● Independent ambulation is achieved on a straight path while turning her head without symptoms (eg, scanning for something in a grocery aisle while walking) in 2 to 3 weeks.
  ● Independent standing is achieved with narrow base of support for 20 to 30 seconds in 2 to 4 weeks.
  ● Positions are changed without dizziness.
◆ Impact on functional limitations
  ● Ability to perform activities related to self-care, home management, work, community, and leisure is improved.
  ● Balance is maintained when walking to the bathroom at night on plush carpeting with a nightlight in 2 to 4 weeks.
  ● Going quickly from supine to sit, rolling left, and sitting to standing without dizziness is achieved in 2 to 3 weeks.
  ● Self-care and home management activities (ADL and IADL) are performed with minimal vertigo.
◆ Impact on disabilities
  ● Participation in preferred community activities is resumed.
◆ Risk reduction/prevention
  ● Risk of falls or injury is reduced.
  ● Safe techniques are demonstrated when performing self-care, home management, work, community, and leisure actions, tasks, and activities.
◆ Impact on health, wellness, and fitness
  ● Physical function is improved and will continue to improve.

◆ Impact on societal resources
  ● Available resources are maximally utilized.
  ● Documentation occurs throughout patient management in all settings and follows APTA's *Guidelines for Physical Therapy Documentation*.[110]
  ● Utilization of physical therapy services is optimized.
◆ Patient/client satisfaction
  ● Case is managed throughout the episode of care.
  ● Patient and family understanding of anticipated goals and expected outcomes is increased.
  ● Patient and family verbalize awareness of the diagnosis, prognosis, interventions, and anticipated goals and expected outcomes.
  ● Patient able to identify relevant community resources.
  ● Sense of well-being is improved.

REEXAMINATION

Reexamination is performed throughout the episode of care. It is anticipated that patients placed in this pattern may require multiple episodes of care over the lifetime. Periodic reexamination and initiation of new episodes of care should occur to allow the patient to continue to be safe and effectively adapt to any changes in physical status, environment, or task demands.

DISCHARGE

Mrs. Richards is discharged from this episode of care after a total of eight physical therapy visits over a 5-week period of time and attainment of her goals. As Mrs. Richards has a condition that may require multiple episodes of care throughout her life span, she and her husband received education regarding factors that may trigger a call to her physical therapist for a reexamination and new episode of physical therapy care.

PSYCHOLOGICAL ASPECTS

The patient with Meniere's disease must understand that it is important to reproduce the symptoms of vertigo, nausea, and/or imbalance during exercise interventions. To get a patient to move into a position that may make him or her dizzy and nauseated may be difficult and requires support and encouragement. Physical therapists need to understand that fear could be a big barrier to the interventions.[141]

Case Study #3C: Benign Paroxysmal Positional Vertigo

Mrs. Jones is a 55-year-old female complaining of dizziness that has been going on now for 1 week.

PHYSICAL THERAPIST EXAMINATION

HISTORY

◆ General demographics: Mrs. Jones is a 55-year-old white female whose primary language is English. She is a college graduate.

◆ Social history: Mrs. Jones is married to an office manager and is the mother of four teenage children.

◆ Employment/work: She works part-time at a retail store, where she helps out with the decorations and needs to be on a ladder part of the time, frequently reaching up and down. She is very busy driving her children to and from practices and other school, athletic, and social events. She does most of her own housework.

◆ Living environment: She lives in a two-story home with a basement. All stairs have a rail. There are two steps to get in from the garage with no rail.

◆ General health status
  ● General health perception: Mrs. Jones feels that she is in good health.
  ● Physical function: Normal.
  ● Psychological function: Normal.
  ● Role function: Wife, mother, chauffeur, neighbor, employee.
  ● Social function: She is very involved in her children's activities, and she is also active in neighborhood functions and activities. She loves to play the piano and read books.

◆ Social/health habits: Mrs. Jones quit smoking 10 years ago. She was a pack-a-day smoker prior to that. She is a social drinker, usually only wine.

◆ Family history: Noncontributory.

◆ Medical/surgical history: There is no significant medical history. She denies any hearing problems and denies any neck or back problems.

◆ Prior hospitalizations: She was hospitalized for the delivery of her four children.

◆ Preexisting medical and other health-related conditions: None.

◆ Current condition(s)/chief complaint(s): One week ago she was getting out of bed (she rolls out onto her right side), and she experienced dizziness that she rated a 4/10 (on a VAS with 0=no dizziness and 10=the worst dizziness). She stated that it was a spinning sensation that lasted approximately 40 seconds. The dizziness passed, and she was symptom free until later in the week. At that time she was reaching up to dust a high shelf when she got another more severe spinning sensation, this time rated as an 8/10 that lasted about a minute. She was unsure if there was a latency period. "It seemed rather fast." Mrs. Jones noted that she has had similar episodes periodically throughout the week both at home and at work. She also reported that a dizzy sensation occurred with bending down to pick up her purse or other objects from the floor. She reported that with all of these events she was able to stop the sensation by closing her eyes and sitting very still. She reported that she now avoids looking up and rolling to the right, and she now moves very slowly to get out of bed. Mrs. Jones does not want this to get any worse, and she and her family are afraid that it will occur when she is up on the ladder at work.

◆ Functional status and activity level: Mrs. Jones does not exercise, but she keeps very active with her ADL and IADL. She gets a massage once a week.

◆ Medications: Mrs. Jones takes a multivitamin and a calcium supplement. She also had been prescribed meclizine by her physician, but she had not taken it since she has not had a bad "dizzy spell."

◆ Other clinical tests: Review of Mrs. Jones's online physician's notes indicated orthostatic testing, which was negative, and no concerns or history of BP or cardiac symptoms. No other clinical tests were performed for this patient.

SYSTEMS REVIEW

◆ Cardiovascular/pulmonary
  ● BP: 128/70 mmHg
  ● Edema: None
  ● HR: 72 bpm
  ● RR: 13 bpm
◆ Integumentary
  ● Presence of scar formation: None
  ● Skin color: WNL
  ● Skin integrity: WNL
◆ Musculoskeletal
  ● Gross range of motion
    ▪ WNL
    ▪ Some directions of the cervical ROM testing resulted in dizziness (see Tests and Measures)
  ● Gross strength: WNL
  ● Gross symmetry: Symmetrical

- Height: 5'6" (1.68 m)
- Weight: 140 lbs (63.50 kg)
- ◆ Neuromuscular
  - Balance: Slight stagger when looking to the right
  - Locomotion, transfers, and transitions
    - Ambulated into the physical therapy clinic independently
    - Transitional movements performed independently, but some movements resulted in dizziness
- ◆ Communication, affect, cognition, language, and learning style
  - Communication, affect, and cognition: All WNL
  - Learning style: Mixed

TESTS AND MEASURES

- ◆ Anthropometric characteristics
  - Body mass index=weight divided by height^2=22.6
  - Mrs. Jones is normal weight (normal=18.5 to 24.9; overweight=25 to 29.9; obese=30 to <40)
- ◆ Cranial and peripheral nerve integrity
  - Positional tests[7] (see Other Clinical Tests, Vestibular Dysfunction, pages 175 and 176)
    - Note: If equipment, such as Frenzel glasses or infrared goggles, to prevent visual fixation are not available, the nystagmus may not be seen or the eyes may be seen to jump for a brief moment; if this is the case then the patient may still be treated based on the symptoms
    - Cervical rotation left: Negative
    - Cervical rotation right: Slight start of dizziness rated as 1/10 lasting less than 3 seconds
    - Cervical flexion: Negative
    - Cervical extension: 5-second latency and was positive for spinning sensation rated as 4/10 lasting 35 seconds
    - Sit to supine: Negative
    - Rolling left: Negative
    - Rolling right: 5-second latency and was positive for spinning sensation rated as 5/10 lasting 40 seconds
    - Supine to sit: 8-second latency and positive for spinning sensation rated as 5/10 lasting 38 seconds
  - Dix-Hallpike[33] (see Other Clinical Tests, Vestibular Dysfunction) (see Figure 6-8)
    - Note: Prior to testing always clear the cervical spine and instruct the patient that you will be positioning her head
    - Left: Negative
    - Right
      - ▶ 5-second latency and positive for spinning

sensation rated as 8/10 lasting 45 seconds
    - ▶ Positive for nystagmus
  - Coming up from supine to sitting, she experienced a 3-second latency and positive dizziness sensation rated as 3/10 lasting 15 seconds (see Figure 6-8)[142]
- ◆ Gait, locomotion, and balance
  - Slight stagger when looking to the right during ambulation
- ◆ Self-care and home management
  - Avoids looking up and rolling to the right
  - Moves slowly getting out of bed
- ◆ Work, community, and leisure integration or reintegration
  - Avoids looking up and bending down at work

EVALUATION

Mrs. Jones is a healthy woman who has a busy lifestyle. She had a sudden onset of dizziness described as spinning with no associated history of trauma. The dizziness occurred with return to upright from supine, rolling right, looking up, and bending over. These are some classic complaints with BPPV. She had a positive right Dix-Hallpike that is diagnostic for BPPV. She avoids rolling to the right and looking up, and she moves slowly to get out of bed. She is cautious with bending down.

DIAGNOSIS

Mrs. Jones was referred with a diagnosis of dizziness and has been further diagnosed as having BPPV. She has impaired: cranial and peripheral nerve integrity and gait, locomotion, and balance. She is functionally limited in self-care and home management and in work, community, and leisure actions, tasks, and activities. These findings are consistent with placement in the Pattern F: Impaired Peripheral Nerve Integrity and Muscle Performance Associated With Peripheral Nerve Injury. The identified impairments and functional limitations will be addressed in determining the prognosis and the plan of care.

PROGNOSIS AND PLAN OF CARE

Over the course of the visits, the following mutually established outcomes have been determined:

- ◆ Ability to perform physical activities related to self-care, home management, work, community, and leisure is improved
- ◆ Balance is improved
- ◆ Knowledge of behaviors that foster prevention is increased

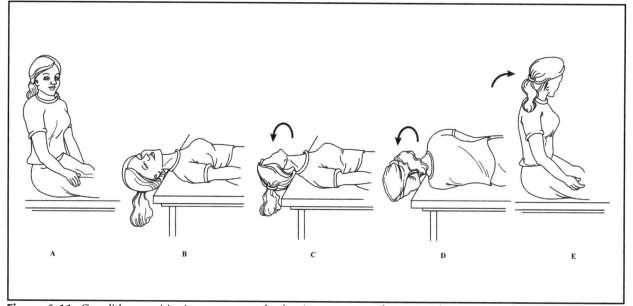

Figure 6-11. Canalith repositioning maneuver for benign paroxysmal positional vertigo involving the right posterior semicircular canal. (A) The patient should be long sitting on the table/plinth with her head rotated to the right (the affected side) to about 45 degrees of rotation. (B) The patient is rapidly moved into the Dix-Hallpike position with the affected ear down. The patient should stay in this position for about 20 seconds or until the dizziness stops, whichever is longer. (C) With the neck still in extension, rotate the head to the other side so the opposite ear is down. The patient should stay in this position for about 20 seconds or until the dizziness stops, whichever is longer. (D) Roll the patient onto the left side with her head in the same position resulting in the patient looking down toward the floor halfway or more. The patient should stay in this position for about 20 seconds or until the dizziness stops, whichever is longer. (E) Assist the patient to sitting, keeping the head turned to the left. Once the patient is up, then she can straighten her head. Adapted from Herdman SJ. Treatment of benign paroxysmal positional vertigo. *Phys Ther.* 1990;70(6):384, with permission of the American Physical Therapy Association. This material is copyrighted, and any further reproduction or distribution is prohibited. Original figure first published in *Arch Otolaryngol.* 1980;106:484-485. Copyright © 1980, American Medical Association. All rights reserved.

To achieve these outcomes, the appropriate interventions for this patient are determined. These will include: coordination, communication, and documentation; patient/client-related instruction; therapeutic exercise; and functional training in self-care and home management.

It is anticipated that Mrs. Jones with a clear-cut diagnosis of BPPV will require two to eight visits over 2 to 4 weeks. Mrs. Jones is healthy, has good social support, and is very motivated.

INTERVENTIONS

RATIONALE FOR SELECTED INTERVENTIONS

Two treatment options exist for this patient: a canalith repositioning maneuver and Brandt-Daroff habituation exercises. Free-floating otoconia in the posterior semicircular canal are believed to be displaced from the utricle making the

posterior semicircular canal sensitive to gravity. Greater than 90% of the patients diagnosed with BPPV can be successfully treated with the canalith repositioning maneuver (Figure 6-11) that moves the otoconia from the semicircular canal back to the utricle.[35,143-154]

Mild nausea or continued feeling of disequilibrium may continue for 24 to 48 hours after the canalith repositioning maneuver, and this occurrence is no indication of success or failure of the maneuver.[7,142] When the maneuver was initially developed, it was felt that it was necessary to impose movement restrictions to keep the otoconia from going back into the semicircular canals. These movement restrictions included keeping one's head in an upright position for the rest of the day, sleeping with an extra pillow at night, and avoiding lying on the affected side.[34,142,155,156]

Research has shown no difference in outcome for patients who are or are not given movement restrictions after the canalith repositioning maneuver.[144,145,155-160]

Brandt-Daroff habituation exercises (Figure 6-12) are used when the canalith repositioning maneuver is not suc-

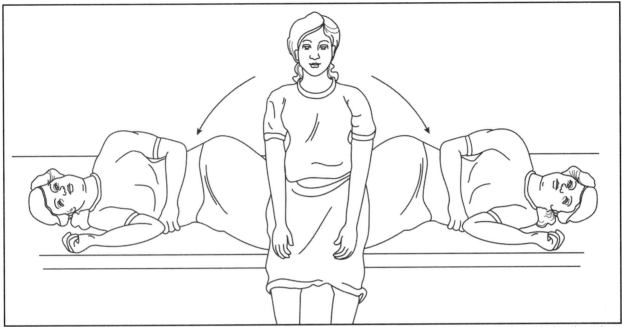

Figure 6-12. Brandt-Daroff exercises. Adapted from Herdman SJ. Advances in the treatment of vestibular disorders. *Phys Ther*. 1997;77:612, with permission of the American Physical Therapy Association. This material is copyrighted, and any further reproduction or distribution is prohibited. Original figure first published in *Arch Otolaryngol*. 1996;122:281-286. Copyright © 1996, American Medical Association. All rights reserved.

cessful in fully decreasing or eliminating the symptoms.[146,161] Two possible theories are put forth as to why habituation exercises decrease the nystagmus and vertigo.[142] One thought is that the Brandt-Daroff exercises work to dislodge the otoconia from the cupula so they no longer have an effect during head movement. A second possibility is that central adaptation occurs reducing the nervous system response to the signal from the posterior canal.[35,162]

The reoccurrence rate for BPPV is 40% to 50%.[34,142] It is also possible to have bilateral BPPV, anterior or horizontal semicircular canal dysfunction, and a vestibular hypofunction all at the same time. If all are present, the BPPV is treated first.[35,162]

COORDINATION, COMMUNICATION, AND DOCUMENTATION

Communication will occur with the patient, both in written and verbal forms. Communication will also occur with the physician regarding the diagnosis and the plan of care. All elements of the patient's management will be documented.

PATIENT/CLIENT-RELATED INSTRUCTION

Mrs. Jones will be provided with information about the anatomy, physiology, pathology, and classic symptoms of BPPV and its affect on her function. The patient and her family will be taught the canalith repositioning maneuver to be used if the symptoms reoccur. Any habituation exercises given will be provided in a home exercise program with complete instructions in writing with pictures.

Mrs. Jones and her family will be instructed to call her physical therapist if she has any questions or concerns or to schedule an appointment if necessary.

THERAPEUTIC EXERCISE

- ◆ Session 1
  - Canalith repositioning maneuver for the right inner ear (see Figure 6-11)[7,142]
- ◆ Session 2
  - Sometime after the 48 hours when the patient may feel some mild nausea or continued disequilibrium
  - If patient has no symptoms
    - Perform the Dix-Hallpike
    - If negative, discontinue the patient
  - If patient has continued symptoms
    - Perform the Dix-Hallpike
    - If positive, perform the canalith repositioning maneuver again
    - Have patient return for another session after the 48-hour period
- ◆ Session 3
  - If patient has no symptoms
    - Perform the Dix-Hallpike
    - If negative, discontinue the patient

- If patient has continued symptoms still pointing to right BPPV, then begin Brandt-Daroff exercises (see Figure 6-12)[142]
  - Performed three to four times a day with three to five repetitions each session
  - Each exercise is held as long as the symptom is present, or to 30 seconds, before moving to the next exercise
  - Exercises are continued until the patient has 2 consecutive days without any symptoms
  - May take up to 2 weeks before symptoms disappear
- Begin habituation exercises that target the positive positional tolerance tests
  - Include a position change that triggered the dizziness
  - Patient performs the position change with the same frequency and duration as the Brandt-Daroff exercises
  - In this case it would be rolling right and supine to sit
- Session 4
  - 1 week or more from third appointment
    - Perform the Dix-Hallpike
    - If negative, discontinue the patient
  - If patient has continued symptoms, perform canalith repositioning maneuver for the right inner ear
  - Note: Patients with BPPV may complain of postural instability that does not immediately resolve with resolution of the vertigo and that may require continued vestibular rehabilitation

FUNCTIONAL TRAINING IN SELF-CARE AND HOME MANAGEMENT

- Self-care and home management
  - Recommend as a safety precaution that patient does not drive to or from the first session

ANTICIPATED GOALS AND EXPECTED OUTCOMES

- Impact on pathology/pathophysiology
  - Canalith debris in the right inner ear is repositioned.
- Impact on impairments
  - Dizziness when looking up or bending down while performing activities is reduced to 0-2/10 in 1 to 2 weeks.
  - Dizziness when performing ADL and IADL is eliminated in 2 to 4 weeks.
  - Dizziness when rolling right is eliminated in 1 to 2 weeks.

- Dizziness with supine to sit is reduced to 0-2/10 in 1 week.
- Impact on functional limitations
  - Ability to perform physical actions, tasks, and activities is improved.
- Risk reduction/prevention
  - Safety is improved.
- Impact on societal resources
  - Documentation occurs throughout patient management and follows APTA's *Guidelines for Physical Therapy Documentation.*[110]
- Patient/client satisfaction
  - Patient and family knowledge and awareness of the diagnosis, prognosis, interventions, and anticipated goals and expected outcomes are increased.
  - Sense of well-being is improved.

REEXAMINATION

Reexamination is performed throughout the episode of care. The intervention plan is modified in accordance with changes in symptoms reported by the patient and with the results of the vestibular reexamination at each visit.

DISCHARGE

Mrs. Jones is discharged from physical therapy after a total of two visits over 2 weeks for a very clear-cut case of BPPV. If habituation exercises had been needed, then six physical therapy visits would have been needed to attain the goals. Mrs. Jones received education regarding factors that may trigger a call to her physical therapist for a new examination and new episode of physical therapy care.

PSYCHOLOGICAL ASPECTS

It is important with vestibular rehabilitation that the patient understands that the physical therapist and the exercises need to reproduce the symptoms, vertigo, nausea, and/or imbalance. To get a patient to move into a position that may make him or her dizzy and nauseated may be difficult and requires support and encouragement. Physical therapists need to understand that fear could be a barrier to the interventions.[141]

Case Study #3D: Unilateral Peripheral Hypofunction

Ms. Susie Smith is a 40-year-old female who had a bout of dizziness and now has feelings of imbalance.

PHYSICAL THERAPIST EXAMINATION

HISTORY

♦ General demographics: Susie Smith is 40-year-old white female whose primary language is English. She is a college graduate with a master's degree.

♦ Social history: Susie is a single mom with a 5-year-old daughter.

♦ Employment/work: She is a first grade teacher.

♦ Living environment: Susie lives in a one-level home with her daughter and two cats. There are two steps to enter with a hand rail.

♦ General health status
  ● General health perception: Susie reports that her health has been good until about 4 weeks ago when she developed an upper respiratory tract infection.
  ● Physical function: Normal for her age.
  ● Psychological function: Normal.
  ● Role function: Mother, teacher.
  ● Social function: She is involved with a summer sand volleyball team and volunteers at the local humane society one to two times per month. She likes to take walks on a regular basis, and if she has a babysitter for her daughter, she works out at a local fitness club.

♦ Social/health habits: At one time Susie smoked, but she reports that she quit prior to becoming pregnant with her daughter. She smoked half a pack per day for about 15 years.

♦ Family history: Her father, who is 67 years of age, has a history of coronary artery disease that has been managed with BP and cholesterol-lowering medications. Her mother, who is 63 years of age, is healthy with no known medical history.

♦ Medical/surgical history: Susie has no significant medical or surgical history.

♦ Current condition(s)/chief complaint(s): Susie awoke 2 weeks ago with dizziness and was unable to get out of bed without "tipping over." She also reported nausea at that time. These symptoms got better over approximately 4 days, but she continued to experience feelings of imbalance, and she has been unable to return to all previous activities.

♦ Functional status and activity level: She continued to teach, but she has been unable to participate in volleyball and at times struggles with playing with her daughter due to the feeling of disequilibrium. Quick turns seem to cause the most unsteadiness.

♦ Medications: Currently she is taking no medications.

♦ Other clinical tests
  ● An MRI of her brain was normal.
  ● Caloric testing demonstrated a diminished response in her right ear.

SYSTEMS REVIEW

♦ Cardiovascular/pulmonary
  ● BP: 110/64 mmHg
  ● Edema: None observed
  ● HR: 65 bpm
  ● RR: 13 bpm

♦ Integumentary
  ● Presence of scar formation: None
  ● Skin color: Normal
  ● Skin integrity: Intact

♦ Musculoskeletal
  ● Gross range of motion: Normal
  ● Gross strength: Good
  ● Gross symmetry: Normal
  ● Height: 5'10" (1.78m)
  ● Weight: 145 lbs (65.77kg)

♦ Neuromuscular
  ● Balance: Mildly impaired
  ● Locomotion, transfers, and transitions: Ambulates without an assistive device but guarded when turning and in crowded halls

♦ Communication, affect, cognition, language, and learning style
  ● Communication, affect, and cognition: Normal
  ● She reports that she is a visual learner

TESTS AND MEASURES

Prior to initiation of the tests and measures the patient was informed that it is important with vestibular examination to reproduce the symptoms.

♦ Aerobic capacity/endurance
  ● She had been walking 10 to 25 minutes each day at approximately a 17-minute mile

♦ Assistive and adaptive devices: None

♦ Anthropometric characteristics
  ● Body mass index=weight divided by height^2=22.6
  ● Susie is normal weight (normal=18.5 to 24.9; overweight=25 to 29.9; obese=30 to <40)

- ◆ Circulation
  - No change in BP in supine and standing
- ◆ Cranial and peripheral nerve integrity
  - Visual tests[32] (see Other Clinical Tests, Vestibular Dysfunction, pages 175 through 177)
    - Eye tests revealed no nystagmus when Susie looked straight ahead
    - She reported "My doctor saw my eyes move" when Susie first developed the dizziness
    - Saccades: Intact
    - Smooth pursuit: Intact
    - VOR/head thrust test: Positive on the right indicating an abnormal VOR
    - VOR cancellation: Normal
  - Positional tolerance (see Other Clinical Tests, Vestibular Dysfunction, pages 175 through 177)
    - All positional tests completed and no nystagmus noted
    - Very mild (1/10) dizziness noted by patient for all position changes except sit to supine
    - Sit to supine she rated as a 2/10
- ◆ Gait, locomotion, and balance
  - Able to perform Romberg with eyes open and with mild sway
  - Loss of balance when performing Romberg with eyes closed
  - Dynamic Gait Index: 20/24[32,137,163]
  - Walks independently without an assistive device but has occasional mild loss of balance with self-recovery
  - Was reluctant to try ambulating with head turns
- ◆ Muscle performance: Muscle strength is WNL in all four extremities
- ◆ Self-care and home management
  - DHI: Scored 40/100
- ◆ Work, community, and leisure integration or reintegration
  - Avoids looking up and bending down at work
  - Fearful of climbing ladder at work

EVALUATION

Susie is a healthy female who 4 weeks ago developed an upper respiratory infection. Two weeks later she developed dizziness and imbalance. Her main deficit is an unsteady gait that is worse with her eyes closed, with an increased pace, and with head turns. She shows an impaired VOR. Because of these difficulties, Susie has modified her lifestyle. She continues to work, but she appears to be participating less in her other activities.

DIAGNOSIS

Susie has symptoms consistent with an uncompensated unilateral peripheral hypofunction of her right ear. She has impaired: cranial and peripheral nerve integrity and gait, locomotion, and balance. She is functionally limited in self-care and home management and in work, community, and leisure actions, tasks, and activities. These findings are consistent with placement in Pattern F: Impaired Peripheral Nerve Integrity and Muscle Performance Associated With Peripheral Nerve Injury. The identified impairments and functional limitations will be addressed in determining the prognosis and the plan of care.

PROGNOSIS AND PLAN OF CARE

Over the course of the visits, the following mutually established outcomes have been determined:
- ◆ Gait and balance is improved
- ◆ Return to her previous activity level is achieved
- ◆ Risk for falls is decreased
- ◆ Safety awareness is improved
- ◆ Sensation of imbalance is decreased
- ◆ Understanding of anticipated goals and outcomes is increased

To achieve these outcomes, the appropriate interventions for this patient are determined. These will include: coordination, communication, and documentation; patient/client-related instruction; therapeutic exercise; functional training in self-care and home management; and functional training in work, community, and leisure integration or reintegration.

Susie is expected to need about between 8 and 12 visits over a 3-month period of time. She has good social support, is motivated, and will follow through with her home exercise program. She is not severely impaired and is healthy.

INTERVENTIONS

RATIONALE FOR SELECTED INTERVENTIONS

After damage to the peripheral components of the vestibular system, a person will have symptoms of vertigo, imbalance, and even nausea. The symptoms that this patient experiences are caused by a sensory mismatch.[32] Along with these symptoms a person can develop psychological symptoms including depression, anxiety, and fears. Many times these psychological and physical symptoms can contribute to an individual's decreasing social and functional activities.

A patient with a diagnosis of unilateral hypofunction is a

good candidate for vestibular rehabilitation, which is targeted at improving symptoms through three mechanisms: adaptation, substitution, and habituation (as described in pathophysiology of hypofunction). Another key component of the rehabilitation program for this patient is the initiation of a walking program to counteract the decreased activity level. Many patients with unilateral hypofunction will be able to return to all previous activities after rehabilitation.[32,139]

The outcome of interventions has been shown to be better if the patient complies with the home exercise program, receives early intervention after onset, does not limit stimulation, and has less initial vestibular deficit.[32]

COORDINATION, COMMUNICATION, AND DOCUMENTATION

Communication will occur with Susie in verbal and written form. Communication will occur with the physician. All elements of the patient's management will be documented.

PATIENT/CLIENT-RELATED INSTRUCTION

Susie will be educated on her current condition. She will have an understanding of the plan of care. She will be instructed both verbally and in writing on her home exercise program. Susie will also be instructed to turn lights on at night when getting up.

THERAPEUTIC EXERCISE

- ◆ Aerobic capacity/endurance conditioning
  - Initiate a walking program daily for 20 minutes
- ◆ Balance, coordination, and agility training
  - Head turn activities
    - Initiate head turning while standing with normal base of support
    - Progress the activity to performing head turns with walking
    - As the task becomes easier and less challenging, vary the head speed and the direction of head turns (from lateral head turns to vertical)
    - Try head turns in a stimulating environment (eg, store)
  - Standing activities
    - Static stance on solid surface with eyes closed (and supervision of another individual for safety) with a goal of 30 seconds
    - Progression
      - ▶ Standing with a narrow base of support
      - ▶ Standing on a piece of foam
- ◆ Vestibular training: Exercises to enhance the VOR for adaptation
  - Vestibular stimulation exercises[32]
    - Sit facing a wall with a plain background and focus on a target taped on the wall that can be

clearly seen or read
    - Turn head from side to side for 30 seconds and gradually progress to a duration of 2 minutes of head turns still focusing on the target
    - Advance the exercise by increasing the speed of head turns, putting the target on a busy background, or standing or marching in place while turning the head
  - Visuovestibular interactions[32]
    - Sit facing a wall with a plain background and hold the target (ie, business card) so it can be read
    - Move the target and head back and forth horizontally in opposite directions keeping the target in focus for 30 seconds and gradually progress to a duration of 2 minutes
    - Further progression would be the same as in vestibular stimulation exercise
- ◆ Habituation exercises
  - Sit to supine
  - Performed three to four times per day
  - Five repetitions each

FUNCTIONAL TRAINING IN SELF-CARE AND HOME MANAGEMENT

- ◆ Self-care and home management
  - Safety awareness training during functional tasks (eg, dark places turn on a light)

FUNCTIONAL TRAINING IN WORK, COMMUNITY, AND LEISURE INTEGRATION OR REINTEGRATION

- ◆ Work
  - Increase her movement around classroom
  - Observe children during recess break
- ◆ Leisure
  - Watch a full volleyball match
  - Toss volleyball with one person
  - Participate for part of a volleyball game

ANTICIPATED GOALS AND EXPECTED OUTCOMES

- ◆ Impact on impairments
  - Ability to perform movement tasks is improved.
  - Balance returns to baseline with daily tasks, and she is able to perform the Romberg with eyes closed for 30 seconds.
  - Dynamic Gait Index score is 24/24.
  - Walking the length of a hallway at a moderate pace with head turns and no loss of balance or symptoms is achieved.

- Impact on functional limitations
  - Return to her previous self-care and home management activity level is achieved.
  - Symptom-free return to her previous activities of volleyball and playing with her daughter is achieved.
- Impact on disabilities
  - Subjective feelings of imbalance and its impact on her life are decreased as shown by a decreased DHI score.
- Risk reduction/prevention
  - Safety awareness is improved.
  - Self-management of symptoms is improved.
- Impact on health, wellness, and fitness
  - Behaviors that foster healthy habits, wellness, and prevention are acquired.
- Impact on societal resources
  - Collaboration and coordination occur as needed.
  - Documentation occurs throughout patient management and follows APTA's *Guidelines for Physical Therapy Documentation.*[110]
- Patient/client satisfaction
  - Patient knowledge and awareness of the diagnosis, prognosis, interventions, and anticipated goals and expected outcomes are increased.
  - Patient understanding of anticipated goals and expected outcomes is increased.
  - Patient is independent in her home exercise program.

REEXAMINATION

Reexamination is performed throughout the episode of care, and the intervention plan is modified in accordance with changes in symptoms reported by the patient and the results of vestibular reexamination at each visit.

DISCHARGE

Susie is discharged from physical therapy after a total of 14 visits over a 3-month period of time for unilateral peripheral hypofunction. She received education regarding factors that may trigger a call to her physical therapist for a new examination and new episode of physical therapy care.

PSYCHOLOGICAL ASPECTS

See Case Study #3C for psychological considerations for this patient.

Case Study #3E: Bilateral Vestibular Hypofunction

Mr. John Miller is a healthy 52-year-old male who complains of dizziness and movement of his visual field as he walks.

PHYSICAL THERAPIST EXAMINATION

HISTORY

- General demographics: Mr. Miller is a healthy 52-year-old white male. He speaks English and is a college graduate.
- Social history: Mr. Miller is married and has two grown children.
- Employment/work: He works in middle management at a publishing company. Although he primarily sits at a desk, he also moves about the office and building.
- Living environment: He lives in a two-story house with four steps to enter and one full flight of stairs to the second floor, both of which have hand rails.
- General health status
  - General health perception: He reports good health with no major illnesses.
  - Physical function: His function is normal without any change noted in his hearing. He had no specific illness preceding the onset of these symptoms.
  - Psychological function: Normal.
  - Role function: Husband, father, manager, outdoorsman.
  - Social function: Mr. Miller enjoys boating, camping, and doing yard work.
- Social/health habits: Mr. Miller reported drinking occasional alcohol, and he is a nonsmoker.
- Family history: He reports no similar problems with dizziness in the family and no other significant family history.
- Medical/surgical history: He reports no significant history and specifically no cardiac or BP problems.
- Prior hospitalizations: None.
- Preexisting medical and other health-related conditions: Noncontributory.
- Current condition(s)/chief complaint(s): Mr. Miller feels dizzy most of the time, but especially with head movements. The problem began 1 month ago. He feels off balance when walking. He has difficulty walking at night. He reports that he is uncomfortable walking around the office at work and has had to leave work

because of dizziness. As he walks, he feels like he is watching a home movie where the person shooting the video was not holding the camera still. When he looks from his computer to items on his desk, objects seem to move, and this makes him feel dizzy. He wants to understand the dizziness that he is experiencing and the prognosis. He hopes to eliminate all symptoms.

♦ Functional status and activity level: He is independent in all ADL. Since the onset of these symptoms, he feels most activities are more difficult, and he is fatigued.

♦ Medications: None.

♦ Other clinical tests: Review of notes from the physician visit prior to physical therapy showed no abnormalities in any system including cardiovascular, pulmonary, or neuromuscular.

SYSTEMS REVIEW

♦ Cardiovascular/pulmonary
  • BP: 110/64 mmHg
  • Edema: None noted
  • HR: 65 bpm
  • RR: 13 bpm

♦ Integumentary
  • Presence of scar formation: None
  • Skin color: Normal
  • Skin integrity: WNL

♦ Musculoskeletal
  • Gross range of motion: WNL
  • Gross strength: WNL
  • Gross symmetry: Symmetrical
  • Height: 5'10" (1.77m)
  • Weight: 170 lbs (77.112 kg)

♦ Neuromuscular
  • Transfers: Independent
  • Locomotion: Walks with wide base of support and guarded gait, and he slows down for turns

♦ Communication, affect, cognition, language, and learning style
  • Communication, affect, and cognition: WNL
  • Learning style: Visual and auditory

TESTS AND MEASURES

♦ Anthropometric characteristics
  • Body mass index=weight divided by height²=24.4
  • Mr. Miller is normal weight (normal=18.5 to 24.9; overweight=25 to 29.9; obese=30 to <40)

♦ Cranial and peripheral nerve integrity
  • Note: Prior to vestibular testing, always clear the cervical spine for vertebral artery compression and

inform the patient that you will be turning his head side to side

  • Spontaneous nystagmus: None noted in any eye position
  • Visual tracking[32] (see Other Clinical Tests, Vestibular Dysfunction, pages 175 through 177)
    ▪ Pursuits: Normal
    ▪ VOR cancellation: Normal
    ▪ VOR
      ▸ Head thrust test: Positive right and left
    ▪ Saccadic eye movements: Normal
  • Positional tolerance (see Other Clinical Tests, Vestibular Dysfunction, pages 175 through 177)
    ▪ Dix-Hallpike[33]: Mild complaints of dizziness, but no nystagmus

♦ Gait, locomotion, and balance
  • BBS[126] score reveals 50/56, which indicated that he has a 12% probability of falling
  • Gait analysis
    ▪ Walks with slightly wide base of support
    ▪ Staggers and weaves while walking with head turns and slows his pace
    ▪ Rates dizziness symptoms as 4/10 with 10 being the worst
    ▪ Able to go up and down stairs without a rail and step over 3-inch obstacles without loss of balance
  • Tandem: Unable to perform tandem stance or tandem gait
  • Romberg eyes open: WNL
  • Romberg eyes closed: Loss of balance after 10 seconds
  • Altered surface: Able to stand on 5-inch thick foam with eyes open with effort, but loss of balance with eyes closed

♦ Self-care and home management and work, community, and leisure integration or reintegration
  • DHI[127]: Scored 56/100, which indicated difficulty with functional activities

EVALUATION

Mr. Miller is a healthy male who is now experiencing dizziness throughout most of his day. His balance is mildly altered, especially in conditions with decreased visual input and/or decreased proprioceptive input. His VOR is impaired bilaterally resulting in decreased ability to stabilize his gaze during head movements. As a result, he has difficulty performing duties at work and home, as well as participating in his hobbies.

Diagnosis

Mr. Miller is a client whose symptoms are consistent with a bilateral vestibular hypofunction. He has impaired: cranial and peripheral nerve integrity and gait, balance, and locomotion. He is functionally limited in self-care and home management and in work, community, and leisure actions, tasks, and activities. These findings are consistent with placement in Pattern F: Impaired Peripheral Nerve Integrity and Muscle Performance Associated With Peripheral Nerve Injury. The identified impairments and functional limitations will be addressed in determining the prognosis and the plan of care.

Prognosis and Plan of Care

Over the course of the visits, the following mutually established outcomes have been determined:

♦ Balance is improved

♦ Gait and locomotion are improved

♦ Participation in work, community, and leisure actions, tasks, and activities is enhanced

♦ Performance of ADL and IADL is improved

To achieve these outcomes, the appropriate interventions for this patient are determined. These will include: coordination, communication, and documentation; patient/client-related instruction; therapeutic exercise; functional training in self-care and home management; and functional training in work, community, and leisure integration or reintegration.

Mr. Miller is expected to need 6 to 10 visits over 8 to 10 weeks. He has good social support, is motivated, and will follow through with his home exercise program. While at slight risk for falls, he is not severely impaired and is healthy.

Interventions

RATIONALE FOR SELECTED INTERVENTIONS

Patients with bilateral vestibular hypofunction or bilateral vestibular loss are at increased risk for falls. Twenty-one percent of all patients with bilateral vestibular loss have multiple falls.[164-166] Seventy percent of individuals under the age of 65 report falls. Fifty-seven percent of individuals age 65 to 74 years report falls, and 18% of patients over 75 report falls. The decreased number of falls with increased age is thought to be due to greater use of assistive devices and being more cautious during activities. Physical therapy can determine the need for assistive devices, provide balance retraining, and educate patients about situations that will put them at risk for falls. It also enables patients to learn to rely more on somatosensory input than on visual input.[7,166,167]

Vestibular rehabilitation has been shown to improve postural stability and decrease the sense of disequilibrium by improving the function of the remaining vestibular system.[133,168-172] Recovery of gaze and postural stability are well documented in humans with vestibular deficits via tonic rebalancing of neural activity, VOR/VSR adaptation, and/or substitution strategies. Adaptation is the capability of the vestibular system to make long-term plastic changes in neuronal responses to head movement. This adaptation decreases retinal slip during head movements, increases postural stability, and helps reduce symptoms. Substitution involves teaching alternative strategies to replace lost or compromised function. Central preprogramming of compensatory eye movements helps maintain gaze stability in predictable tasks.[7,167]

Patients should be instructed in strategies to compensate for permanent risks due to a bilateral vestibular hypofunction including decreased balance on alternative surfaces (uneven, compliant, and graded), decreased balance in the dark, a very poor ability to orient oneself in water, limited ability to participate in sports, and limitations in the ability to drive.[165,173]

COORDINATION, COMMUNICATION, AND DOCUMENTATION

Communication will occur with the patient, both in written and verbal format. The physical therapist will communicate with the physician about the patient's diagnosis and plan of care. All elements of the patient's management will be documented.

PATIENT/CLIENT-RELATED INSTRUCTION

The patient will be instructed in the functional results of a bilateral vestibular hypofunction. He will be educated in the role of the vestibular system in balance and as a motion sensor. The patient will also be provided information about the permanent risks due to a bilateral vestibular hypofunction, including decreased balance on alternative surfaces (uneven, compliant, and graded), decreased balance in the dark, and very poor ability to orient oneself in water.

THERAPEUTIC EXERCISE

♦ Balance, coordination, and agility training
  • Balance training
    ▪ Static balance using progressively narrower base of support until doing tandem
    ▪ Single leg stance
    ▪ Progress to a variety of surfaces
    ▪ Practice eyes open, eyes closed, and with head turns
  • Vestibular training
    ▪ VOR exercises for adaptation if there is any remaining vestibular function and for maximizing

the use of the cervico-ocular reflex

- ▶ Start in sitting with the patient focusing on one point on a plain background for 30 seconds
- ▶ Slowly turn head from side to side keeping the target in focus for 30 seconds
- ▶ Increase the time as tolerated with the long-term goal of 2 minutes
- ▶ Progression of the exercise
  - ○ Vary the speed of head turn
  - ○ Go from sitting to standing
  - ○ Modify background to provide more stimulation
  - ○ March in place
  - ○ Walk to and from the target
- ■ Compensatory saccade exercise for substitution
  - ▶ Place two targets on the wall approximately 4 feet apart
  - ▶ Patient starts with eyes and head turned toward one target, and then turns his eyes toward the other target, followed by turning his head
  - ▶ Repeat for 30 seconds, progressing to a duration of 2 minutes
  - ▶ Once able to perform the exercise, have him carryover the activity to daily functional activities
- ■ Imaginary targets exercise for central preprogramming
  - ▶ Patient chooses two targets on a wall approximately 4 feet apart with eyes and head turned toward one target
  - ▶ Patient shuts his eyes and turns his eyes, while shut, toward the other target, and then open eyes to see if he has accurately estimated the target placement
  - ▶ Then turn head toward target
  - ▶ Finally patient shuts his eyes again and repeats the activity toward the first target
  - ▶ Perform for 30 seconds and gradually progress to a duration of 2 minutes

- ◆ Gait and locomotion training
  - ● Variations in gait speed
  - ● Walking while turning head
  - ● Tandem gait
  - ● Gait with 180-degree turns, 360-degree turns, and Figure 8's
  - ● Stepping over obstacles

FUNCTIONAL TRAINING IN SELF-CARE AND HOME MANAGEMENT

- ◆ Home management

- ● Use nightlights or turn on lights when up at night
- ● Emergency lighting in case of a power failure

FUNCTIONAL TRAINING IN WORK, COMMUNITY, AND LEISURE INTEGRATION OR REINTEGRATION

- ◆ Work
  - ● Use compensatory saccades when looking between the computer and other items in the office in order to better stabilize gaze
- ◆ Leisure
  - ● Use a flashlight or headlamp when walking outside at night when camping
  - ● Choose a level path instead of an uneven surface when walking in dim light or darkness
  - ● Always use a personal flotation device while in the water
  - ● Driving
    - ■ With an incomplete bilateral vestibular hypofunction, driving at night may be possible
    - ■ With a complete bilateral loss, driving at night or possibly at all may not be possible
    - ■ It is anticipated that he will be able to drive at night

ANTICIPATED GOALS AND EXPECTED OUTCOMES

- ◆ Impact on impairments
  - ● Gait and balance are improved.
  - ● Tandem stance with eyes open for 10 seconds is achieved.
  - ● Walking and turning his head without loss of balance with only mild symptoms (2/10) is achieved.
- ◆ Impact on functional limitations
  - ● Ability to perform activities related to self-care, home management, work, community, and leisure is improved.
  - ● Performance and safety levels in self-care, home management, work, community, and leisure activities are improved.
  - ● Return to 8-hour workdays with minimal symptoms is attained.
  - ● Tolerance to activities is increased.
- ◆ Impact on disabilities
  - ● Subjective feelings of dizziness are decreased as shown by an improved DHI score.
- ◆ Risk reduction/prevention
  - ● Knowledge of deficits and safety precautions is verbalized.

- Risk of falls or injury is reduced.
- Risk of secondary impairments is reduced, and safety is improved during performance of all ADL and IADL.
  - Safety is improved.
- Impact on health, wellness, and fitness
  - Behaviors that foster healthy habits, wellness, and prevention are acquired.
  - Patient knowledge of personal and environmental factors associated with the condition is increased.
  - Physical function is improved.
- Impact on societal resources
  - Documentation occurs throughout patient management and follows APTA's *Guidelines for Physical Therapy Documentation*.[110]
  - Resources are used in a cost-effective manner.
- Patient/client satisfaction
  - Knowledge and awareness of the diagnosis, prognosis, interventions, and anticipated goals and expected outcomes are increased.
  - Sense of well-being is improved.
  - Understanding of anticipated goals and expected outcomes is increased.

REEXAMINATION

Reexamination is performed throughout the episode of care.

DISCHARGE

Mr. Miller is discharged from physical therapy after a total of nine physical therapy visits over a 10-week period of time and attainment of his goals. Mr. Miller received education regarding factors that may trigger a call to his physical therapist for a new examination and new episode of physical therapy care.

REFERENCES

1. Moore KL, Dalley AF. *Clinically Oriented Anatomy.* 4th ed. Philadelphia, PA: Lippincott Williams & Williams; 1999.
2. Singhi P, Jain V. Bell's palsy in children. *Semin Pediatr Neurol.* 2003; 10(4):289-297.
3. Ulug T, Ulubil SA. Management of facial paralysis in temporal bone fractures: a prospective study analyzing 11 operated fractures. *American Journal of Otolaryngology—Head and Neck Medicine and Surgery.* 2005:26:230-238.
4. Rahman I, Sadiq SA. Ophthalmic management of facial nerve palsy: a review. *Surv Ophthalmol.* 2007;52(2):121-144.
5. Agur A, Dalley AF. *Grant's Atlas of Anatomy.* 11th ed. Philadelphia, PA: Lippincott Williams & Wilkins; 2005.
6. Gill-Body KM. Current concepts in the management of patients with vestibular dysfunction. *PT-Magazine of Physical Therapy.* 2001;9(12);40-56.
7. Herdman SJ. *Vestibular Rehabilitation.* Philadelphia, PA: FA Davis; 1994.
8. Baloh RW. *Dizziness, Hearing Loss, and Tinnitus: The Essentials of Neurotology.* Philadelphia, PA: FA Davis Co; 1984.
9. Adams GL, Boies LR, Hilger P. *Boies Fundamentals of Otolaryngology.* Philadelphia, PA: WB Saunders Co; 1989.
10. Barr ML, Kiernan JA. *The Human Nervous System: An Anatomical Viewpoint.* Philadelphia, PA: Harper and Row; 1983.
11. Herdman SJ. Physical therapy management of vestibular disorders in older patients. *Phys Ther.* 1992;1(1):77-87.
12. Nashner LM. A model describing vestibular detection of body sway motion. *Acta Otolaryngol.* 1971;72:429-436.
13. Szabo RM, Chidgey LK. Stress carpal tunnel pressures in patients with carpal tunnel syndrome and normal patients. *J Hand Surg (Am).* 1989;14:624-627.
14. Campbell WW. Diagnosis and management of common compression and entrapment neuropathies. *Neurol Clin.* 1997; 15:549-567.
15. Gelberman G, Hergenroeder PT, Hargens AR, et al, The carpal tunnel syndrome. A study of carpal canal pressures. *J Bone Joint Surg Am.* 1981;63:380-383.
16. Tanaka S, Wild D, Seligman P, et al. The US prevalence of self reported carpal tunnel syndrome: 1988 national health interview survey data. *Am J Public Health.* 1994;84:1846-1848.
17. MacKinnon SE. Pathophysiology of nerve compression. *Hand Clin.* 2002;18:231-241.
18. Lee MJ, LaStayo PC. Pronator syndrome and other nerve compressions that mimic carpal tunnel syndrome. *J Orthop Sports Phys Ther.* 2004;34:601-609.
19. Eversmann WW. Proximal median nerve compression. *Hand Clin.* 1992;8:307-315.
20. Rehak DC. Pronator syndrome. *Clin Sports Med.* 2001;20:531-540.
21. Nadler SF. Distal upper-extremity nerve injuries. In: Feinberg JH, Spielholz NI, eds. *Peripheral Nerve Injuries in the Athlete.* Champaign, IL: Human Kinetics; 2003.
22. Peitersen E. Bell's palsy: the spontaneous course in 2500 peripheral facial nerve palsies of different aetiologies. *Acta Otolaryngol.* 2002;549(Suppl):S4-S30.
23. Gurwood AS, Drake J. Guillain-Barre syndrome. *Optometry.* 2006;77:540-546.
24. Ulku CH, Uyar Y, Acar O, et al. Facial nerve schwannomas: a report of four cases and a review of the literature. *Am J Otolaryngol.* 2004;25(6):426-431.
25. Napoli AM, Panagos P. Delayed presentation of traumatic facial nerve paralysis. *J Emerg Med.* 2005;29(2):421-424.
26. Evans AK, Licameli G, Brietzke S, et al. Pediatric facial nerve paralysis: patients, management and outcomes. *Int J Pediatr Otorhinolaryngol.* 2005;69:1521-1528.
27. Murakami S, Mizobuchi M, Nakashiro Y, et al. Bell palsy and herpes simplex virus: identification of viral DNA in endoneurial fluid and muscle. *Ann Intern Med.* 1996;124:27-30.
28. Quinn F. Facial nerve paralysis. *Otolaryngol.* 1996;1:1-13.
29. Bergstralh MS, Erik J, Wiederhold WC, et al. Incidence, clinical features and prognosis in Bell's palsy. *Ann Neurol.* 1986;20(5):622-627.
30. Seddon H. *Surgical Disorders of the Peripheral Nerve.* 2nd ed.

New York, NY: Churchill Livingstone; 1975.

31. Sunderland S. *Nerves and Nerve Injuries.* 2nd ed. New York, NY: Churchill Livingstone; 1978.

32. Herdman SJ. *Vestibular Rehabilitation.* Philadelphia, PA: FA Davis; 2000.

33. Dix MR, Hallpike CS. Pathology, symptomatology and diagnosis of certain disorders of the vestibular system. *Proceedings of the Royal Society of Medicine.* 1952;45:341.

34. Eply JM. New dimensions of benign paroxysmal positional vertigo. *Otolaryngol Head Neck Surg.* 1980;88:599-605.

35. Parnes LS, Agrawal SK, Atlas J. Diagnosis and management of benign paroxysmal positional vertigo (BPPV). *CMAJ.* 2003; 169(7):1-21.

36. Washko NL, Gilbert J. *Balance Retraining: A Comprehensive Approach to Treatment of Patients with Dizziness and Imbalance.* New York, NY: Thieme Medical Publishers; 1991.

37. Zee D. The management of patients with vestibular disorders. In: Barber H, Sharp JA, eds. *Vestibular Disorders.* Chicago, IL: Year Book Medical Publishers; 1988.

38. Shumway-Cook A, Horak FB. Rehabilitation strategies for patients with vestibular deficits. *Neurol Clin.* 1990;8:441-457.

39. Norre ME, De Weerdt W. Treatment of vertigo based on habituation. 1. Physio-pathological basis. *J Laryngol Otol.* 1980;94:689-696.

40. Herdman SJ. Assessment and treatment of balance disorders in the vestibular-deficient patient. In: Duncan P, ed. *Balance: Proceedings of the APTA Forum.* Alexandria, VA: American Physical Therapy Association; 1990:87-94.

41. Herdman SJ, Clendaniel RA, Mattox DE, et al. Vestibular adaptation exercises and recovery: acute stage after acoustic neuroma resection. *Otolaryngol Head Neck Surg.* 1995;113:77-87.

42. Cohen H, Ewell CR, Jenkins HA. Disability in Meniere's disease. *Archives of Otolaryngology.* 1995;121:29-33.

43. Gibson W, Arenberg IK. Pathophysiologic theories in the etiology of Meniere's disease. *Otolaryngol Clin North Am.* 1997;30(6):961-967.

44. Slattery WH, Fayad JN. Medical treatment of Meniere's disease. *Otolaryngol Clin North Am.* 1997;30(6):1027-1037.

45. Silverstein H, Rosenberg S, Arruda J, Isaacson JE. Surgical ablation of the vestibular system in the treatment of Meniere's disease. *Otolaryngol Clin North Am.* 1997;30(6):1075-1095.

46. Hoffer ME, Balough B, Henderson J, et al. Use of sustained release vehicles in the treatment of Meniere's disease. *Otolaryngol Clin North Am.* 1997;30(6):1159-1166.

47. Katsarkas A. Benign paroxysmal positional vertigo (BPPV): idiopathic versus post-traumatic. *Acta Otolaryngol.* 1999; 119(7):745-749.

48. Mizukoshi K, Watanabe Y, Shojaku H, et al. Epidemiological studies on benign paroxysmal positional vertigo in Japan. *Acta Otolaryngol Suppl.* 1988;447:67-72.

49. Oas JG. Benign paroxysmal positional vertigo: a clinician's perspective. *Ann N Y Acad Sci.* 2001;942:201-209.

50. Uno A, Moriwaki K, Kato T, et al. Clinical features of benign paroxysmal positional vertigo. *Nippon Jibiinkoka Gakkai Kaiho.* 2001;104:9-16.

51. Wrisley DM, Sparto PJ, Whitney SL, Furman JM. Cervicogenic dizziness: a review of diagnosis and treatment. *J Orthop Sports Phys Ther.* 2000;30:755-766.

52. Murphy TP. Mal de debarquement syndrome: a forgotten entity? *Otolaryngol Head Neck Surg.* 1993;109:10-13.

53. Bikhazi P, Jackson C, Ruckenstein MJ. Efficacy of antimigrainous therapy in the treatment of migraine-associated dizziness. *Am J Otolaryngol.* 1997;18:350.

54. Johnson GD. Medical management of migraine-related dizziness and vertigo. *Laryngoscope.* 1998;108:1-28.

55. Jacob RG, Furman JM, Durrant JD, Turner SM. Panic, agoraphobia, and vestibular dysfunction. *Am J Psychiatry.* 1996; 153:503-512.

56. Stein MB, Asmundson GJ, Ireland D, Walker JR. Panic disorder in patients attending a clinic for vestibular disorders. *Am J Psychiatry.* 1994;151:1697-1700.

57. Asmundson GJG, Larsen DK, Stein MB. Panic disorder and vestibular disturbance: an overview of empirical findings and clinical implications. *J Psychosom Res.* 1998;44:107-120.

58. Watson D, Clark LA, Carey G. Positive and negative affectivity and their relations to anxiety and depressive disorders. *J Abnorm Psychol.* 1988;97:346-353.

59. Jenkins HA, Furman JM, Gulya AJ, Honrubia R, Linthicum FH, Mirka A. Dysequilibrium of aging. *Otolaryngol Head Neck Surg.* 1989;100:272-282.

60. Ross MD, Peacor D, Johnsson LG, Allard LF. Observations on normal and degenerating human otoconia. *Ann Otol Rhinol Laryngol.* 1976;85:310-326.

61. Baloh RW, Spain S, Socotch TM, Jacobson KM, Bell TS. Posturography and balance problems in older people. *J Am Geriatr Soc.* 1995;43:638-644.

62. Chang H, Krebs DE. Dynamic balance control in elders: gait initiation assessment as a screening tool. *Arch Phys Med Rehabil.* 1999;80:490-494.

63. Kensalo DR. Age changes in touch, vibration, temperature, kinesthesia and pain sensitivity. In: Birren JE, Schaie KW, eds. *Handbook of the Psychology of Aging.* New York, NY: Van Notrand Reinhold; 1977:562-579.

64. Lord SR, Ward JA. Age-associated differences in sensori-motor function and balance in community dwelling women. *Age Ageing.* 1996;25:292-299.

65. Kumar A, Mafee MF, Mason T. Value of imaging in disorders of the facial nerve. *Top Magn Reson Imaging.* 2000;11:38-51.

66. Van den Hauwe L, Bernaerts A, Van Goethem JW, et al. Imaging in patients with vertigo. *JBR-BTR.* 1999;82:241-244.

67. Keles I, Kendi ATK, Aydin G, et al. Diagnostic precision of ultrasonography in patients with carpal tunnel syndrome. *Am J Phys Med Rehabil.* 2005;84:443-450.

68. Jordan R, Carter T, Cummins C. A systemic review of the utility of electrodiagnositic testing in carpal tunnel syndrome. *Br J Gen Pract.* 2002;52:670-673.

69. May M, Harvey JE, Marovitz WF, et al. The prognostic accuracy of the maximal stimulation test compared with that of the nerve excitability test in Bell's palsy. *Laryngoscope.* 1971; 81:931-938.

70. Kimura J. *Electrodiagnosis in Diseases of Nerve and Muscle.* 3rd ed. New York, NY: Oxford University Press; 2001.

71. Coker NJ, Fordice JO, Moore S. Correlation of the nerve excitability test and electroneurography in acute facial paralysis. *Am J Otolaryngol.* 1992;13:127-133.

72. Overholt SM. Bell's palsy. Grand rounds presentation Baylor College of Medicine, July 20, 1995. Available at: http://www.bcm.edu/oto/grand/72095.html. Accessed August 21, 2007.

73. Sittel C, Stennert E. Prognostic value of electromyography in acute peripheral facial nerve palsy. *Otol Neurotol.* 2001;22:100-104.

74. Huffman MD, Baker RS, Stava MW, et al. Kinematic analysis of eyelid movements in patients recovering from unilateral facial nerve palsy. *Neurology.* 1996;46:1079-1085.

75. Ruckenstein MJ, Shepard NT. Balance function testing, a rational approach. *Otolaryngol Clin North Am.* 2000;33:3:507-517.

76. Monsell EM, Furman JM, Herdman SJ, et al. Computerized dynamic platform posturography. *Otolaryngol Head Neck Surg.* 1997;117:394.

77. Della Santina CC, Cremer PD, Carey JP, Minor LB. Comparison of head thrust test with head autorotation test reveals that the vestibulo-ocular reflex is enhanced during voluntary head movements. *Arch Otolaryngol Head Neck Surg.* 2002;128:1044-1054.

78. Adour KK, Ruboyianes JM, Von Doersten PG, et al. Bell's palsy treatment with acyclovir and prednisone compared with prednisone alone: a double-blind, randomized, controlled trial. *Ann Otol Rhinol Laryngol.* 1996;105:371-378.

79. Takahashi H, Hato N, Honda N, et al. Effects of acyclovir on facial nerve paralysis induced by herpes simplex virus type 1 in mice. *Auris Nasus Larynx.* 2003;30:1-5.

80. Kinishi M, Amatsu M, Mohri M, et al. Acyclovir improves recovery rate of facial nerve palsy in Ramsay Hunt syndrome. *Auris Nasus Larynx.* 2001;28:223-226.

81. Hato N, Matsumoto S, Kisaki H, et al. Efficacy of early treatment of Bell's palsy with oral acyclovir and prednisolone. *Otol Neurotol.* 2003;24:948-951.

82. Zuccaro TA. Pharmacological management of vertigo. *Journal of Neurologic Physical Therapy.* 2003;27(3):118-121.

83. *Mosby's Nursing Drug Reference.* St. Louis, MO: Mosby Inc; 2001.

84. Thomson Healthcare Inc. *Physician's Desk Reference.* 59th ed. Montvale, NJ: Thomson PDR; 2005.

85. Rice GPA, Ebers GC. Ondansetron for intractable vertigo complicating acute brainstem disorders. *Lancet.* 1995;345:1182-1183.

86. Macleod A. Ondansetron in multiple sclerosis. *J Pain Symptom Manage.* 2000;20(5):388-391.

87. Black FO, Pesznecker SC, Stallings V. Permanent gentamicin vestibulotoxicity. *Otol Neurotol.* 2004;25(4):559-569.

88. Minor LB. Gentamicin–induced bilateral vestibular hypofunction. *JAMA.* 1998;279(7):541-544.

89. Callahan AD. Sensibility testing. In: Hunter J, Schneider LH, Jackin EJ, Callahan AD, eds. *Rehabilitation of the Hand: Surgery and Therapy.* St. Louis, MO: CV Mosby; 1990.

90. Strauch B, Lang A, Ferder M, et al. The ten test. *Plast Reconstr Surg.* 1997;99(4):1074-1078.

91. Levin DW, Simmons BP, Koris MJ, et al. A self-administered questionnaire for the assessment of severity of symptoms in functional status in carpal tunnel syndrome. *J Bone Joint Surg Am.* 1993;75:1585-1592.

92. Nadler S. Distal upper extremity nerve injuries. In: Feinberg JH, Spielholtz NI, eds. *Peripheral Nerve Injuries in the Athlete.* Champaign, IL: Human Kinetics; 2003.

93. Jensen MP, Karoly P, Braver S. The measurement of clinical pain intensity: a comparison of six methods. *Pain.* 1986;27(1):117-126.

94. Magee D. *Orthopedic Physical Assessment.* 3rd ed. Philadelphia, PA: WB Saunders Co; 1997.

95. Jebsen RH, Taylor N, Trieschmann RB, et al. An objective and standardized test of hand function. *Arch Phys Med Rehabil.* 1969;50:311-319.

96. Burke FD, Ellis J, McKenna H, Bradley MJ. Primary care management of carpal tunnel syndrome. *Postgrad Med J.* 2003; 79;433-437.

97. Seradge H, Jia YC, Owens W. In vivo measurement of carpal tunnel pressure in the functioning hand. *J Hand Surg (Am).* 1995;20:855-859.

98. Akalin E, El O, Peker O, et al. Treatment of carpal tunnel syndrome with nerve and tendon gliding exercises. *Am J Phys Med Rehabil.* 2002;81:108-113.

99. Rozmaryn LM, Dovelle S, Rothman ER, et al, Nerve and tendon gliding exercises and the conservative management of carpal tunnel syndrome. *J Hand Ther.* 1998;11:171-179.

100. Seradge H, Bear C, Bithell D. Preventing carpal tunnel syndrome and cumulative trauma disorder: effect of carpal tunnel decompression exercises: an Oklahoma experience. *J Okla State Med Assoc.* 2000;93:150-153.

101. Seradge H, Parker W, Baer C, et al. Conservative treatment of carpal tunnel syndrome: an outcome study of adjunct exercises. *J Okla State Med Assoc.* 2002;95:7-14.

102. Michlovitz S. Conservative interventions for carpal tunnel syndrome. *J Orthop Sports Phys Ther.* 2004;34:589-600.

103. Gerristen AA, de Vet HC, Scholten RJ, et al. Splinting vs surgery in the treatment of carpal tunnel syndrome: a randomized controlled trial. *JAMA.* 2002;288:1245-1251.

104. Werner RA, Franzblau A, Gell N. Randomized controlled trial of nocturnal splinting for active workers with symptoms of carpal tunnel syndrome. *Arch Phys Med Rehabil.* 2005;86:1-7.

105. Manente G, Torrieri F, DiBlasio F, et al. An innovative hand brace for carpal tunnel syndrome: a randomized controlled trial. *Muscle Nerve.* 2001;24:1020-1025.

106. Walker WC. Mettzler M, Cifu DX, Swarth Z. Neutral wrist splinting in carpal tunnel syndrome: a comparison of night-only versus full-time wear instructions. *Arch Phys Med Rehabil.* 2000;81:424-429.

107. Gokoglu F, Fndkoglu G, Yorgancoglu ZR, et al. Evaluation of iontophoresis and local corticosteroid injection in the treatment of carpal tunnel syndrome. *Am J Phys Med Rehabil.* 2005;84(2):92-96.

108. Ebenbichler GR, Resch KL, Nicolakis P, et al. Ultrasound treatment for treating the carpal tunnel syndrome: randomized "sham" controlled trial. *BMJ.* 1988;316:731-735.

109. Oztas O, Turan B, Bora I, Karakaya MK. Ultrasound therapy effect in carpal tunnel syndrome. *Arch Phys Med Rehabil.* 1988; 79:1540-1544.

110. American Physical Therapy Association. Guide to physical therapist practice. 2nd ed. *Phys Ther.* 2001;81:9-744.

111. House JW, Brackmann DE. Facial nerve grading system. *Otolaryngol Head Neck Surg.* 1985;93:146-147.

112. Ho K, Spence J, Murphy MF. Review of pain management tools. *Ann Emerg Med.* 1996;27:427-432.

113. Brach JS, VanSwearingen JM. Physical therapy for facial paralysis: a tailored treatment approach. *Phys Ther.* 1999;79:397-404.

114. Krasilovsky G. Biofeedback. In: Hecox B, Mehreteab TA, Weisberg J, Sanko J, eds. *Integrating Physical Agents in Rehabilitation.* 2nd ed. Upper Saddle River, NJ: Pearson Prentice Hall; 2006:459-481.

115. Carr J, Shepherd R. *Movement Science, Foundations for Physical Therapy in Rehabilitation.* 2nd ed. Gaithersburg, MD: Aspen; 2000.

116. Kisner C, Colby LA. *Therapeutic Exercise.* 5th ed. Philadelphia, PA: FA Davis; 2007.

117. Cronin GW, Steenerson RL. The effectiveness of neuromuscular facial retraining combined with electromyography in facial paralysis rehabilitation. *Otolaryngol Head Neck Surg.* 2003;128:534-538.

118. Basmajian JV, ed. *Biofeedback, Principles and Practice for Clinicians.* 3rd ed. Baltimore, MD: Williams & Wilkins; 1989.

119. Adler SS, Beckers D, Buck M. *PNF in Practice: An Illustrated Guide.* Berlin, Germany: Springer-Verlag; 2000.

120. Rogers RG. Mental practice and acquisition of motor skills: examples from sports training and surgical education. *Obstet Gynecol Clin North Am.* 2006;33(2):297-304.

121. Seiff SR. Surgical management of seventh nerve paralysis and floppy eyelid syndrome. *Curr Opin Ophthalmol.* 1999;10:242-246.

122. Zwick O, Seiff S. Supportive care of facial nerve palsy with temporary external eyelid weights. *Optometry.* 2006;77:340-342.

123. Ohtake PJ, Zafron ML, Poranki LG, Fish DR. Does electrical stimulation improve motor recovery in patients with idiopathic facial palsy? *Phys Ther.* 2006;86(11):1558-1564.

124. Jansen J, Lomo T, Nicolaysen K, Westgaard R. Hyperinnervation of skeletal muscle fibers: dependence on muscle activity. *Science.* 1973;181:559-561.

125. Lomo T. The role of activity in the control of membrane and contractile properties of skeletal muscle. In: Thesleff S, ed. *Motor Innervation of Muscle.* New York, NY: Academic Press; 1976:289-321.

126. Berg KO, Wood-Dauphinee SL, Williams JI, Maki B. Measuring balance in the elderly: validation of an instrument. *Can J Public Health.* 1992;(Suppl 2):S7-S11.

127. Jacobson GP, Newman CW. The development of the Dizziness Handicap Inventory. *Arch Otolaryngol Head Neck Surg.* 1990; 116:424-427.

128. Judge JO, Lindsey C, Underwood M, Winsemius D. Balance improvements in older women: effects of exercise training. *Phys Ther.* 1993;73:254-262.

129. Hauer K, Rost B, Rutschle K, et al. Exercise training for rehabilitation and secondary prevention of falls in geriatric patients with a history of injurious falls. *J Am Geriatr Soc.* 2001;49:10-20.

130. Schlicht J, Camaione DN, Owen SV. Effect of intense strength training on standing balance, walking speed, and sit-to-stand performance in older adults. *J Gerontol A Biol Sci Med Sci.* 2001;56:M281-M286.

131. Williams GN, Higgins MJ, Lewek MD. Aging skeletal muscle: physiologic changes and the effects of training. *Phys Ther.* 2002;82:62-68.

132. Shumway-Cook A, Gruber W, Baldwin M, Liao S. The effect of multidimensional exercises on balance, mobility, and fall risk in community-dwelling older individuals. *Phys Ther.* 1997;77:46-57.

133. Yardley L, Beech S, Zander L, Evans T, Weinman J. A randomized controlled trial of exercise therapy for dizziness and vertigo in primary care. *Br J Gen Pract.* 1998;48:1136-1140.

134. Rizzo JA, Baker DI, McAvay G, Tinetti ME. The cost-effectiveness of a multifactorial targeted prevention program for falls among community elderly persons. *Med Care.* 1996; 34:954-969.

135. Day L, Fildes B, Gordon I, et al. Randomized factorial trial of falls prevention among older people living in their own homes. *BMJ.* 2002;325(7356):128-131.

136. Campbell AJ, Robertson MC, Gardner MM, et al. Falls prevention over 2 years: a randomized controlled trial in women 80 years and older. *Age Ageing.* 1999;28:513-518.

137. Shumway-Cook A, Baldwin M, Polissar NL, Gruber W. Predicting the probability for falls in community dwelling older adults. *Phys Ther.* 1997;77:812-819.

138. Thorbahn LD, Newton RA. Use of the Berg Balance test to predict falls in elderly persons. *Phys Ther.* 1996;76(6):576-583.

139. Whitney SL, Metzinger RM. Efficacy of vestibular rehabilitation. *Otolaryngol Clin North Am.* 2000;33(3):659-672.

140. Meissner I. Natural history of drop attacks. *Neurology.* 1986; 36:1029-1986.

141. Yardley L, Kirby S. Eval of booklet-based self management of symptoms in Meniere's disease: a randomized controlled trial. *Psychosom Med.* 2006;68:762-769.

142. Herdman SJ. Treatment of benign paroxysmal positional vertigo. *Phys Ther.* 1990;70(6):381-388.

143. Eply JM. The canalith repositioning procedure: for treatment of benign paroxysmal positional vertigo. *Otolaryngol Head Neck Surg.* 1992;107:399-404.

144. Nuti D, Nati C, Passali D. Treatment of benign paroxysmal positional vertigo: no need for post-maneuver restrictions. *Otolaryngol Head Neck Surg.* 2000;122:440-444.

145. Massoud EA, Ireland DJ. Post-treatment instructions in the non-surgical management of benign paroxysmal positional vertigo. *J Otolaryngol.* 1996;25:121-125.

146. Brandt T, Daroff RB. Physical therapy for benign paroxysmal positional vertigo. *Arch Otolaryngol.* 1980;106:484-485.

147. Atlas JT, Parnes LS. Benign paroxysmal positional vertigo: mechanism and management. *Curr Opin Otolaryngol Head Neck Surg.* 2001;9:284-289.

148. Parnes LS, Price-Jones RG. Particle repositioning maneuver for benign paroxysmal positional vertigo. *Ann Otol Rhinol Laryngol.* 1993;102:325-331.

149. Parnes LS, Robichaud J. Further observations during the particle repositioning maneuver for benign paroxysmal positional vertigo. *Otolaryngol Head Neck Surg.* 1997;116:238-243.

150. LeLiever WC. Comparative repositioning maneuvers for benign paroxysmal positional vertigo. Proceedings from the COSM meeting, Palm Beach, Florida, May 7-13; 1994. From Furman JM, Cass SP. *Balance Disorders. A Case Study Approach.* Philadelphia, PA: FA Davis; 1996.

151. Pollak L, Davies RA, Luxon LL. Effectiveness of the particle repositioning maneuver in benign paroxysmal positional vertigo with and without additional vestibular pathology. *Otol Neurotol.* 2002;23:79-83.

152. Fung K, Hall SF. Particle repositioning maneuver: effective treatment for benign paroxysmal positional vertigo. *J*

Otolaryngol. 1996;25:243-248.

153. O'Reilly RC, Elford B, Slater R. Effectiveness of the particle repositioning maneuver in subtypes of benign paroxysmal positional vertigo. *Laryngoscope.* 2000;110:1385-1388.

154. Korres SG, Balatsouras DG, Papoullakos S, Ferekidis E. Benign PPV and its management. *Med Sci Monit.* 2007;13(6): CR275-CR282.

155. Simoceli L, Moreira Bittar RS, Greters ME. Posture restrictions do not interfere in results of canalith repositioning maneuver. *Revista Brasileira de Otorrinolaringologia.* 2005;71(1):55-59.

156. Roberts R, Gans R, Deboodt J, Lister J. Treatment of benign paroxysmal positional vertigo: necessity of postmaneuver patient restrictions. *J Am Acad Audiol.* 2005;16:357-366.

157. Marciano E, Marcelli V. Postural restrictions in labyrintholithiasis. *Eur Arch Otorhinolaryngol.* 2002;259:262-265.

158. Ireland D. *The Semont Maneuver.* Proceedings of the XVIth Barany Society Meeting, Prague, Czechoslovakia; 1994:367-370.

159. Gordon CR, Gadoth N. Repeated vs single physical maneuver in benign paroxysmal positional vertigo. *Acta Neurol Scand.* 2004;110:166-169.

160. Seo T, Miyamoto A, Saka N, et al. Immediate efficacy of the canalith repositioning procedure for the treatment of benign paroxysmal positional vertigo. *Otol Neurol.* 2007;28(7):917-919.

161. Shepard NT, Telian SA. Programmatic vestibular rehabilitation. *Otolaryngol Head Neck Surg;* 1995;112:173-182.

162. Rahko T. The test and treatment methods of benign paroxysmal positional vertigo and an addition to the management of vertigo due to the superior vestibular canal (BPPV-SC). *Clin Otolaryngol.* 2002;27:392-395.

163. Whitney SL, Hudak MT, Marchetti GF. The dynamic gait index relates to self-reporting fall history in individuals with vestibular dysfunction. *J Vestib Res.* 2000;10:99-105.

164. Herdman SJ, Blatt P, Schubert MC, Tusa RJ. Falls in patients with vestibular deficits. *American Journal of Otology.* 2000;21(6):847-851.

165. Gillespie MD, Minor LB. Prognosis in bilateral vestibular hypofunction. *Laryngoscope.* 1999;109:35-41.

166. Krebs DE, Gill-Body KM, Riley PO, Parker SW. Double-blind, placebo-controlled trial of rehabilitation for bilateral vestibular hypofunction: preliminary report. *Otolaryngol Head Neck Surg.* 1993;109:735-741.

167. Cohen H. Vestibular rehabilitation reduces functional disability. *Otolaryngol Head Neck Surg.* 1992;107:638.

168. Cass SP, Borello-France D, Furman JM. Functional outcome of vestibular rehabilitation in patients with abnormal sensory organization testing. *American Journal of Otology.* 1996;17:581-594.

169. Horak FB, Jones-Rycewicz C, Black FO, Shumway-Cook A. Effects of vestibular rehabilitation on dizziness and imbalance. *Otolaryngol Head Neck Surg.* 1992;106:175-180.

170. Szturm T, Ireland DJ, Lessing-Turner M. Comparison of different exercise programs in the rehabilitation of patients with chronic peripheral vestibular dysfunction. *J Vestib Res.* 1994;4: 461-479.

171. Shepard NT, Smith-Wheelock M, Telian S, Raj A. Vestibular and balance rehabilitation therapy. *Ann Otol Rhinol Laryngol.* 1993;102:198-205.

172. Herdman SJ. Advances in the treatment of vestibular disorders. *Phys Ther.* 1997;77:602.

173. Goebel J, Highstein S. Strategies for balance rehabiliation. *The Vestibularlabyrinth in Health and Disease.* 2001;942:394-412.

CHAPTER SEVEN

Impaired Motor Function and Sensory Integrity Associated With Acute or Chronic Polyneuropathies (Pattern G)

Laura Gilchrist, PT, PhD
Marilyn Woods, PT[†]

ANATOMY

The PNS includes all nervous system structures that lie outside of the cranium or vertebral column and includes the spinal and cranial nerves. The cell bodies for these neurons may lie in the periphery (ie, autonomic ganglia), in the spinal column (sensory neurons in dorsal root ganglia and motor neurons in the spinal cord), or in the brainstem (cranial nerves). Motor neurons within the PNS innervate both somatic muscles (through spinal and cranial nerves) and visceral structures (via autonomic ganglia and nerves). Sensory information from peripheral structures, such as the skin, joints, muscles, and visceral organs, also travels through peripheral nerves, and these neurons have cell bodies located in sensory ganglia/nuclei.

Peripheral axons are bundled together into nerves that may have purely sensory or motor axons, but many times have a mixture of axon types. The axons within the nerves have supporting cells, called glia, that protect axons and promote cellular function. In the PNS, Schwann cells serve as the glial support cells. Many Schwann cells in succession create a myelin sheath that wraps each axon. Some axons have only minimal coverage by the Schwann cell and are called unmyelinated axons. Others are wrapped by numerous layers of the Schwann cell membrane and are termed myelinated axons. On each axon a small gap in myelination occurs between successive Schwann cells. This gap is a small unmyelinated segment called the node of Ranvier. While these small nodes do not impede electrical conduction and in fact regenerate the electrical impulse, large segments of completely unprotected axon can prevent electrical conductance and inhibit neuron communication.

An example of the number of Schwann cells needed to assist a single neuron's function is described by Kandel and associates.[1] In the femoral nerve, sensory axons mediating the stretch reflex are 0.5 meter long. Each sensory axon in this example has approximately 500 internode segments (myelinated segments with nodes of Ranvier on each side). Since each Schwann cell wraps only one internode segment of an axon, approximately 500 Schwann cells are needed to insulate that single axon.

PHYSIOLOGY

The key to neuronal communication is each nerve cell's ability to undergo rapid changes in electrical potential and conduct those changes along an axon. The distribution of electrical charge via unequal distribution of charged ions across the neuron's membrane sets up an electrical potential. In healthy neurons the resting potential of the cell is approximately -65 mV.[1] Ion channels in the neural membrane can open and close, thus altering the resting membrane potential of the cell. When a channel opens, ions flow across the membrane according to their concentration and electrical gradients and lead to either cellular excitation (depolariza-

[†]Deceased.

tion) or inhibition (hyperpolarization). Ion channels are initially opened in neurons by activation of modality-gated or ligand-gated channels. Modality-gated channels are specific to sensory neurons and open in response to mechanical (touch, pressure), temperature, or chemical stimuli. Ligand-gated channels open when a neurotransmitter released from an adjacent neuron interacts with a neurotransmitter receptor on the target neuron. This is the mechanism for induction of electrical signals at interneuronal synapses (ie, excitation of an alpha motor neuron by a sensory neuron).

Once the signal has been initiated either by the modality- or ligand-gated channels, it spreads passively to the axon hillock, at which point an action potential is generated by the opening of voltage-gated channels if the cell membrane is sufficiently depolarized. The action potential is propagated along the axon by passive transmission along myelinated segments. At each node of Ranvier, the action potential is actively regenerated when voltage-gated channels clustered there open due to the passively propagated depolarization. When the action potential reaches the end of the axon or the synapse, the electrical signal is converted to a chemical signal. Electrical depolarization causes a release of a chemical neurotransmitter by the presynaptic neuron, which diffuses across the synaptic cleft to the postsynaptic neuron's membrane. This chemical neurotransmitter then interacts with ligand-gated ion channels in the post-synaptic cell to begin the signaling process over again. Thus, information is carried along the axon by electrical signaling and passed on to the next neuron in the circuit by chemical signaling.

Myelination of the axon is critical in the process of action potential propagation. Although some axons are termed unmyelinated (such as C-fiber nociceptors), they still are ensheathed but not tightly wrapped by Schwann cells.[2] Other axons, such as alpha motor neurons and axons from muscle and joint receptors, have multiple layers of myelin provided by Schwann cells. The myelin coating acts as insulation around an axon, which prevents the leakage of ions across the membrane that would decrease the amplitude of the action potential. The greater the myelin coating around the axon, the fewer times the action potential needs to be regenerated, and the faster the action potential travels along the axon. When axons lack a tight myelin coating, as is seen in unmyelinated axons, the action potential needs to be regenerated at all points along the axon for the signal to be propagated, thus decreasing the speed of transmission. For a more detailed description of action potential propagation and electrochemical signaling in neurons, refer to Kandel, Schwartz, and Jessell's *Principles of Neural Science*.[1]

PATHOPHYSIOLOGY

Peripheral polyneuropathies occur when neurons or their myelin sheath are disturbed by metabolic, infectious, toxic, or autoimmune disorders.[3,4] In contrast to injuries of a single nerve bundle (mononeuropathies) that frequently occur due to compression or traumatic injury, peripheral polyneuropathies occur in multiple nerve bundles simultaneously and often have a symmetric presentation. Damage to the myelin sheath alone may be rapidly reversed as remyelination by Schwann cells occurs.[5] Damage to a peripheral axon is repaired through regeneration or sprouting from the intact cell body and axon, yet may take months; recovery may be incomplete.[1] If the cell body of the peripheral neuron is irreparably damaged, cellular regeneration will not occur.[6] Some common causes of peripheral polyneuropathy include diabetes mellitus, alcoholic neuropathy, chemotherapy-induced peripheral neuropathy (CIPN), post-polio syndrome, reflex sympathetic dystrophy (RSD, known now as complex regional pain syndrome [CRPS]), and Guillain-Barré syndrome (GBS). The reader is referred to *Musculoskeletal Essentials: Applying the Preferred Physical Therapist Practice Patterns*[SM7] (Chapter Three, Impaired Muscle Performance [Pattern C] for description and case study of diabetes mellitus and Chapter Four, Impaired Joint Mobility, Motor Function, Muscle Performance, and Range of Motion Associated With Connective Tissue Dysfunction [Pattern D] for description and case study of CRPS [or RSD]). To illustrate the assessment of and intervention for peripheral polyneuropathies, two cases involving GBS and CIPN will be discussed.

GUILLIAN-BARRÉ SYNDROME

GBS is an acute polyneuropathy considered to be an autoimmune disease triggered by a preceding viral or bacterial infection.[8] Now that polio infections have been dramatically reduced by vaccination, GBS is the most common cause of acute flaccid paralysis in developed countries.[9,10] Estimates of the incidence of GBS range from 0.4 to 4.0 cases per 100,000, with a median of 1.3 cases.[10,11] These estimates have been completed in geographically diverse regions of the world with little variation, indicating no geographical clustering of incidence.

GBS is reported to have a heterogeneous clinical presentation and a wide range of severity.[12] Clinical subtypes of GBS have been identified with differing pathogenesis that may account for this variable clinical picture.[8,13] The most common form of GBS in Western countries is acute inflammatory demyelinating polyneuropathy (AIDP).[14] AIDP is thought to be an autoimmune-related disorder, where the Schwann cell is attacked by the immune system resulting in demyelination of peripheral axons. Most commonly, both motor and sensory functions are involved. Acute motor axonal neuropathy (AMAN) is a subtype of GBS most common in China and Japan, although some cases have been identified in Europe and North America.[8] Pathophysiological and electrodiagnostic studies have demonstrated that AMAN is an autoimmune attack on motor neurons, with axonal degeneration as the prominent feature.[15] GBS subtypes of lesser frequency, acute motor and sensory axonal neuropathy (AMSAN) and Miller-Fisher syndrome (a triad of ophthalmoplegia, ataxia, and areflexia), have also been reported in the clinical literature.[15,16]

Two thirds of patients with GBS have an antecedent viral or bacterial infection, most commonly of the upper respiratory or gastrointestinal tracts. Some common infectious agents include *Campylobacter jejuni*, Epstein-Barr virus, and cytomegalovirus.[13,17,18] In the demyelinating form of GBS, induction of antiganglioside antibodies from the primary infection is thought to initiate neuronal damage.[8,13] The antibodies originally developed against the invading infection are thought to bind to the surface of myelin, leading to an inflammatory response. Macrophages infiltrate the layers of myelin and eventually ingest and digest the myelin layers.[19] Demyelination of the axon can lead to slowing of action potential propagation and, if extensive, can lead to the failure of the action potential to conduct all together.[20] Initial signs of demyelination include weakness and/or sensory abnormalities with slowed conduction on NCV testing. When the Schwann cells divide and repair the myelin sheath, the number of nodes increases as compared to pre-insult, and thus a slowed conduction velocity will remain.[21]

Axonal damage may occur secondary to demyelination, but in the case of AMAN it is thought that axonal damage occurs in the absence of demyelination. Simple conduction blocks may occur within intact axons that may lead to rapid patient recovery, or immune complexes may target the axon membrane itself causing axon degeneration and long-term dysfunction. In AMAN, electrodiagnostic testing often reveals no slowing of conduction velocities, but instead decreased compound muscle action potentials indicating conduction block or axon degeneration.[14,22] Degenerated axons in the PNS may be repaired by sprouting and regrowth, but this recovery is often incomplete.[1] The reader is referred to Chapter Three, Impaired Muscle Performance (Pattern C) in *Musculoskeletal Essentials: Applying the Preferred Physical Therapist Practice Patterns*[SM7] for the anatomy, physiology, and pathophysiology of muscle and the motor unit.

Clinical manifestations include an ascending progressive paralysis, areflexia, and distal sensory impairments. Presentation is often an acute fulminate progression, where in extreme cases a person may go from experiencing minor numbness or tingling in the feet or hands to being bedridden with flaccid paralysis in a period of 2 to 3 days.[23] In severe cases, external respiratory support is needed and approximately 10% of patients succumb to this illness.[24] As the disease progresses over the first few days, patients typically develop symmetrical weakness in the LEs, that may progress into the UEs and face, and have decreased or absent deep tendon reflexes. Although paresthesias are a common feature, clinical sensory testing is often intact. Pain and fatigue are also common components that may persist. Disturbances of autonomic function include hyper- and hypotension, tachy- and bradycardia, and diaphoresis. The progression generally lasts for 10 to 12 days before it plateaus, and the disease often resolves within 12 weeks.[25]

CHEMOTHERAPY-INDUCED PERIPHERAL NEUROPATHY

CIPN is a disorder of the PNS incurred by patients who have received chemotherapeutic agents known to be neurotoxic. Treatment for cancer is designed to suppress cell growth and to eliminate the malignancy, and as such, has the potential to damage or interfere with function in essential organ systems. While multiple systems, including the cardiac, pulmonary, and renal systems, may be impacted by chemotherapeutic agents, peripheral nerves are especially susceptible to the toxic effects of chemotherapy.

The mechanism of cell damage is believed to be a result of the interaction of the chemical with the metabolic structures in the neuron. For example, Flatters and Bennett[26] demonstrated mitochondrial dysfunction in peripheral nerves induced by paclitaxel, a common chemotherapeutic agent for breast, ovarian, and non-small cell lung carcinomas. Vincristine, another commonly used agent, has been shown to cause impairments in retrograde and anterograde axonal transport in myelinated axons resulting in axonal swelling.[27] Without metabolic support for the axons, the nerve fibers degenerate, resulting in neuropathy.

Most often, these neuropathic changes occur in the distal portions of the PNS first, such as in the nerves to the feet and hands. Often there is a delay between the onset of the chemotherapy and the onset of symptoms. Indeed there is a dose-dependent relationship between neuropathy and chemotherapeutic agent use, so that development of neuropathy may require reaching a specific cumulative threshold.[28] The incidence of CIPN appears to be greater in patients who have previous conditions that predispose them to neurologic disease, such as diabetes and alcoholism.[28]

Specific chemotherapeutic agents are associated with peripheral neuropathy. Table 7-1 describes the commonly used drugs that are associated with neuropathy, in addition to the specific symptoms noted with each class of agents. Incidence of clinically detected neuropathy varies from 4% to 74% of patients,[29-36] but few long-term follow-up studies exist that investigate the incidence and potential resolution of these symptoms.

IMAGING

CHEMOTHERAPY-INDUCED PERIPHERAL NEUROPATHY

Imaging of the brain and spinal cord for patients with CIPN may be obtained to ensure that neurologic changes are not a result of tumor infiltration into the CNS or PNS.

Table 7-1

CHEMOTHERAPEUTIC AGENTS AND ASSOCIATED NEUROPATHY AND SYMPTOMS

Agent	Sensory Symptoms	Motor Symptoms	Other Effects

Taxanes
  Paclitaxel[26]
  Docetaxel
	Mild to moderate numbness and tingling
	Burning/stabbing pain
		Weakness of distal muscles	Neutropenia, anemia, myalgia/arthralgia, nausea, alopecia

Vinca alkaloids
  Vincristine[33]
  Vinorelbine
	Mild to moderate numbness and tingling
	Burning/stabbing pain
		Weakness of distal muscles, decreased deep tendon reflexes, foot drop	Granulocytopenia, leukocytopenia, anemia, fatigue, nausea, alopecia

Platinum compounds
  Carboplatin[34]
  Oxaliplatin[35]
  Cisplatin[36]
	Mild to moderate numbness and tingling	Weakness is rare	Ototoxicity, vestibular toxicity, anemia, neutropenia, leukocytopenia, thrombocytopenia, nausea

OTHER CLINICAL TESTS

GUILLAIN-BARRÉ SYNDROME

Electromyography

The most sensitive and specific findings in GBS are found via serial electrodiagnostic testing. Specific criteria for the demyelinating forms of GBS have been published.[37] According to the proposed criteria, three of the four following conditions need to be met:

1. Reduction in NCV in two or more nerves

2. Conduction block or abnormal temporal dispersion in one or more motor nerves

3. Prolonged distal latencies in two or more nerves

4. Absent or prolonged F-waves in two or more motor nerves[37]

Gordon and Wilbourn[38] published results of a retrospective analysis of electrodiagnostic studies of patients with GBS. They found that an absent H reflex was the most sensitive electrodiagnostic measure of early GBS. If the lesion impacts the axon itself, other electrodiagnostic findings can be present, such as fibrillation potentials and/or positive sharp waves in EMG recordings from paralyzed muscles.[39] In the demyelinating forms of the syndrome, definitive diagnosis by electrodiagnostic studies is possible in approximately half of patients, but not until the fifth day after onset.[38]

Cerebrospinal Fluid

CSF is also assessed in potential cases of GBS. Results consistent with the diagnosis of GBS include normal pressure, few to no cells, and an elevated concentration of protein.[40]

PHARMACOLOGY

GUILLAIN-BARRÉ SYNDROME

Medical interventions for GBS have improved with the introduction of plasma exchange (PE) and IVIg that attempt to decrease the immune attack on the nervous system. Both PE and IVIg have been shown to be superior to supportive care alone in terms of time to return to independent ambulation.[41-43] While PE is provided mainly at large hospitals, IVIg therapy can be used in most hospitals where an intensive care unit (ICU) is available and thus, there has been a shift in the hospital types treating patients with GBS.[44] Whichever treatment is chosen, earlier initiation improves outcomes.[43,45]

Corticosteroid therapy alone has been found to be ineffective in preventing disability in patients with GBS and is no longer recommended as a lone medical therapy in these cases.[46] Some physicians still use methylprednisone as an adjunct therapy to other interventions due to potential positive synergistic effects.[12] Despite the advances, GBS can still be a severe disease with resultant disability. Other pharmacologic and medical therapies continue to be investigated including interferon, cyclooxygenase-2 inhibitors, and CSF filtration.[12]

Because pain can be a feature of GBS, a variety of medications may be used. Gabapentin is a drug that decreases the abnormal excitement of the brain and is utilized to relieve pain, especially burning, stabbing pain. Side effects of the drug may include drowsiness, headache, nausea, constipation, back or joint pain, rash, and itching. Fentanyl is one of the opioid narcotic drugs that acts on the CNS to relieve pain. Side effects of the drug may include dizziness, light-headedness, and anxiety.

Patients will likely also be taking other medications to treat co-morbid conditions or treatment-related side effects, such as headache or constipation.

CHEMOTHERAPY-INDUCED PERIPHERAL NEUROPATHY

Because peripheral neuropathy is a dose-limiting side effect of chemotherapeutic agents, recent research has focused on neuroprotective medications. A variety of substances continue to be investigated for their ability to protect the nervous system from oxidative stress during use of the chemotherapeutic agents. Substances in clinical trials include vitamin E, glutamine, glutathione, amofostine, and neurotrophic factors.[47]

Patients experiencing neuropathic pain symptoms may also be treated with tricyclic antidepressants, anticonvulsants (such as gabapentin), and opioid medications.[48] The following pharmacological agents for use with these patients are detailed below.

- Cyclobenzaprine
  - Actions: Muscle relaxant and pain relief
  - Administered: By mouth
  - Side effects: Drowsiness, dizziness, dry mouth, upset stomach
- Gabapentin
  - Actions: Pain relief of neuralgia by altering patient perception of pain
  - Administered: By mouth
  - Side effects: Drowsiness, dizziness, headache, tiredness, blurred or double vision, unsteadiness, anxiety, nausea, diarrhea, weight gain
- Oxycodone
  - Action: Relief of moderate to moderate-to-severe pain
  - Administered: By mouth
  - Side effects: Upset stomach, constipation, dry mouth, rapid heart beat, rash

Patients will likely be taking other medications for co-morbid conditions.

Case Study #1: Guillain-Barré Syndrome

Mr. Thomas Stone is a 57-year-old male with Guillain-Barré syndrome and acute inflammatory demyelinating polyneuropathy who has just entered a subacute rehabilitation facility.

PHYSICAL THERAPIST EXAMINATION

HISTORY

- General demographics: Mr. Stone is a 57-year-old white male whose primary language is English. He is right handed. He is a college graduate.
- Social history: Mr. Stone is married and the father of two grown daughters ages 30 and 34. His daughters live nearby.
- Employment/work: Mr. Stone works in the banking industry.
- Living environment: He lives in a one-level ranch-style home with his wife. His home has three steps with a hand rail to enter in the front and one step with no hand rail from the garage to the kitchen. There is one flight of stairs with a hand rail to the family room in the basement.
- General health status
  - General health perception: His health had been generally good, but he is anxious about what is happening to him now.
  - Physical function: Normal for age.
  - Psychological function: No reported issues.
  - Role function: Husband, father, grandfather, banker, volunteer.
  - Social function: He attends church, likes to play recreational golf, and is an active member of several community organizations.
- Social/health habits: He is a nonsmoker and occasionally drinks alcohol.
- Family history: His parents are deceased. His mother died of a myocardial infarction, and his father from natural causes.
- Medical/surgical history: He reports no significant medical or surgical issues in the past.
- Prior hospitalizations: None.
- Preexisting medical and other health-related conditions: No significant conditions.
- Current condition(s)/chief complaint(s): Mr. Stone reports that he was healthy until 11 days ago, when he began to have some minor numbness and tingling in his feet. This rapidly got worse with numbness and

tingling moving up his legs and beginning in his hands. He also started to have weakness in the legs, feet, and hands. He reports extreme fatigue. He was unable to walk without help, had difficulty with self-care, and was unable to work. Mr. Stone was hospitalized 10 days ago with initial progression of weakness and fatigue that has plateaued. Over the course of the hospitalization, he was given five rounds of therapeutic plasmaphoresis (a type of blood cleansing in which damaging antibodies are filtered from the blood, blood cells are then returned to the patient's body to maintain hematologic function, and the patient's body also produces plasma to restore the fluid that is removed).

♦ Functional status and activity level: He has been unable to independently ambulate due to weakness, and he reports mild back and bilateral foot pain. Mr. Stone is unable to perform his normal ADL or IADL.

♦ Medications
  • Preadmission: Tylenol for pain.
  • Current and hospital admission
    ▪ Prednisone (40 mg/day for the first week and will continue to be tapered over 4 weeks).
    ▪ High doses IVIg, now complete.
    ▪ For bowel and esophageal function: Colace 100 bid, Senokot two to four tablets by mouth bid, and Protonix 40 mg qd.
    ▪ For pain management: Gabapentin, Tylenol, and fentanyl as needed.
    ▪ Patient allergic to sulfa drugs.

♦ Other clinical tests
  • Lumbar puncture failed to disclose evidence of any infectious process. Oligoclonal bands on the CSF were negative, as were all bands on CSF studies. Elevated protein in CSF was reported with normal cells.
  • EMG was performed disclosing evidence of neurologic changes, specifically reduced muscle unit potentials and decreased recruitment in multiple muscles of the distal LEs and UEs.

SYSTEMS REVIEW

♦ Cardiovascular/pulmonary
  • BP: 138/69 mmHg
  • Edema: None observed
  • HR: 80 bpm
  • RR: 18 bpm

♦ Integumentary
  • Presence of scar formation: None
  • Skin color: Normal
  • Skin integrity: Intact

♦ Musculoskeletal
  • Gross range of motion: WFL passively; moderate limitations with active movement
  • Gross strength: Decreased in bilateral UEs and LEs, greater loss distally than proximally
  • Gross symmetry: No asymmetry noted
  • Height: 5'10" (1.78 m)
  • Weight: 168 lbs (76.2 kg)

♦ Neuromuscular
  • Balance: Impaired sitting and standing balance observed
  • Locomotion, transfers, and transitions: Requires assistance with all transitions, unable to ambulate without assistance
  • Dysaesthesia reported in distal portions of hands and legs

♦ Communication, affect, cognition, language, and learning style
  • Communication, affect, cognition: WFL
  • Learning style: Visual learner

TESTS AND MEASURES

♦ Aerobic capacity/endurance
  • Endurance not formally assessed at this time, see functional activities for endurance limitations during activity
  • 5.2/7.0 in Fatigue Severity Scale,[49] representing severe fatigue

♦ Anthropometric characteristics
  • BMI=705 x (body weight [in pounds] divided by height^2 [in inches])
  • Mr. Stone's BMI=24.17, which is WNL[50]

♦ Arousal, attention, and cognition
  • Oriented x3 but lethargic
  • Follows two-step verbal commands
  • Is cooperative and motivated

♦ Assistive and adaptive devices
  • None currently used
  • Will need assistive device for ambulation
  • Will need assistive and adaptive devices for ADL

♦ Cranial and peripheral nerve integrity
  • Decreased temperature sensation at ankle and wrist bilaterally
  • Light touch sensation mildly impaired at both feet, ankles, lower legs, and hands
  • Previous EMG testing indicated reduced muscle unit potentials and decreased recruitment in multiple muscles in the distal LEs and UEs

♦ Environmental, home, and work barriers
  • Home has three steps with hand rail to enter front entrance and one step without hand rail in the back entrance, full flight with hand rail to basement area
  • Floors are mostly carpeted

- Owns large sport utility vehicle
- Patient reports he thinks work area is accessible with wide power doors and elevator

♦ Gait, locomotion, and balance
- Sitting balance: Required minimal assist of one to maintain balance without back or UE support
- Patient fatigues as evidenced by increased left lean with >5 minutes of sitting, appears unaware of lean to left and has difficulty correcting lean
- Transfers/transitions
  - Sit to/from supine: Minimal assistance of one for LE assistance
  - Sit to/from stand: Moderate assistance of one for LE stabilization and balance
  - Bed to/from wheelchair: Moderate assistance of one for LE stabilization and balance
- Standing balance
  - Moderate assistance of one to maintain static balance
  - Assist at knees required to prevent buckling
- Unable to ambulate due to poor balance and weakness

♦ Integumentary integrity
- No evidence of points of increased pressure at sacrum, heels, scapulae, elbows, or occiput

♦ Motor function
- Unable to perform grasp with either hand
- Fine motor skills of UE severely limited due to weakness
- Coordination limited in LEs movements due to weakness
- Coordination limited in UEs due to weakness

♦ Muscle performance
- MMT revealed the following deviations from normal
  - Shoulder flexion=3/5 bilateral
  - Shoulder abduction=3/5 bilateral
  - Elbow flexion=3-/5 bilateral
  - Elbow extension=3-/5 bilateral
  - Wrist flexion=2/5 bilateral
  - Wrist extension=2/5 bilateral
  - Finger flexion=1/5 bilateral
  - Finger extension=1/5 bilateral
  - Hip flexion=3-/5 bilateral
  - Hip extension=3-/5 bilateral
  - Knee flexion=3/5 bilateral
  - Knee extension=3/5 bilateral
  - Ankle dorsiflexion=1/5 bilateral
  - Ankle plantarflexion=1/5 bilateral
  - Eversion=0/5 bilateral
  - Inversion=0/5 bilateral

- Trunk flexion=3/5
- Trunk extension=3/5

♦ Orthotic, protective, and supportive devices
- Needs to be monitored for potential resting splints or orthotics for hands and feet
- Needs to be monitored for abdominal binder and supportive stockings

♦ Pain
- Initially, 3-4/10 at rest in the low back and posterior thighs on the NPS where 0=no pain and 10=worst possible pain[51]
- 1-2/10 since initiating gabapentin therapy
- Eases with repositioning and stretching of LEs

♦ Posture
- Unable to stand independently
- When sitting unsupported leans to the left

♦ Range of motion
- PROM: WFL throughout bilateral UEs and LEs
- Mild tightness in hamstrings bilaterally

♦ Reflex integrity
- Deep tendon reflexes
  - Absent at the ankle bilaterally
  - Diminished (1+/4) at the patellar tendon bilaterally
  - Intact at biceps and triceps bilaterally
- Babinski reflex: Toes down going bilaterally indicated normal response

♦ Self-care and home management
- Observed unable to brush teeth and comb hair
- All other self-care required assistance

♦ Sensory integrity
- Absent vibratory sensation hand and wrist bilaterally
- Decreased joint position sense at great toe and ankle bilaterally

♦ Ventilation and respiration/gas exchange
- Cough assessment: Weak cough production
- Oxygen saturation: 98% at rest, 97% in sitting
- Chest wall excursion
  - Patient has symmetrical excursion
  - He has decreased chest wall expansion during deep inhalation
- Lung sounds: All lung fields were clear to auscultation

♦ Work, community, and leisure integration or reintegration
- Unable to do any work activities and is on medical leave
- Needs to be able to drive to work, walk from parking area, and maneuver through building to office on fifth floor
- Job includes: Sitting at a desk for extended periods

working at a computer terminal, retrieving files, dealing with customers in person and on the phone, interacting with staff, frequent evening meetings, and work hours vary from 8 to 12 hours per day

EVALUATION

Mr. Stone was an active, right-handed male prior to onset of the current episode of care. He was hospitalized 10 days ago with symptoms of numbness, sensory loss, and weakness bilaterally in hands and feet that resulted in a medical diagnosis of GBS. Upon admission to a subacute rehabilitation facility, he is totally dependent for all self-care activities and is unable to ambulate due to weakness. He is breathing on his own, but he has difficulty with cough production. He is unable to work and is on medical leave. He has decreased strength and endurance, cutaneous sensation, proprioception, and balance affecting the LEs greater than the UEs and distal more than proximal. He is unable to sit or stand without assistance, unable to ambulate independently, and requires assistance with all bed mobility, transfers, and self-care. Mr. Stone also presents a safety risk due to his increased risk of falls. If early mobility is not initiated, he will be additionally at risk for skin breakdown and other complications due to inactivity and impaired sensation. He is unable to manage independently or participate in his previous roles in church and community.

DIAGNOSIS

Mr. Stone has GBS, AIDP type with pain. He has impaired: aerobic capacity/endurance; cranial and peripheral nerve integrity; gait, locomotion, and balance; motor function; muscle performance; posture; reflex integrity; sensory integrity; and ventilation and respiration/gas exchange. He is functionally limited in self-care and home management and in work, community, and leisure actions, tasks, and activities. He has environmental, home, and work barriers. He will need assistive, adaptive, orthotic, protective, and supportive devices and equipment. These findings are consistent with placement in Pattern G: Impaired Motor Function and Sensory Integrity Associated With Acute or Chronic Polyneuropathies. The identified impairments, functional limitations, barriers, and device and equipment needs will be addressed in determining the prognosis and the plan of care.

PROGNOSIS AND PLAN OF CARE

Over the course of the visits, the following mutually established outcomes have been determined:
♦ Balance is improved
♦ Cough is improved
♦ Endurance is improved

♦ Functional independence in ADL and IADL is increased
♦ Gait, locomotion, and balance are improved
♦ Independent ambulation and stair climbing with appropriate assistive device are achieved
♦ Motor function is increased
♦ Muscle performance is increased
♦ Pain is decreased or eliminated
♦ Performance levels in self-care are improved
♦ Physical capacity is improved
♦ Physical function is improved
♦ Postural control is improved
♦ Relevant community resources to meet his discharge needs are identified
♦ Risk factors are reduced
♦ Weightbearing status is improved
♦ Work, community, and leisure activities are resumed

To achieve these outcomes, the appropriate interventions for this patient are determined. These will include: coordination, communication, and documentation; patient/client-related instruction; therapeutic exercise; functional training in self-care and home management; functional training in work, community, and leisure integration or reintegration; prescription, application, and, as appropriate, fabrication of devices and equipment; airway clearance techniques; and electrotherapeutic modalities.

Based on the diagnosis and prognosis, Mr. Stone is expected to require 20 to 24 visits over the next 3 to 6 months. Mr. Stone is expected to regain functional independence through his subacute rehabilitation facility and will return home with transition to home care and outpatient physical therapy. The above outcomes cover his entire episode of care that includes all of these settings.

Many factors may influence the frequency and duration of physical therapy intervention including the patient's level of initial impairment,[52] the patient's response to exercise therapy, recurrence of symptoms, and adherence to the intervention plan. Mr. Stone is very motivated and his prognosis for rehabilitation is good to excellent.

INTERVENTIONS

RATIONALE FOR SELECTED INTERVENTIONS

Research on patients with GBS indicates improvement after rehabilitation,[53-55] although long-term disability has been noted in some cases.[56] Common residual impairments have been found to be fatigue, decreased strength, and mild sensory loss.[57-59]

Therapeutic Exercise

Following GBS, patients consistently demonstrate decreased strength in the UEs and LEs distally greater than proximally[53,58,60,61] and decreased cardiorespiratory fitness.[61] Fatigue is an additional impairment thought to be related to decreased strength and endurance.[61] While aerobic and strength training are the preferred methods to increase strength and endurance, there is some concern that exercise therapy may inhibit recovery of injured neurons.[62] One animal study revealed that intensive exercise performed during the early stages of reinnervation may inhibit nerve sprouting,[63] yet other studies have shown either no effect[64,65] or a beneficial effect on functional recovery when exercise is performed during reinnervation.[66,67] Thus, judicious use of exercise therapy while monitoring the patient's response for adverse effects appears to be supported in the early stages of recovery for this patient. Even in the initial, acute phases of GBS, PROM exercise should be initiated to maintain muscle length and joint health. Once neurological status has stabilized, exercise therapy can be initiated with close monitoring for increasing fatigue or worsening symptoms.

Exercise therapy is also indicated in later stages of recovery from GBS, as the residual effects on strength and endurance may be long lasting. A small-scale exercise trial has been completed in the chronic phase of GBS recovery. A bike ergometry program of 12 weeks in length demonstrated significant improvements in cardiorespiratory function, isokinetic strength, and fatigue,[61] with few minor and transient side effects that did not require cessation of the training program. These results support a previous case report of a patient recovering from severe GBS who improved muscular strength and endurance with a bike ergometry program.[68] Importantly, in the bike ergometry trial, Garssen and associates[61] also demonstrated functional improvement in patients with GBS on the 36-Item Short Form Health Survey (SF-36) physical performance subscale, although they remained below the levels reported for healthy individuals.

Focus on compensatory strategies (use of adaptive and assistive devices) should be done in conjunction with supporting restorative functional reinnervention and preservation of central neural circuits. An example of supported functional retraining is the use of body-weight supported gait training as described by Tuckey and Greenwood.[69] Such training could theoretically support functional reinnervation and retention of central neural mechanisms for gait, while preventing overfatigue for the impacted nerves and muscles. A patient's functional mobility should also be supported during the recovery stage with the use of assistive/adaptive devices, such as a power wheelchair.

Functional Training in Self-Care and Home Management

Training in various conditions related to the patient's functional goals and discharge needs should be stressed. Pacing of activities must be considered due to the increased fatigability of the affected muscles. As functional innervation is recovered, decreased use of adaptive and assistive equipment should be stressed to allow for full recovery by challenging the nervous system.

Functional Training in Work, Community, and Leisure Integration or Reintegration

Reintegration into work, community, and leisure activities should occur in a phased in manner, increasing patient participation and motivation, yet preventing overfatigue. Due to the long-term effects of GBS, education and development of a health, wellness, and fitness plan is critical.[54-57] The patient needs to identify preferred activities and community resources as part of this plan.

Prescription, Application, and, as Appropriate, Fabrication of Devices and Equipment

Given decreased strength, sensation, endurance, and loss or impaired balance, gait, and aerobic capacity, patients with GBS may require assistive, adaptive, orthotic, protective, or supportive devices and equipment throughout the course of recovery. It is important to improve mobility prior to the return of motor and sensory function. Therefore, for longer distances, wheelchair (power) use may be necessary in the short term to allow for energy conservation and accessing home and preferred community settings.

Airway Clearance Techniques

Given the loss of functional muscle strength in the LEs and UEs, musculature of the trunk is also likely to be involved and dynamic lung volumes are likely decreased. Decreased trunk muscle strength has been linked to increased risk of respiratory compromise.[70] Use of mechanical ventilation during hospitalization would further the risk for pulmonary infection and compromise. As many as 25% of patients requiring mechanical ventilation will develop pneumonia.[40] In patients not on mechanical ventilation, coughing should be assessed for adequate airway clearance capability. Positioning and breathing exercises should be initiated to improve cough effectiveness and assist in preventing further complications from occurring. Supportive devices, such as an abdominal binder, may also be necessary during the early stages.

Electrotherapeutic Modalities

Pain can be a major finding related to GBS.[71] Advances in pain management via use of pharmacologic agents have been well described.[8,72,73] Physical therapists need to be aware of both the neuropathic features associated with GBS and also the possibility of generalized pain from muscle tightness related to inactivity. This pain is amenable to other modalities, such as stretching and possibly electrotherapy. In one case report, a patient with GBS was reported to benefit from the adjunct use of transcutaneous electrical nerve stimulation (TENS) for pain management.[74]

COORDINATION, COMMUNICATION, AND DOCUMENTATION

Communication will occur with Mr. Stone, his family members, and all members of the multidisciplinary rehabilitation team. Interdisciplinary teamwork will be demonstrated in patient-family conferences and patient care rounds. The family will be provided with information on transitioning from subacute care to home care and outpatient services. Information on community resources will also be provided to the patient and his family. All elements of the patient's management will be documented.

PATIENT/CLIENT-RELATED INSTRUCTION

The patient and family will be educated and instructed in the current condition and its sequelae and reasons for his current impairments, functional limitations, disabilities, and risk factors. He will be instructed in the need to reposition his body throughout the day to prevent skin breakdown. He will also be provided instruction about safety issues, such as checking temperatures on intact areas of skin and checking shoes and skin for possible skin irritation.

The patient and his family will also be provided with information regarding community resources for additional support. Mr. Stone and his family will be consulted in creating the plan of care. They will be taught techniques to enhance his independent function and activities.

THERAPEUTIC EXERCISE

- ◆ Aerobic capacity/endurance conditioning
  - Initiated in the later stages to improve cardiovascular/pulmonary function
  - Mode
    - Cycle ergometry is added once tolerated by patient, starting with interval training
      - ‣ Sitting arm ergometry
      - ‣ Sitting leg ergometry
      - ‣ Cycle ergometry
  - Intensity: 60% MHR
  - Duration: Working up to 20 to 25 minutes continuous exercise
  - Frequency: Three to four times per week
- ◆ Balance, coordination, and agility training
  - Static balance exercises sitting
    - Training will begin in sitting supported due to his balance and LE strength deficits
    - Work on maintaining trunk stability during static

sitting increasing endurance as able
  - Sitting on firm and then compliant surfaces with and without UE support will be added as patient tolerance allows
  - Dynamic balance exercises
    - Head turns
    - Weight shifting in all planes
    - Rhythmic stabilization to the trunk
    - Reaching activities out of base of support
  - Static standing balance
    - Start in parallel bars for safety using transfer belt
    - Work on maintaining upright posture and extended hips and knees
    - Work on increasing standing time and decreasing rest time
    - Progress to standing with assistive devices and standing to perform functional activities including self-care
    - Dynamic standing balance exercises with and without UE support
    - Head turns
    - Weight shifting in all planes
    - Rhythmic stabilization
    - Reaching activities
    - Stepping activities
    - Progress to assistive devices
    - Practice during functional tasks, such as transfers and self-care activities
- ◆ Flexibility exercises
  - All motions should occur in pain-free range
  - Begin with PROM progressing to AAROM
  - Stretching
    - Initially stretching exercises will be performed on the patient, and stretching should be done using a slow and steady stretch, holding at end range for 30 to 60 seconds
    - As patient is able to participate in stretches, they should be done after warming up or following functional activities or therapy session if fatigue is an issue
      - ‣ Ankle dorsiflexors, knee extensors, hamstrings, and hip flexors in the LEs should be monitored and stretched as appropriate
  - Positioning for muscle lengthening
    - Positioning schedule should be developed to include prone, supine, side-lying, and sitting with follow-up with staff and family as appropriate
    - Resting splints may be used for prolonged stretch to the ankle plantarflexors
    - Supportive standing, as with a tilt table, may also be used for prolonged stretching in a weightbearing position

- Gait and locomotion training
  - Instruction and training in proper and safe use of a manual or power wheelchair for use in the early stages in the hospital, subacute nursing facility, and home and for later stages for energy conservation in work or community settings if needed
  - Gait training should begin with standing balance tasks, as described above, incorporating weight shifting
  - Both forward and backward steps should be taught to allow safe stand to sit transition
  - BWSTT will be utilized early in the rehabilitation process in conjunction with the above methods
  - Instruction in proper use and sequencing of assistive devices with ambulation should begin when the patient is ready to progress outside of the parallel bars
- Strength and endurance training
  - Initially, endurance training can be accomplished by decreasing the rest time during functional training and strength training
    - Begin by increasing time sitting up in bed, progressing to chair with arms
    - While sitting in chair begin activities that require use of one or both arms
    - Complete functional tasks and self-care activities while sitting
    - Progress to standing activities
    - Decrease amount of time doing activity while decreasing amount of rest between activities
  - The initiation of a more formalized strength and endurance exercise program will be added as Mr. Stone's symptoms and functional independence stabilize
    - Begin strengthening with use of body weight performing AAROM progressing to AROM, focusing on proximal muscle groups, such as the shoulder girdle and hip, as well as the trunk, to promote stability
    - Begin in planes that eliminate or reduce gravity, progress to movement against gravity as strength increases
    - Use of resistance should begin gradually using manual resistance, low weights, or elastic bands
    - Critical to monitor level of fatigue during and after exercise periods and determine rate of recovery following exercise periods
    - Need to recognize the amount of exercise and energy consumed through completion of daily routine
    - Use of variable-resistance machines with low weights may be beneficial to help retrain the

motor pathways, as well as strengthen the muscles
  - Tai Chi or yoga should be considered as a part of Mr. Stone's long-term health, wellness, and fitness program

FUNCTIONAL TRAINING IN SELF-CARE AND HOME MANAGEMENT

- Self-care and home management
  - Many of the therapeutic exercises described in the previous section will help support ADL training (ie, seated and standing reaching exercises will help with grooming/hygiene tasks)
  - A home evaluation would be ideal in order to provide the most task-specific assessment of readiness of the patient and family to manage at home
  - Support through compensated functional mobility through use of a wheelchair during his recovery phase
  - Pacing of activities will be considered due to the increased fatigability of the affected muscles
  - As functional innervation is recovered, decreased use of adaptive and assistive equipment for self-care and home management will be stressed
- Injury prevention or reduction
  - Mr. Stone and his family will be instructed, with opportunities for return demonstration, in safe techniques to assist with ambulation and transfers during functional recovery
  - A task-specific environment in the therapeutic setting will be created that mirrors the patient's home as it pertains to ambulation surfaces, stairs, and bathroom situations to prevent/reduce the likelihood of injury upon return home
- Development of a plan for energy management that provides for energy conservation so Mr. Stone is able to complete daily routine
  - Identify high and low energy activities
  - Identify times of day where energy is high and low
  - Identify rest times
  - Identify daily routine for home noting high and low energy activities
  - Develop plan for activities and rest for a typical week

FUNCTIONAL TRAINING IN WORK, COMMUNITY, AND LEISURE INTEGRATION OR REINTEGRATION

- Devices and equipment use and training
  - Initial use of a power wheelchair or scooter in preferred community settings based on the requirements

of the activity and his level of energy

- As his strength increases, his fatigue lessens, and his energy level increases, may progress to a manual wheelchair
- Refer for a driving evaluation to determine need for adaptations for his car

♦ IADL training

- Reintegration into his work activities will occur in a phased manner, increasing his participation and motivation, yet preventing overfatigue
- Refer for a driving evaluation to determine safety and potential supportive needs for driving
- A visit with the physical therapist will be made to his work site to evaluate job requirements and potential environmental barriers

♦ Injury prevention or reduction

- Instructions in how to safely progress his work, community, and leisure activities to prevent injury

♦ Development of a plan for energy management that provides for energy conservation so Mr. Stone is able to complete work and community activities (see Functional Training in Self-Care and Home Management)

- Identify daily routine for work noting high- and low-energy activities

♦ Leisure and play

- Reintegration into community and leisure activities will occur in a phased manner, increasing his participation and motivation, while preventing overfatigue

PRESCRIPTION, APPLICATION, AND, AS APPROPRIATE, FABRICATION OF DEVICES AND EQUIPMENT

♦ Assistive devices

- A walker or cane may be used until strength and endurance improve, working toward independent ambulation
- A walker or cane used for mobility will enhance his performance and independence in home and community and will increase mobility and stability and reduce risk of falls
- Instructions given in the use and care of the device

♦ Protective devices

- Pressure-relieving devices for bed and for wheelchair to prevent skin breakdown

♦ Supportive devices

- May benefit from an abdominal binder for support to aid in breathing and coughing and general trunk support

AIRWAY CLEARANCE TECHNIQUES

♦ Breathing strategies

- Breathing exercises to improve cough effectiveness and to assist in preventing further complications from occurring
- Pair inhalation with trunk extension and exhalation with trunk flexion
- Diaphragmatic breathing in a variety of positions progressing as his strength and endurance increase, such as from supine to sitting and standing
- Active assistive cough techniques, such as therapist-assisted abdominal support during cough
- Self-assisted cough techniques

♦ Manual/mechanical techniques (see Pattern C: Impaired Ventilation, Respiration/Gas Exchange, and Aerobic Capacity/Endurance Associated With Airway Clearance Dysfunction in *Cardiovascular/Pulmonary Essentials: Applying the Preferred Physical Therapist Practice Patterns*[SM75] for further information related to manual/mechanical techniques)

- Chest percussion, shaking, and vibration in combination with pulmonary postural drainage
- Use of Acapella device to assist airway clearance by providing positive expiratory pressure and oscillations in the airway while exhaling

♦ Positioning

- Instructions provided in the importance of positioning to enhance breathing and cough production
- Positioning will allow for movement from trunk extension for inhalation to trunk flexion for exhalation based on need of patient
- Positioning will take into account how gravity is assisting or inhibiting ability of patient to use active diaphragmatic movement
- Instructions in good postural positioning to aid breathing

ELECTROTHERAPEUTIC MODALITIES

♦ Electrical stimulation

- If Mr. Stone's current regime of gabapentin and the rescue pain drug fentanyl as needed are not effective in managing generalized pain from muscle tightness related to inactivity, then TENS may be tried

ANTICIPATED GOALS AND EXPECTED OUTCOMES

♦ Impact on pathology/pathophysiology

- Pain is decreased to 0-1/10 during rest and activity.
- Physiological response to increased oxygen demand is improved.

♦ Impact on impairments

- Balance control is improved demonstrating independence in static and dynamic sitting balance, as well as independence in static standing with an assistive device.

- Cardiovascular and muscular endurance are increased, allowing for 15 to 20 minutes of activity before the onset of fatigue.
- Energy expenditure per unit of work is decreased.
- Fatigue is reduced to a score of lower than 3.0, indicating no significant fatigue.
- Muscle performance is increased in UEs and LEs and trunk to WFL.
- Pain is independently self-managed.
- Postural control is improved as demonstrated through independent sitting control during dynamic activity for ADL.

♦ Impact on functional limitations
- Ambulation with an assistive device and contact guard is achieved in a variety of settings.
- Bed mobility is performed independently.
- Climbing up and down curbs with minimal assist of one in a variety of settings is attained.
- Functional independence in ADL and IADL is increased.
- Self-care and home management activities (ADL and IADL) are performed with minimal assistance or supervision and use of appropriate assistive device.
- Stair climbing with minimal assist of one up and down a full flight of steps with use of a hand rail and single-end cane is attained.
- Standing independently is achieved with use of a single UE for support for 5 minutes to perform daily grooming tasks.
- Transfers from bed to/from chair with supervision are achieved.
- Unsupported sitting is achieved without loss of balance for 30 minutes to perform simple hygiene and ADL tasks independently.
- Wheelchair mobility is achieved in the household to ensure safe mobility when unsupervised.

♦ Impact on disabilities
- Participation in preferred community activities is resumed.
- Role of bank manager returning to work and performing all job requirements is resumed.
- Roles of adult, husband, father, grandfather, and volunteer with support of spouse are resumed.

♦ Risk reduction/prevention
- Risks for skin damage due to loss of sensory integrity and movement are fully understood.
- Safe techniques are demonstrated when assisting patient in self-care, transitions, and community activities.
- Safety of patient and family is improved through

demonstration by patient and family of safe techniques for assisted ambulation and stair climbing.

♦ Impact on health, wellness, and fitness
- Exercise and increased activity are incorporated in his daily routine.
- Fitness and health are improved.
- Physical capacity is improved.
- Physical function is improved and will continue to improve.

♦ Impact on societal resources
- Available resources are maximally utilized.
- Documentation occurs throughout patient management in all settings and follows APTA's *Guidelines for Physical Therapy Documentation.*[76]
- Utilization of physical therapy services is optimized.

♦ Patient/client satisfaction
- Admission data and discharge planning are completed.
- Care is coordinated with patient, family, and other professionals.
- Discharge needs are determined.
- Interdisciplinary collaboration occurs through patient care rounds and patient family meetings.
- Patient and family understanding of anticipated goals and expected outcomes is increased.
- Patient and family will verbalize an awareness of the diagnosis, prognosis, interventions, and anticipated goals and expected outcomes.
- Patient will be able to identify relevant community resources to meet his discharge needs.
- Referrals are made to other professionals or resources whenever necessary and appropriate.

REEXAMINATION

Reexamination is performed throughout the entire episode of care, especially at times of medical status change or transfer of care to home care or outpatient physical therapy. In addition, periodic reexamination of the patient's functional limitations and impairments should occur to monitor progress toward his goals. This is very important in patients with GBS as their status can change quite quickly, both for the better or worse.

DISCHARGE

Mr. Stone would be discharged from this physical therapy episode of care after attainment of his goals in a total of 22 physical therapy visits spread across acute, subacute, and outpatient settings over a period of 5 months, with eight visits occurring in subacute care. Since any residual effects of GBS may influence Mr. Stone's function in the future, he would receive education regarding factors that may trigger a call to his physical therapist for a reexamination and new episode of physical therapy care. Mr. Stone would be discharged from this episode of care after attaining the identified goals and placed on an episode of physical therapy prevention. The episode of physical therapy prevention will focus on Mr. Stone's health, wellness, and fitness program and will monitor changes in his functional status. As Mr. Stone continues to make functional improvements as innervation continues, it is important for him to have periodic contact with his physical therapist to discuss changes and, if necessary, return for further examination.

Case Study #2: Chemotherapy-Induced Peripheral Neuropathy

June Fredrick is a 49-year-old female who began treatment for breast cancer 6 months ago. She began to feel unsteady while walking approximately 4 months ago, and because it has not resolved after the cessation of chemotherapy, she has begun outpatient physical therapy.

PHYSICAL THERAPIST EXAMINATION

HISTORY

- General demographics: The patient is a 49-year-old female. She is college educated, with an MBA. She is of English and German descent.
- Social history: The patient is unmarried and usually lives alone with her two dogs. Her sister lives in the same town, and she has been staying with her sister's family during her cancer treatment.
- Employment/work: She is a self-employed businesswoman, who owns her own consulting firm. Her job is primarily sedentary and requires much computer work. She has eight employees. Her business is located on the ground level of an office complex, and she drives a car to work.
- Living environment: She lives in a condominium complex with an elevator to access her fourth floor home. There are no steps once she is inside the building, but she needs to ascend/descend two stairs with a railing for access to the building. There is an accessible entrance at the rear of the building. She has been living with her sister for support since 1 week after the start of chemotherapy. Her sister's home has two levels, but Ms. Fredrick is using a bedroom and bathroom on the main floor. There are three steps with a railing to enter the home.

- General health status
  - General health perception: Prior to her cancer diagnosis, she reports that health issues did not negatively impact her life.
  - Physical function: Prior to her cancer diagnosis, she was independent in all activities, but she now relies on minimal assistance from family.
  - Psychological function: She feels that she is coping well with support from family and a cancer support group.
  - Role function: Since beginning chemotherapy, she has cut back on her work schedule to 75% of full time. She reports that she is unable to fulfill her role as a business owner.
  - Social function: Prior to onset, she was active in competitive obedience trials for her dogs. She reports being unable to train her dogs at this time due to her unsteadiness.
- Social/health habits: She admits to working too much and exercising too little. She reports walking one or two times a week for exercise prior to her diagnosis, as well as working with her dogs in obedience training four to five times per week, but she has not exercised since beginning treatment. She is a nonsmoker and only has occasional alcoholic drinks (one or two per week). She reports that her diabetes has been fairly well controlled, but has had some issues controlling blood sugars during the chemotherapy treatments.
- Family history: There is no family history of cancer, but both her father and sister have HTN and type 2 diabetes.
- Past medical history: She has had type 2 diabetes mellitus for 15 years that is controlled by diet and medication. She also has HTN and hypercholesterolemia, both of which are treated with medications.
- History of current cancer treatment: Ms. Fredrick was diagnosed 6 months ago with invasive ductal carcinoma, clinical stage III, that was found on the left breast by needle biopsy. Confirmation was made by MRI of a 5.5 x 5.2 x 6.7 cm mass and axillary lymphadenopathy. Her bone scans were negative. Chemotherapy was instituted prior to surgery and consisted of the AC/T protocol (Adriamycin [doxorubicin] and cyclophosphamide followed by taxane [docetaxel or paclitaxel]). Neoadjuvant therapy consisted of two phases: Phase 1—four cycles of doxorubicin and cyclophosphamide for a total of 12 weeks of treatment and Phase 2—four cycles of docetaxel, one cycle every 3 weeks for 12 weeks. The patient noted symptoms of numbness and tingling within 2 weeks of initiating docetaxel, but at that time the symptoms were transient. After 24 weeks of chemotherapy, the patient underwent surgical removal of the tumor, as well as lymph node dissection. Postsurgically

the patient complained of pain in her LEs and incisional pain, which were treated with oxycodone and gabapentin with limited relief. Two weeks post surgery, her medications were changed to include oxycodone, gabapentin, hydrocodone/acetaminophen, and cyclobenzaprine. These provided some additional pain relief, but the patient continued to complain of unsteadiness. Three weeks later she received a consult to outpatient physical therapy.

♦ Medications: Gabapentin, oxycodone, cyclobenzaprine, captopril, glyburide, lovastatin.

♦ Other clinical tests: CT scan of the brain and spine were negative.

SYSTEMS REVIEW

♦ Cardiovascular/pulmonary
  ● BP: 110/84 mmHg
  ● Edema: None observed
  ● HR: 86 bpm
  ● RR: 18 bpm
♦ Integumentary
  ● Presence of scar formation: Reports healed incisional scar on left breast
  ● Skin color: Normal
  ● Skin integrity: Intact
♦ Musculoskeletal
  ● Gross range of motion
    ▪ AROM WFL through all LEs and RUE bilaterally
    ▪ Mild decrease in shoulder flexion and abduction on left
  ● Gross strength: Mild decrease in bilateral UEs and LEs
  ● Gross symmetry: No asymmetry noted
  ● Height: 5'6" (1.68 m)
  ● Weight: 158 lbs (71.67 kg)
♦ Neuromuscular
  ● Balance
    ▪ Intact sitting balance
    ▪ Impaired standing balance observed
  ● Locomotion, transfers, and transitions
    ▪ Sit to stand transitions with assist of arms, ambulates independently
    ▪ Displays slight unsteadiness and prefers to hold onto nearby objects
  ● Paresthesia and numbness reported in distal portions of hands and legs
♦ Communication, affect, cognition, language, and learning style
  ● Communication, affect, cognition: WFL
  ● Learning style: Visual learner

TESTS AND MEASURES

♦ Aerobic capacity and endurance
  ● Endurance not formally assessed at this time, see functional activities for endurance limitations during activity
  ● 3.6/7.0 in Fatigue Severity Scale[49] representing mild fatigue
♦ Anthropometric characteristics
  ● BMI=705 x (body weight [in pounds] divided by height^2 [in inches])
  ● Ms. Fredrick's BMI=25.5 which is in the overweight category[50]
♦ Arousal, attention, and cognition
  ● Oriented x3
  ● Follows three-step verbal commands
  ● The patient is cooperative and motivated
♦ Assistive and adaptive devices
  ● None currently used
  ● May require assistive device for safe ambulation
♦ Cranial and peripheral nerve integrity
  ● Decreased temperature sensation at ankle and wrist bilaterally
  ● Light touch sensation mildly impaired at both feet, ankles, lower legs, and hands, but intact to the 5.07 Semmes-Weinstein monofilament indicating protective sensation[77]
  ● Visual field screening intact
  ● Reports no auditory disturbance
  ● Intact visual tacking
♦ Environmental, home, and work barriers
  ● Home has two steps with hand rail to enter front entrance, elevator access to her fourth floor condominium
  ● Primarily wood floors, except tile in bathroom
  ● Has mid-sized sedan for transportation to work, no permit for accessible parking
  ● Patient reports that her work area is accessible, but she needs to be able to walk one block from parking area and she needs to ascend and descend curbs
♦ Gait, locomotion, and balance
  ● Sitting balance: Independent in static and dynamic tests
  ● Transfers/transitions
    ▪ Sit to/from supine: Independent
    ▪ Sit to/from stand: Modified independent with use of hands, minimal assist needed when asked to not use arms
  ● Standing balance
    ▪ Maintains static balance for 25 seconds, but only 5 seconds with eyes closed
    ▪ Standing reach 4 inches

- BBS[78]: 39/56, indicating high risk of falls
- ◆ Integumentary integrity
  - Skin on feet and hands intact, with no areas of concern
  - Well-healed incision on left anterior chest wall and axilla, scar tissue mobile
- ◆ Motor function
  - Coordination
    - Heel-shin slide: Smooth movement with no sign of incoordination
    - Finger-nose: Smooth and precise movements at normal speed
- ◆ Muscle performance
  - MMT revealed the following deviations from normal[78]
    - Shoulder flexion=4+/5 R, 4/5 L
    - Shoulder abduction=4+/5 R, 4/5 L
    - Elbow flexion=4+/5 bilateral
    - Elbow extension=4+/5 bilateral
    - Wrist flexion=5/5 bilateral
    - Wrist extension=5/5 bilateral
    - Finger flexion=5/5 bilateral
    - Finger extension=5/5 bilateral
    - Hip flexion=4+/5 bilateral
    - Hip extension=5/5 bilateral
    - Knee flexion=5/5 bilateral
    - Knee extension=4+/5 bilateral
    - Ankle dorsiflexion=4/5 bilateral
    - Ankle plantarflexion=4+/5 bilateral
    - Grip strength
      - ‣ R=67 lbs and L=55 lbs
      - ‣ WNL for age and gender[79]
- ◆ Orthotic, protective, and supportive devices
  - None
- ◆ Pain
  - Currently 1-2/10 in both feet since initiating gabapentin/oxycodone therapy (10 is worst pain ever)[51]
- ◆ Posture
  - No major deviations noted
- ◆ Range of motion
  - PROM: WFL throughout RUE and bilateral LEs
  - LUE: All motions WNL except
    - Shoulder flexion=108 degrees
    - Shoulder abduction=110 degrees
    - Shoulder external rotation=70 degrees
    - Shoulder internal rotation=60 degrees
- ◆ Reflex integrity
  - Deep tendon reflexes
    - Absent at the ankle bilaterally
    - Patellar tendon bilaterally: Normal

- Biceps, brachioradialis, and triceps bilaterally: Normal
- Babinski reflex: Toes down going bilaterally indicated normal response
- ◆ Self-care and home management
  - Reports independence in self-care including dressing and bathing with use of a chair or stool
  - Has been having sister assist with laundry and meal preparation
- ◆ Sensory integrity
  - Decreased vibratory sensation in feet, ankles, hands, and wrists bilaterally[80]
  - Decreased joint position sense at great toe and ankle bilaterally[80]
  - Michigan Neuropathy Score[81]: 26/46, indicating moderate neuropathy
  - Negative response to Dix-Hallpike maneuver for BPPV[82]
- ◆ Ventilation and respiration/gas exchange
  - No complaint of cough or dyspnea
- ◆ Work, community, and leisure integration or reintegration
  - Able to complete approximately 75% of work activities, some difficulty with fatigue
  - Able to drive to work, but difficulty walking from parking area
  - Job includes sitting at a desk for extended periods, facilitating office meetings, supervising employees, and dealing with customers in person and on the phone, and work hours vary from 8 to 12 per day
  - Unable to participate in leisure activity of obedience training for her dogs

EVALUATION

Ms. Fredrick was an active, right-handed female prior to onset of her cancer diagnosis and treatment. She has symptoms of peripheral neuropathy (sensory symptoms greater than motor symptoms) resulting from chemotherapeutic intervention leading to balance dysfunction and mild fatigue. She requires assistance for some household tasks and is at increased risk for falls. She has cut back to approximately 75% of full-time employment. She has impairments in cutaneous sensation, proprioception, strength, ROM, and balance affecting the LEs greater than the UEs and distal more than proximal. She is independent in transfers, but requires assistance for curbs and stairs without railings. She is at risk for skin breakdown in her hands and feet and other complications due to inactivity and impaired sensation. She is unable to manage her household independently or participate in her previous roles in the community.

Diagnosis

Ms. Fredrick has CIPN with pain in both feet. She has impaired: aerobic capacity/endurance; cranial and peripheral nerve integrity; gait, locomotion, and balance; muscle performance; range of motion; reflex integrity; and sensory integrity. She is functionally limited in self-care and home management and in work, community, and leisure actions, tasks, and activities. She has environmental, home, and work barriers. She will require assistive and adaptive devices and equipment. These findings are consistent with placement in Pattern G: Impaired Motor Function and Sensory Integrity Associated With Acute or Chronic Polyneuropathies. The identified impairments, functional limitations, barriers, and device and equipment needs will be addressed in determining the prognosis and the plan of care.

Prognosis and Plan of Care

Over the course of the visits, the following mutually established outcomes have been determined:
♦ Balance is improved
♦ Functional independence in ADL and IADL is increased
♦ Gait, locomotion, and balance are improved
♦ Independent ambulation and stair climbing with appropriate assistive device are achieved
♦ Pain is decreased or eliminated
♦ Performance levels in self-care are improved
♦ Physical capacity is improved
♦ Physical function is improved
♦ Relevant community resources to meet her needs are identified
♦ Risk factors are reduced
♦ Work, community, and leisure activities are resumed

To achieve these outcomes, the appropriate interventions for this patient are determined. These will include: coordination, communication, and documentation; patient/client-related instruction; therapeutic exercise; functional training in self-care and home management; functional training in work, community, and leisure integration or reintegration; prescription, application, and, as appropriate, fabrication of devices and equipment; and electrotherapeutic modalities.

Based on the diagnosis and prognosis, Ms. Fredrick is expected to require 5 to 10 visits over the course of the next 2 to 3 months. Ms. Fredrick is expected to regain functional independence. It is anticipated that she will be able to return to independent living in her own home.

Many factors may influence the frequency and duration of physical therapy intervention including the patient's level of initial impairment,[52] the patient's response to exercise therapy, recurrence of symptoms, and adherence to the intervention plan. Ms. Fredrick is very motivated, and her prognosis for rehabilitation is good to excellent.

Interventions

RATIONALE FOR SELECTED INTERVENTIONS

Therapeutic Exercise

Research on patients with peripheral neuropathy due to chemotherapy is sparse. Improvement after rehabilitation has been reported in a case study,[83] although long-term impairments may remain.

Resistance and endurance exercise could theoretically improve strength and balance in patients with metabolic or toxic peripheral neuropathy. Theoretically, improved circulation from endurance exercise could also improve sensory function if the neuronal environment is improved to allow regeneration. Unfortunately, few clinical studies of exercise for patients with toxic or metabolic neuropathies have been conducted.[62] Focus on compensatory strategies (use of adaptive and assistive devices) should be done in conjunction with supporting restorative functional reinnervation or adaptive changes in body systems.

Challenging the patient's balance system to allow her to rely on the available information (vestibular and visual) to compensate for the lack of appropriate somatosensory information from her feet will be a key feature of her rehabilitation. The loss of somatosensory information from her feet and ankles may be permanent or temporary, thus adapting the CNS's motor planning to the intact sensations may result in improved balance. This adaptation will require repetition of challenging balance tasks to produce a change in function.

Although Ms. Fredrick's fatigue is mild, it may inhibit her from participating in her home, work, and leisure activities. Cancer-related fatigue is defined as "persistent, subjective sense of tiredness related to cancer or cancer treatment that interferes with usual functioning."[84] Moderate aerobic exercise has been described to be the "treatment of choice" for cancer-related fatigue.[85] Aerobic exercise has shown to be helpful in reducing fatigue in patients post-breast cancer treatment.[86]

Functional Training in Self-Care and Home Management

Functional training in home management will be a critical factor in assisting Ms. Fredrick to return to independent living at home. Improving balance through therapeutic exercise will assist in this endeavor, but training in specific situations that mimic her home situation will also be important. Specifically, she will need strategies to manage tasks that challenge her balance capabilities, including meal preparation, laundry, and caring for her dogs. An assistive device, as will be discussed below, may be important in this functional training.

Fatigue is often seen in patients post-cancer treatment, and it may impede her ability to return to all of her home activities. Education on pacing of activities may need to be addressed with Ms. Fredrick before she is able to independently manage her home situation. Additional equipment (such as a robotic vacuum) or outside assistance (from a cleaning person) may assist her in her home management.

Functional Training in Work, Community, and Leisure Integration or Reintegration

Ms. Fredrick continues to work, but is currently not participating in her regular leisure activities. Adaptation of her work site may be appropriate to enhance function and reduce risks of falls. A work site visit by the physical therapist could be helpful in this area. Reintegration to her hobby of dog training may be enhanced by use of an assistive device (see below).

Prescription, Application, and, as Appropriate, Fabrication of Devices and Equipment

Given her decreased sensation, decreased strength, impaired balance, impaired gait, and fatigue, Ms. Fredrick may require assistive, adaptive, orthotic, or supportive equipment. It is important to improve mobility prior to the return of balance function. Ms. Fredrick may benefit from use of a cane for early mobility, then reducing her reliance on the cane in comfortable and nonchallenging environments as her balance improves. She may need to continue to use the cane in challenging environments, such as when walking her dogs or during periods of increased fatigue.

Electrotherapeutic Modalities

Neuropathic pain, such as is seen in some patients with CIPN, could theoretically be assisted by electrotherapeutic modalities such as TENS. Indeed, some patients with diabetic neuropathic pain find that TENS is helpful. In a patient with cancer, the decision to use an electrotherapeutic or deep heating modality needs to be carefully considered. Physical modalities, such as electrical stimulation, have the potential to break down the cell membranes of abnormal tissues, and thus could potentially increase the risk of metastasis.[87] Since this patient is in the subacute phase of her cancer, she is considered to be a high-risk patient for modality use, and it is not recommended to use electrotherapeutic or deep heating agents if other pain-reducing methods are available.[87]

COORDINATION, COMMUNICATION, AND DOCUMENTATION

Communication will occur with Ms. Fredrick, her physician, and any other members of the rehabilitation team. Interdisciplinary teamwork will be demonstrated through communication and coordination with other team members. Information on community resources will also be provided to the patient. All elements of the patient's management will be documented.

PATIENT/CLIENT-RELATED INSTRUCTION

The patient will be provided instruction about her current condition and potential complications. She will be educated on the reasons for her current impairments, functional limitations, disabilities, and risk factors. She will be instructed in the need to protect her hands and feet due to decreased protective sensation leading to an increased risk of skin breakdown. She will also be provided instruction about safety issues, such as reducing the risk for falls through behavioral and environmental modifications.

The patient will also be provided with information regarding community resources for additional support. Ms. Fredrick will be consulted in the creation of the plan of care. She will be taught techniques to enhance her independent function.

THERAPEUTIC EXERCISE

♦ Aerobic capacity/endurance conditioning
  ● Initiated to improve cardiovascular/pulmonary function and decrease fatigue
  ● Mode
    ▪ Cycle ergometry
    ▪ Swimming
  ● Intensity: Moderate
  ● Duration: Working up to 30 minutes of activity
  ● Frequency: Three to five times per week
♦ Balance, coordination, and agility training
  ● Static and dynamic standing balance
    ▪ Dynamic standing balance exercises with and without UE support
    ▪ Head turns
    ▪ Weight shifting in all planes
    ▪ Rhythmic stabilization
    ▪ Reaching activities
    ▪ Stepping activities
    ▪ Progress to assistive devices
    ▪ Practice during functional tasks, such as self-care and household activities
    ▪ Tai Chi or yoga should be considered as a part of Ms. Fredrick's long-term health, wellness, and fitness program to continue to challenge balance
♦ Flexibility exercises
  ● Stretching exercises should be done after warming up, using a slow and steady stretch accompanied by deep breathing, and progressing hold up to 60 seconds

- Gentle stretching to increase ROM in left shoulder flexion, abduction, internal rotation, and external rotation
- Gait and locomotion training
  - Gait training should begin with standing balance tasks, as described above, incorporating weight shifting
  - Both forward and backward steps should be taught to allow safe stand to sit transition
  - Instruction in the use of a cane during functional ambulation
- Strength, power, and endurance training
  - Patient should not become fatigued during these exercises, therefore, begin with lower repetitions
  - Active exercises emphasizing low repetition strengthening of muscles of left shoulder and elbow
  - Functional strengthening of LE muscles (eg, sit to stand, standing plantar and dorsiflexion, wall slides)

FUNCTIONAL TRAINING IN SELF-CARE AND HOME MANAGEMENT

- Self-care and home management
  - Many of the therapeutic exercises described in the previous section will help support ADL training (ie, standing reaching exercises will help with household activities)
  - A home evaluation would be ideal in order to provide the most task-specific assessment of readiness of the patient to manage at home
  - As return of sensory function occurs or compensatory strategies allow, she will decrease use of adaptive and assistive equipment for self-care and home management
- Injury prevention or reduction
  - A task-specific environment in the therapeutic setting will be created that mirrors the patient's home as it pertains to ambulation surfaces, stairs, and bathroom situations to prevent/reduce the likelihood of injury upon return to her home
- Energy management
  - Development of a plan for energy management that provides for energy conservation if fatigue is impacting her daily routine

FUNCTIONAL TRAINING IN WORK, COMMUNITY, AND LEISURE INTEGRATION OR REINTEGRATION

- IADL training
  - Reintegration into her work activities will occur in a phased manner, increasing her independence and allowing her to return to work
  - A visit with the physical therapist will be made to her

work site to evaluate job requirements and potential environmental barriers
- Injury prevention or reduction
  - Instructions will be given in how to safely progress her work, community, and leisure actions, tasks, and activities to prevent any injury
- Energy management
  - Development of a plan for energy management that provides for energy conservation if fatigue is impacting her work and community activities
- Leisure and play
  - Reintegration into community and leisure activities will occur in a phased manner, increasing her participation and motivation

PRESCRIPTION, APPLICATION, AND, AS APPROPRIATE, FABRICATION OF DEVICES AND EQUIPMENT

- Assistive devices
  - An assistive device, such as cane, will be used since her sensory deficits may or may not improve over time
    - The use of a cane for mobility will enhance her performance and independence in home and community and will increase mobility and stability and reduce risk of falls
    - Instructions will be given in the use and care of the device
- Supportive devices
  - Enhance her access to her work environment by the use of a handicap parking permit until her independent mobility improves

ELECTROTHERAPEUTIC MODALITIES

- Electrical stimulation
  - If Ms. Fredrick's current regime of gabapentin and opioids as needed are not effective in managing the LE pain, then TENS may be tried, only as long as she is cleared for metastatic spread of cancer and potential risks have been thoroughly discussed with the patient

ANTICIPATED GOALS AND EXPECTED OUTCOMES

- Impact on pathology/pathophysiology
  - Peripheral nerve function is improved as measured by improvement on the Michigan Neuropathy Scale.
- Impact on impairments
  - Fatigue is decreased to 2.0/7.0 on the Fatigue Severity Scale.

♦ Impact on functional limitations
  ● Independent and safe community ambulation is achieved.
  ● Independent transfers from sit to stand from chair without assistance of arms are achieved.
♦ Impact on disabilities
  ● Independent living is achieved.
  ● Meal preparation and laundry are independently performed.
♦ Risk reduction/prevention
  ● Risk of falls is reduced to low risk category as measured by a score of >45/56 on the BBS.
♦ Impact on health, wellness, and fitness
  ● Fitness and health are improved.
  ● Physical capacity is improved.
  ● Physical function is improved and will continue to improve.
  ● Return to active leisure activities including walking and training her dogs is achieved.
♦ Impact on societal resources
  ● Available resources are maximally utilized.
  ● Documentation occurs throughout patient management in all settings and follows APTA's *Guidelines for Physical Therapy Documentation*.[76]
  ● Utilization of physical therapy services is optimized.
♦ Patient/client satisfaction
  ● Patient and family understanding of anticipated goals and expected outcomes is increased.

REEXAMINATION

Reexamination is performed throughout the entire episode of care, especially at times of medical status change or transfer of care. In addition, periodic reexamination of the patient's functional limitations and impairments should occur to monitor progress toward her goals.

DISCHARGE

Ms. Fredrick is discharged from this physical therapy episode of care after attainment of her goals in a total of eight physical therapy visits in an outpatient setting over a period of 3 months. Since any residual effects of CIPN may influence Ms. Fredrick's function in the future, she will receive education regarding factors that may trigger a call to her physical therapist for a reexamination and new episode of physical therapy care. Ms. Fredrick would be discharged from this episode of care after attaining the identified goals and placed on an episode of physical therapy prevention. The episode of physical therapy prevention will focus on Ms. Fredrick's health, wellness, and fitness program and will monitor changes in her functional status.

REFERENCES

1. Kandel ER, Schwartz JH, Jessell TM. *Principles of Neural Science.* 4th ed. New York, NY: McGraw Hill; 2000.
2. Kiernan JA. *Barr's The Human Nervous System: An Anatomical Viewpoint.* 8th ed. Philadelphia, PA: Lippincott Williams & Wilkins; 2005.
3. England JD, Asbury AK. Peripheral neuropathy. *Lancet.* 2004;363:2151-2161.
4. Younger DS. Peripheral nerve disorders. *Primary Care: Clinics in Office Practice.* 2004;31:67-83.
5. Waxman SG, Degroot J. *Correlative Neuroanatomy.* 22nd ed. Norwalk, CT: Appleton and Lange; 1995.
6. Nadeau SE, Ferguson TS, Valenstein E, et al. *Medical Neuroscience.* Philadelphia, PA: Saunders; 2004.
7. Moffat M, Rosen E, Rusnak-Smith S, eds. *Musculoskeletal Essentials: Applying the Preferred Physical Therapist Practice Patterns.*[SM] Thorofare, NJ: SLACK Incorporated; 2006.
8. Kuwabara S. Guillain-Barre syndrome: epidemiology, pathophysiology, and management. *Drugs.* 2004;64:597-610.
9. Olive JM, Castillo C, Castro RG et al. Epidemiologic study of Guillain-Barre syndrome in children < 15 years in Latin America. *J Infect Dis.* 1997;175(Suppl 1):S160-S164.
10. Hahn AF. Guillain-Barre syndrome. *Lancet.* 1998;352:635-641.
11. Hughes RA, Rees JH. Clinical and epidemiologic features of Guillain-Barre syndrome. *J Infect Dis.* 1997;176(Suppl 2):S92-S98.
12. Van Doorn P. Treatment of Guillain-Barre syndrome and CIDP. *J Peripher Nerv Syst.* 2005;10:113-127.
13. Hughes RA, Hadden RDM, Gregson NA, Smith KJ. Pathogenesis of Guillain-Barre syndrome. *J Neuroimmunol.* 1999;100:74-97.
14. Hadden RD, Cornblath DR, Hughes RA, et al. Electrophysiological classification of Guillain-Barre syndrome: clinical associations and outcomes: plasma exchange/Sandglobulin Guillain-Barre syndrome trial group. *Ann Neurol.* 1998;44:780-788.
15. Griffin JW, Li CY, Macko C, et al. Early nodal changes in the acute motor axonal neuropathy pattern of Guillain-Barre syndrome. *J Neurocytol.* 1996;25:33-51.
16. Fisher CM. An unusual variant of acute idiopathic polyneuritis (syndrome of ophthalmoplegia, ataxia, and areflexia). *N Engl J Med.* 1956;225:57-75.
17. Jacobs BC, Rothbarth PH, van der Meche FG, et al. The spectrum of antecedent infections in Guillain-Barre syndrome: a case control study. *Neurology.* 1998;51:1110-1115.
18. Ogawara K, Kuwabara S, Mori M, et al. Axonal Guillain-Barre syndrome: relation to anti-ganglioside antibodies and Campylobacter jejuni infection in Japan. *Ann Neurol.* 2000;48:624-631.
19. Prineas JW. Acute idiopathic polyneuritis. An electromicroscope study. *Lab Invest.* 1972;26:133-147.
20. Hafer-Macko C, Hsieh ST, Li CY, et al. Acute motor axonal neuropathy: an antibody mediated attack on axolemma. *Ann Neurol.* 1996;40:635-644.
21. Smith KJ, Hall SM. Nerve conduction during peripheral demyelination and remyelination. *J Neurol Sci.* 1980;48:201-219.
22. Ho TW, Mishu B, Li CY, et al. Guillain-Barre syndrome in

northern China: relationship to Campylobacter jejuni infection and anti-glycolipid antibodies. *Brain*. 1995;118:597-605.

23. Meythaler JM. Rehabilitation of Guillain-Barre syndrome. *Arch Phys Med Rehabil*. 1997;78:872-879.

24. Winer JB, Hughes RAC, Osmond C. A prospective study of acute idiopathic neuropathy: clinical features and prognostic value. *J Neurol Neurosurg Psychiatry*. 1988;51:605-612.

25. Alter M. The epidemiology of Guillain-Barre syndrome. *Ann Neurol*. 1990;27:S7-S12.

26. Flatters SJL, Bennett GJ. Studies of peripheral sensory nerves in paclitaxel-induced painful peripheral neuropathy: evidence for mitochondrial dysfunction. *Pain*. 2006:122:245-57.

27. Tanner KD, Levine JD, Topp KS. Microtubule disorientation and axonal swelling in unmyelinated sensory axons during vincristine-induced painful neuropathy in the rat. *J Comp Neurol*. 1998;395:481-492.

28. Visovsky C. Chemotherapy-induced peripheral neuropathy. *Cancer Invest*. 2003;21(3):439-451.

29. Taxol prescribing information. Bristol Myers Squibb. Available at: www.accessdata.fda.gov/scripts/cder/onctools/labels.cfm?GN=paclitaxel. Accessed February 2, 2007.

30. Taxotere prescribing information. Aventis. Available at: www.adventis-us.com/Pis/taxotere TXT.html. Accessed February 2, 2007.

31. Abraxane prescribing information. Abraxis. Available at: www.fda.gov/cder/foi/label/2005/021660lbl.pdf. Accessed February 2, 2007.

32. Navelbine prescribing information. GalaxoSmithKline. Available at: www.accessdata.fda.gov./scripts/cder/onctools/labels.cfm?GN=vinorelbine. Accessed February 2, 2007.

33. Vincristine prescribing information. Eli Lilly. Available at: www.accessdata.fda.gov/scripts/cder/onctools/labels.cfm?GN=vincristine. Accessed February 2, 2007.

34. Carboplatin prescribing information. Bristol Myers Squibb. Available at: www.accessdata.fda.gov/scripts/cder/onctools/labels.cfm?GN=carboplatin. Accessed February 2, 2007.

35. Oxaliplatin prescribing information. Sanfi Sythelabo Onc. Available at: www.accessdata.fda.gov/scripts/cder/onctools/labels.cfm?GN=oxaliplatin. Accessed February 2, 2007.

36. Cisplatin prescribing information. Bristol Myers Squibb. Available at: www.accessdata.fda.gov/scripts/cder/onctools/labels.cfm?GN=cisplatin. Accessed February 2, 2007.

37. Asbury AK, Cornblath DR. Assessment of current diagnostic criteria for Guillain-Barre syndrome. *Ann Neurol*. 1990;27(Suppl):S21-S24.

38. Gordon PH, Wilbourn AJ. Early electrodiagnostic findings in Guillain-Barre syndrome. *Arch Neurol*. 2001;58:913-917.

39. Miller RG, Peterson GW, Daube JR, Albers JW. Prognostic value of electrodiagnosis in Guillain-Barre syndrome. *Muscle Nerve*. 1988;11:769-774.

40. Ropper AH. The Guillain-Barre syndrome. *N Engl J Med*. 1992;326:1130-1136.

41. The Guillain-Barre Study Group. Plasmapheresis and acute Guillain-Barre syndrome. *Neurology*. 1985;35:1096-1104.

42. Plasma Exchange/Sandoglobulin Guillain-Barre Syndrome Trial Group. Randomised trial of plasma exchange, intravenous immunoglobulin, and combined treatments in Guillain-Barre syndrome. *Lancet*. 1997;349:225-230.

43. Hughes RA, Raphael JC, Swan AV, Doorn PA. Intravenous immunoglobulin for Guilian-Barre syndrome. *Cochrane Database Syst Rev*. 2004;CD002063.

44. Van Koningsveld R, van Doorn PA, Schmitz PI, van der Meche FG. Changes in referral pattern and its effect on outcome in patients with Guillain-Barre syndrome. *Neurology*. 2001;56:564-566.

45. Hughes RA, Wijdicks EF, Baron R, et al: Quality Standards Subcommittee of the American Academy of Neurology. Practice Parameter: immunotherapy for Guillain-Barre syndrome—report of the quality standards subcommittee of the American Academy of Neurology. *Neurology*. 2003;61:736-740.

46. Guillian-Barre Syndrome Steroid Trial Group. Double-blind trial of intravenous methylprednisone in Guillain-Barre syndrome. *Lancet*. 1993;341:586-590.

47. Albers J, Chaudry V, Cavaletti G, Donehower R. Interventions for preventing neuropathy caused by cisplatin and related compounds. *Cochrane Database Syst Rev*. 2007;Jan 24(1): CD005228.

48. Cavaletti G, Zanna C. Current status and future prospects for the treatment of chemotherapy-induced peripheral neurotoxicity. *Eur J Cancer*. 2002;38(14):1832-1837.

49. Krupp LB, LaRocca NG, Muir-Nash J, Steinberg AD. The fatigue severity scale. Applications to patients with multiple sclerosis and systemic lupus erythematous. *Arch Neurol*. 1989;46:1121-1123.

50. *ACSM's Guidelines for Exercise Testing and Prescription*. 6th ed. Philadelphia, PA: American College of Sports Medicine; 2000.

51. Jensen MP, Karoly P, Braver S. The measurement of clinical pain intensity: a comparison of six methods. *Pain*. 1986;27(1):117-126.

52. Foster EC, Mulroy SJ. Muscle belly tenderness, functional mobility, and length of hospital stay in the acute rehabilitation of individuals with Guillain-Barre syndrome. *Journal of Neurologic Physical Therapy*. 2004;28:154-160.

53. Meythaler JM, DeVivo MJ, Braswell WC. Rehabilitation outcomes of patients who have developed Guillain-Barre syndrome. *Am J Phys Med Rehabil*. 1997;76:411-419.

54. Nichols R, Playford ED, Thompson AJ. A retrospective analysis of outcome in severe Guillain-Barre syndrome following combined neurological and rehabilitation management. *Disabil Rehabil*. 2000;22:451-455.

55. Prasad R, Hellawell DJ, Pentland B. Usefulness of the Functional Independence Measure (FIM), its subscales and individual items as outcome measures in Guillain-Barre syndrome. *Int J Rehabil Res*. 2001;24:59-64.

56. Bersano A, Carpo M, Allaria S, et al. Long term disability and social status change after Guillain-Barre syndrome. *J Neurol*. 2005 (E-pub).

57. Bernsen RA, de Jager AE, Schmitz PI, van der Meche FG. Long-term sensory deficit after Guillain-Barre syndrome. *J Neurol*. 2001;248:483-486.

58. Forsberg A, Press R, Einarsson U, Pedro-Cuesta J, Holmqvist LW, Network Members of the Swedish Epidemiological Study Group. Impairment in Guillain-Barre syndrome during the first 2 years after onset: a prospective study. *J Neurol Sci*. 2004;227:131-138.

59. Vajsar J, Fehlings D, Stephens D. Long-term outcomes in children with Guillain-Barre syndrome. *J Pediatr*. 2003;142:305-309.

60. Fehlings D, Vajsar J, Wilk B, Stephens D, Bar-Or O. Anaerobic muscle performance of children after long-term recovery from Guillain-Barre syndrome. *Dev Med Child Neurol.* 2004;46:689-693.

61. Garssen MP, Bussman JB, Schmitz PI, et al. Physical training and fatigue, fitness, and quality of life in Guillain-Barre syndrome and CIDP. *Neurology.* 2004;63:2393-2395.

62. White CM, Pritchard J, Turner-Stokes L. Exercise for people with peripheral neuropathy. *Cochrane Database Syst Rev.* 2004;4:CD003904.pub2. DOI:10.1002/14651858. CD003904.pub2.

63. Tam SL, Archibald V, Jassar B, et al. Increased neuromuscular activity reduces sprouting in partially denervated muscles. *J Neurosci.* 2001;21:654-657.

64. Gardiner PF, Faltus RE. Contractile responses of rat plantaris muscles following partial denervation and the influence of daily exercise. *Pfleugers Arch.* 1986;406:51-56.

65. Sebum KL, Gardiner PF. Properties of sprouted motor units: effect of period of enlargement and activity level. *Muscle Nerve.* 1996;19:1100-1109.

66. Einseidel LF, Ruff AR. Activity and motor unit size in partially denervated rat medial gastrocnemius. *J Appl Physiol.* 1994;76(6):2663-2671.

67. Ribchester RR. Activity-dependent and -independent synaptic interactions during reinnervation of partially denervated rat muscle. *J Physiol.* 1988;401:53-75.

68. Pietti K, Barrett PJ, Abbas D. Endurance exercise training in Guillain-Barre syndrome. *Arch Phys Med Rehabil.* 1993;74:761-765.

69. Tuckey J, Greenwood R. Rehabilitation after severe Guillain-Barre syndrome: the use of partial body weight support. *Physiother Res Int.* 2004;9:96-103.

70. Hillegass EA, Sadowsky HS. *Essentials of Cardiopulmonary Physical Therapy.* 2nd ed. Philadelphia, PA: WB Saunders Co; 2001.

71. Ropper AH, Shahani BT. Pain in Guillain Barre syndrome. *Arch Neurol.* 1984;41:511-514.

72. Hughes RA, Wijdicks EF, Benson E, et al. Multidisciplinary Consensus Group. Supportive care for patients with Guillain-Barre syndrome. *Arch Neurol.* 2005;62:1194-1198.

73. Pandey CK, Raza M, Tripathi M, et al. The comparative evaluation of gabapentin and carbamazepine for pain management in Guillain-Barre syndrome patients in the intensive care unit. *Anesth Analg.* 2005;101:220-225.

74. McCarthy JA, Zigenfus RW. Transcutaneous electrical nerve stimulation: an adjunct in the pain management of Guillain-Barre syndrome. *Phys Ther.* 1978;58(1):23-24.

75. Stackowicz DM, Moffat M, Frownfelter D, Butler McNamara SM. Impaired ventilation, respiration/gas exchange, and aerobic capacity/endurance associated with airway clearance dysfunction (pattern C). In: Moffat M, Frownfelter D, eds. *Cardiovascular/Pulmonary Essentials: Applying the Preferred Physical Therapist Practice Patterns.SM* Thorofare, NJ: SLACK Incorporated; 2007:83-112.

76. American Physical Therapy Association. Guide to physical therapist practice. 2nd ed. *Phys Ther.* 2001;81:9-744.

77. Shy ME, Frohman EM, So YT, et al. Quantitative sensory testing: report of the Therapeutics and Technology Assessment Subcommittee of the American Academy of Neurology. *Neurology.* 2003;6:898-904.

78. Berg K, Wood-Dauphinee S, Williams JI, Maki B. Measuring balance in the elderly: validation of an instrument. *Can J Public Health.* 1992;2(Suppl):S7-S11.

79. Mathiowetz V. Grip and pinch strength: normative data for adults. *Arch Phys Med Rehabil.* 1985;66:69-74.

80. Reese N. *Muscle and Sensory Testing.* 2nd ed. St. Louis, MO: Elsevier Saunders; 2005.

81. Feldman EL, Stevens MJ, Thomas PK, et al. A practical two-step quantitative clinical and electrophysiological assessment for the diagnosis and staging of diabetic neuropathy. *Diabetes Care.* 1994;17:1281-1289.

82. Shumway-Cook A, Woollacott MH. *Motor Control: Translating Research into Clinical Practice.* 3rd ed. Philadelphia, PA: Lippincott Williams & Wilkins; 2007.

83. Wampler MA, Hamolsky D, Hamel K, et al. Case report: painful peripheral neuropathy following treatment with docetaxel for breast cancer. *Clin J Oncol Nurs.* 2005;9(2):189-193.

84. Mock V, Atkinson A, Barsevick A, et al. Cancer-related fatigue clinical practice guidelines in oncology. *J Natl Comp Cancer Network.* 2003;1(3):308-331.

85. Watson T, Mock V. Exercise as an intervention for cancer-related fatigue. *Phys Ther.* 2004;84(8):736-743.

86. Mock V, Fragakis C, Davidson NE, et al. Exercise manages fatigue during breast cancer treatment: a randomized controlled trail. *Psychooncology.* 2005;14(6):464-477.

87. Goodman CC, Boissonault WF, Fuller KS. *Pathology: Implications for the Physical Therapist.* 2nd ed. Philadelphia, PA: Elsevier Saunders; 2003.

CHAPTER EIGHT

Impaired Motor Function, Peripheral Nerve Integrity, and Sensory Integrity Associated With Nonprogressive Disorders of the Spinal Cord (Pattern H)

Barbara Garrett, PT

ANATOMY

The spinal cord is the conduit for sensory information from the body to higher brain structures and also for the signals from the brain that regulate motor and autonomic functions. Spinal reflexes are incorporated in the spinal cord as part of the involuntary reflex arc to regulate various body functions. The spinal cord is protected and surrounded by the vertebral column. It begins rostrally at the medulla and terminates at the second lumbar vertebra. A transection of the spinal cord reveals central gray matter containing nerve cell bodies and the surrounding white matter containing the spinal tracts. A pair of spinal nerves emerges from the spinal cord through the intervertebral foramina at each of the 31 spinal segments (8 cervical, 12 thoracic, 5 sacral, 5 lumbar, and 1 coccygeal). Each spinal nerve is composed of a dorsal root of afferent fibers carrying sensory information (dermatomes) from the body and a ventral root of efferent fibers to innervate groups of muscles (myotomes). The spinal cord has an enlargement in the cervical region and fibers originating from this area form the brachial plexus that innervates the UE. A similar enlargement in the lumbar region sends fibers to form the lumbar plexus to innervate the LE. The autonomic nervous system also transmits information to and from the brain via the spinal cord and also through sympathetic pre- and post-ganglionic neurons situated on either side of the vertebral column. Parasympathetic ganglia are located next to or within the organ being innervated. The blood supply of the spinal cord is provided primarily by the single anterior and two posterior spinal arteries originating from the vertebral arteries in the neck and segmentally by the radicular arteries originating from the thoracic and abdominal aorta.[1]

PHYSIOLOGY

The spinal cord is primarily responsible for transmitting sensory information to the brain and subsequently sending the neural signals to regulate motor and autonomic functions. Nerves traveling in the spinal cord regulate volitional movements of the trunk and extremities. The cortico-spinal tract (pyramidal tract) is the descending motor tract responsible for voluntary motor control. These neurons originate in the motor area of the cerebral cortex and cross over in the medulla before descending to the appropriate spinal segment. Impulses are then transmitted to the lower motor neurons to directly innervate striated muscle. Spinal reflexes also utilize the spinal cord to facilitate a variety of body functions. A spinal reflex is an involuntary response to a stimulus, involving a sensory receptor, afferent or sensory neuron, possible interneurons, a reflex center, efferent neurons, and an effector organ. The autonomic nervous system also utilizes the spinal cord as a conduit for its maintenance of homeostasis of the body. Stimulation of the sympathetic nervous system produces general responses of "fight or flight." The parasympathetic nervous system balances these responses, often producing the opposite effect.[1]

SUPPORT CELLS

The spinal cord is a continuation of the CNS and has numerous cells that provide support for its function. Glial cells produce myelin, guide neural cell migration, respond to injury, and provide support to the internal environment of the spinal cord. Cells that surround the blood vessels in the spinal cord form a "blood-spinal cord barrier" that protects the spinal cord from potentially harmful substances by restricting entry through the circulatory system.

NEURAL CONTROL OF LOCOMOTION

The spinal cord receives projections from supraspinal pathways originating in the cortex, cerebellum, and brainstem. These pathways provide input for the initiation, modulation, and control of locomotion. It is also believed that a spinal network or spinal CPGs, or central pattern generators, are located in the spinal cord that are able to produce rhythmic stepping without supraspinal input.[2] Research in animal models supports the concept of CPGs located in the spinal cord that produce coordinated stepping movements. The strongest evidence that CPGs exist in human infants is the observation of stepping movements in children born with anecephaly.[3] These spinal CPGs appear to be dependent on stimulation to initiate stepping. In the absence of supraspinal input the spinal CPGs will initiate stepping in response to afferent input.[4,5] This activity-dependent plasticity appears to be in response to specific afferent input from the stretch of hip extensors and loading of the LE.[2,6,7]

PATHOPHYSIOLOGY

The incidence of spinal cord injury (SCI) is approximately 11,000 new cases per year.[8] For the reporting period ending June 2006, the National Spinal Cord Injury Statistical Center (NSCISC) Database[9] found the average age at injury to be 28.7 years with 77.8% of new injuries being male. Among those injured since 2000, 63% are white, 22.7% are black, and 11.89% are of Hispanic ethnicity. There are numerous causes of SCI that result in impaired motor function and disrupted sensory integrity. SCI can be of traumatic or nontraumatic etiology. Traumatic SCI is often the result of motor vehicle accidents (MVAs) (46.9%), falls (23.7%), violence (13.7%) with gunshot wound or stab wound most common, and sporting injuries (8.7%).[9] Traumatic SCI accounts for the majority of all new cases enrolled in the NSCISC each year.

Nontraumatic SCI can be further divided into a variety of etiologies[10,11] including:

♦ Ischemia secondary to vascular lesion including spinal arteriovenous malformation (AVM), thrombosis, aneurysm, and hemorrhage
♦ Myelopathy of various causes including inflammatory demyelinating processes, radiation, nutritional deficiency, and toxicity
♦ Compression of the spinal cord caused by spinal stenosis, infection, or tumor

The NSCISC[8] data of neurologic level at discharge indicates incomplete tetraplegia (34.1%) as the most common type of SCI. Other levels are as follows: complete paraplegia (23.0%), complete tetraplegia (18.3%), and incomplete paraplegia (18.5%). Since 2000, those that have a complete recovery by discharge are less than 1%.

Primary damage from the injury occurs within the first 18 hours.[5] Secondary pathological changes occur over the next days and weeks after injury.[5,12] Secondary damage is also caused by immune reactions, oxidative damage, and excitotoxicity. Within the first hours of injury, cell injury and death occurs with multifocal hemorrhages and inflammatory changes including edema. Cell injury is the result of loss of myelin or degeneration of the axon. Cell death can occur through necrosis, where the cells break open releasing their contents, or apoptosis in which the cells appear to be programmed to die. While necrosis has the ability to increase neighboring cell death due to the release of their contents that may be toxic, apoptosis does not as the cells do not break open.

MEDICAL MANAGEMENT OF ACUTE SPINAL CORD INJURY

Medical treatment of acute SCI is aimed at preventing the secondary injury process related to the immune system response and inflammation. When given within 8 hours of injury, methylprednisone, a steroid, has been shown to decrease secondary damage to the neurons and the size of the lesion.[5,13] Surgical or nonsurgical stabilization techniques are employed to restore the bony structural alignment and achieve decompression of the spinal cord.[14]

CLASSIFICATION OF SPINAL CORD INJURY

Classification of SCI is determined by assessing the structural damage and functional limitations of the neurological system. Segments of the spinal column are used to determine the neurologic level of the injury and type of injury. Tetraplegia includes injury to one of the eight cervical segments, while paraplegia includes injury to the remaining segments (thoracic, lumbar, and sacral). Structural damage looks at damage to the vertebral column and zone of interruption. Functional limitations include assessment of the level of sensory and motor impairment, as well as the completeness of the injury.

Structural Classification

Denis' three-column (zone) concept of vertebral stability can be utilized to assess the degree of structural damage to the vertebral column.[15] The vertebral column can be divided into the following three zones:

Table 8-1
FIVE RADIOGRAPHIC SIGNS THAT DETERMINE WHICH ZONES ARE INTERRUPTED

Radiographic Sign	Zones Interrupted
Displacement	Zones A, M, P
Wide interlaminar space	Zones M, P
Wide facet joint	Zones M, P
Wide vertebral canal	Zones A, M, P
Disrupted posterior vertebral body line	Zones A, M

A=anterior zone, M=middle zone, P=posterior zone.

Reprinted with permission from Kirshblum S, Campagnolo DI, Delisa JA, eds. *Spinal Cord Medicine*. Philadelphia, PA: Lippincott Williams & Wilkins; 2002:33-34.

1. An anterior zone (zone A), formed by the anterior longitudinal ligament and the anterior part of the annulus fibrosis and anterior wall of the vertebral body
2. The middle zone (zone M), formed by the posterior longitudinal ligament, the posterior annulus fibrosis, and the posterior wall of the vertebral body
3. The posterior zone (zone P), formed by the posterior bony neural arch and a posterior ligamentous complex

The middle zone with its osteoligamentous complex determines the pattern of structural spinal injury. If it has not failed, operative fixation is rarely indicated. The five radiographic signs used to determine a diagnosis of instability include:

1. Displacement that implies injury of major ligamentous and articular structures
2. Wide interlaminar space that implies injury to posterior ligamentous structures and facet joints
3. Wide facet joint that implies injury to posterior ligamentous structures
4. Wide vertebral canal that implies injury to the entire vertebra in the sagittal plane
5. Disrupted posterior vertebral body line that implies burst injury with disruption of anterior bony and posterior ligamentous structures (Table 8-1)[15]

Functional Classification

The clinical method to assess the functional degree of SCI utilizes the International Standards for Neurological Classification of Spinal Cord Injury as designed by the American Spinal Injury Association (ASIA).[16] The neurological examination is comprised of motor and sensory testing, which will determine the sensory, motor, and neurological levels, as well as the completeness of the injury.

The motor level is determined by testing key muscles at the 10 right and left myotomes and grading them on a scale of 0 (total paralysis) to 5 (normal). The motor level is deter-

mined as the most caudal segment of the spinal cord with a grade of 3/5 in the key muscle on both sides of the body with a grade of 5/5 in the next most rostral key muscle. Table 8-2 provides an overview of selected myotomes and associated major muscle group that are easily tested in the clinic. Levels that are not easily tested in the clinic with MMT include C1-C4, T2-L1, and S2-S5, and these levels are tested by determining only the sensory level.

The sensory level is determined as the most caudal segment of the spinal cord with normal sensory function on both sides of the body. It is determined by testing each of the 28 sensory key points within the dermatomes on each side of the body for sensitivity to pinprick and light touch on a scale of 0 (absent) to 2 (normal). The dermatomes run from C2 (tested at the occipital protuberance) throughout the UEs, trunk, and LEs to S4-S5 (tested in the perianal region). Table 8-3 provides the ASIA key sensory levels that are tested.

Completeness of the injury is determined by the presence or absence of sensory and motor function in the lowest sacral segments. The ASIA impairment scale grades the level of impairment as listed in Table 8-4. To be classified as incomplete (ASIA B through E) there must be some sensory and motor function at S4-S5, without this the patient is classified as complete (ASIA A). Neurological level is then determined as the most caudal level of the spinal cord with normal motor and sensory function on both sides of the body.[16]

Table 8-5 provides a brief overview of the expected functional outcomes for each spinal level based on a motor complete injury that is 1-year post-traumatic injury. Actual ability is very individualized, but these outcomes will provide a beginning framework when working with the newly injured as to what he or she may expect. The reader is encouraged to access the Consortium for Spinal Cord Medicine Clinical Practice Guidelines' *Outcomes Following Traumatic Spinal Cord Injury: Clinical Practice Guidelines for Health-Care Professionals*[17] for more detail.

Table 8-2

MYOTOMES AND MUSCLES USED FOR DETERMINATION OF MOTOR LEVEL

Myotome	Major Muscle Tested
C5	Elbow flexors (biceps, brachialis)
C6	Wrist extensors (extensor carpi radialis longus and brevis)
C7	Elbow extensors (triceps)
C8	Finger flexors (flexor digitorum profundus) to the middle finger
T1	Small finger abductors (abductor digiti minimi)
L2	Hip flexors (iliopsoas)
L3	Knee extensors (quadriceps)
L4	Ankle dorsiflexors (tibialis anterior)
L5	Long toe extensors (extensor hallicus longus)
S1	Ankle plantarflexors (gastrocnemius, soleus)

SECONDARY IMPAIRMENTS

Secondary impairments associated with SCI are numerous, and many are preventable. Impairments include autonomic dysreflexia (AD), cardiovascular deconditioning, deep vein thrombosis (DVT), depression, heterotopic ossification (HO), muscular changes,[18] neurogenic pain, spasticity, OH, osteoporosis, respiratory complications, skin breakdown, and urinary tract infections (UTIs). Three secondary impairments—AD, HO, and OH—are further described below.

Autonomic Dysreflexia

AD is a sudden severe rise in BP that can be life threatening. It can occur in individuals with SCI at or above T6 but has been reported to occur in those with lesions as low as T8.[19,20] AD occurs as a result of a noxious stimulus below the level of lesion, which triggers sympathetic hyperactivity. The most common triggers are related to bowel or bladder problems. However, triggers can be any irritant to the body, such as a pressure sore or aggressive stretching of the legs.

The Paralyzed Veterans of America[21] developed clinical guidelines for the acute management of AD. The identified symptoms of AD may include a sudden, significant increase in both systolic and diastolic BP (systolic increases over baseline of 20 to 40 mmHg in adults, 15 to 20 mmHg in adolescents, and 15 mmHg in children), pounding headache, bradycardia, profuse sweating above the level of lesion, piloerection or goose bumps, cardiac arrhythmias, flushing of skin above the level of lesion, blurred vision, appearance of spots in the visual fields, nasal congestion, feelings of apprehension or anxiety over an impending physical problem, or minimal or no symptoms despite significantly elevated BP (silent AD). Individuals may have one or more of these symptoms and intervention is required immediately. If the BP is elevated, treatment includes immediately sitting the person up if not already sitting, loosening clothing or constrictive devices, monitoring BP and pulse, and looking

Table 8-3

AMERICAN SPINAL INJURY ASSOCIATION KEY SENSORY LEVELS TESTED[16]

C2	Occipital protuberance
C3	Supraclavicular fossa
C4	Superior acromioclavicular joint
C5	Lateral side of the antecubital fossa
C6	Thumb (and index finger)
C7	Middle finger
C8	Little finger
T1	Medial (ulnar) side of antecubital epicondyle
T2	Apex of axilla
T3	Third IS
T4	Nipple line—fourth IS
T5	Fifth IS
T6	Xiphoid—sixth IS
T7	Seventh IS
T8	Eighth IS
T9	Midway between T8 and T10—ninth IS
T10	Umbilicus—tenth IS
T11	Eleventh IS
T12	Inguinal ligament at midpoint
L1	Half the distance between T12 and L2
L2	Mid-anterior thigh
L3	Medial femoral condyle
L4	Medial malleolus
L5	Dorsum of foot at third MTP joint
S1	Lateral heel
S2	Popliteal fossa in the midline
S3	Ischial tuberosity
S4/S5	Perianal area (taken as one level)

IS=intercostal space.

for and eliminating any potential irritant beginning with the urinary system. If the source of irritation is not found

Table 8-4
AMERICAN SPINAL INJURY ASSOCIATION IMPAIRMENT CLASSIFICATION SCALE

A=Complete	No sensory or motor function preserved in sacral segments S4-S5
B=Incomplete	Sensory but no motor is preserved below the neurological level and includes the sacral segments S4-S5
C=Incomplete	Motor function is preserved below the neurological level, and more than half of key muscles below the neurological level have a muscle grade less than 3
D=Incomplete	Motor function is preserved below the neurological level and at least half of key muscles below the neurological level have a muscle grade greater than or equal to 3
E=Normal	Sensory and motor function are normal

Reprinted with permission from American Spinal Injury Association: International Standards for Neurological Classification of Spinal Cord Injury, revised 2002; Chicago, IL, American Spinal Injury Association, 2002.

Table 8-5
EXPECTED FUNCTIONAL OUTCOMES BASED ON LEVEL OF INJURY

Level	Transfers	Wheelchair Propulsion	Ambulation	Personal Assistance Required per Day
C1-C4	Dependent	Power w/c: Independent	Not indicated	24-hour care
C5	Some to total assistance	Power w/c: Independent Manual w/c: Independent to some assist indoors; some assist to total assist outdoors	Not indicated	Personal care: 10 hours Home care: 6 hours
C6	Level transfers: Some assist to independent Uneven: Some to total assist	Power w/c: Independent Manual w/c: Independent indoors; some to total assist outdoors	Not indicated	Personal care: 6 hours Home care: 4 hours
C7-C8	Level transfers: Independent Uneven: Independent to some assist	Manual w/c: Independent indoors and level outdoors, some assist uneven terrain	Not indicated	Personal care: 6 hours Home care: 2 hours
T1-T9	Independent	Manual w/c: Independent all terrains	Typically not functional	Homemaking: 3 hours
T10-L1	Independent	Manual w/c: Independent all terrains	Functional: Some assist to independent	Homemaking: 2 hours
L2-S5	Independent	Manual w/c: Independent all terrains	Functional: Independent to some assist	Homemaking: 0 to 1 hour

w/c=wheelchair.

Adapted from Consortium for Spinal Cord Medicine Clinical Practice Guidelines. *Outcomes Following Traumatic Spinal Cord Injury: Clinical Practice Guidelines for Health-Care Professionals.* Washington, DC: Paralyzed Veterans of America; July 1999:13-20.

immediately, medical management including medication administration must begin.[21]

Heterotopic Ossification

HO is the most common orthopedic complication after SCI, occurring in up to 50% of adult patients with SCI. With HO, bone forms at ectopic sites with the majority of the cases occurring at the hips and much less often at the knee, elbow, or shoulder. Factors contributing to this bone formation include trauma, spasticity, tissue hypoxia, and necrosis. Early symptoms include fever, joint swelling, pain, and edema in the involved limb and within weeks, significant reduction of joint mobility occurs in 10% to 20% of patients.[22]

The medical goal is to diagnose and treat HO in the initial stage typically with epidronate prior to the formation of mineralized tissue. In the later stages, when significant extra-articular bone formation has formed that limits functional mobility, surgical resection may become an option.

Orthostatic Hypotension

OH is a decrease in BP from a change in body position toward upright. This secondary impairment is most common in the first few weeks after SCI, especially in individuals with high cervical complete injuries. It is caused by pooling of blood in the LEs and viscera, coupled with the impairment of sympathetic arterial vasoconstriction. OH is helped by repeated postural challenges. In addition, abdominal binders, elastic stockings, Ace wrapping of the legs, proper hydration, salt tablets, and other pharmacological interventions are typically prescribed to address this condition.[23] Elokda and associates[24] reported that functional neuromuscular stimulation was effective in reducing OH when progressing to standing in patients with acute SCI.

IMAGING

A variety of imaging techniques are utilized to determine which elements of the spinal cord and surrounding structures are involved in the injury. These may include:

♦ CT
  ● Beneficial in detecting subtle fractures that may be difficult to visualize with radiographs
♦ MRI
  ● Noninvasive
  ● Able to obtain images of soft tissue and to provide complementary information regarding the surrounding joint
♦ Radiographs (x-ray or plain films)
  ● Most common method and is usually the first attempt to assess disorders of the skeletal system
♦ Spinal angiography
  ● May be helpful in showing the blood flow and the size, location, or configuration of a malformation

Each of the imaging techniques has its benefits for assessment. However, MRI provides the best means of evaluating the type of SCI and its evolution including prognosis for recovery.

PHARMACOLOGY

The following pharmacological agents, grouped by function, are utilized in the management of patients with SCI.[25-27]

♦ Analgesia, anti-inflammatory
  ● Examples: NSAIDs, ibuprofen (Advil, Motrin)
  ● Actions: Analgesic, anti-inflammatory
  ● Side effects: Headache, nausea, anorexia, cholestatic hepatitis, nephrotoxicity, blood dyscrasias
♦ Anticoagulation
  ● Heparin
    ■ Example: Warfarin (Coumadin)
    ■ Action: Inhibits synthesis of vitamin K dependent clotting factors
    ■ Side effects: Diarrhea, hepatitis, hematuria, rash, fever, hemorrhage, agranulocytosis, leukopenia, eosinophilia
  ● Low molecular weight heparin
    ■ Example: Dalteparin (Fragmin)
      ▸ Action: Believed to enhance inhibitory effects of antithrombin III
      ▸ Side effects: Intracranial bleeding, hemorrhage, anaphylaxis, thrombocytopenia
    ■ Example: Enoxaparin (Lovenox)
      ▸ Action: Believed to enhance inhibitory effects of antithrombin III
      ▸ Side effects: Hypochromic anemia, thrombocytopenia, cardiac toxicity
♦ Antidepression[28] (caution should be used when prescribing these medications to the elderly, to individuals with hepatic or renal insufficiency, and to patients with CNS compromise)
  ● Selective serotonin reuptake inhibitors (SSRIs)
    ■ Examples: Fluoxetine, paroxetine, sertraline
    ■ Action: Facilitate neurotransmission of serotonin and/or norepinephrine
    ■ Side effects: Greater risk than with tricyclic antidepressants (TCAs) for anticholinergic side effects and OH due to SCI, sedation
  ● TCAs
    ■ Examples: Amitriptyline, desipramine, doxepin, imipramine, nortriptyline, protriptyline, trimipramine
    ■ Action: Facilitate neurotransmission of serotonin and/or norepinephrine
    ■ Side effects: Great risk for anticholinergic side effects and OH due to SCI, sedation

- Other antidepressants
  - Examples: Amoxapine, bupropion, maprotiline nefazodone, trazodone, venlafaxine
  - Action: Facilitate neurotransmission of serotonin and/or norepinephrine
  - Side effects: Sedation, slight risk of OH
- Antihypertension
  - Example: Clonidine
  - Action: Inhibits sympathetic vasomotor center resulting in decreased BP, pulse rate, and cardiac output
  - Side effects: Congestive heart failure, OH, palpitations, drowsiness, sedation, headache, fatigue, nausea, vomiting, malaise, impotence, nocturia, rash
  - Studies: Conflicting results on the impact of clonidine on locomotor abilty,[2] with it appearing effective in the acute phase but interfering with locomotor ability in the chronic phase[4]
- AD (elevated BP) acute management
  - Example: Nifedipine
  - Action: Inhibits the transmembrane influx of calcium ions into smooth muscle, thus relaxing coronary smooth muscle and dilating coronary and peripheral arteries
  - Side effects: Congestive heart failure, myocardial infarction, pulmonary edema, nocturia, polyuria
- Bladder management
  - Example: Oxybutynin chloride (Ditropan)
    - Action: Relaxation of bladder muscles by inhibiting uptake of Ach at post-ganglionic sites
    - Side effects: Anxiety, restlessness, dizziness, convulsions, palpitations, sinus tachycardia, nausea, vomiting, anorexia
  - Example: Tamsulosin (Flomax)
    - Action: Relaxation of smooth muscles in the bladder by blocking of adrenoceptors
    - Side effects: Chest pain, dizziness, headache, nausea, diarrhea
- Bowel management
  - Examples: Senna (Senokot), docusate calcium (Colace), bisacodyl (Dulcolax suppositories, Ducolax tabs), lactulose
  - Actions: Stimulate peristalsis, soften stools, increase water
  - Side effects: Nausea, vomiting, anorexia, cramps, tetany
- Coronary vasodilation
  - Example: Topical nitroglycerin ointment 2%
  - Actions: Relaxes coronary vascular smooth muscle, dilates coronary and peripheral arteries
  - Side effects: Postural hypotension, collapse, headache, flushing, dizziness
- Heterotopic ossification

- Example: Etidronate disodium (Didronel)
- Actions: Prevents HO, decreases bone resorption and formation of new bone
- Side effects: Nephrotoxicity, seizures
- Neurogenic pain[29]
  - Example: Gabapentin (Neurontin)
    - Action: Exact mechanism of action is unknown
    - Side effects: Somnolence and dizziness
  - Example: Amitriptyline
    - Action: A TCA, it is thought to block reuptake of a variety of neurotransmitters, particularly serotonin
    - Side effects: Anticholinergic and CNS effects, such as dry mouth and somnolence
  - Example: Acetaminophen (paracetamol, Tylenol)
    - Action: Analgesic effect is believed to be comparable with aspirin but there is little or no anti-inflammatory effect
    - Side effects: Chronic ingestion and large doses can cause kidney and liver damage and effect bone marrow production, should not be taken with alcohol
- Orthostatic hypotension
  - Example: Ephedrine sulfate
    - Actions: Acts on alpha and beta receptors to increase contractility of heart and vasoconstriction of blood vessels
    - Side effects: Cerebral hemorrhage, tremors, anxiety, dizziness, palpitations, tachycardia, dysrhythmias, anorexia, nausea, vomiting, dyspnea
  - Example: Fludrocortisan
    - Actions: Acts to increase reabsorption of sodium and loss of potassium, water, and hydrogen from renal tubes
    - Side effects: Circulatory collapse, thrombophlebitis, embolism, flushing, sweating, HTN
  - Example: Midodrine
    - Actions: Acts on alpha-adrenergic receptors to increase vascular tone and BP
    - Side effects: Paresthesia, pain
- Pulmonary management
  - Example: Albuterol sulfate (Proventil nebulizer or multi-dose inhaler [MDI])
    - Action: Bronchial dilation through action on pulmonary receptors relaxing smooth muscle
    - Side effects: Pulmonary edema, hypotension, erratic pulse, tachycardia
  - Example: Ipratropium (Atrovent nebulizer or MDI)
    - Action: Bronchial dilation as a result of inhibition of Ach at receptor sites
    - Side effects: Dry mouth, constipation, urinary

retention, urinary hesitancy, headache, dizziness, paralytic ileus

- Example: Salmeterol (Serevent MDI Diskus)
  - Action: Bronchial dilation through action on pulmonary receptors relaxing smooth muscle
  - Side effects: Bronchospasm, tremors, anxiety, dry mouth
- Examples: Fluticasone propionate and salmeterol (Advair MDI Diskus)
  - Actions: Bronchial dilation through action on pulmonary receptors relaxing smooth muscle, corticosteroid decreases inflammation in lungs
  - Side effects: Bronchospasm, tremors, anxiety, dry mouth, increased BP, fast or irregular HR, chest pain, headache, lowers bone density

- ◆ Spasticity
  - Example: Baclofen
    - Actions: Inhibits synaptic responses by decreasing GABA
    - Side effects: Seizures, dizziness, weakness, fatigue, drowsiness, disorientation, nausea, vomiting
  - Example: Dantrolene sodium (Dantrium)
    - Action: Inhibits contraction of muscle by interfering with the intercellular release of calcium
    - Side effects: Seizures, eosinophilia, hepatic injury, hypotension, dizziness, weakness, fatigue, drowsiness, urinary frequency, nausea
  - Example: Diazepam (Valium)
    - Action: Facilitates presynaptic inhibition
    - Side effects: OH, neutropenia, respiratory depression, ECG changes, tachycardia, dizziness, drowsiness, blurred vision
  - Example: Tizanidine (Zanaflex)
    - Action: Acts on motor neurons by increasing presynaptic inhibition
    - Side effects: UTI infection, urinary frequency, dizziness, speech disorder, dyskinesia
- ◆ Chemical denervation commonly done with phenol, alcohol, or botulinum toxin (Botox) injection
  - Example: Phenol
    - Action: A chemodenervator or neuromuscular blocking agent that destroys the protein to decrease spasticty
    - Side effects: Transient dysaesthesias and numbness, hematomas possible, with large intravascular injection, systemic effects may include muscle tremors, convulsions, and depressed cardiac activity, BP, and respiration
  - Examples: Botulinum toxin type A (Botox, Dysport), botulinum toxin type B (Myobloc)
    - Action: Chemodenervators that block Ach releases

at the neuromuscular junction to decrease spasticity in a specific muscle group[30]

- Side effects: Pain with injection, hematoma, transient fatigue, nausea[31]

Case Study #1: Cervical Spinal Cord Injury

John Smith is a 17-year-old healthy male with a spinal cord injury resulting in C5 motor and sensory ASIA A tetraplegia secondary to a motor vehicle accident 2 weeks ago. John also has a Stage 3 sacral decubitus and Stage 1 bilateral heel decubiti.

PHYSICAL THERAPIST EXAMINATION

HISTORY

- ◆ General demographics: John Smith is a 17-year-old white male whose primary language is English. He is right-hand dominant. He is a senior in high school.
- ◆ Social history: John is single and lives with his parents and younger sister. He has a girlfriend of 1 year and also has many friends in high school. He had been involved in sports and other activities at school.
- ◆ Employment/work: He attends high school full time as a senior and has had weekend employment as a busboy in a local restaurant. He has been a member of the varsity football and baseball teams.
- ◆ Living environment: John lives in a bi-level home with six single-railed stairs to enter and eight double-railed stairs to his bedroom and bathroom. His parents plan to make their home accessible for him to return after inpatient rehabilitation.
- ◆ General health status
  - General health perception: He reports the status of his health to be good, calling himself athletic.
  - Physical function: His reported physical function had been normal for his age.
  - Psychological function: His parents report that he seems anxious and depressed since his accident.
  - Role function: High school honor student, son, boyfriend, varsity football and baseball player, drama club member, employee.
  - Social function: John has participated in high school activities, such as varsity sports, the drama club, and the National Honor Society. He is preparing for college in the fall. He enjoys socializing with his girlfriend and friends. He has his driver's license.

♦ Social/health habits: John has enjoyed skiing and running in addition to his high school sports. He denies smoking or drug use and admits to occasional alcohol consumption at school parties.

♦ Family history: His father has a history of a myocardial infarction 5 years ago, and his mother and sister are in good health.

♦ Medical/surgical history: John had an anterior cruciate ligament (ACL) repair to his left knee 2 years ago and wears contact lenses for nearsightedness.

♦ Prior hospitalizations: ACL repair 2 years ago.

♦ Preexisting medical and other health-related conditions: Noncontributory.

♦ Current condition(s)/chief complaint(s): John was an unrestrained front seat passenger in an MVA that occurred 2 weeks ago. MRI revealed C5-C6 bilateral jumped facets, and his injury was determined to be C5 sensory and motor ASIA A. He underwent a C5-C7 cervical fusion with a left iliac bone graft and anterior/posterior plating. He also received a Greenfield filter in his inferior vena cava, has a Foley catheter, and a hard cervical collar. His goals are to walk again and go to college in the fall. His parents state he has been positive in his outlook with occasional anxious and depressed periods. They express the expectation that their son "will return to normal."

♦ Functional status and activity level: John was independent in all functional activities including ADL and IADL prior to his MVA. He is currently dependent in ADL and IADL and has only been sitting in a recliner wheelchair at 50 degrees for 1 to 2 hours daily in the week since his MVA. He has tolerated 45 degrees on the tilt table for 15 minutes. He is dependent for mobility, including wheelchair propulsion and management, weight shifts, transfers, and mat mobility.

♦ Medications: John is taking the following medications daily: Percocet, heparin 5, Colace, Dulcolax suppository, Senokot, Pepcid, and Ativan.

♦ Other clinical tests
  • Doppler scan of the LEs was negative for DVT.
  • Video fluoroscopy swallow study revealed no swallowing difficulties.
  • Hip x-ray was negative for HO.
  • Urinalysis and urine culture were negative for UTI.
  • Baseline blood levels were normal.
  • Vital capacity in supine was 0.9 L (900 cc) compared to 4 liters (4000 cc) normal value.

SYSTEMS REVIEW

♦ Cardiovascular/pulmonary: All measurements were taken when John was in reclined sitting in his wheelchair while wearing an abdominal binder and compres-

sion stockings
  • BP: 100/60 mmHg
  • Edema: None noted while wearing compression stockings
  • HR: 70 bpm
  • RR: 16 bpm
♦ Integumentary
  • Presence of scar formation
    ▪ Anterior and posterior cervical surgical site with steristrips, dry and intact
    ▪ Left iliac crest scar with steristrips, dry and intact
    ▪ Abdominal surgery scar with steristrips, dry and intact
    ▪ Healed surgical incision on left knee from previous ACL repair
  • Skin color: WNL
  • Skin integrity: Sacral decubitus and bilateral posterior calcaneus decubiti present
♦ Musculoskeletal
  • Gross range of motion
    ▪ Cervical not examined secondary to medical precautions and hard collar
    ▪ UEs and LEs WFL
  • Gross strength: Limited in shoulders and elbows, absent in wrist and fingers, absent in trunk and LEs
  • Gross symmetry: Symmetrical in supported sitting
  • Height: 6'1" (1.85 m)
  • Weight: 180 lbs (81.648 kg)
♦ Neuromuscular
  • Balance: Dependent in unsupported sitting, standing not applicable
  • Locomotion, transfers, and transitions: Dependent
♦ Communication, affect, cognition, language, and learning style
  • Communication, affect, and cognition: WNL but concerned about his future
  • Learning style: John reports learning best with visual aids

TESTS AND MEASURES

♦ Aerobic capacity/endurance
  • Only tolerates sitting in reclined wheelchair at 50 degrees with head rest
  • Only tolerates standing on tilt board at 45 degrees for 15 minutes
  • Becomes short of breath with work of transfers, sitting, standing, and self-care
♦ Assistive and adaptive devices
  • Currently has the following devices and equipment
    ▪ Reclining wheelchair with elevating leg rests, head rest, specialty wheelchair seat cushion with gel

insert, foam back cushion with sacral cutout, and a lap tray

- Specialty air mattress on hospital bed
- Tilt-in-space shower commode chair
- Transfer board
- Skin inspection mirror

- John will need power wheelchair for future independent mobility

◆ Circulation
- Uses abdominal binder and compressive stockings to prevent OH
- Vital signs (taken while wearing abdominal binder and compression stockings)
  - Sitting in wheelchair: BP 100/60 mmHg, HR 70 bpm, RR 16 bpm
  - At 45 degrees on tilt table: BP 90/55 mmHg, HR 72 bpm, RR 18 bpm
- John had an episode of AD with BP 200/110 mmHg, HR 60 bpm, RR 18 bpm secondary to blockage in Foley catheter; BP back to 100/60 mmHg after catheter unblocked

◆ Cranial and peripheral nerve integrity
- Passed video fluoroscopy swallow study
- Absent sensation to pinprick and light touch below the C5 dermatome on the right and left and absent sensation in the S4-S5 dermatome, which results in a complete C5 ASIA A sensory classification based on ASIA standards[16]
- Absent motor function below the C5 myotome on the right and left and absent voluntary anal contraction, which results in a complete C5 ASIA A motor classification based on ASIA standards[16]

◆ Environmental, home, and work barriers
- His home has six single-railed stairs to enter and eight double-railed stairs to his bedroom and bathroom
- His school has 10 stairs to enter

◆ Ergonomics and body mechanics
- Body mechanics
  - John requires total assistance for functional tasks including weight shifts in wheelchair, transfer board, or mechanical lift transfers; mat mobility; and wheelchair management and propulsion secondary to decreased strength and balance
  - Caregivers will need instruction in proper body mechanics and safe ways of assisting patient

◆ Gait, locomotion, and balance
- Currently using a manual wheelchair for positioning and unable to propel
- Dependent in balance activities in sitting with no postural reactions noted below level of shoulders and elbows
- Cervical collar does not allow for head righting

◆ Integumentary integrity
- John has a 2 cm x 3 cm Stage III sacral decubitus and Stage I decubiti posteriorly on both heels
- He has several dry and intact surgical scar sites (anterior and posterior cervical, abdominal, and left iliac crest) all with steristrips
- John is utilizing a wheelchair cushion with pressure-relieving gel
- He has been instructed to request weight shifts (tilting wheelchair back) every half hour for a minute when sitting in the wheelchair and is on limited sitting schedule of 2 hours twice a day at this time secondary to sacral decubitus
- Every 2 hours, he will be turned in his hospital bed with its specialty air mattress to prevent excessive pressure when recumbent
- John has a skin inspection mirror with adapted quad handle and requires total assistance to utilize it to inspect bony prominences and other areas prone to breakdown

◆ Motor function
- His injury is at the C5 level with limited shoulder active motion, and he is not demonstrating any motor activity in wrist or fingers and no zone of partial preservation noted in trunk or LEs
- Limited neck movement at this time due to hard cervical collar and precautions to avoid AROM
- John has control over speech and facial and eye movements

◆ Muscle performance
- MMT revealed the following deviations from normal
  - Cervical: Not tested secondary to hard collar and precautions to avoid AROM
  - Shoulder flexion: R=3/5, L=3/5
  - Shoulder abduction: R=3/5, L=3/5
  - Shoulder extension: R=3/5, L=3/5
  - Elbow flexion: R=5/5, L=5/5
  - No motor activity in elbow extensors, wrist, hand, trunk, and LEs bilaterally
  - No voluntary anal contraction

◆ Orthotic, protective, and supportive devices
- John is using the following orthotic, protective, and supportive devices
  - Abdominal binder and compressive stockings when out of bed
  - Bilateral wrist supports and universal cuff to assist with feeding and basic grooming skills
  - Bilateral resting hand splints worn at night for positioning
  - Bilateral resting AFOs used in bed to prevent foot drop and skin breakdown
  - Hard cervical collar

- He is dependent for donning and doffing all devices
- John requires cueing to inspect skin for redness after use
♦ Pain
  - NPS with 0=no pain and 10=worst possible pain[32]
  - John reports pain 2/10 in the posterior cervical region at rest, 5/10 with position changes
  - He reports diffuse "burning pain" in the trunk and legs, 6/10, in the evenings (characteristic of neurogenic pain)
♦ Posture
  - Unsupported short sitting on mat: Forward head and shoulders, increased thoracic kyphosis, absent lumbar lordosis with maximal assistance required to maintain the position
  - Sitting in wheelchair: Symmetrical weightbearing on ischia and symmetrical trunk alignment
♦ Range of motion (all motions PROM)
  - Cervical not tested secondary to cervical collar and precaution to avoid cervical ROM
  - Shoulder
    - Flexion: R=160 degrees, L=165 degrees
    - Abduction: R=145 degrees, L=145 degrees
    - Extension: R=20 degrees, L=25 degrees
    - External rotation: R=50 degrees, L=55 degrees
    - Internal rotation: R=65 degrees, L=65 degrees
  - Elbow and wrist: WFL
  - Trunk: WFL
  - Hip
    - Straight leg raise: R=60 degrees, L=65 degrees
    - All other joints: WFL
  - Knee and ankle: WFL
♦ Reflex integrity
  - Increased resistance to passive stretch noted in LEs, especially in flexor musculature
  - Flexor spasms noted in both LEs with position changes and PROM
♦ Self-care and home management
  - He requires total assistance of one for transfer board placement and requires cueing to instruct others
  - He requires total assistance for transfers to shower chair, commode chair, hospital bed, and recliner wheelchair
  - His home, job, and school have stairs, which will need to be navigated with use of the wheelchair
  - John is currently dependent for all functional activities, including ADL and IADL, and he needs cueing to give instructions to caregivers
  - He is learning to use devices and equipment to assist in performance of functional activities
♦ Ventilation and respiration/gas exchange
  - John did not require intubation or ventilatory support at the time of his injury
  - His vital capacity is 900 cc (0.9 liters) in supine and 800 cc (0.8 liters) in sitting
  - He is a diaphragmatic breather with some accessory muscle usage (upper trapezius, anterior scalene, and sternocleidomastoid muscles) noted with deep inspiratory effort
  - No intercostal muscle activity noted
  - His cough is weak and nonproductive secondary to absent abdominal musculature
  - He requires cueing to instruct others in an assisted cough to remove secretions
♦ Work, community, and leisure integration or reintegration
  - His home, school, and work environments will need to be evaluated to determine how to allow wheelchair accessibility (stairs, doorways, bathroom, shower, etc) either through a home evaluation form filled out by the family or through a site visit by both the physical and occupational therapists
  - John's weekend job at the restaurant requires clearing of tables and lifting of trays
  - John had been driving a car
    - A driver training evaluation may become appropriate in the future
    - He will be referred to a driving specialist for accessible van prescription
  - He is concerned about finishing high school and attending college

EVALUATION

John is a previously healthy 17-year-old male who is 2 weeks post MVA. He is a high school senior and was involved in athletic and scholastic activities. His driving accident resulted in a C5 ASIA A (sensory and motor complete) SCI. He underwent a C5-C7 cervical fusion with left iliac crest graft and anterior and posterior plating. He also received a Greenfield filter in the inferior vena cava and has a Foley catheter. He has a Stage III sacral decubitus and bilateral Stage I decubiti on his heels. He is currently wearing a hard cervical collar and has restrictions for active movement. He tolerates reclined supported sitting at 45 degrees at this time. He is dependent for functional activities, such as ADL, wheelchair management and propulsion, weight shifts, transfers, and mat mobility. His home and school will require modifications to allow wheelchair accessibility. His goals are to walk again and go to college in the fall.

DIAGNOSIS

John is a patient with C5 ASIA A (sensory and motor complete) tetraplegia due to MVA that resulted in SCI with cervical vertebra dislocation 2 weeks ago. He now has a Stage III sacral ulcer and Stage I bilateral heel ulcers. He is currently experiencing pain. He has impaired: aerobic capacity/endurance; circulation; cranial and peripheral nerve integrity; ergonomics and body mechanics; gait, locomotion, and balance; integumentary integrity; motor function; muscle performance; posture; range of motion; reflex integrity; and ventilation and respiration/gas exchange. He is functionally limited in self-care and home management and in work, community, and leisure actions, tasks, and activities. He has environmental, home, and work barriers. He is also in need of assistive, adaptive, orthotic, protective, and supportive devices and equipment. These findings are consistent with placement in Pattern H: Impaired Motor Function, Peripheral Nerve Integrity, and Sensory Integrity Associated With Nonprogressive Disorders of the Spinal Cord. Due to the presence of decubitus ulcers on John's sacrum and heels, classification in an additional integumentary pattern is required. Based on the stages of his ulcers, John is also placed in Integumentary Pattern D: Impaired Integumentary Integrity Associated With Full-Thickness Skin Involvement and Scar Formation.[33] The identified impairments, functional limitations, barriers, and device and equipment needs will be addressed in determining the prognosis and the plan of care.

PROGNOSIS AND PLAN OF CARE

Over the course of the inpatient and outpatient visits, the following mutually established outcomes have been determined:
- ♦ Ability to instruct others in his care including management of power wheelchair and equipment, assistance with bed mobility and transfers, and home management is improved
- ♦ Ability to perform physical activities (with assistive and adaptive devices as needed) related to self-care, home management, work, community, and leisure is improved
- ♦ Ability to tolerate upright sitting and balance in this position is improved
- ♦ Aerobic capacity is increased
- ♦ Devices and equipment are issued, and patient is able to provide instruction in their usage and maintenance
- ♦ Environmental barriers at home, school, and play are addressed and overcome
- ♦ Knowledge is gained of behaviors that address precautions related to SCI including skin breakdown, HO, osteoporosis, DVT, AD, respiratory complications, and OH
- ♦ Muscle performance is increased in UE, cervical, and respiratory musculature to allow performance of ADL
- ♦ ROM is increased to allow functional activities
- ♦ Wound healing is enhanced

To achieve these outcomes, the appropriate interventions for this patient are determined. These will include: coordination, communication, and documentation; patient/client-related instruction; therapeutic exercise; functional training in self-care and home management; functional training in work, community, and leisure integration and reintegration; manual therapy techniques; prescription, application, and, as appropriate, fabrication of devices and equipment; airway clearance techniques; integumentary repair and protection techniques; electrotherapeutic modalities; and physical agents and mechanical modalities.

John is expected to need about 150 visits over a 2-month period of time. Based on the diagnosis of C5 ASIA A tetraplegia, John is expected to require moderate to total assist for transfers in and out of bed, can be modified independent for power wheelchair mobility, and may require care in the home up to 16 hours per day. Follow-up visits are anticipated after discharge from inpatient care.

INTERVENTIONS

RATIONALE FOR SELECTED INTERVENTIONS

Therapeutic Exercise

Following SCI, the exercise program must address strengthening of existing musculature, increasing flexibility of the joints and the paralytic muscles, and training in balance and coordination so that daily activities are most easily accomplished in light of the neuromuscular deficits. According to Nash,[34] an exercise program for a person with a SCI should follow guidelines to minimize certain inherent health-related consequences of SCI, including alterations in adrenergic regulation and thermal regulation, increased risk of fractures and musculoskeletal injury, and accelerated cardiovascular disease. For example, UE pain is common after SCI and is often due to insufficient shoulder strength and ROM coupled with strenuous functional activities, such as transfers and wheelchair propulsion.[35] Specific exercises and activities, including practicing proper wheelchair propulsion, should be included in the exercise program to address and prevent shoulder dysfunction.

In addition, patients with SCI often have thermal dysregulation due to impaired vasomotor and sudomotor responses below the level of the injury and must keep hydrated and avoid extremes of temperature.[36] Patients with high level injuries are more susceptible to AD and should be educated to empty their bladder and urine bags before exercising.[37] OH is also a concern for high level injuries. Ditor and associates[38] found that measures of HR variability and BP variability are reliable and valid and may be used in the clinic to monitor the patient's response to interventions. They also found that patients with SCI were able to lower their HR and BP following 6 months of BWSTT.

Duran and colleagues[39] found that patients with SCI demonstrated improved measures of physical function after a program of directed physical exercise including muscle strength, power, and endurance training. Diaphragmatic strengthening and general inspiratory muscle training have been described as effective treatment interventions by Frownfelter and Dean[40] for patients with SCI and even shown by Sprague and Hopkins[41] to assist in the weaning of six patients who were ventilator dependent. Stowell and colleagues[42] suggested that the clinical aquatic environment is an efficient method of incorporating multiple therapeutic activities.

BWSTT has been researched and clinically tried with subjects with SCI.[2,7,38,43-50] Behrman and Harkema[46] found that locomotor training that was designed to optimize sensory cues related to locomotion in order to facilitate more normal stepping on a treadmill and overground resulted in improved performance in patients with both complete and incomplete SCI. In the clinical setting, more typically the patient with incomplete tetraplegia or paraplegia utilizes the BWSTT system in a progression toward more independent ambulation.[12] Studies have demonstrated that the predictor for overground walking following BWSTT is whether the injury is complete vs incomplete, not the neurological level of the injury.[2,4,5,12,43] Individuals with incomplete SCI, regardless of neurological level, appear to be able to benefit from BWSTT. Individuals with complete injury were able to perform stepping on the treadmill with assistance but were unable to transfer stepping to overground stepping and lost stepping ability once training stopped.[12,43] This patient with a complete injury is not a candidate for BWSTT for ambulation but may benefit from it for other therapeutic reasons. Therapeutic benefits of BWSTT include increased ability to bear weight on legs, improved trunk posture, improved balance in standing,[5,43,46,47] improved cardiovascular function, and decreased severity of spastic symptoms.[2] The reader is referred to Case Study #2 in this chapter for additional information on BWSTT.

Functional Training in Self-Care and Home Management

As a result of the SCI and resulting tetraplegia, patients with level C5 ASIA A will need to learn how to perform self-care activities with a variety of compensatory techniques and equipment including durable medical equipment and orthoses. Assistive technology equipment and product systems including electronic aids to daily living will be ordered as needed to improve the patient's functional capabilities.[51] At John's level of injury, with absent elbow extensors and wrist/finger musculature, he will be taught how to instruct others in his care, since he will need assistance with most self-care and mobility activities.[17] John will be taught compensatory movement patterns and methods so that he can maximize

his mobility.[52] For example, by locking out his elbows with shoulder external rotation and relative flexion with weight-bearing on palms of hands in wrist extension, he can be taught to bear weight on them. In addition, using momentum to initiate movement and incorporating the strategy that "head goes opposite the hips" can both assist with functional mobility activities, such as transfers.

Functional Training in Work, Community, and Leisure Integration or Reintegration

Reintegration into the community, school, and leisure activities is challenging for a patient with a SCI, especially with locomotion at the wheelchair level. NSCISC data for employment 10 years post injury is only 24.2% for individuals with tetraplegia.[13] A wide variety of assistive and adaptive devices and equipment is available, and trial usage of all appropriate devices and equipment with John should be undertaken in order to maximize his capabilities.[52,53] The equipment and product systems, whether commercially acquired or customized for this patient, fall under the title of "assistive technology" and will improve his functional capabilities outside of the home.[51]

Manual Therapy Techniques

Soft tissue dysfunction is common following SCI with neurological deficits. With decreased AROM in the UEs and absent musculature in the trunk and LEs, this patient is likely to develop joint and soft tissue limitations. Specifically, Curtis and associates[54] found shoulder pain in two thirds of the sample of patients with SCI who used manual wheelchairs. In another study, Curtis and associates[55] suggested that a standard exercise protocol consisting of flexibility and strengthening interventions could decrease the intensity of shoulder pain that interferes with functional activity in wheelchair users. John will be most likely utilizing a power wheelchair but can still experience shoulder pain with functional activities secondary to muscle imbalance and limitations in shoulder ROM.

Manual therapy techniques may include massage, PROM, joint mobilization for the glenohumeral and scapular joints, and soft tissue mobilization.

Prescription, Application, and, as Appropriate, Fabrication of Devices and Equipment

John has already been provided with the following devices and equipment: a reclining wheelchair with elevating leg rests, head rest, a specialty wheelchair seat cushion with gel insert, foam back cushion with sacral cutout, and a lap tray; a specialty type mattress on his hospital bed; a shower chair; a commode chair; a transfer board; a skin inspection mirror with quad adapted handle; an abdominal binder; and compressive stockings. He will also need a power wheelchair with possible joystick control for future independent mobility.

Patients with neurological impairment often benefit from devices that provide a more stable alignment, protect joints and skin, or assist functional activities. A patient with limited UE use will require not only the appropriate wheelchair seating system and cushion, but also devices and equipment to assist in self-care and other daily tasks.[52,53] This patient with a neurological level of C5 ASIA A and limited shoulder and elbow strength and absent wrist and finger strength will require wrist splints and perhaps a cuff around the hand to hold utensils and devices to assist with feeding, writing, and typing. His wheelchair may be fitted with an adaptation, typically known as a balanced forearm orthosis (BFO), to support and position his arm to assist with feeding.

He may also be appropriate for a cough-assist modality, known as mechanical in-exsufflation that can be augmented with timed Heimlich maneuver manual assist (see section on airway clearance for more details).

Airway Clearance Techniques

A SCI involving the cervical spine will impair the patient's ventilatory function in varying degrees depending on the severity of neurological damage. An injury at a cervical level will definitely affect the intercostals (with a role in both inhalation and exhalation), the abdominals (needed for effective cough), and the diaphragm (the main muscle of inspiration) with its innervation at C3, C4, and C5. It is crucial for this patient with absent intercostals and abdominals to maximize his ventilatory capacity to avoid life-threatening complications. Interventions will include teaching John how to utilize postural drainage positions to centralize secretions and then how to instruct an assisted cough. In addition, diaphragmatic strengthening, as described by Frownfelter and Dean,[40] can improve his vital capacity and has been reported by Sprague and colleagues[41] to assist in improving respiratory function enough to wean from a ventilator, in those who are ventilator dependent. An inspiratory training device will also enhance maximum inspiration.

Cough may be improved by manually assisting the patient in a Heimlich maneuver type of thrust to the abdomen on the exhalation phase and/or by means of a mechanical insufflation/exsufflation device.[56] This mechanical device applies a positive pressure breath (insufflation) followed by negative pressure (exsufflation) in order to stimulate a cough to facilitate secretion clearance. The device is intended to aid individuals whose cough function is ineffective.[57]

Integumentary Repair and Protection Techniques

Presence of a decubitis ulcer requires placement in the appropriate integumentary pattern. The reader is referred to *Integumentary Essentials: Applying the Preferred Physical Therapist Practice Patterns*[SM58] for the anatomy, physiology, pathophysiology, and rationale for interventions of the integument. For specific rationale for Stage I pressure ulcers refer to

Chapter 2, Impaired Integumentary Integrity Associated With Superficial Skin Involvement (Pattern B) in *Integumentary Essentials*.[59] For specific rationale for Stage III pressure ulcers refer to Chapter 4, Impaired Integumentary Integrity Associated With Full-Thickness Skin Involvement and Scar Formation (Pattern D) in *Integumentary Essentials*.[60]

Electrotherapeutic Modalities

Therapeutic programs of functional electrical stimulation (FES) for patients with a cervical SCI may enhance UE function[61] either in a muscle reeducation format or within a neuroprosthesis. A neuroprosthesis uses implanted electrodes in UE muscles below the level of the injury that are stimulated by contractions of intact muscles above the level of injury. An implanted neuroprosthetic system for the LEs to facilitate ambulation is also an option for LE muscles of patients with incomplete SCI and therefore is not appropriate for this patient.[62] Diaphragmatic or phrenic nerve pacing is not an appropriate intervention for this patient with an intact diaphragm but is typically considered for patients on ventilators with partial or absent diaphragmatic innervation to allow for degrees of weaning from the ventilator with electrodes surgically placed on the motor point of the diaphragm.[63] Other potential therapeutic uses of electrical stimulation may include stimulation of exhalation muscles to facilitate improved cough effectiveness, stimulation of intact sacral nerves to stimulate bowel and bladder function as well as ejaculation,[64] and stimulation of knee extensors and plantarflexors during standing to minimize effects of postural related orthostatic stress.[24]

John is also a possible candidate for one of the computer-mediated FES cycle ergometry programs for the LEs. These ergometry programs have been shown to result in various physiologic benefits, including increased blood flow to the LEs[65] and increased muscle mass.[66] Bickel and colleagues[67] found that muscle was able to respond to electromyostimulation-induced resistance exercise in individuals with complete SCI.

High-volt electrical stimulation has been shown to result in enhanced healing of decubitus ulcers and should be considered for management of John's sacral decubitus.[68] TENS may also be utilized to decrease pain.[69]

Physical Agents and Mechanical Modalities

To decrease musculoskeletal pain, modalities such as hot packs and cold packs may be helpful. Tolerance to upright can be improved by utilizing a tilt table at gradually increasing degrees of inclination or with a standing frame as a progression.

COORDINATION, COMMUNICATION, AND DOCUMENTATION

Communication will occur with John, his family members, and his girlfriend to engender support for his therapy program and home exercise program. Interdisciplinary team-work will occur as needed including case conferences and family meetings. Collaboration and coordination will occur with agencies including equipment suppliers, home care agencies, schools, and transportation agencies. Referrals will be made to other professionals or resources to ensure that all of the patient's needs are being met. All elements of the patient's management will be documented.

PATIENT/CLIENT-RELATED INSTRUCTION

John will be instructed in the precautions related to his SCI and in behaviors to prevent or address complications including skin breakdown, DVT, respiratory dysfunction, OH, HO, AD, and osteoporosis. John's family will also be instructed in how to assist John with the behaviors that can prevent or address these complications.

He will also be taught how to instruct others to assist him in his care, as he learns the compensatory techniques for mobility. These may include weight shifts, transfers to various surfaces, mat and bed mobility, and wheelchair maneuvering on stairs, curbs, and ramps. His family will be instructed in how to assist John with these activities.

John will also be instructed in a home exercise program of therapeutic exercises including PROM, stretching of his limbs and trunk, and muscle strengthening for his UEs, neck, and respiratory musculature (diaphragm and accessory muscles).

THERAPEUTIC EXERCISE

- ◆ Aerobic conditioning/endurance conditioning
  - Mode
    - Aerobic using UE and cervical muscles
    - Continuous or for prolonged period
  - Examples
    - Upper body cycle: With hands secured to handles of upper body cycle and possible chest strap, patient cycles forward or backward or both
    - Arm exercises: Use elastic band or cuff weights as tolerated on wrists for various UE movement patterns
    - Swimming in pool: Use flotation devices on trunk and legs as needed, patient lying on his back and performing arm strokes in the water
  - Duration
    - 15 to 20 minutes initially and work up to 30 minutes of continuous activity
    - Increase duration progressively
  - Intensity
    - Determine appropriate perceived exertion using the modified Borg scale[70] so that he is working in the aerobic or training zone
    - The patient would rate his effort between 3 and 7 on a scale of 1 to 10

- Frequency
  - Start with two to three times per week and progress to three to four times per week
- ◆ Balance, coordination, and agility training
  - Short and long sitting balance activities on mat, sitting in wheelchair, or in short sitting on tilt board
  - Using UE support: Practice anterior, lateral, and posterior weightbearing and weight shifts with instruction to lock out elbows utilizing shoulder musculature (shoulder external rotation and relative flexion with weightbearing on palm in wrist extension) in absence of triceps muscles
  - Without UE support: John will be instructed in how his head and UEs can be used to assist in maintaining midline
  - In modified kneeling on an inclined bench with full knee flexion and approximately 90 degrees hip flexion with buttocks on bench: Practice balance with and without UE support
- ◆ Body mechanics and postural stabilization
  - In the absence of trunk and lower body AROM, John will utilize his arms and vision (and head/neck when cervical collar removed) to facilitate postural alignment
- ◆ Flexibility exercises
  - Cervical ROM when cleared by surgeon
  - PROM and stretching of shoulder, elbow, wrist, and fingers with emphasis on anterior shoulder stretch, elbow extension, and wrist extension with finger flexion to maintain tenodesis
  - Full shoulder external rotation and extension, elbow extension, supination, and wrist extension with finger flexion needed to lock out and bear weight on hands
  - Trunk PROM and stretching
  - LE PROM and stretching of hips, knees, and ankles with emphasis on hamstring, hip adductor, and ankle plantarflexor muscle groups
  - Straight leg raise of approximately 90 degrees recommended for long sitting position and full hip external rotation needed to don/doff shoes
- ◆ Gait and locomotion training
  - With a complete high cervical injury, John is not a candidate for traditional gait training but may be appropriate for BWSTT for therapeutic purposes according to the following four locomotor training principles[6,27]
    - Maximize weightbearing on the legs: Harness system provides support of body weight allowing maximum to no support; amount of support is decreased as John is able to take more weight and continue to step using appropriate pattern
    - Optimize sensory cues: Orthotics are not used in

order to allow sensory input through the foot and ankle; loading of LE and hip extension are critical for sensory input

- Optimize kinematics for each motor task: Manual assistance is provided to each leg to ensure appropriate stepping and alignment of legs; the amount of manual assistance is decreased as John demonstrates the ability to perform the step appropriately

- Maximize recovery and minimize compensation: BWSTT provides for neuroplasticity within the spinal cord; allows for John to actively participate in movement; limit the use of arms for weight-bearing and encourage arm swing during gait cycle

- Training in use and safety of a power wheelchair with joystick control for indoor and community use

- Trial use in manual wheelchair mobility with power-assist wheels or possible modifications on push rims, such as raised projections, to facilitate propulsion

♦ Strength, power, and endurance training

- Instruct in position changes with compensatory techniques
  - Head and shoulders move opposite of hips and lower trunk
  - Lock out elbows in absence of triceps with shoulder flexors and external rotators
  - Weight shifts in wheelchair anteriorly, tilting back, and laterally

- Gross and fine motor tasks for UE to be done in conjunction with occupational therapy

- UE program includes active assistive, active, and resistive exercises with emphasis on balanced shoulder and increased elbow strength (eg, scapular retraction, protraction, and elevation; shoulder flexion, abduction, and extension; internal rotation and external rotation; forearm supination; and elbow flexion)

- Weightbearing exercises including prone on elbows, supine on elbows, and long and short sitting with weightbearing on hands with elbows locked out or elbows positioned anteriorly, posteriorly, or laterally

- Diaphragmatic and accessory muscle strengthening, including deep breathing, controlled exhalation, and use of an inspiratory muscle trainer

FUNCTIONAL TRAINING IN SELF-CARE AND HOME MANAGEMENT

♦ Self-care and home management

- Self-care including bathing, dressing, eating, grooming, toileting
  - John will be instructed in the utilization of appropriate assistive technology to improve his

functional ability in these areas

- Refer to Devices and Equipment Use and Training section
- Transfers to various surfaces including bed, car, toilet, wheelchair
- Bed mobility including sitting to and from supine, rolling left and right, and supine to and from prone
- Devices and equipment use and training
  - Dressing aids including loops sewn in clothing and/or Velcro closures and techniques for patient to assist with upper body dressing
  - Electronic aids to daily living including phone system, call bells, computer access, and environmental control units with possible house wiring
  - Mechanical lifts may be necessary depending on caregiver ability
  - Shower/commode chair with back rest, head rest, and lateral supports as needed
  - Transfer board to assist with transfers
- Various splints to assist with fine motor tasks including wrist supports, typing pegs, cuff to hold utensils

- Wheelchair management and propulsion (manual and power)

♦ IADL training

- Simple meal preparation, shopping, and limited household chores can be tried to determine if possible

- Instruction in how to direct caregivers and use technology to assist with completion of tasks

- Injury prevention or reduction

- Instruction in prevention of injury when performing self-care and mobility activities with neurological deficits including measures to protect skin and joints with impaired sensation and motor control[53,54]

- Instruction of caregivers in prevention of injury when assisting John in ADL

FUNCTIONAL TRAINING IN WORK, COMMUNITY, AND LEISURE INTEGRATION OR REINTEGRATION

♦ Device and equipment use and training will require John to instruct others

- Wheelchair mobility on stairs, curbs, and ramps

- Use of computer/writing devices during school

- Accessible van usage with lift or car transfers with transfer board

♦ Functional training programs

- Travel training[53] in wheelchair includes skills neces-

sary to move from one place to another safely and efficiently
- May include indoor and outdoor mobility as well as use of transportation
- Simulated environments and tasks

◆ Work, community, and leisure activities with instruments and equipment as needed at wheelchair level
- IADL training
- Injury prevention and reduction
- Instructing others to assist as needed to maintain safety during school, leisure, and community activities
- Instruction of caregivers in prevention of injury when assisting patient in IADL
- Leisure activities including sports at wheelchair level

MANUAL THERAPY TECHNIQUES

◆ Massage
- Connective tissue and therapeutic massage with emphasis on cervical (within surgical precautions) and shoulder regions
◆ Mobilization of soft tissue
- Emphasis on shoulder region with goal of balanced shoulder which can reduce pain and overuse
- Stretch anterior shoulder soft tissue structures and scapular region
◆ PROM
- Maximize and maintain ROM of limbs and trunk to allow function

PRESCRIPTION, APPLICATION, AND, AS APPROPRIATE, FABRICATION OF DEVICES AND EQUIPMENT

◆ Adaptive devices
- Assessment and prescription of environmental controls, typically in collaboration with occupational therapy and speech therapy
- Seating system in wheelchair to achieve optimal postural alignment
◆ Assistive devices
- Power wheelchair with appropriate mode of control (possibly joystick) and weight shift capability
- Manual wheelchair as back up with aids for propulsion, such as power-assisted wheels or modifications on push rims
- Shower chair and commode chair
- Hospital bed with specialty mattress
- Consider mechanical lift at home for ease of transfers
- Wrist supports for motor tasks and positioning

◆ Orthotic devices
- Positioning braces to prevent foot drop and heel decubiti when in bed
- Dynamic UE or LE splints to decrease contracture as needed
◆ Protective devices
- Mattress topper or specialty bed as needed to prevent skin breakdown
- Elbow pads to prevent breakdown with weightbearing on elbows
- Heel protectors or positioning boots
- Specialized cushion for wheelchair to distribute weight in sitting
◆ Supportive devices
- Compressive stockings and possibly Ace wraps for LEs to decrease edema and prevent OH
- Abdominal binder to enhance diaphragmatic breathing and to prevent OH
- Cervical collar
- Therapeutic taping techniques: Support taping may be tried as a means of shoulder realignment to facilitate muscle retraining of the shoulder

AIRWAY CLEARANCE TECHNIQUES

◆ Breathing strategies
- Techniques to maximize diaphragmatic breathing
- Techniques to improve use of accessory muscles of breathing
- Techniques to maximize ventilation including maximum inspiratory hold and staircase breathing (several inhalation efforts in a row without exhalation)
◆ Manual/mechanical techniques
- Assisted cough by patient and by assistant
- Chest percussion and vibration
- Chest wall stretch and rib mobilization
- Mechanical in-exsufflation
◆ Positioning
- Positioning to alter the work of breathing (eg, position to enhance diaphragmatic action typically with trunk reclined to lessen working against gravity)
- Positioning to maximize ventilation and perfusion
- Pulmonary postural drainage to centralize secretions

INTEGUMENTARY REPAIR AND PROTECTION TECHNIQUES

◆ For specific intervention techniques for Stage I ulcers, see Case Study #2 in Impaired Integumentary Integrity Associated With Superficial Skin Involvement (Pattern B) in *Integumentary Essentials*[59]
◆ For specific intervention techniques for Stage III ulcers,

see Case Study #3 in Impaired Integumentary Integrity Associated With Full-Thickness Skin Involvement and Scar Formation (Pattern D) in *Integumentary Essentials*[60]

ELECTROTHERAPEUTIC MODALITIES

♦ FES
  ● UEs: Enhance active contraction of the existing musculature including the biceps, deltoids, and rotator cuff
  ● LE strengthening program of specific muscles with electrical current of an adequate amplitude to allow for contraction for typically a 20- to 30-minute session as tolerated
  ● LEs: ERGYS Rehabilitation System—computerized FES program of cycling
  ● Evaluate for appropriateness of neuroprostheses for UEs and/or LEs to enhance function
♦ High voltage pulsed current
  ● For enhanced healing of pressure ulcers
    ■ Duration up to 60 minutes
    ■ Applied typically with an active electrode positioned at the wound and a dispersive electrode positioned at a distance from the wound
    ■ Use continuous mode
    ■ Frequency of 30 to 200 pulses per second and an amplitude of 1 to 500 volts[71]
♦ TENS
  ● For decreasing pain via triggering complex physiological systems of the PNS and CNS
    ■ For shoulder pain
    ■ For neurogenic pain

PHYSICAL AGENTS AND MECHANICAL MODALITIES

♦ Physical agents
  ● Cryotherapy
    ■ Cold packs and ice massage for shoulder pain and inflammation
  ● Hydrotherapy
    ■ Pool therapy for UE strengthening, relaxation of tone, balance, and body awareness
  ● Thermotherapy
    ■ Hot packs for UE and cervical pain
    ■ Paraffin and fluidotherapy for finger/hand flexibility
♦ Mechanical modalities
  ● Standing frame and tilt table to address OH and increase tolerance to upright

ANTICIPATED GOALS AND EXPECTED OUTCOMES

♦ Impact on pathology/pathophysiology
  ● Atelectasis is prevented, and John will demonstrate improved ability to perform diaphragmatic breathing and improve vital capacity to 1500 cc.
  ● Pain is decreased, and John will instruct others independently in proper wheelchair positioning to avoid shoulder impingement with functional tasks.
  ● Pressure on body tissues is reduced, so that John will independently instruct in techniques for skin inspection and pressure relieving in bed and in the wheelchair.
  ● Wound healing is enhanced such that John will achieve closure of the sacral decubitus and be independent with performing tilt back pressure relief while in power wheelchair.
♦ Impact on impairments
  ● Ability to perform movement tasks is improved.
  ● Aerobic capacity is increased to point where John will achieve 15 to 20 minutes of UE cycling to improve endurance for functional tasks.
  ● Cough is improved, and John will independently instruct others in how to perform assisted cough maneuver.
  ● Flexibility is increased to allow functional activities that include positions, such as long sitting on mat or bed (at a range of at least 90 degrees passive straight leg raise), prone on elbows, and weightbearing on extended arms behind him (will have full shoulder extension and external rotation, elbow extension, supination, and wrist extension).
  ● Joint restrictions are reduced, and John will achieve increased scapular mobility to facilitate shoulder movements needed for feeding himself with equipment as needed with supervision.
  ● Joint stability is improved with optimized alignment so that John will independently instruct others in donning of wrist support splints bilaterally to assist with fine motor tasks including typing, and donning of positional boots to be worn in bed to prevent foot drop and pressure sores.
  ● Motor function is improved, so that John will demonstrate improved ability to reposition upper body in the wheelchair with appropriate UE motions on arm rests.
  ● Muscle performance is increased, and John will demonstrate improved shoulder and elbow strength to allow 10 minutes of typing on the computer with adaptive UE splints.
  ● Muscle performance of the diaphragm and accessory muscles of respiration is improved, and John will

perform deep breathing exercises using his diaphragm to facilitate improved vital capacity up to 1500 cc.

- Muscle performance of UEs is enhanced with increased biceps and deltoid strength of his RUE to allow independent feeding with wrist support splint.
- Physical function is improved.
- Postural control is improved, and John will independently instruct others and himself in proper positioning in his wheelchair to allow optimal function and pressure relief.
- ROM is improved, and dorsiflexion ROM is to 5 degrees to allow proper positioning on foot rest of wheelchair, and shoulder extension and external rotation, elbow extension, and wrist extension ROM are full to allow propping on extended arms behind him as a position of improved sitting balance.
- Sitting balance is improved in wheelchair and in unsupported long and short sitting on mat, and John will demonstrate ability to independently reach for objects on table with right arm with left arm hooking around push handle of wheelchair for stability.
- Tolerance to upright is increased, so that he is able to sit in his wheelchair 4 to 5 hours with 70-degree wheelchair back support position.
- Ventilation and respiration/gas exchange are improved.
- Ventilatory muscles are strengthened to allow for increased vital capacity to 1500 cc, decreased work of breathing, and improved airway clearance.

♦ Impact on functional limitations
- Ability to instruct others to assist in his care is improved, and John will independently instruct his caregivers in techniques of assisted cough, turning in bed, positioning in the wheelchair, and stretching of his extremities.
- Ability to perform or instruct others in physical tasks and activities related to self-care (including toileting, taking a shower, and transfers in and out of bed with mechanical lift) and home management is improved.
- Ability to perform physical tasks and activities related to work, community, and leisure is improved, so that John will independently instruct others in wheelchair mobility techniques on stairs and curbs and how to load the wheelchair into a vehicle, and he will independently access transportation including knowing transportation options, schedules, and processes in order to attend medical appointments and school and leisure activities.
- Performance of these activities with equipment and adaptive devices is improved, and John will independently utilize a power wheelchair with joystick control in his school setting and will instruct his caregivers as needed.

♦ Impact on disabilities
- John resumes his role of student.
- John returns to school.
- Performance levels in self-care, home management, work, community, and leisure activities are improved.

♦ Risk reduction/prevention
- Complications of immobility are reduced, so that John independently instructs caregivers in PROM of his extremities and trunk to maintain functional ROM.
- Prevention or healing of skin breakdown is achieved, and John will independently instruct caregivers in skin inspection and pressure-relieving techniques in the bed and wheelchair.
- Risk of secondary impairment, such as shoulder pain, is reduced through performance of a home exercise program that includes shoulder stretches and exercises and through independent instruction of others in how to assist with this program to minimize risk of shoulder pain secondary to poor alignment with activities.
- Risk of secondary impairments is reduced and safety is improved during performance of self-care activities, and John will be able to independently instruct his parents to safely perform self-care activities including showering, toileting, dressing, and transfers with mechanical lift or transfer board.

♦ Impact on health, wellness, and fitness
- Behaviors that foster healthy habits, wellness, and prevention are acquired, and John will independently instruct others to perform skin inspections, assisted cough, turning in bed, and stretching his extremities and trunk.
- Health status is improved.
- John will be able to recognize and verbalize signs and treatment of AD, pressure sores, HO, and bowel and bladder dysfunction.

♦ Impact on societal resources
- Collaboration and coordination occurs with agencies as needed.
- Communication occurs across settings through case conferences, education plans, and documentation.
- Decision making is enhanced regarding John's health and the use of health care resources.
- Documentation occurs throughout patient management and follows APTA's *Guidelines for Physical Therapy Documentation.*[33]
- Referrals are made to other professionals or resources when appropriate.

♦ Patient/client satisfaction
- John's and family's knowledge and awareness of the

diagnosis, prognosis, interventions, and anticipated goals and expected outcomes are increased.

REEXAMINATION

Reexamination is performed throughout the episode of care. It is anticipated that patients placed in this pattern will require multiple episodes of care over their lifetime. Periodic reexamination and initiation of new episodes of care should occur as the patient's functional limitations or disabilities change and as the need for secondary prevention arises. This will allow the patient to continue to be safe and effectively adapt as a result of changes in multiple factors including his own physical status, caregivers, environment, or task demands.

DISCHARGE

John is discharged from physical therapy after a total of 130 visits over 2 months and attainment of his goals and expectations. As John's SCI may impact his future function, he received education regarding factors that may trigger a call to his physical therapist for a reexamination and new episode of physical therapy care. John is discharged from this episode of care after attaining the identified goals and placed on an episode of physical therapy prevention. This is a series of unspecified visits or contacts that allows John to continue to utilize the expertise of his physical therapist while he continues his home program. The episode of physical therapy prevention will focus on John's prevention and risk management program. As John has a chronic condition, it is important for him to have periodic contact with his physical therapist to discuss changes and if necessary return for a new examination. As a part of this episode of prevention, John's physical therapist will contact him one time per month to check on his home program, any changes in status, and any other needs he may have.

PSYCHOLOGICAL ASPECTS

A SCI changes an individual's life profoundly and typically induces a period of enforced helplessness post injury followed by a gradual resumption of limited independence. Depression is a common post-injury diagnosis that compounds disability, usually appearing within the first month, more frequently in those with complete injuries than with incomplete injuries. Individuals with SCI should be periodically screened for depression including an assessment of their social support system and receive a treatment plan including patient and family education and referrals to mental health services and community resources.[72]

Case Study #2: Thoracic Spinal Cord Injury

Juan Lopez is a 40-year-old male with a spinal cord injury resulting in T11 sensory and motor incomplete ASIA C paraplegia secondary to a fall.

PHYSICAL THERAPIST EXAMINATION

HISTORY

♦ General demographics: Mr. Lopez is a 40-year-old Hispanic male whose primary language is Spanish, and he is also fluent in English. He is a high school graduate. He is right-hand dominant.

♦ Social history: Mr. Lopez is divorced and has a 20-year-old son and an 18-year-old daughter who live with his ex-wife in a nearby town. He socializes with his coworkers and a brother frequently.

♦ Employment/work: He is a self-employed roofer with two assistants. He has a home office.

♦ Living environment: The patient lives alone on the seventh floor of an apartment building with an elevator. His brother lives in the same apartment building on the first floor.

♦ General health status
  ● General health perception: He reports the status of his health had been good.
  ● Physical function: He reported that his physical function prior to the accident had been normal for his age.
  ● Psychological function: Mr. Lopez reports being "in shock" about the accident and resulting disability. His brother states that he seems to be "coping as well as he could be but doesn't talk much about it."
  ● Role function: Employer, father, roofer, brother, uncle, recreational sports team member.
  ● Social function: He played in a summer baseball league and has been a member of a winter bowling league. He enjoys spending time with his children and often socializes on the weekends with friends.

♦ Social/health habits: He smokes two packs of cigarettes per week. He denies drug use and admits to drinking five to six bottles of beer per week. He reports having little time for exercise other than his baseball and bowling, claiming that his work is "enough exercise."

♦ Family history: His father is deceased secondary to cancer, and his mother is in good health.

♦ Medical/surgical history: Mr. Lopez had a left inguinal hernia surgical repair 4 years ago.

♦ Prior hospitalizations: He was hospitalized for the surgery to repair the hernia.

♦ Preexisting medical and other health-related conditions: Mr. Lopez has HTN, which was diagnosed 5 years ago and is regulated with medication.

♦ Current condition(s)/chief complaint(s): Mr. Lopez fell from a second-story roof and landed on his back 4 weeks ago. He experienced no loss of consciousness. A CT scan of his thoracic spine revealed a comminuted fracture of the T10 spinous process and subluxation of T9 on T10. MRI indicated bony fragments impinging on the spinal cord at the level of T10. Mr. Lopez underwent surgery to remove the fragments and to receive T7-T12 instrumentation to restore alignment. He is wearing a thoraco-lumbo-sacral orthosis (TLSO) when out of bed. He has HO in the region of his left hip as revealed on x-ray. Mr. Lopez expects to return to his prior functional status. It is now 4 weeks since his accident, and he is in the acute rehabilitation setting (after having received physical therapy in the acute care hospital).

♦ Functional status and activity level: The following status was reported in the physical therapy notes received from the acute care hospital. Mr. Lopez currently is sitting for up to 3 hours at a time, and he is able to propel his manual wheelchair with supervision up to 200 feet. His transfers to the mat require a transfer board and moderate assistance. Mat mobility, including sitting to and from supine and rolling, requires moderate assist with a strap for leg management. He has had trials of standing and ambulation in the parallel bars with long leg bracing, which have been limited by decreased strength and OH.

♦ Medications: He is taking oral baclofen, Lotensin, Colace, Dulcolax suppositories, Percocet, Didronel, and amitriptyline.

♦ Other clinical tests
  • Baseline blood levels were WNL.
  • A Doppler scan of his LEs was negative for DVT.
  • Urinalysis and urine cultures were negative.
  • X-ray of his hips revealed HO of the left hip.
  • Vital capacity was 2 liters (2000 cc) in supine.

SYSTEMS REVIEW

♦ Cardiovascular/pulmonary (taken while sitting in manual wheelchair while wearing abdominal binder, TLSO, and compression stockings)
  • BP: 105/65 mmHg
  • Edema: None since wearing compression stockings
  • HR: 80 bpm at rest
  • RR: 18 bpm
♦ Integumentary
  • Presence of scar formation
    ▪ Posterior thoracic surgery scar, 22 cm, dry and intact

    ▪ Left inguinal hernia repair scar well healed
  • Skin color: WNL
  • Skin integrity: Intact
♦ Musculoskeletal
  • Gross range of motion
    ▪ Bilateral UEs: WFL
    ▪ Bilateral LEs: WFL except left hip flexion
    ▪ Trunk not evaluated secondary to thoracic brace and medical restrictions
  • Gross strength
    ▪ Bilateral UEs: WFL
    ▪ Bilateral LEs: Limited
  • Gross symmetry: Symmetrical posture while sitting in wheelchair
  • Height: 5'8" (1.47 m)
  • Weight: 170 lbs (77.12 kg)
♦ Neuromuscular
  • Balance
    ▪ Sitting unsupported with assistance
    ▪ Standing supported with assistance
    ▪ Impaired postural reactions of trunk and LEs due to TLSO and muscle weakness
  • Locomotion, transfers, and transitions
    ▪ Ambulation in parallel bars with bracing and moderate to maximal assistance
    ▪ Wheelchair propulsion with supervision
    ▪ Wheelchair to mat with transfer board with moderate assistance
    ▪ Sitting to and from supine with moderate assistance
♦ Communication, affect, cognition, language, and learning style
  • Communication, affect, and cognition: WNL
  • Learning style: Mr. Lopez is fluent in English, although he occasionally prefers explanations in Spanish

TESTS AND MEASURES

♦ Aerobic capacity/endurance
  • Mr. Lopez demonstrates fatigue and decreased balance during propulsion of manual wheelchair, but is able to propel wheelchair 200 feet with supervision
  • He becomes short of breath when working on transfers, ADL, and mobility
♦ Assistive and adaptive devices
  • A strap is utilized to assist leg management with bed/mat mobility and self-stretch secondary to limited mobility with TLSO
  • He is using a manual wheelchair with seat cushion
  • He uses a transfer board to assist with transfers between wheelchair and bed or mat

- Mr. Lopez uses a tub bench and requires moderate assistance to transfer on and off the bench with a transfer board
♦ Circulation
  - Mr. Lopez occasionally experiences OH with position change from supine to sitting (BP 80/50 mmHg), which can be prevented with gradual transition from supine to sitting
  - He utilizes an abdominal binder and compressive stockings to prevent OH
♦ Cranial and peripheral nerve integrity
  - Sensory level
    - Mr. Lopez has intact sensation to light touch and pinprick to T11 halfway between umbilicus and inguinal ligament and impaired sensation at T12 and below
    - Mr. Lopez has intact sensation at the perianal area
    - These findings indicate a sensory level of T11 incomplete
  - Motor level
    - Mr. Lopez's trunk was not evaluated secondary to the TLSO
    - Mr. Lopez has generally 4/5 strength in his UEs
    - In his LEs, his hip flexors were 3/5 and all other muscles were 2 or less (see Muscle Performance results for specifics)
    - Mr. Lopez has voluntary contraction of the external anal sphincter
    - These findings indicate a motor level of L2 incomplete
  - Based on ASIA classification standards,[16] Mr. Lopez is classified as T11 ASIA C incomplete paraplegia
♦ Environmental, home, and work barriers
  - Mr. Lopez's apartment is on the seventh floor of a building with one stair to enter and an elevator to his floor
  - Housing forms will be filled out by his brother as he assesses doorway widths, accessibility of the bathroom, and other potential barriers
  - Mr. Lopez was a self-employed roofer
  - He may be able to return as a supervisor
♦ Ergonomics and body mechanics
  - Mr. Lopez is limited by his TLSO and decreased strength in his LEs during functional activities including transfers and mat/bed mobility
  - The TLSO affects typical mobility strategies for a patient with paraplegia, including initiating movement with momentum and moving head/shoulders opposite the direction of the hips
♦ Gait, locomotion, and balance
  - Sitting balance on mat

- Static with UE support: Independent
- Dynamic without UE support: Minimal assist needed as postural reactions limited due to TLSO and muscle weakness in LEs
- Standing balance in parallel bars with bilateral long leg splints
  - Static with UE support: Minimal assist
  - Dynamic with UE support: Moderate assist
- Mr. Lopez is able to ambulate 10 feet in the parallel bars with bilateral long leg training braces with a reciprocal pattern requiring moderate to maximal assistance to maintain balance and advance his LEs
- Balance needed for weight shifts in wheelchair
  - Anterior: Not evaluated secondary to TLSO
  - Lateral: Independent
  - Push-up: Contact guard for balance
  - Weight shifts during propulsion of manual wheelchair
  - Independent indoors
  - Contact guard outdoors on uneven surfaces
- Wheelchair on stairs, ramps, and curbs: Maximal assist and verbal cueing to instruct others to assist him
♦ Integumentary integrity
  - Thoracic surgery scar: Vertical in orientation, 22 cm, dry, and intact
  - Mr. Lopez is utilizing a pressure-relieving mattress on his bed and is being turned every 2 hours
  - He is also utilizing a wheelchair with a gel cushion and a back cushion with a sacral cutout
  - He is able to perform push-up weight shifts with contact guard and lateral weight shifts independently every half hour while in wheelchair
  - He is able to utilize an inspection mirror on a long handle with verbal cueing to check his skin for areas of redness and breakdown
♦ Joint integrity and mobility
  - LE joint mobility
    - WNL except left hip flexion to 85 degrees with hard end feel secondary to HO
    - Straight leg raise to 60 degrees bilaterally (90 degrees needed for long sitting position)
♦ Muscle performance
  - Bilateral shoulder flexion, extension, and abduction=5/5
  - Bilateral elbow flexion and extension=5/5
  - Bilateral wrist flexion and extension=5/5
  - Bilateral forearm supination and pronation=5/5
  - Hip flexion=R 3/5, L 3/5
  - Hip abduction=R 2-/5, L 2-/5
  - Bilateral hip extension=1+/5

- Knee extension=R 2/5, L 2+/5
- Bilateral knee flexion=1+/5
- Bilateral ankle dorsiflexion=2-/5
- Ankle plantarflexion=R 1/5, L 1+/5
- Trunk not evaluated secondary to TLSO
- Voluntary contraction of external anal sphincter

♦ Orthotic, protective, and supportive devices
- Mr. Lopez requires moderate assistance to don and doff the TLSO, which he is utilizing when the head of the bed is greater than 30 degrees and when he is out of bed
- With maximal assist, he can don and doff his positioning bilateral AFOs, which he uses when in bed to prevent foot drop and skin breakdown
- He wears long leg braces to assist with gait training, which he can don and doff with max assist

♦ Pain
- NPS with 0=no pain and 10=worst possible pain[32]
- Mr. Lopez reports pain in the area of his thoracic surgery site
- 2/10 pain at rest
- 6/10 with movement of UEs or change in body position

♦ Posture
- Mr. Lopez exhibits symmetrical alignment in sitting, with equal weightbearing on his ischia both in his wheelchair and in unsupported sitting on the mat
- In standing, Mr. Lopez has equal weight distribution on his LEs
- He stands with long leg braces in a "para stance" position for stability (in bilateral hip extension resting on his "Y" ligaments with shoulders posterior to his hips secondary to hip extensor weakness)

♦ Range of motion
- Cervical ROM: WFL
- Trunk ROM: Not evaluated secondary to his TLSO and medical restrictions
- UE ROM: WNL except bilateral shoulder flexion and abduction to 160 degrees secondary to thoracic surgery site causing discomfort
- LE ROM: WNL except left hip flexion to 85 degrees with hard end feel secondary to HO and straight leg raise to 60 degrees bilaterally (90 degrees needed for long sitting position)

♦ Self-care and home management
- Transfers with transfer board
  - Wheelchair to and from mat with moderate assistance
  - Wheelchair to and from bed with moderate assistance
  - Wheelchair to and from toilet with moderate assistance

- Upper body dressing and basic hygiene: Independent except moderate assist to don and doff TLSO
- Lower body dressing: Minimal assist secondary to TLSO
- Shower chair transfer moderate assistance and bathing contact guard secondary to TLSO

♦ Ventilation and respiration/gas exchange
- TLSO has cut out to allow abdominal excursion needed for diaphragmatic breathing
- Vital capacity
  - 2 liters in supine and 1.9 liters in sitting
  - Mr. Lopez reports difficulty taking deep breath secondary to thoracic discomfort
- RR is 18 bpm with diaphragmatic breathing pattern
- Cough is effective for airway clearance

♦ Work, community, and leisure integration or reintegration
- Mr. Lopez will not be able to resume former occupation (roofer) due to significant LE weakness
- He may be able to return as a supervisor and visit job sites at wheelchair level at this time
- Mr. Lopez is in need of driver training evaluation
- Mr. Lopez's apartment building has one step in the front and a ramp to a side entrance
- His apartment is on the seventh floor of an elevated building
- It is recommended that he move to the first floor if possible in case an emergency evacuation is required or if elevator breaks down
- His leisure activities include bowling and baseball
- Bowling and other sports can be accessed with adaptive devices using his wheelchair

EVALUATION

Mr. Lopez is a previously healthy and independent 40-year-old male who was self-employed and enjoyed an active lifestyle. Four weeks ago he fell off a roof while working and sustained a SCI resulting in T11 ASIA C (incomplete) paraplegia. He has impaired motor performance in his LE muscles and a TLSO preventing trunk ROM. He requires hands-on assistance at this time for most functional activities at the wheelchair level. Standing at this time requires assistance and LE bracing in the parallel bars. He is using a manual wheelchair with custom seating. He plans to return to his roofing business and return to pre-injury activities.

DIAGNOSIS

Mr. Lopez is a patient with T11 ASIA C (incomplete) paraplegia as a result of a fall 4 weeks ago. He has pain around the thoracic surgical site. He has impaired: aerobic capacity/endurance; circulation; cranial and peripheral nerve integrity; ergonomics and body mechanics; gait, locomotion, and balance; integumentary integrity; joint integrity and mobility; motor function; muscle performance; posture; range of motion; and ventilation and respiration/gas exchange. He is functionally limited in self-care and home management and in work, community, and leisure actions, tasks, and activities. He has home and work barriers. He is also in need of assistive, adaptive, orthotic, protective, and supportive devices and equipment. These findings are consistent with placement in Pattern H: Impaired Motor Function, Peripheral Nerve Integrity, and Sensory Integrity Associated With Nonprogressive Disorders of the Spinal Cord. The identified impairments, functional limitations, barriers, and device and equipment needs will be addressed in determining the prognosis and the plan of care.

PROGNOSIS AND PLAN OF CARE

Over the course of the visits, the following mutually established outcomes have been determined:
♦ Ability to instruct others in his care including management of wheelchair on curbs, ramps, and stairs is improved
♦ Ability to perform physical activities (with assistive and adaptive devices as needed) related to self-care, home management, work, community, and leisure is improved
♦ Assistive, adaptive, orthotic, protective, and supportive devices are issued, and Mr. Lopez is independent in their usage and maintenance
♦ Environmental barriers at home, work, and play are addressed and overcome
♦ Gait and locomotion are improved
♦ Knowledge of behaviors that address precautions related to SCI including skin breakdown, HO, osteoporosis, DVT, AD, respiratory dysfunction, and OH is enhanced
♦ Knowledge of safety needs in a variety of settings with a plan for evacuation from home and work is enhanced
♦ Muscle performance is increased in UEs and LEs and trunk musculature
♦ ROM is increased to allow functional activities
♦ Wound healing is enhanced

To achieve these outcomes, the appropriate interventions for this patient are determined. These will include: coordination, communication, and documentation; patient/client-related instruction; therapeutic exercise; functional training in self-care and home management; functional training in work, community, and leisure integration or reintegration; manual therapy techniques; prescription, application, and, as appropriate, fabrication of devices and equipment; airway clearance techniques; electrotherapeutic modalities; and physical agents and mechanical modalities.

Mr. Lopez is expected to need 90 to 100 visits over a 4- to 8-week period of time. Based on the diagnosis of T11 ASIA C paraplegia, Mr. Lopez will require modified independence for manual wheelchair propulsion, transfers, and bed mobility and will possibly be a household or community ambulator with appropriate assistive device and orthoses.

INTERVENTIONS

RATIONALE FOR SELECTED INTERVENTIONS

Therapeutic Exercise

See Rationale for Seletected Interventions, Therapeutic Exercise in Case Study #1.

BWSTT has been researched and has undergone clinical trials with subjects with acute and chronic SCI.[2,7,38,43-50] Behrman and Harkema[46] found that locomotor training, designed to optimize sensory cues related to locomotion in order to facilitate a more coordinated and normal stepping pattern on a treadmill and overground, has resulted in improved performance in both complete and incomplete injuries. Locomotor training has been termed a "recovery"-based approach to ambulation training, as opposed to the traditional "compensatory" approach that relies more on bracing and assistive devices.[5-7,45-48] By providing BWS with a harness system as needed in the presence of absent or weak LE muscles, the patient's steps on the treadmill can initially be facilitated manually or mechanically with maximal sensory cues. As the patient improves, BWS is decreased and cadence is increased. Each session includes treadmill training with progression to overground and community training components. BSWTT is based on the theory that the spinal cord can learn. BSWTT is used to facilitate reorganization of the spinal cord below the level of lesion by providing external sensory stimulation and loading of the LEs to generate stepping.[2,7,12,43] Behrman and Harkema[46] describe the required sensory cues used in their research with BSWTT:
♦ Generating stepping speeds approximating normal walking speeds (0.75 to 1.25 m/s)
♦ Providing the maximum sustainable load on the stance limb
♦ Maintaining an upright and extended trunk and head
♦ Approximating normal hip, knee, and ankle kinematics for walking
♦ Synchronizing timing of extension of the hip in stance and unloading of limb with simultaneous loading of the contralateral limb
♦ Avoiding weightbearing on the arms and facilitating reciprocal arm swing
♦ Facilitating symmetrical interlimb coordination
♦ Maximizing cutaneous stimulation from the sole of the

foot by wearing lightweight tennis shoes with thin soles and low cut ankles and not wearing orthoses

BWSTT requires specialized equipment and, if the extremities are moved manually, it is labor intensive for the physical therapist. The assistance of two or three physical therapists is needed, one for each leg and one to assist with arm swing. Appropriate kinematics are facilitated for each step with the patient providing as much active movement as possible. Active participation from the patient is essential for enhancing neuroplasticity at the spinal cord level, since passive movement does not enhance neural reorganization. Robotic-assisted BWSTT was developed to decrease the labor required by physical therapists while providing appropriate kinematics for stepping. Hornby and associates[73] described the use of a robotic device or driven gait orthosis (DGO) with patients with incomplete SCI. They found that while the DGO was less labor intensive and allowed patients to begin to develop appropriate kinematic movement patterns there were limitations of the device that necessitated transition to therapist-assisted BSWTT. These limitations included lack of active movement by the patient, limited speed of the device, and conflicting sensory input due to the attachment of the DGO to the body. Israel and colleagues[74] studied the metabolic costs and muscle activity patterns during robotic- and therapist-assisted treadmill walking in patients with incomplete SCI. They found that the metabolic costs for robotic-assisted treadmill walking were less than for therapist-assisted treadmill walking; however, the costs became similar when the patients were asked to put forth maximum effort while using the robotic device. They also found that activity patterns for muscle activation were different between the two methods with more normal pattern activation and use occurring when performing therapist-assisted walking. While robotic-assisted training does not replicate therapist-assisted training it does reduce therapist labor and may be beneficial in the early stages of locomotor training.[73-75]

Gait training can also be addressed in the parallel bars with LE orthotics as needed for this patient and can progress to gait training with an assistive device, such as a walker or forearm crutches and LE orthoses as needed. This compensatory type of training is based on assessing the remaining muscle function. Then support is provided through equipment (eg, tilt table, standing frame, parallel bars, walkers, etc) and orthotics.[6,42] Behrman and coworkers[47] provided a review of the science and evidence for compensatory and recovery models, as well as a comparison of the two models. Dobkin and associates[44,45] recently completed a multi-site randomized clinical trial comparing the effectiveness of recovery training using BWSTT with overground training with a more traditional compensatory overground training method in acute SCI. Their findings suggest that there is no significant difference in the training methods. There is currently discussion regarding these findings and the appli-

cation of this random clinical trial[44,45] to practice.[76,77] One factor that may have influenced the results is the intensity of training for both groups, which was 1 hour per week, 5 days a week, for 12 weeks with a recommended total number of sessions of 45 to 60.[44,45] While this intensity is more common for BWSTT,[44-48] it appears to be higher than would be expected in traditional therapy.[6,45]

This patient with an incomplete SCI is a candidate for BSWTT. At this time there are no standard guidelines for use or progression of patients using locomotor training. Behrman and associates[47] provide an example of a locomotor progression program and a decision-making algorithm that may be used for standing and walking progression and is a good resource for clinicians. Studies have varied in the dosage of BSWTT[44,46,47,49] and there is discussion regarding the necessary components.[2,7,76-79]

Functional Training in Self-Care and Home Management

As a result of the SCI and resulting incomplete paraplegia, this patient will need to learn how to perform self-care activities with a variety of compensatory techniques and equipment. When patients use a TLSO, self-care activities, especially bed mobility and dressing, are more difficult. Using momentum to initiate movement and remembering that "head goes opposite the hips" are two principles that can assist his mobility. Patients should initially be taught how to instruct others to assist in their care until gains in strength, balance, and agility allow them to perform independently.[17] It is expected that patients with this level of involvement will be independent in self-care, but they may need some assistance with heavy housekeeping activities.[17]

Functional Training in Work, Community, and Leisure Integration or Reintegration

Reintegration into school, community, and leisure activities is challenging for a patient with a SCI, especially at the wheelchair level. A wide variety of assistive and adaptive devices and equipment is available. Mr. Lopez must be given trial uses of these devices and equipment in order to maximize his capabilities.[52,53] The equipment and product systems, whether commercially acquired or customized for this patient, fall under the title of "assistive technology" and will improve his functional capabilities outside of the home.[51]

This patient will receive training using a manual wheelchair. The training will include instructions and practice on how to negotiate the environment, propulsion on even and uneven surfaces, wheelchair use on stairs and curbs, door management, and possibly a work site evaluation with appropriate recommendations. Mr. Lopez is a candidate for a driving evaluation and may benefit from vehicle modification, including hand controls for an appropriate car or van.

With improvements in LE strength, he may be a candidate for household ambulation with appropriate bracing and orthotic devices and may possibly be able to perform limited community ambulation. Functional training at the ambulatory level will include ambulation on a variety of surfaces, stair/curb/ramp negotiation, and floor transfer and fall techniques.

Manual Therapy Techniques

Soft tissue dysfunction is common following SCI with neurological deficits. With decreased AROM in the UEs secondary to thoracic surgery limitations and pain and impaired musculature in the LEs, patients are likely to have joint and soft tissue limitations. Specifically, Curtis and associates[54] found shoulder pain present in two thirds of a sample of patients with SCI who used manual wheelchairs. In another study, Curtis and associates[55] suggested that a standard exercise protocol consisting of flexibility and strengthening interventions could decrease the intensity of shoulder pain that interferes with functional activity in wheelchair users. Massage, soft tissue mobilization, and PROM within surgical precautions may be utilized to address trunk ROM limitations.

Prescription, Application, and, as Appropriate, Fabrication of Devices and Equipment

Patients with neurological impairment often benefit from devices that provide a more stable alignment, protect joints and skin, or assist functional activities. A patient with limited lower body strength will benefit not only from an appropriate wheelchair seating system and cushion, but also from devices and equipment to assist in self-care and other daily tasks.[17,51] This patient with a TLSO and limited leg strength could benefit from dressing aids, including a mechanical reacher and sock donning device to help with lower body dressing. He utilizes bilateral positioning ankle boots in bed to prevent skin breakdown on bony prominences and to also prevent foot drop.

The degree of use of LE orthotic devices, such as KAFOs or AFOs, will depend on the model followed in rehabilitation for retraining ambulation.[6,47] In the compensatory model, LE orthotics would be used to provide stability and limit degrees of freedom for more proximal control of the limb during standing and ambulation. The patient will be taught compensatory movement patterns to perform daily tasks with his lessened degree of motor function. For example, a patient with a long leg brace with a locked knee is taught to hip hike in order to facilitate swing phase. In the recovery model, LE orthoses and assistive devices are minimized to facilitate proper limb/trunk kinematics and increased LE weightbearing.[2,7,47] Studies have demonstrated that the motor patterns used for walking were not the same when using assistive devices or when holding onto parallel bars.[2,7,47] By optimizing the sensory cues given to the patient during gait training, recovery of normal movement patterns is facilitated.[6]

Airway Clearance Techniques

A SCI involving the thoracic spine will impair the patient's ventilatory function in varying degrees, depending on the neurological level and severity of neurological damage. An upper thoracic injury can result in limited or absent intercostal and abdominal strength. A lower thoracic injury will result in less intercostal involvement with their segmental innervations and less abdominal muscle weakness with innervation from T5-T12. Even an incomplete injury at a thoracic level (as with this case study) with subsequent surgical intervention may affect the degree of thoracic expansion and the strength of the cough, which are secondary to the pain and physical restriction imposed by the surgery and the thoracic orthosis. It is crucial for this patient to maximize his ventilatory capacity to avoid life-threatening complications.

Interventions will include teaching the patient how to perform a self-assisted cough. In addition, diaphragmatic strengthening, as described by Frownfelter and Dean[40] can improve his vital capacity. Intercostal facilitation may enhance his thoracic expansion during inspiration. An inspiratory training device may also facilitate deep breathing.

Electrotherapeutic Modalities

Patients with a thoracic SCI are candidates for one of the computer-mediated cycle ergometry FES programs for the LEs with various physiologic benefits including increased blood flow to the LEs[65] and increased muscle mass.[66] Bickel and associates[67] found that muscle was able to respond to electromyostimulation-induced exercise. In addition, neuroprosthetic systems with either surface or implanted electrodes may provide an opportunity for ambulation for patients with significant motor deficits. The Parastep I System,[80] a surface FES system with a microcomputer-controlled neuromuscular stimulation unit, has allowed patients to take steps though stimulation of the LE sensory nerves to initiate swing by means of a reflex flexor contraction and to facilitate stance through stimulation of the quadriceps. The user controls stimulation through a keypad on the stimulator unit or via control switches mounted on the electronically modified walker. Ambulation may also be facilitated with implanted muscle- or nerve-based multichannel electrodes, which are put in place surgically and then connected to an implanted stimulation device.[81] Field-Fote and Tepavac[48] found that electrical stimulation combined with BWSTT was effective in improving interlimb coordination in patients with incomplete SCI. TENS may be utilized to decrease pain.[69]

Physical Agents and Mechanical Modalities

Physical agents, such as hot packs and cold packs, may be helpful as means to decrease musculoskeletal pain. Caution must be taken to inspect skin in areas of incomplete sensation to prevent injury from these modalities.

COORDINATION, COMMUNICATION, AND DOCUMENTATION

Communication will occur with Mr. Lopez and appropriate family members to engender support for his therapy program and home exercise program. Interdisciplinary teamwork will occur as needed including case conferences and family meetings. Collaboration and coordination with agencies including equipment suppliers, home care agencies, and transportation agencies will occur. Referrals to other professionals or resources will be made to ensure all of the patient's needs are being met. All elements of the patient's management will be documented.

PATIENT/CLIENT-RELATED INSTRUCTION

Mr. Lopez will be instructed in the precautions related to his SCI and in behaviors to prevent or address complications including skin breakdown, DVT, respiratory dysfunction, OH, HO, AD, and osteoporosis. Mr. Lopez's family will also be instructed in how to assist Mr. Lopez with the behaviors that can prevent or address these complications.

He will also be taught various recovery and compensatory techniques for mobility. These may include weight shifts, transfers to various surfaces, mat and bed mobility, ambulation and elevation training, and wheelchair management on stairs, curbs, and ramps. His family will be instructed in how to assist Mr. Lopez with these activities.

Mr. Lopez will also be instructed in a home exercise program of therapeutic exercises, including PROM, stretching of his limbs, and muscle strengthening for his UEs and LEs. His trunk will be stretched and strengthened with physician clearance after his TLSO is removed.

THERAPEUTIC EXERCISE

- ◆ Aerobic capacity/endurance conditioning
  - Mode
    - Aerobic using UE and LE muscles
    - Continuous or for prolonged period
    - Upper body ergometer
    - UE exercises (eg, light weights/high reps, cardio body blade)
    - Swimming in pool
    - Leg equipment, such as bicycle, as leg strength improves or with a computer-mediated cycle ergometry FES program for the LEs
  - Duration
    - 15 to 20 minutes initially and work up to 30 minutes
    - Increase duration progressively
  - Intensity
    - Determine appropriate perceived exertion with modified Borg scale[70] so that he is working in the aerobic or training zone
      - The patient effort should be between 3 and 7 on a scale of 1 to 10
  - Frequency
    - Start with two to three times per week and progress to three to four times per week
- ◆ Balance, coordination, and agility training
  - Short and long sitting balance activities on mat
  - Sitting in wheelchair using static and dynamic balance activities
  - With initial UE support, practice balance with transitioning UE position to anteriorly, laterally, and posteriorly
  - Without UE support, practice the technique of how his head and UEs assist in maintaining midline (in presence of TLSO and weakness in LE musculature)
  - Without UE support can progress to tilt board and other uneven surfaces including sitting on exercise ball, inflated cushions, or straddling a bolster
  - In side sitting, weightbear on elbows laterally
  - In quadruped, kneel, and half kneel positions, balance (with physician clearance secondary to TLSO) with focus on weight shifting and upper body assisting lower body to maintain midline
  - Practice assuming and maintaining quadruped, kneel, and half kneel positions
  - In standing, practice balance using static and dynamic activities with appropriate assistive devices and LE orthoses
    - In parallel bars with and without bracing as appropriate
    - In standing frame
    - Progression to assistive device (eg, walker) and bracing (eg, KAFOs or AFOs) as needed
  - Pool therapy for balance training with patient in sitting or standing with flotation devices as needed
- ◆ Flexibility exercises
  - Cervical ROM
  - Trunk ROM (after TLSO is removed and with physician clearance)
  - PROM/stretch of hips, knees, and ankles with emphasis on hip extension, knee extension, and dorsiflexion in preparation for gait
  - PROM/stretch of UEs with emphasis on shoulder extension and external rotation stretches since Mr. Lopez will be utilizing anterior shoulder muscles for wheelchair propulsion, transfers, and mat and bed mobility
  - Mr. Lopez will be instructed in self-PROM of his LEs with or without leg loops to assist
- ◆ Gait and locomotion training
  - Standing balance activities as listed above

- Assess periodically for bracing needs
- Orthoses may not be prescribed until motor recovery plateaus
- Mr. Lopez may progress from long leg braces to short leg braces and possibly to no brace as knee and ankle control return
- With an incomplete thoracic injury, Mr. Lopez may also be a candidate for BWSTT
- Manual wheelchair management and propulsion
- Emphasize independence at the wheelchair level with ergonomically correct wheelchair propulsion style and include advanced wheelchair skills when out of the TLSO as a prerequisite or as a concurrent goal
- Advanced wheelchair skills including wheelies, door management, floor transfers, and wheelchair management on curbs, stairs, ramps, and uneven surfaces
- ◆ Strength, power, and endurance training
  - UE program including active and resistive exercises utilizing cuff weights, elastic bands, and/or weight machines with emphasis on exercises and activities performed with ergonomically correct mechanics to avoid undue stress on UE joints
  - Push-ups and lateral weight shifts in wheelchair
  - Weightbearing exercises for UEs and LEs, including prone on elbows, quadruped, kneeling, and standing with activities including weight shifting, lifting an extremity, reaching, and resisted extremity motions
  - LE exercises including active, active assisted, and resisted exercises in a variety of gravity-eliminated to against-gravity positions utilizing cuff weights, elastic bands, weight machines, and closed- and open-chain activities in standing
  - Diaphragmatic and accessory muscle strengthening, including deep breathing, controlled exhalation, and use of an inspiratory muscle trainer
  - Pool therapy (when TLSO is removed and wounds are healed) for UE and LE strengthening including exercises in standing and while floating with flotation devices as needed

FUNCTIONAL TRAINING IN SELF-CARE AND HOME MANAGEMENT

- ◆ ADL training
  - Transfers to various surfaces including bed, car, toilet, tub, and wheelchair beginning at wheelchair level with possibility of being at ambulatory level in the future
  - Bed mobility, including sitting to and from supine and rolling
  - Instruction in position changes with compensatory techniques including utilizing momentum to initiate movement and head/shoulders moving opposite hips (limited by TLSO)

- Self-care activities including bathing, dressing, eating, grooming, and toileting
- Mr. Lopez is independent with feeding and grooming and may need dressing aids, including reachers and a sock aid as a result of his TLSO and limited leg strength
- He could utilize a shower/commode chair in an accessible stall shower
- ◆ Devices and equipment use and training
  - Transfer board to assist with transfers (may not need in the future)
  - Equipment and devices to assist with bathing, toileting, and dressing
  - Assistive device for ambulation and LE orthoses
  - Manual wheelchair for mobility
- ◆ Functional training program
  - Simulated environment to return to home and perform all self-care activities (eg, some inpatient rehabilitation sites offer a room to simulate overnight stay with significant other)
- ◆ IADL training
  - Home maintenance and household chores to be practiced at wheelchair level and possibly at ambulatory level
  - Shopping and yard work also simulated and practiced at wheelchair and ambulatory levels
- ◆ Injury prevention or reduction
  - Instruction in risk factors of performing self-care, home management, shopping, and other ADL and IADL at wheelchair or ambulatory levels
  - Awareness of injury prevention/reduction with the use of devices or equipment

FUNCTIONAL TRAINING IN WORK, COMMUNITY, AND LEISURE INTEGRATION OR REINTEGRATION

- ◆ Device and equipment use and training
  - Wheelchair training on stairs, curbs, and ramps
    - Instruction on how to negotiate a curb, ramp, and stairs in the wheelchair in a wheelie including techniques to perform the tasks himself and how to instruct others to assist
    - Instruction on how to perform wheelchair transfer to and from floor
  - Work site evaluation and recommendations
  - Car transfers with transfer board including loading and unloading of wheelchair or options with modified van
- ◆ Functional training programs
  - Travel training[33] in wheelchair including skills necessary to move from one place to another safely and efficiently

- May include indoor and outdoor mobility and use of transportation
- Simulated environments and tasks

♦ IADL training
  - Work and leisure activities with instruments and equipment as needed including sports at wheelchair level, such as tennis, basketball, bowling, and wheelchair racing with a progression to activities at ambulatory level if leg strength improves
♦ Injury prevention and reduction
  - During leisure and community activities instruction in maintaining safety including wheelchair management, practicing falls, and floor transfers at wheelchair and ambulatory level
  - During leisure and community activities instructing others in maintaining safety

MANUAL THERAPY TECHNIQUES

♦ Massage
  - Connective tissue and therapeutic massage with emphasis on shoulder region as needed for pain relief and flexibility
  - Thoracic region may be addressed after TLSO removal within surgical precautions
♦ Mobilization of soft tissue
  - Emphasis on shoulder region with goal of balanced shoulder, which can reduce pain and overuse
  - Stretch of anterior shoulder structures
♦ PROM
  - Maximize and maintain ROM of limbs and trunk to allow function

PRESCRIPTION, APPLICATION, AND, AS APPROPRIATE, FABRICATION OF DEVICES AND EQUIPMENT

♦ Adaptive devices
  - Appropriate cushion in wheelchair to achieve optimal postural alignment and disperse pressure
♦ Assistive devices
  - Manual wheelchair
  - Hospital bed (may not be needed after TLSO is removed and mobility is improved)
  - Commode chair
  - Tub bench
♦ Orthotic devices
  - Positioning AFOs to prevent foot drop and skin breakdown in bed
  - KAFOs or AFOs may be given a trial use for gait training depending on degree of LE musculature recovery

♦ Protective devices
  - Specialized mattress for bed to prevent skin breakdown
  - Specialized cushion for wheelchair to distribute weight in sitting
♦ Supportive devices
  - Compressive stockings and possibly Ace wraps for LEs to prevent edema and OH

AIRWAY CLEARANCE TECHNIQUES

♦ Breathing strategies
  - Techniques to maximize diaphragmatic muscle strength including inspiratory muscle trainer
  - Techniques to maximize ventilation (eg, maximum inspiratory hold, staircase breathing with several inhalations without exhalation)
♦ Manual/mechanical technique
  - Chest percussion and vibration after TLSO removal when precautions are lifted
  - Chest wall stretch and rib mobilization after TLSO removal when precautions are lifted
♦ Positioning
  - Pulmonary postural drainage may be needed secondary to recent thoracic surgery and immobility so patient is taught to vary position in bed in degrees of side-lying

ELECTROTHERAPEUTIC MODALITIES

♦ FES systems
  - LE strengthening program of specific muscles with electrical current of an adequate amplitude to allow for contraction (typically 20- to 30-minute session as tolerated)
  - A surface FES system for ambulation with a microcomputer-controlled neuromuscular unit with a key pad or control switches mounted on the walker[80]
  - A neuroprosthesis option for ambulation with implanted muscle or nerve-based multichannel electrodes with an implanted stimulation device[81]
  - A computer-mediated FES cycle ergometry program for the LE with stimulation of quadriceps, hamstrings, and gluteal muscles that results in various physiologic benefits, including increased blood flow to the LEs[65] and increased muscle mass[66]
♦ TENS
  - For decreasing pain via triggering complex physiological systems of the PNS and CNS
    - For shoulder or thoracic pain
    - For neurogenic pain

PHYSICAL AGENTS AND MECHANICAL MODALITIES

- ♦ Physical agents
  - Cryotherapy
    - Cold packs and ice massage for possible pain and inflammation, commonly for the shoulder from overuse
  - Thermotherapy
    - Hot packs for relaxation and pain relief of trunk and limb

ANTICIPATED GOALS AND EXPECTED OUTCOMES

- ♦ Impact on pathology/pathophysiology
  - Atelectasis is prevented, and Mr. Lopez demonstrates a diaphragmatic breathing pattern with intercostals providing chest expansion during inhalation.
  - Edema is prevented and is enhanced by patient's ability to independently don and doff compressive stockings to reduce LE edema.
  - Pain is decreased, and Mr. Lopez is able to independently position himself in the wheelchair to best propel his wheelchair without shoulder impingement.
  - Pressure on body tissues is reduced in that he independently performs anterior weight shifts in the wheelchair to relieve pressure every half hour for 2 minutes, and he can independently turn in bed every 2 hours.
- ♦ Impact on impairments
  - Ability to perform movement tasks is improved, in that he demonstrates lateral transfer from wheelchair to and from mat with supervision, performs bed mobility with leg loops with supervision, and increases strength in legs to allow household ambulation with orthoses and forearm crutches with supervision up to 100 feet.
  - Aerobic capacity is increased so that Mr. Lopez performs 30 minutes on UE cycle and has improved endurance for manual wheelchair propulsion.
  - Airway clearance is improved, and a strong effective cough is achieved to allow secretion removal.
  - Airway clearance is improved when the TLSO is removed so that there is better recruitment of intercostals and diaphragm for inspiration.
  - Balanced shoulder is attained to decrease the possibility of chronic shoulder pain in the future, and Mr. Lopez will perform his home exercise program of appropriate shoulder stretches and exercises independently.
  - Diaphragmatic strength is maximized to attain vital capacity of 4000 cc.

- Dynamic sitting balance is independently achieved on mat to facilitate improved functional mobility including dressing and transfers from wheelchair to and from bed.
- Flexibility is increased to allow functional activities requiring positions such as long sitting, standing, and prone; straight leg raise range is increased to 90 degrees; and patient performs self-stretching of legs with loops as needed secondary to limited flexibility with TLSO to allow full knee extension, ankle dorsiflexion, and hip extension for postural alignment in standing.
- Joint restrictions are prevented.
- Joint stability is improved with optimized alignment, and Mr. Lopez will independently don and doff positioning boots in bed to prevent foot drop.
- Motor function is improved to allow trunk stability and mobility when TLSO is removed.
- Muscle performance is increased, upper body strength is increased to allow independent lift-up pressure relief technique while sitting in wheelchair, and LE strength is increased to allow ambulation up to 150 feet with bracing and forearm crutches with modified independence.
- Muscle performance of diaphragm and accessory muscles is improved.
- Physical function is improved so that Mr. Lopez performs bed mobility and wheelchair transfers to and from bed independently using loops for leg management when the TLSO is on
- Postural control is improved so that he can correctly position himself in the wheelchair without cueing to maximize function of UEs during propulsion, and he achieves upright posture with center of gravity over base of support in standing to facilitate modified independent ambulation.
- ROM is improved so that his shoulder flexion ROM is to 160 degrees to allow reaching into upper shelf of his closet and his straight leg ROM allows long sitting in bed to assist with independent dressing.
- Standing balance is achieved with long leg braces and walker.
- Standing using a standing frame is achieved for 30 minutes with UE exercise as lead up to gait activities.
- Ventilation and respiration/gas exchange is improved.
- ♦ Impact on functional limitations
  - Ability to instruct others to assist with transfer from floor to wheelchair or standing in case of a fall and with performance of physical actions, tasks, and activities is achieved.
  - Performance levels in self-care (including shower-

ing, dressing, eating, toileting, and bowel/bladder management techniques), home management, work, community, and leisure actions, tasks, and activities (including independent wheelchair propulsion on all surfaces, ambulation in the community up to 500 feet with bracing and assistive device with supervision, driving a modified van, and both performing and instructing others in wheelchair navigation on stairs and curbs) are improved.

  • Performance of these activities with equipment and adaptive devices (including shower/commode chair, modified van, leg orthoses, assisitive devices, and wheelchair for long distance locomotion) is improved.

♦ Impact on disabilities

  • Ability to perform physical tasks and activities related to work, community, and leisure is improved.

  • Ability to resume required self-care, home management, work, community, and leisure roles is improved.

  • Negotiation takes place with his office to see if he can return in a supervisory position at a wheelchair and ambulatory level.

♦ Risk reduction/prevention

  • Complications of immobility are reduced, and he performs self-stretching of legs with loops independently.

  • Prevention of skin breakdown is achieved by independently performing lift-up or anterior pressure relief maneuvers when in sitting and by turning in bed every 2 hours independently.

  • Risk of secondary impairments is reduced, and safety is improved during performance of self-care, home management, work, community, and leisure activities using assistive technology with precautions to avoid secondary impairment, such as skin breakdown or contractures.

♦ Impact on health, wellness, and fitness

  • Behaviors that foster healthy habits, wellness, and prevention are acquired including Mr. Lopez independently performing stretches and exercises to maintain strength and flexibility in his extremities and trunk.

  • Health status is improved.

♦ Impact on societal resources

  • Collaboration and coordination occurs with agencies as needed.

  • Communication occurs across settings through case conferences and documentation.

  • Decision making regarding his health and the use of health care resources is improved.

  • Documentation occurs throughout patient management and follows APTA's *Guidelines for Physical*

Therapy Documentation.[33]

  • Referrals are made to other professionals or resources when appropriate.

♦ Patient/client satisfaction

  • Knowledge and awareness of the diagnosis, prognosis, interventions, and anticipated goals and expected outcomes are increased.

REEXAMINATION

It is anticipated that patients placed in this pattern will require multiple episodes of care over their lifetime. Periodic reexamination and initiation of new episodes of care should occur as the patient's functional limitations or disabilities change and the need for secondary prevention is identified. These visits will allow Mr. Lopez to continue to be safe and effectively adapt as a result of changes in multiple factors including his own physical status, caregivers, environment, or task demands.

DISCHARGE

Mr. Lopez is discharged from physical therapy after a total of 95 physical therapy visits over 5 weeks and attainment of his goals. As Mr. Lopez has a condition that may require multiple episodes of care throughout his life span, Mr. Lopez received education regarding factors that may trigger a call to his physical therapist for reexamination and a possible new episode of care. Mr. Lopez is placed on an episode of prevention to monitor progress of his home program and transition to home and community. As a part of this episode of prevention the physical therapist will contact Mr. Lopez one time per month to review his current status and any potential needs.

PSYCHOLOGICAL ASPECTS

See Psychological Aspects in Case Study #1 for additional information. Hicks and associates[49] found that individuals that participated in BWSTT had improved life satisfaction levels. Latimer and colleagues[82] observed that regular exercise improved psychological well-being and resolved pain and stress with stress mediating change in depression.

REFERENCES

1. Sapru HN. Spinal cord: anatomy, physiology, and pathophysiology. In: Kirshblum S, Campagnolo DI, Delisa JA, eds. *Spinal Cord Medicine.* Philadelphia, PA: Lippincott Williams & Wilkins; 2002.

2. Dietz V, Wirz M, Jensen L. Locomotion in patients with spinal cord injuries. *Phys Ther.* 1997;77:508-516.

3. Andres T, Autgaerden S. Locomotion from pre to post-natal life. In: *Clinics in Developmental Medicine.* No 24. London,

England: Medical Books Ltd; 1966.

4. Field-Fote EC. Spinal cord control of movement: implications for locomotor rehabilitation following spinal cord injury. *Phys Ther.* 2000;80:477-484.

5. Basso DM. Neuroanatomical substrates of functional recovery after experimental spinal cord injury: implications of basic science research for human spinal cord injury. *Phys Ther.* 2000;80:808-817.

6. Behrman AL, Bowden MG, Nair PM. Neuroplasticity after spinal cord injury and training: an emerging paradigm shift in rehabilitation and walking recovery. *Phys Ther.* 2006;86:1406-1425.

7. Barbeau H. Locomotor training in neurorehabilitation: emerging rehabilitation concepts. *Neurorehabil Neural Repair.* 2003;17:3-11.

8. Spinal Cord Injury Information Network. Facts and figures at a glance. Birmingham, AL: National Spinal Cord Injury Statistical Center, UAB; June 2006. Available at: http://www.spinalcord.uab.edu/show.asp?durki=21446. Accessed August 4, 2006.

9. The 2005 Annual Statistical Report for the Model Spinal Cord Injury Care Systems. Public Version. Birmingham, AL: National Spinal Cord Injury Statistical Center; 2005.

10. McKinley WO. Nontraumatic spinal cord injury: etiology, incidence, and outcome. In: Kirshblum S, Campagnolo DI, Delisa JA, eds. *Spinal Cord Medicine.* Philadelphia, PA: Lippincott Williams & Wilkins; 2002.

11. Kamin SS. Vascular, nutritional, and other diseases of the spinal cord. In: Kirshblum S, Campagnolo DI, Delisa JA, eds. *Spinal Cord Medicine.* Philadelphia, PA: Lippincott Williams & Wilkins; 2002.

12. Ramer LM, Ramer MS, Steeves JD. Setting the stage for functional repair of spinal cord injuries: a cast of thousands. *Spinal Cord.* 2005;43:134-161.

13. National Institute of Neurologic Disorders and Stroke. Spinal cord injury: emerging concepts, September 30-October 1, 1996. NINDS. Last updated 8/5/2005. Available at: http://www.ninds.hih.gov/news_and_events/proceedings/sci_report.htm#Summary. Accessed August 4, 2006.

14. DeVivo MJ. Epidemiology of traumatic spinal cord injury. In: Kirshblum S, Campagnolo DI, Delisa JA, eds. *Spinal Cord Medicine.* Philadelphia, PA: Lippincott Williams & Wilkins; 2002.

15. Schneck CD. Anatomy, mechanics, and imaging of spinal injury. In: Kirshblum S, Campagnolo DI, Delisa JA, eds. *Spinal Cord Medicine.* Philadelphia, PA: Lippincott Williams & Wilkins; 2002.

16. American Spinal Injury Association. *International Standards for Neurological Classification of Spinal Cord Injury.* 5th ed. Chicago, IL: American Spinal Injury Association; 2002.

17. Consortium for Spinal Cord Medicine Clinical Practice Guidelines. *Outcomes Following Traumatic Spinal Cord Injury: Clinical Practice Guidelines for Health-Care Professionals.* Washington, DC: Paralyzed Veterans of America; 1999.

18. Shields RK. Muscular, skeletal, and neural adaptations following spinal cord injury. *J Orthop Sports Phys Ther.* 2002;32:65-74.

19. Kurnick NB. Autonomic hyperreflexia and its control in patients with spinal cord lesions. *Ann Intern Med.* 1956;44:678-686.

20. Erickson RP. Autonomic hyperreflexia: pathophysiology and medical management. *Arch Phys Med Rehabil.* 1980;61:431-440.

21. Consortium for Spinal Cord Medicine Clinical Practice Guidelines. *Acute Management of Autonomic Dysreflexia.* 2nd ed. Washington, DC: Paralyzed Veterans of America; 2005.

22. Banovac K, Banovac F. Heterotrophic ossification. In: Kirshblum S, Campagnolo DI, Delisa JA, eds. *Spinal Cord Medicine.* Philadelphia, PA: Lippincott Williams & Wilkins; 2002.

23. Campagnolo D, Merli G. Autonomic and cardiovascular complications of spinal cord injury. In: Kirshblum S, Campagnolo DI, Delisa JA, eds. *Spinal Cord Medicine.* Philadelphia, PA: Lippincott Williams & Wilkins; 2002.

24. Elokda AS, Neilsen DH, Shields RK. Effect of functional neuromuscular stimulation on postural related orthostatic stress in individuals with acute spinal cord injury. *J Rehabil Res Dev.* 2000;37:535-542.

25. Barker E, Captain C, Chase T, et al. *Nursing Practice Related to Spinal Cord Injury and Disorders: A Core Curriculum.* Jackson Heights, NY: Eastern Paralyzed Veterans Association; 2001.

26. Skidmore-Roth L. *Mosby's 2001 Nursing Drug Reference.* St. Louis, MO: Mosby; 2001.

27. *Physician's Desk Reference.* Montvale, NJ: Thomason PDR; 2005.

28. Consortium for Spinal Cord Medicine Clinical Practice Guidelines. *Depression Following Spinal Cord Injury.* Washington, DC: Paralyzed Veterans of America; 2005.

29. Mense S, Simons DG. *Muscle Pain: Understanding Its Nature, Diagnosis, and Treatment.* Philadelphia, PA: Lippincott, Williams & Williams; 2001.

30. Butler C, Campbell S. Evidence of the effects of intrathecal baclofen for spastic and dystonic cerebral palsy. *Dev Med Child Neurol.* 2000;42:634-645.

31. Albright AL, Gilmartin R, Swift D, et al. Long-term intrathecal baclofen therapy for severe spasticity of cerebral origin. *J Neurosurg.* 2003;98:291-295.

32. Jensen MP, Karoly P, Braver S. The measurement of clinical pain intensity: a comparison of six methods. *Pain.* 1986;27(1):117-126.

33. American Physical Therapy Association. Guide to physical therapist practice. 2nd ed. *Phys Ther.* 2001;81:9-744.

34. Nash M. Exercise as a health-promoting activity following spinal cord injury. *Journal of Neurologic Physical Therapy.* 2005;29:87-96.

35. Boninger ML, Souza AL, Fitzgerald SG, et al. Propulsion patterns and pushrim biomechanics in manual wheelchair propulsion. *Am J Phys Med Rehabil.* 2002;83:718-723.

36. Nash M, Horton J. Recreational and therapeutic exercise after spinal cord injury. In: Kirshblum S, Campagnolo DI, Delisa JA, eds. *Spinal Cord Medicine.* Philadelphia, PA: Lippincott Williams & Wilkins; 2002.

37. Ditor DS, Kamath MV, MacDonald MJ, et al. Reproducibility of heart rate variability and blood pressure variability in individuals with spinal cord injury. *Clin Auton Res.* 2005;15:387-393.

38. Ditor DS, Kamath MV, MacDonald MJ, et al. Effects of body weight-supported treadmill training on heart rate variability and blood pressure variability in individuals with spinal cord injury. *J Appl Physiol.* 2005;98(4):1519-1525.

39. Duran FS, Lugo L, Ramirez L, et al. Effects of an exercise program on the rehabilitation of patients with spinal cord injury. *Arch Phys Med Rehabil.* 2001;82(10):1349-1354.

40. Frownfelter DL, Dean E. *Cardiovascular and Pulmonary Physical Therapy: Evidence and Practice.* 4th ed. St. Louis, MO: Mosby Elsevier; 2006.

41. Sprague S, Hopkins P. Use of inspiratory strength training to wean 6 patients who were ventilator dependent. *Phys Ther.* 2003;83(2):171-181.

42. Stowell T, Fuller R, Fulk G. An aquatic and land-based physical therapy intervention to improve functional mobility for an individual after an incomplete C6 spinal cord lesion. *Journal of Aquatic Physical Therapy.* 2001;9(1):27-32.

43. Wirz M, Colombo G, Dietz V. Long term effects of locomotor training in spinal humans. *J Neurol Neurosurg Psychiatry.* 2001;71:93-96.

44. Dobkin BH, Apple D, Barbeau H, et al. Spinal Cord Injury Locomotor Trial Group. Methods for a randomized trial of weight-supported treadmill training versus conventional training for walking during inpatient rehabilitation after incomplete traumatic spinal cord injury. *Neurorehabil Neural Repair.* 2003;17:153-167.

45. Dobkin BH, Apple H, Barbeau H, et al. Spinal Cord Injury Locomotor Trial Group. Weight-supported treadmill training vs over-ground training for walking after acute incomplete SCI. *Neurorehabil Neural Repair.* 2006;66:484-493.

46. Behrman AL, Harkema SJ. Locomotor training after human spinal cord injury: a series of case studies. *Phys Ther.* 2000;81(7):688-700.

47. Behrman AL, Lawless-Dixon AR, Davis SB, et al. Locomotor training progression and outcomes after incomplete spinal cord injury. *Phys Ther.* 2005;85:1356-1371.

48. Field-Fote EC, Tepavac D. Improved intralimb coordination in people with incomplete spinal cord injury following training with body weight support and electrical stimulation. *Phys Ther.* 2002;82:707-715.

49. Hicks AL, Adams MM, Martin Ginis K, et al. Long-term body-weight-supported treadmill training and subsequent follow-up in persons with chronic SCI: effects on functional walking ability and measures of subject well-being. *Spinal Cord.* 2005;43:291-298.

50. Adams MM, Ditor DS, Tarnopolsky MA, et al. The effect of body weight-supported treadmill training on muscle morphology in an individual with chronic, motor-complete spinal cord injury: a case study. *J Spinal Cord Med.* 2006;29(2):167-171.

51. Cook AM, Hussey SM. *Assistive Technologies: Principles and Practice.* 2nd ed. St. Louis, MO: Mosby; 2002.

52. Kirshblum S, House JG, Druin E, et al. Rehabilitation of spinal cord injury. In: Kirshblum S, Campagnolo DI, Delisa JA, eds. *Spinal Cord Medicine.* Philadelphia, PA: Lippincott Williams & Wilkins; 2002.

53. Salerno S, Kirshblum S. Wheelchairs/adaptive mobility equipment and seating. In: Kirshblum S, Campagnolo DI, Delisa JA, eds. *Spinal Cord Medicine.* Philadelphia, PA: Lippincott Williams & Wilkins; 2002.

54. Curtis KA, Drysdale GA, Lanza RD, et al. Shoulder pain in wheelchair users with tetraplegia and paraplegia. *Arch Phys Med Rehabil.* 1999;80(4):453-457.

55. Curtis KA, Tyner TM, Zachary L, et al. Effect of a standard exercise protocol on shoulder pain in long-term wheelchair users. *Spinal Cord.* 1999;37(6):421-429.

56. Chatwin M, Ross E, Hart N, et al. Cough augmentation with muscular insufflation/exsufflation in patients with neuromuscular weakness. *Eur Respir J.* 2003;21:502-508.

57. Fink JB, Hess DR. Secretion clearance techniques. In: Hess DR, MacIntyre NR, Mishoe SC, et al, eds. *Respiratory Care; Principles & Practice.* Philadelphia, PA: WB Saunders; 2002:665-693.

58. Moffat M, Biggs Harris K, eds. *Integumentary Essentials: Applying the Preferred Physical Therapist Practice Patterns.*^{SM} Thorofare, NJ: SLACK Incorporated; 2006.

59. Sussman C. Impaired integumentary integrity associated with superficial skin involvement (Pattern B). In: Moffat M, Biggs Harris K, eds. *Integumentary Essentials: Applying the Preferred Physical Therapist Practice Patterns.*^{SM} Thorofare, NJ: SLACK Incorporated; 2006:17-39.

60. Myers BA. Impaired integumentary integrity associated with full-thickness skin involvement and scar formation. (Pattern D). In: Moffat M, Biggs Harris K, eds. *Integumentary Essentials: Applying the Preferred Physical Therapist Practice Patterns.*^{SM} Thorofare, NJ: SLACK Incorporated; 2006:71-98.

61. Degnan GG, Wind TC, Jones EV, et al. Functional electrical stimulation in tetraplegic patients to restore hand function. *Journal of Long-Term Effects of Medical Implants.* 2002;12(3):175-188.

62. Kobetic R, Triolo RJ, Pinault G, et al. Facilitating ambulation after incomplete spinal cord injury with implanted FES system. 10th Annual IFFESS Conference, Montreal, Canada, July 2005.

63. Onders RP, Diamarco AF, Ignagni AR, et al. Mapping the phrenic nerve motor point: the key to a successful laparoscopic diaphragm pacing system in the first human series. *Surgery.* 2004:136;819-826.

64. Creasey GH, Ho CH, Triolo RJ, et al. Clinical applications of electrical stimulation after spinal cord injury. *J Spinal Cord Med.* 2004;27(4):365-375.

65. Gerrits HL, de Haan A, Sargeant AJ, et al. Peripheral vascular changes after electrically stimulated cycle training in people with spinal cord injury. *Arch Phys Med Rehabil.* 2001;82(6):832-839.

66. Scremin AM, Kurta L, Gentili A, et al. Increasing muscle mass in spinal cord injured persons with a function electrical stimulation exercise program. *Arch Phys Med Rehabil.* 1999;80(12):1531-1536.

67. Bickel CS, Slade JM, Hadda F, et al. Acute molecular responses of skeletal muscle to resistance exercise in able-bodied and spinal cord-injured subjects. *J Appl Physiol.* 2003;94:2255-2262.

68. Gardner SE, Frantz RA, Schmidt FL. Effect of electrical stimulation on chronic wound healing: a meta-analysis. *Wound Repair Regen.* 1999;7(6):495-503.

69. Cheing GLY, Hui-Chan C. Transcutaneous electrical nerve stimulation: nonparallel antinociceptive effects on chronic clinical pain and active experimental pain. *Arch Phys Med Rehabil.* 1999;80:305-312.

70. Wilson RC, Jones PW. Long-term reproducibility of Borg scale estimates of breathlessness during exercise. *Clin Sci.* 1991;80:309-312.

71. Belanger A. *Evidence-Based Guide to Therapeutic Physical Agents.* Philadelphia, PA: Lippincott Williams & Wilkins;

2003.

72. Consortium for Spinal Cord Medicine: A Clinical Practice Guideline for Primary Care Physicians. *Depression Following Spinal Cord Injury.* Washington, DC: Paralyzed Veterans of America; August 1998.

73. Hornby TG, Zemon DH, Campbell D. Robotic-assisted, body-weight-supported treadmill training in individuals following motor incomplete spinal cord injury. *Phys Ther.* 2005;85:52-66.

74. Israel JF, Campbell DD, Kahn JH, Hornby TG. Metabolic costs and muscle activity patterns during robotic- and therapist-assisted treadmill walking in individuals with incomplete spinal cord injury. *Phys Ther.* 2006;86:1466-1478.

75. Winchester P, Querry R. Robotic orthoses for body weight-supported treadmill training. *Phys Med Rehabil Clin N Am.* 2006;17(1):159-172.

76. van Hedel HJ. Letter to the editor. *Phys Ther.* 2006;86:1444-1445.

77. Behrman A. Editorial board response. *Phys Ther.* 2006;86:1445-1447.

78. Wernig A. Letter to the editor. *Spinal Cord.* 2006;44:265-266.

79. Hicks AL, Adams MM. Letter to the editor. *Spinal Cord.* 2006;44:267-268.

80. Chaplin E. Functional neuromuscular stimulation for mobility in patients with spinal cord injuries. The Parastep I System. *J Spinal Cord Med.* 1996;19(2):99-105.

81. Stein RB, Belanger M, Wheeler G, et al. Electrical systems for improving locomotion after incomplete spinal cord injury: an assessment. *Arch Phys Med Rehabil.* 1993;74:954-959.

82. Latimer AE, Martin Ginis KA, Hicks AL, et al. An examination of the mechanisms of exercise-induced change in psychological well-being among people with spinal cord injury. *J Rehabil Res Dev.* 2004;41(5):643-652.

CHAPTER NINE

Impaired Arousal, Range of Motion, and Motor Control Associated With Coma, Near Coma, or Vegetative State (Pattern I)

Laura Gilchrist, PT, PhD
Marilyn Woods, PT[†]
Joanell A. Bohmert, PT, MS
Janice B. Hulme, PT, MS, DHSc
Anne-Marie Dupre, PT, DPT, MS, NCS

ANATOMY

The regions of the CNS responsible for alertness and arousal are located in the brainstem and diffusely throughout the thalamus and cerebral cortex. The cerebral cortex has been described in earlier patterns (see Pattern B: Impaired Neuromotor Development, Pattern C: Impaired Motor Function and Sensory Integrity Associated With Nonprogressive Disorders of the Central Nervous System—Congenital Origin or Acquired in Infancy or Childhood, and Pattern D: Impaired Motor Function and Sensory Integrity Associated With Nonprogressive Disorders of the Central Nervous System—Acquired in Adolescence or Adulthood), and the brainstem will be detailed here. There are three major anatomical divisions of the brainstem.[1] Starting inferiorly and working superiorly, the brainstem consists of the medulla oblongata, pons, and midbrain. A wide variety of structures are located within the three regions of the brainstem, in addition to the neural tracts that run through the brainstem on their way to or from the spinal cord, cerebrum, and/or cerebellum. For example, the corticospinal tract controlling voluntary movement passes through the ventral aspect of the brainstem, and the spinothalamic tract carrying pain and temperature sensation runs through the dorsal aspect of the brainstem.[1]

MEDULLA

The medulla oblongata is the most inferior portion of the brainstem and is contiguous with the spinal cord.[1] Within the medulla, most of the corticospinal tract axons cross the midline at the pyramidal decussation. Sensory information regarding proprioception and light touch from the dorsal column medial lemniscal pathway synapses in the gracile and cuneate nuclei and then crosses the midline before ascending to the thalamus. Numerous cranial nerve nuclei connect to the brain and have nuclei in the medulla (Table 9-1), including the following cranial nerves: XII (hypoglossal), XI (accessory), X (vagus), and IX (glossopharyngeal). Due to the influence of the 10th cranial nerve (vagus), the medulla modulates HR, vasoconstriction, and vasodilation. Respiratory control is shared between the medulla and pontine regions. Portions of the nuclei for cranial nerves VII (facial) and V (trigeminal) also reside in the medulla.

[†]Deceased.

Table 9-1 CRANIAL NERVE LOCATION AND FUNCTION			
Number	*Name*	*Connecting Region*	*Function*
I	Olfactory	Frontal lobe	Smell
II	Optic	Diencephalon	Vision
III	Oculomotor	Midbrain	Eye movements, upper eyelid raising, pupillary constriction
IV	Trochlear	Midbrain	Eye movement
V	Trigeminal	Pons	Sensation of the face and TMJ, chewing
VI	Abducens	Pontomedullary junction	Eye movement
VII	Facial	Pontomedullary junction	Muscles of facial expression, salivation, taste
VIII	Vestibulocochlear	Pontomedullary junction	Hearing, vestibular function
IX	Glossopharyngeal	Medulla	Swallowing, salivation, taste
X	Vagus	Medulla	Visceral control, swallowing, speech
XI	Accessory	Spinal cord and medulla	Shoulder elevation, head turning
XII	Hypoglossal	Medulla	Tongue control

Modified from Lundy-Ekman L. *Neuroscience: Fundamentals for Rehabilitation*. 2nd ed. Philadelphia, PA: WB Saunders; 2002.

Another medullary structure, the inferior olive, receives information from the spinal cord and brain relaying this to the cerebellum for detection of movement errors.

PONS

The pons is located between the medulla and midbrain and connects to the cerebellum.[1] A number of cranial nerves enter or exit the brainstem at the junction between the medulla and the pons. Cranial nerves VI (abducens), VII (facial), and VIII (vestibulocochlear) all connect with the brainstem at the pontomedullary junction. Cranial nerve V (trigeminal) also connects with the brainstem in the pons, but it has nuclei in all three regions of the brainstem. Cortical fibers carrying information about motor planning synapse in the pons. This information is then relayed to the cerebellum through pontocerebellar fibers in the middle cerebellar peduncles. Thus, the cerebellum can compare information about the actual movement and the intended movement.[1]

MIDBRAIN

The midbrain connects the pons and the diencephalons.[1] Two cranial nerves, III (oculomotor) and IV (trochlear), control all eye movements except lateral gaze (controlled by cranial nerve VI [abducens]) and reside in the midbrain. Additional structures in the midbrain include: 1) the sub-

stantia nigra, a nucleus of the basal ganglia complex; 2) cerebral peduncles containing axons ascending and descending to/from the cerebrum; 3) the oculomotor complex that controls pupillary response to light; 4) the superior and inferior colliculi that control head movements toward sound and motion; and 5) the red nucleus, which will be discussed in the next section on posture and gross motor function.[1]

POSTURE AND GROSS MOTOR CONTROL BY THE BRAINSTEM

Motor tracts that control posture and gross motor function reside in the brainstem regions. Starting superiorly in the brainstem, the midbrain contains two motor pathways. The tectospinal tract originates in the superior colliculi and generates an orienting response that directs the head and eyes toward sounds and motion.[1] The rubrospinal tract originates in the red nucleus of the midbrain and innervates contralateral UE flexor motor neurons.[1] In the pons, the medial reticulospinal tract activates postural muscles including the extensor muscle groups of the trunk and LEs. The vestibulospinal tracts also originate in the pons and medulla and assist postural recovery by facilitating extension in the neck, trunk, and hips after imbalance is detected by the vestibular system.[1] In the medulla, the lateral reticulospinal tract acts to facilitate the flexor muscle groups.[1]

When evaluating a comatose patient, the level of lesion may be hypothesized at times in accordance with the posturing of the patient. In patients with lesions involving the cortex and subcortical regions, but not the brainstem, all of the above discussed brainstem motor tracts will be intact, except the descending control from the corticospinal tract. Thus, the patient will display decorticate rigidity consisting of UE flexion and LE extension.[1] If the lesion includes the midbrain, the rubrospinal tract will not be active, and thus UE flexion will not be seen. As a result, the posturing will be decerebrate rigidity, consisting of extension of the limbs and trunk.[1]

RETICULAR NUCLEI

A large net-like group of nuclei, named the reticular nuclei, exists throughout the brainstem. This system has wide distribution of axons both ascending to the cerebrum and descending to the spinal cord, and thus has a wide modulatory influence on activity of neural function.[2] The reticulospinal tracts, as noted above, modulate motor neuron activity in the spinal cord. Other reticular nuclei are responsible for collecting information about homeostasis and then regulating cardiac and respiratory function accordingly. The third major function of the reticular system is to modulate arousal and attention.

There is not one single nucleus in the brainstem that is responsible for alertness. Multiple nuclei in the pons and midbrain, including the Raphe nuclei, the locus coeruleus, the tuberomamillary nuclei, and the cholenergic nuclei at the pons-midbrain junction, are all active when a person is awake.[3] These same nuclei are in varying states of activation during sleep, depending on if the person is in REM or non-REM sleep.[3] Together, these nuclei act to stimulate the thalamus and other cortical regions, inducing alertness, and have collectively been termed the reticular-activating system.

PATHOPHYSIOLOGY

Consciousness has two clinical features: wakefulness and awareness.[4] Wakefulness is a function of the reticular system and its projections to the thalamus, while awareness requires not only a functioning reticular system but also a functioning thalamus and cerebral cortical regions and projections.[4] Coma is a pathological state of "eyes-closed unconsciousness from which patients cannot be aroused to wakefulness by stimuli."[4(p 1181)]

Coma can be due to a variety of causes including both intracranial and extracranial disorders. The most prevalent cause of coma comes from an intracranial disorder as a result of a TBI.[4] When cerebral trauma occurs, often there is resulting cerebral edema and/or intracranial bleeding. Both of these types of injuries lead to increased ICP, which has a twofold effect. First, increased ICP and swelling places pressure

on the compressible brain tissues and may lead to decreased arousal by compression of the brainstem through the foramen magnum, termed a brainstem herniation.[1] Direct pressure of the brainstem on the surrounding bone leads to decreased blood flow in the region and decreased function of the brainstem tissues. Second, increasing ICP may also decrease the ability of blood to flow into the cerebral vessels, even without the direct compression of brain tissue against bone or meningeal tissues (see Pattern D: Impaired Motor Function and Sensory Integrity Associated With Nonprogressive Disorders of the Central Nervous System—Acquired in Adolescence or Adulthood for further discussion of the meninges).

To supply the CNS with adequate oxygen and glucose, the brain requires adequate perfusion as measured by the cerebral perfusion pressure (CPP).[5] The CPP is the difference between the arterial pressure that is supplying blood to the cerebrum minus the ICP. The ICP would prevent the flow of blood into the brain if it is too high.[5] If the CPP is inadequate due to high ICP, both the function of the brainstem and the cerebral cortex can be diminished.[6]

Other space-occupying lesions in the CNS may lead to decreased consciousness in the absence of trauma. Both benign (such as meningeoma) and malignant (gliomas or metastatic cancers) tumors can compress or destroy brain tissue. This growth of a tumor in the CNS may invade the brain tissues responsible for consciousness and lead to decreased consciousness.[7] Alternately, a meningeoma will not invade the brain tissue but will cause compression of brain tissue leading to CNS ischemia and possible increases in ICP.[7] Intracranial bleeds, such as occur after trauma or from rupture of a cerebral aneurysm, take up space in the cranial vault, resulting in increased ICP and compression of surrounding tissues.[7]

Extracranial disorders may also cause a decrease in consciousness. Since the brain has a large metabolic need for oxygen and glucose, any disorder that disrupts the supply can lead to decreased cortical and subcortical functions. While increased ICP leading to decreased CPP has been discussed as an intracranial reason for coma, any other reason for decreased arterial pressure (such as inadequate oxygen or abnormal levels of glucose in the blood) may also result in poor functioning of CNS tissues.

Hypoxia, a lack of oxygenation of the blood, may be due to pulmonary dysfunction (such as occurs in chronic obstructive pulmonary disease or near drowning) or to anemia (in which case blood does not have adequate carrying capacity for oxygen).[7] Circulatory hypoxia may occur when the cardiovascular system is unable to meet metabolic demands. This commonly occurs during cardiac arrest or as a result of vascular insufficiency.[7] Abnormally high levels of glucose, as is found in severe uncontrolled diabetes, can also lead to coma with or without ketoacidosis. In diabetic ketoacidosis, the patient may become rapidly dehydrated leading to severe electrolyte disturbance.[7] This electrolyte disturbance leads to alterations in neuron function that can lead to coma. Coma may also result from uncontrolled blood sugars even without acidosis, in the form of hyperosmolar, hyperglycemic nonketogenic coma.[7]

Disorders of the liver and kidney may result in impaired consciousness. In end-stage liver disorders, encephalopathy may occur. It is thought that the toxins that are normally cleared by the liver build-up in the blood, alter the blood-brain barrier, and allow electrolytes and proteins into the CSF. This alteration in CSF will eventually cause cerebral edema and a decrease in cerebral and brainstem function.[7] Kidney failure also results in electrolyte disturbance in the blood leading to fluid overload that eventually may result in cerebral edema if not treated.[7] In multi-organ system dysfunction, cardiac failure may result in poor perfusion of the cerebral and brainstem tissues, and liver and kidney failure may result in cerebral edema, again reducing CPP.[7]

CLASSIFICATIONS OF SEVERE BRAIN INJURY

The Brain Injury Association of America Inc has identified six categories of severe brain injury:
1. Coma
2. Vegetative state
3. Persistent vegetative state
4. Minimally responsive state
5. Akinetic mutism
6. Locked-in syndrome[8]

Coma, a deep state of unconsciousness in which the individual is unable to follow commands, speak, open his or her eyes, and respond to his or her environment, usually persists for only a few weeks.[9,10] When some arousal (ie, eye opening, general responses to pain and sleep-wake cycles, and respiratory and digestive functions) is present, but the ability to interact with the environment is not functioning, the individual is said to be in a vegetative state.[9,11] In this condition, hypothalmic and brainstem automatic functions are either completely or partially preserved.[11] There is no test to specifically diagnose vegetative state. The diagnosis is made only by repetitive neurobehavioral assessments.[9]

When a state of wakeful consciousness persists for 1 month in an individual post-acute traumatic or nontraumatic brain injury, it is referred to as a persistent vegetative state (PVS).[11] In a PVS there is a loss of higher brain functions, cognition, and awareness of surroundings, while noncognitive functions, such as breathing, circulation, and normal sleep patterns, remain relatively intact. Individuals in PVS may exhibit spontaneous movements; their eyes may open in response to external stimuli and occasionally they scowl, cry, or laugh. Although they may appear somewhat normal at times, they are unable to respond to commands or verbalize.[12,13]

Patients are described as being in a minimally responsive state (MRS) when they are no longer in a coma or PVS after a severe head injury. They begin to demonstrate an awareness of their surroundings and external stimuli. Patients in this state may still demonstrate primitive reflexes and be able to follow simple commands, but are inconsistent in their ability to follow commands.[8,9,12]

Akinetic mutism is a rare syndrome characterized by pathologically slow bodily movement and loss of speech. In this condition, mental function is reduced, although wakefulness may be preserved.[11] Locked-in syndrome is a condition characterized by paralysis of the voluntary motor system with intact consciousness and cognition.[11] In the absence of all brain functions, including those of the brainstem, patients are declared to be brain dead. These patients are irreversibly comatose and apneic.[11,14]

POST-TRAUMATIC SEIZURES

Seizures are the most extreme form of synchronous brain activity and are always a sign of pathology.[15] Seizures may be the result of many causes, including medications, high fevers, head injuries, and certain diseases. People who have repeated seizures due to a brain disorder have epilepsy that is the result of sudden, abnormal electrical activity in the brain.[15,16]

There are many types of seizures and symptoms vary. Seizures fall into two main groups. A generalized seizure involves the entire cerebral cortex of both hemispheres. A partial seizure involves only a circumscribed area of the cortex. In both, the neurons of the affected areas fire with a synchrony that never occurs in normal behavior. As a result, seizures are usually accompanied by very large EEG patterns.[15] A partial seizure may spread within the brain, a process known as secondary generalization, while generalized seizures are divided according to the effect on the body. Nonetheless, they all involve loss of consciousness. The types of generalized seizures are categorized as absence, myoclonic, clonic, tonic, tonic-clonic, and atonic seizures.[17] Most seizures last from 30 seconds to 2 minutes.[16,18]

Pathophysiological changes in the brain are linked to the severity of injury in TBI and can lead to changes in brain metabolism, blood flow, and homeostasis that are a threat to survival.[19] As a result of the acute injury, seizures may occur at any time from immediately upon injury, which may possibly contribute to the accumulation of blood within the cranium, to within the first 24 hours post injury or even later in the course of the disease. The interval of time from head injury to the development of seizures varies. However, 57% of patients have an onset of seizure within 1 year of injury. The onset of seizures is significant in prognosticating the development of epilepsy.[19]

The risk of developing post-traumatic epilepsy is also directly related to the severity of the brain injury. The incidence of seizures within the first year following head trauma is 12 times greater than that found in the general population. There is a 7% to 39% prevalence of seizures in people with severe cortical injury with neurological deficits but with the dura mater remaining intact. With increased severity of trauma (eg, dural penetration and neurological abnormalities), the range of epilepsy incidence increases to 20% to 57%.[19]

Guidelines have been established for identifying those at risk for developing epilepsy later in the course of the disease. These include the occurrence of an early seizure and factors associated with the severity of the injury, including the presence of an intracerebral hematoma and the need for surgical repair of a depressed skull fracture.[20] Environmental factors that are also associated with an increased likelihood of seizures include being asleep, the transition between sleep and wakefulness, tiredness and sleep deprivation, illness, constipation, menstruation, stress or anxiety, and alcohol consumption.[17]

Many drugs are used to prevent or reduce frequency of seizures (see Anticonvulsant Medications in Pharmacology). All of these medications have possible side effects, however they are usually reversible when the medication is discontinued.[21]

PAIN AND SUFFERING

Whether patients in a PVS can experience pain and suffering has always been questioned. The unpleasant experiences that occur in response to stimulation of peripheral nociceptive receptors and their afferent pathways or that come from deep self-perception are referred to as pain and suffering.[22] The experience of pain is not what is commonly referred to as "nociceptive," the response to noxious stimuli, which can be elicited at every level of the nervous system. The responses in PVS are behaviorally controlled by motor system functions and include flexor spasms and decorticate and decerebrate posturing. None of these necessarily reflect the perception of pain. Nociceptive stimulation elicits unconscious postural responses and other motor, autonomic, and endocrine reflexive responses. These responses do not evoke the experience of pain and suffering if the brain has lost its capacity for self-awareness. The perceptions of pain and suffering are conscious experiences. Coma or a vegetative state is a state of unconsciousness, which, by definition, precludes these experiences.[22,23]

There are four levels of neurologic responses to nociceptive stimuli. The levels range from unconscious responses to the experience of pain and suffering and include monosynaptic reflex responses, simple nociception, subcortical nociceptive responses, and conscious awareness of pain or the experience of suffering, which occurs at a cortical level. The first three responses are commonly seen in patients in a PVS and are mediated at subcortical levels.[22]

Patients in a PVS are unaware, insensate, and lacking the cerebral cortical capacity to be conscious of pain. This belief is supported by PET studies, clinical experience, and neuropathological examination.[11,22] With the exception of someone in a severe locked-in state, almost all patients have

some degree of motor activity and eye movement that could express a behavioral response to signal conscious perception of pain or suffering.[22]

RECOVERY

Prognosis

Coma often persists for a few weeks after injury. There is no spontaneous eye opening and vigorous stimulation does not result in awareness. The vegetative state follows, when there is wakefulness without awareness. In the vegetative state, the function in the ascending reticular activating system is preserved but not in the thalamus or cerebral hemispheres.[24]

Advances in medicine have improved survival, making it possible for the body to remain viable without brain function following severe TBI, as long as proper nursing care is provided.[18,24,25] If the coma is not reversible, the condition has been labeled as cerebral death, or brain death. For a person to be considered brain dead, he or she must meet three neurological criteria: coma, absent brainstem reflexes, and apnea.[26,27] Under such circumstances, it is a legal and ethical question as to whether the person is living or dead. As the allocation of medical funds becomes more selective and the need for donor organs increases, the issue becomes more critical.[18]

Probability

PVS develops in up to 14% of patients in prolonged traumatic coma according to the Multi-Society Task Force. The Task Force reported (from an analysis of 754 published cases) that for those people who were in a vegetative state 1 month post injury, 43% had regained consciousness by 12 months, 34% had died, and 23% were still vegetative.[22,28] A retrospective analysis of numerous adult and children patient records determined that a persistent vegetative condition lasting for 12 months could be judged to be permanent after a traumatic injury. Recovery after this time is extremely rare and nearly always involves a severe disability. In a patient analysis completed by the Multi-Society Task Force, not one case where recovery began after 1 year had a good recovery,[22] and not one case of recovery of any level of consciousness in patients who met the criteria for brain death had been identified.[26] Those cases, who recovered with moderate or severe disability, had shown signs of improvement within 6 months post injury. Later recovery was almost always associated with severe disability.[22,24,29,30] Strauss and colleagues used the Disability Rating Scale to determine long-term mortality after TBI rehabilitation and found clear evidence that the more severe the disability the greater the mortality.[31]

Although a wide range of clinical and laboratory variables have been studied by a number of researchers, no well-established criteria have been established that can accurately predict an outcome for people while they are in a coma.[11]

Some evidence suggests that the presence of ventilatory dysfunction, decorticate posturing, extraneural trauma soon after the insult, older age, pupillary abnormalities, and a low score on a motor response test may be associated with a poor post-traumatic vegetative outcome.[11,22] At 6 months post injury, age and rating on the Glasgow Coma Score are the most dependable predictors of functional recovery in patients with a TBI-related coma.[26] The prognosis for recovery remains unfavorable for patients in a vegetative state as a result of TBI.[22]

Recovery is more likely for patients when the coma is caused by sedatives or low blood sugar if procedures to alleviate the toxic stimuli are performed quickly. Low blood sugar levels should be eliminated through the administration of glucose within 1 hour.[32] There are reports of individuals who have "awakened" following years in a coma and have been able to make some recovery, but statistically this is rare.

Survival and Life Expectancy

The severity of neurological injury required to induce the vegetative state in adults and children imposes a reduction of 2 to 5 years from the average life expectancy despite the preservation of hypothalamic and brainstem function. Survival beyond 10 years is atypical. A review of a database of 251 patients found the mortality rate to be 33% for adults in a vegetative state within 1 year post a traumatic injury, 82% at 3 years, and 95% at 5 years. Mortality was 9% for children in a vegetative state within 1 year post TBI.[22]

A shortened life expectancy for people in a PVS can be attributed to several factors: bladder and other infections, pressure sores, generalized systemic failure, respiratory failure, sudden death of unknown cause, and other disease-related causes, such as recurrent strokes or tumors.[33] Another adverse factor is age. Infants, children, and the elderly have a shorter life expectancy than young or middle-aged adults. It is not known whether this is related to the cause of the vegetative state or to the risks of medical complications. No information exists as to the level of care and its impact on life expectancy of patients in a PVS.[22,34]

ETHICAL ISSUES

Modern medicine has afforded many benefits, but many complex ethical decisions have been brought about in return. The decision to let medical technology keep a loved one alive or to allow him or her to die is one of the hardest to make. Questions about ethical issues, quality of life, appropriate use of resources, beliefs, and wishes of family members and professional responsibilities are raised.[29,35]

The ethical dilemma of withdrawing of food and fluids from patients in a PVS is one of the most challenging.[29,35] When artificial nutrition and hydration are withdrawn from patients in a PVS, they usually die within 10 to 14 days. As patients in a PVS cannot experience thirst or hunger, the immediate cause of death is dehydration and electrolyte imbalance rather than malnutrition. Some patients may die from acute illnesses, such as pneumonia, or from underlying cardiac or renal problems with the discontinuation of medications.[22]

Frequently, technology serves as a "link" between life and death.[35] No ethical difference exists between withholding and withdrawing the same treatment once it has been initiated. Initiation of treatment serves two purposes. It enables the establishment of the prognosis with greater certainty, and it may provide time to clarify the patient's state and in turn clarify the wishes of the family. The fundamental ethical principle surrounding the decision to withdraw life-sustaining treatments once they have been initiated is compounded by the emotional reaction this elicits.[36] The decision to refuse life-sustaining support is another dilemma. The position of medical ethicists supported by many legal decisions is that the difference between cessation and initiation of treatment is not relevant, ethically or legally, if the critical considerations of medical indications, patient preference, and quality of life are the same.[37,38] A decision to withhold or withdraw a treatment should be made openly and communicated with the team and documented in the medical record so that all health professionals involved will be aware of the decision.[29,35]

MEDICAL INTERVENTIONS

ACUTE MANAGEMENT

Initial medical management of the individual who has lost consciousness is to identify if there is an individual who knows the victim or may know what occurred. The airway and breathing are checked followed by pulse and BP. CPR is administered if needed. If not needed, the body temperature is checked as this may indicate an infection if the temperature is abnormally high or may indicate prolonged exposure to cold, an underactive thyroid gland, or alcohol intoxication if the temperature is abnormally low.[32] A low temperature in the elderly may also indicate an infection. The body and head are checked for injury and any signs of allergic reactions or drug injections.

A neurological examination is completed to determine the status of brain function. Signs of significant brain damage include periodic breathing that is rapid then slows, then may stop for several seconds (Cheyne-Stokes respiration); decerebrate rigidity (head tilted back, arms and legs are extended); decorticate rigidity (arms are flexed); or general limpness of the body (indicates extensive damage including brainstem and cerebrum).[32] The position, size, and reaction to light is checked in each pupil, since dilated pupils that do not react to light may indicate pressure on the third cranial nerve or damage to the brainstem. It should be noted that medications for glaucoma may interfere with an accurate response.

Laboratory tests are completed for urine and blood to check levels of sugar, sodium, alcohol, oxygen, carbon dioxides, and toxic substances (see Other Clinical Tests).[32]

NEUROSURGICAL MANAGEMENT

Maintaining blood flow and oxygen to all parts of the brain is essential to minimize damage and enhance the prospect of survival and recovery. Sometimes this requires neurosurgical intervention to remove any hematomas that are pressing on the brain and to surgically repair damaged blood vessels to stop any further bleeding. In severe cases, portions of the brain that are damaged beyond recovery may be removed to increase chances of recovery for the healthy portions of the brain. It may also be necessary to insert a shunt, or ventricular drain, to remove excess fluids.[39]

IMAGING

- ◆ CT scan
  - Utilizes x-rays to take images in slices and allows the user to view the images in sequence recreating the three-dimensional images through a computer program
  - Is particularly useful to image bleeds, ventricular enlargement, and compression of brain tissues, but not all injuries are evident on CT scan[8]
- ◆ CT angiography
  - Requires injection of contrast dye to demonstrate vascular lesions
  - Identifies arterial blood flood
- ◆ MRI
  - Uses magnetic fields to image brain tissues producing increased anatomical detail over CT scans
  - Used to distinguish healthy from injured tissue
  - Although anatomical detail is enhanced with MRI, diffuse lesions may be difficult to image
- ◆ PET scan
  - Sometimes used for showing utilization of oxygen, glucose, and other nutrients by the brain (metabolism)
  - Used to identify areas weakened or damaged
- ◆ SPECT
  - Uses nuclear isotopes to provide a tomographic image of the brain
  - Shows perfusion in the brain

OTHER CLINICAL TESTS

- ◆ Blood tests
  - Arterial blood gas analyses may be used to assess the presence of adequate oxygen in the blood for cerebral perfusion
  - Electrolytes and other blood chemicals (eg, ammonia) may also be measured as altered levels may influence arousal and alertness
- ◆ Electroencephalography
  - Allows an electrical activity assessment of the brain
  - Identifies seizure activity
  - Establishes levels of unconsciousness in unresponsive patients
- ◆ Glasgow Coma Scale[40]
  - Generally administered in the field or emergency room to determine the level of consciousness
  - Patients are scored on their best motor, verbal, and eye responses
  - Three parameters
    - Best eye response (4): 1=No eye opening, 2=Eye opening to pain, 3=Eye opening to verbal command, 4=Eyes open spontaneously
    - Best verbal response (5): 1=No verbal response, 2=Incomprehensible sounds, 3=Inappropriate words, 4=Confused, 5=Orientated
    - Best motor response (6): 1=No motor response, 2=Extension to pain, 3=Flexion to pain, 4=Withdrawal from pain, 5=Localizing pain, 6=Obeys commands
  - Scores of 15 are normal/near normal and 3 is the lowest possible score
- ◆ Urine tests
  - Urine sample is analyzed to assess the presence of chemicals or toxins

PHARMACOLOGY[21,41,42]

- ◆ Anti-anxiety
  - Example: Diazepam (Valium)
  - Actions: Relieves anxiety, muscle spasms, and seizures
  - Side effects: Drowsiness, dizziness, tiredness, weakness, diarrhea, upset stomach
- ◆ Antibiotic medications
  - Examples: Levofloxacin (Levaquin), gentamicin (Garamycin), piperacillin, tazobactam (Zosyn)
  - Action: Eliminate bacteria that cause infections
  - Side effects: Upset stomach, diarrhea, vomiting, headache, restlessness, fatigue, constipation
- ◆ Anticonvulsant medications[43]
  - Examples: Phenytoin (Dilantin), valproic acid (Depakene, Depakote), carbamazepine (Tegretol, Carbatrol), ethosuximide (Zarontin), felbamate (Felbatol), Gabitril, levetiracetam (Keppra), lamotrigine (Lamictal), topiramate (Topamax), gabapentin (Neurontin), oxcarbazepine (Trileptal), clonazepam (Klonopin), clorazepate (Tranxene)

- Actions
  - Act on the brain and nervous system to control convulsions and seizures and treat epilepsy
  - May also block sustained repetitive firing in a frequency dependent manner by: blocking sodium channels; promoting sodium efflux from the neuron; inducing calming effects by acting on parts of the limbic system, the thalamus and hypothalamus; augmenting neurotransmitter GABA activity; antagonizing the AMPA/kainate subtype of the glutamate receptor; and inhibiting the carbonic anhydrase enzyme
  - Valproic acid is thought to increase brain concentrations of GABA
- Side effects: Drowsiness, fatigue, dizziness, redness, irritation of the gums, nausea, constipation, weight loss, heartburn, mental confusion, muscle twitching, headache, blurred or double vision
- Antihypertensive medications
  - Example: Metoprolol (Lopressor, Toprol XL)
  - Action: A beta blocker that slows down the HR and relaxes the blood vessels decreasing the work of the heart
  - Side effects: Dizziness, tiredness, upset stomach, depression, dry mouth, constipation, heartburn, vomiting, rash, cold hands and feet
- Artificial tears[44-46]
  - Examples: Carboxymethyl cellulose, hydroxypropyl cellulose
  - Actions
    - Used as a lubricant in nonvolatile eye drops
    - Stabilize and thicken the precorneal tear film and prolong the tear film breakup time
  - Side effects: Eye pain, irritation, continued redness, hyperaemia, photophobia, stickiness of eyelashes
- Baclofen pump
  - Example: Baclofen (Lioresal)
  - Actions: Acts on the spinal cord nerves to decrease number and severity of muscle spasms and relieves pain and improves muscle movement
  - Side effects: Drowsiness, dizziness, weakness, confusion, upset stomach
- Proton-pump inhibitors
  - Example: Pantoprazole (Protonix)
  - Action: Used to treat gastroesophageal reflux disease
  - Side effects: Diarrhea, headache, stomach pain, bloating
- Stimulant laxatives
  - Examples: Dulcolax, Senokot
  - Action: Treat constipation by increasing the movement of the bowel
  - Side effects: Upset stomach, stomach cramps, diarrhea, vomiting

- Stool softeners
  - Example: Colace
  - Action: Relieves constipation by softening stool
  - Side effects: Upset stomach, stomach or intestinal cramps

Case Study #1: Left Medial Temporal Lobe Infarct

Mrs. Helen Boggs is an 80-year-old female who sustained a left medial temporal lobe infarct and is comatose.

PHYSICAL THERAPIST EXAMINATION

HISTORY

- General demographics: Mrs. Boggs is an 80-year-old female whose primary language is English. She is right handed.
- Social history: Mrs. Boggs is widowed and is the mother of two grown children, both of whom live nearby. Her daughter and son are married, and she has three grandchildren and one great-grandchild.
- Employment/work: She is a homemaker and volunteers at her church.
- Living environment: She lives in a ranch-style home with two steps to enter in the house with railings on both sides.
- General health status (as reported by her family):
  - General health perception: Her health prior to this episode was generally good. Recently she has had some health problems including hypothyroidism, hyperlipidema, HTN, and internal carotid artery stenosis.
  - Physical function: Her function was normal for age.
  - Psychological function: She had some anxiety prior to this stroke.
  - Role function: Mother, grandmother, great-grandmother, volunteer, club member.
  - Social function: She has been active in her church. She belongs to a women's club and a bridge club.
- Social/health habits: Mrs. Boggs is a nonsmoker and does not drink alcohol.
- Family history: Noncontributory.
- Medical/surgical history: She has had several prior surgeries including a hysterectomy (age 55), appendectomy (age 57), bladder suspension (age 72), cataract surgery (age 78), and breast biopsy (age 79). She also has a

history of hypothyroidism, hyperlipidema, HTN, and internal carotid artery stenosis.

♦ Current condition(s)/chief complaint(s): Mrs. Boggs was admitted to the hospital 5 days ago with complaints of difficulty with word finding, confusion, dizziness, and decreased balance. Medical testing revealed a left temporal lobe infarct. Her chest x-ray was negative. Once her medical condition stabilized, rehabilitation was ordered. While getting dressed the third morning in the rehabilitation center, she suffered an extension of the stroke. Mrs. Boggs was hard to arouse at times near coma and is now nonresponsive to noxious stimulus, has no speech, and has no purposeful movement. Her eyes are closed. She was placed in the ICU. Her family is asking about her situation and would like to know when she will "wake up."

♦ Functional status and activity level: Prior to the stroke, she lived alone and was able to manage all of her self-care and home management actions, tasks, and activities independently. She has her own car and was driving to appointments, church, shops, and visit family and friends. Her family reported that she was getting anxious about driving on the freeway and in busy traffic.

♦ Medications: Prior to admission she was on Valium, Dilantin, and Levaquin. Following her first stroke, her preadmission medications were adjusted, and she was provided an antihypertensive medication to decrease the risk of a second stroke.[47] Following her second stroke, medications were again adjusted to address her immediate medical needs. She is receiving artificial tears prn.

♦ Other clinical tests: Following her first stroke the CAT scan revealed a localized left cerebral infarct, and MRI revealed localized left temporal lobe infarct. Her chest x-ray revealed clear lungs. Following her second stroke, the CAT scan revealed a massive hemorrhage in the left temporal lobe with compression of the midbrain and brainstem. Her chest x-ray was normal. The neurologic exam indicated coma with findings consistent with tentorial herniation (ipsilateral temporal lobe herniation that initially causes ipsilateral paresis then progresses to compression of midbrain and brainstem resulting in impaired consciousness and bilateral paresis).[32]

SYSTEMS REVIEW

♦ Cardiovascular/pulmonary
  • BP: 154/76 mmHg
  • Edema: None
  • HR: 80 bpm
  • RR: 18 bpm
♦ Integumentary
  • Presence of scar formation: Healed incisions from hysterectomy, appendectomy, bladder suspension, and breast biopsy

  • Skin color: Normal
  • Skin integrity: Intact
♦ Musculoskeletal
  • Gross range of motion: WFL
  • Gross strength: Unresponsive, unable to test, flaccid UEs and LEs
  • Gross symmetry: Symmetrical while in bed
  • Height: 5'1" (1.55 m)
  • Weight: 124 lbs (56.25 kg)
♦ Neuromuscular
  • Balance: Unresponsive, unable to test
  • Locomotion, transfers, and transitions: Unresponsive, dependent for all transfers and changes of position in bed
♦ Communication, affect, cognition, language, and learning style
  • Communication, affect, and cognition: Unresponsive, unable to determine
  • Learning style: Unresponsive, unable to determine, family would prefer any material in writing

TESTS AND MEASURES

♦ Arousal, attention, and cognition
  • Mrs. Boggs is unresponsive and does not open her eyes
  • Glasgow Coma Score[48]
    ▪ Eye response=1, Motor response=1, Verbal response=1
    ▪ Glasgow Coma Score is scored between 3 and 15 with 3 the worst and 15 the best
    ▪ Glasgow Coma Score composed of three parameters
      ‣ Best eye response (4): 1=No eye opening, 2=Eye opening to pain, 3=Eye opening to verbal command, 4=Eyes open spontaneously
      ‣ Best verbal response (5): 1=No verbal response, 2=Incomprehensible sounds, 3=Inappropriate words, 4=Confused, 5=Orientated
      ‣ Best motor response (6): 1=No motor response, 2=Extension to pain, 3=Flexion to pain, 4=Withdrawal from pain, 5=Localizing pain, 6=Obeys commands
♦ Cranial and peripheral nerve integrity
  • No response to stimulation of cranial nerves (auditory, visual, olfactory, tactile)
    ▪ Pupils are fixed in midposition, do not move in response to head movements (absent oculocephalic reflex)
  • No response to stimulation of peripheral nerves (motor response, tactile, temperature, somatosensory)

♦ Integumentary integrity
  • Skin unremarkable for pressure areas
  • No skin breakdown noted
♦ Motor function
  • No spontaneous movement observed
  • No purposeful movement observed
  • Nursing reports no movement observed
  • Family reports no movement observed
♦ Orthotic, protective, and supportive devices
  • Mrs. Boggs is using a pressure-reducing mattress
  • Will need splints to protect joints and maintain appropriate muscle length
    ▪ UEs: Possible bilateral wrist and hand splints
    ▪ LEs: Possible bilateral ankle splints
♦ Pain
  • Mrs. Boggs does not present with any signs of pain
  • No response to noxious stimulation
♦ Range of motion
  • PROM: WFL in all four extremities
♦ Reflex integrity
  • Will need to monitor tone watching for signs of change
  • Deep tendon reflexes: Absent in all four extremities
♦ Self-care and home management
  • Dependent for all self-care
  • All self-care tasks handled by nursing staff
♦ Ventilation and respiration/gas exchange
  • Breathing on her own
  • Nursing monitoring breathing patterns for Cheyne-Stokes respiration (periodic breathing in which patient will breath rapidly, then more slowly, then stop for several seconds)[32]
  • Will need activities to prevent respiratory complications

EVALUATION

Mrs. Boggs' history and risk factors indicated that she was a previously active, right-handed female who had a stroke, had begun rehabilitation, and then 3 days later suffered an extension of her stroke leaving her comatose. She is now 5 days post her original stroke. Her risk factors for stroke included hyperlipidema, HTN, and internal carotid artery stenosis. She is currently nonresponsive to noxious stimulation, gives no indication of pain, has not opened her eyes, has not followed any commands, and has not demonstrated any purposeful or spontaneous movement. She is currently breathing on her own. She is using a hospital bed with an air mattress for pressure relief and is currently free of skin breakdown. Her family has been present on a regular basis and is concerned about her "waking up."

DIAGNOSIS

Mrs. Boggs sustained an extension of a previous stroke that was diagnosed as a left medial temporal lobe infarct that rendered her comatose. She has impaired: arousal, attention, and cognition; cranial and peripheral nerve integrity; motor function; and reflex integrity. She is functionally limited in all self-care actions, tasks, and activities. She is in need of devices and equipment, and she is at risk for impaired range of motion, integumentary integrity, and ventilation and respiration/gas exchange. These findings are consistent with placement in Pattern I: Impaired Arousal, Range of Motion, and Motor Control Associated With Coma, Near Coma, or Vegetative State. The identified impairments, functional limitations, and device and equipment needs will be addressed in determining the prognosis and the plan of care.

PROGNOSIS AND PLAN OF CARE

Over the course of the visits, the following established outcomes have been determined:
♦ Arousal, attention, and cognition are increased
♦ Caregivers are educated in appropriate management of Mrs. Boggs
♦ Devices and equipment are issued
♦ Joints are protected
♦ Respiratory complications are prevented or minimized
♦ ROM is maintained
♦ Secondary impairments are prevented or minimized
♦ Skin breakdown is prevented

Based on the neurological findings, the prognosis for recovery of consciousness or function for Mrs. Boggs is poor. Fatal or severe brain damage is indicated with a Glasgow Coma Scale score of 3 to 5 and lack of movement with flaccidity.[32] Outcomes are dependent on her neurological and physiological state and will need to be evaluated on an ongoing basis.

To achieve these outcomes, the appropriate interventions for this patient are determined. These will include: coordination, communication, and documentation; patient/client-related instruction; therapeutic exercise; functional training in self-care and home management (staff and family); manual therapy techniques; prescription, application, and, as appropriate, fabrication of devices and equipment; airway clearance techniques; and integumentary repair and protection techniques.

It is anticipated that she will need 15 to 20 visits over 3 weeks. The patient's discharge will be determined by change in status.

INTERVENTIONS

RATIONALE FOR SELECTED INTERVENTIONS

Mrs. Boggs has neurological findings that indicate deep coma in agreement with her CT scan and her Glasgow Coma Score of 3, since a score of 3 to 5 indicates fatal brain damage[32] with a poorer prognosis for recovery.[49,50] Giacino and Whyte described the characteristics of coma as no spontaneous or stimulus-induced eye movements, no ability to follow commands, no intelligible speech, no purposeful movement, and no discrete defensible movements or capacity to localize noxious stimuli.[51] Coma is reported to be short term, lasting from at least 1 hour to 4 weeks[51,52] with progression to either recovery of consciousness, brain death, or death.[32,51] The focus of intervention for the health care team is maintaining a healthy physical state, preventing complications, and providing secondary prevention.

The focus of physical therapy for Mrs. Boggs will be on positioning, ROM, sensory stimulus, prevention of skin breakdown and pulmonary complications, and education to caregivers. She will be monitored for progress or change in status. The plan of care will be modified accordingly. This may result in identification of additional needs or discontinuation of physical therapy services.

Coordination, Communication, and Documentation

Families may have an unrealistic picture of coma as it has been inaccurately portrayed on television and in the movies.[53,54] The health care team needs to coordinate interaction with the family regarding discussions of prognosis. Discussion must also take place concerning decisions that need to be made concerning medical interventions, including use of a ventilator, feeding tube, and medications, that will maintain life[55] and also concerning issues about the possibility of brain death and organ donation.[33] The team needs to determine if there are any medical directives, living will, or durable power of attorney for health care and to identify a surrogate decision maker.[55] The family should be advised to discuss these issues with their attorney.

There are also legal and ethical issues surrounding the use or termination of life support and determination of "brain dead."[51,55,56] The American Academy of Neurology developed *Practice Parameters: Determining Brain Death in Adults*.[57] Brain death is defined as the loss of all brain function including brainstem functioning.[57] Along with clinical indicators of brain death, sensory evoked potentials have been used to determine brain function.[50,58]

Patient/Client-Related Instruction

The family needs to be provided with education about coma, impairments, possible complications, and secondary prevention. It is important to discuss the realistic effects of coma, such as loss of muscle and motor function, changes in breathing, and the possibility of contractures and skin breakdown.[53,54] Families are stressed[33] and may want to participate in the care of the patient. They should be taught appropriate methods for handling, including PROM, and how to apply and remove splints. Nursing staff are the primary caregivers for patients in the ICU and should be taught precautions and specific handling, positioning, PROM, and application and removal of splints.

Therapeutic Exercise

Sensory stimulation for patients in coma may be beneficial.[59] Gruner and Terhaag[60] developed a sensory stimulation program that provides acoustic, tactile, olfactory, gustatory, visual, kinesthetic, and proprioceptive stimulation. They found that tactile and acoustic stimulation were the most effective at changing heart and respiratory functions in patients in deep coma (Glasgow Coma Score 3-4). In patients in medium coma, mimic changes and eye movements were significant following tactile, acoustic, kinesthetic, and proprioceptive stimulation. Their sensory stimulation program was carried out by nursing staff, therapists, and family or caregivers. Mitchell and colleagues[49] stated that coma arousal procedures could also be effective in reducing levels of stress of the patient's family. This patient with a Glasgow Coma Score of 3 may benefit from a sensory stimulation program beginning with tactile and acoustic stimulation. For additional information on sensory programs see Case Study #2 in this pattern.

Manual Therapy Techniques

Activities to prevent contractures and deformities to bones, joints, and muscles are performed. Mrs. Boggs' flaccid limbs will need to be moved to maintain flexibility and to be protected to prevent overelongation of muscles. Case Study #2 in this pattern provides rationale and specific protocols for PROM and stretching.

Integumentary Repair and Protection Techniques

Skin breakdown is a common complication of patients in coma.[32,33,51] Use of a pressure-reducing mattress and positioning is important for secondary prevention. The reader is referred to Chapter One, Primary Prevention/Risk Reduction for Integumentary Disorders (Pattern A) in *Integumentary Essentials: Applying the Preferred Physical Therapist Practice Patterns*[SM61] for further information, interventions, and rationale.

COORDINATION, COMMUNICATION, AND DOCUMENTATION

Communication will occur with family members and all

members of the multidisciplinary rehabilitation team. Care will be coordinated with nursing staff with training provided for positioning and application of splints as needed. Interdisciplinary teamwork will be demonstrated in case conferences and patient care rounds. All elements of the patient's management will be documented.

PATIENT/CLIENT-RELATED INSTRUCTION

The family and caregivers will be instructed in the current condition and reasons for patient's impairments and functional limitations. They will also be provided with information regarding potential recovery and community resources for additional support. Her family will be informed of the plan of care. Techniques will be taught to family and caregivers to prevent secondary impairments.

THERAPEUTIC EXERCISE

♦ Sensory stimulation
  ● Monitor patient prior to beginning to evaluate current status and determine baseline function
  ● Sensory stimulation schedule should be established to work with the regular nursing care, provide times of no stimulation, and allow for family participation[59]
  ● Acoustic stimulation
    ■ Use of low level sound that includes conversation, reading a book out loud, playing a book on tape or CD, singing, or favorite music
    ■ May be carried out by nursing and family/friends
  ● Tactile stimulation
    ■ Use of different forms of touch, such as light, deep, stroking, and massage
    ■ Use of temperature changes, such as warm or cool cloths
    ■ Use of different textures, such as soft, smooth, rough, feathers, etc
    ■ Done by the physical therapist, who then may educate family in application of the different techniques

FUNCTIONAL TRAINING IN SELF-CARE AND HOME MANAGEMENT

♦ Devices and equipment
  ● Staff are educated regarding need for regular positional changes
  ● Positioning schedule is developed with nursing staff
  ● Staff are educated in application, use, and monitoring of splints
  ● Family is educated in application and use of splints
♦ Injury prevention or reduction
  ● Patient is monitored for pressure areas and skin breakdown

● Patient is on a positioning program
● Patient is on a schedule for wearing splints
● Staff are educated in handling and positioning of limbs and trunk for self-care

MANUAL THERAPY TECHNIQUES

♦ PROM
  ● PROM to all joints daily to maintain joint integrity and muscle length
    ■ Due to flaccidity, joints need to be stabilized when providing passive movement
  ● Monitor joint movement and muscle length to prevent loss of muscle length or joint integrity

PRESCRIPTION, APPLICATION, AND, AS APPROPRIATE, FABRICATION OF DEVICES AND EQUIPMENT

♦ Orthotic devices
  ● Application or fabrication of splints to protect wrist, hand, and ankle
♦ Protective devices
  ● Application of specialized air mattress to ensure skin integrity

AIRWAY CLEARANCE TECHNIQUES

♦ Positioning to enhance breathing and prevent pulmonary complications

ANTICIPATED GOALS AND EXPECTED OUTCOMES

♦ Impact on impairments
  ● Integumentary integrity is improved.
  ● Joint integrity is maintained.
  ● Level of arousal is improved.
  ● ROM is maintained.
  ● Sensory awareness is increased.
♦ Impact on functional limitations
  ● Ability of family to perform self-care is improved.
  ● Family is able to perform sensory activities as part of self-care routine for Mrs. Boggs.
♦ Risk reduction/prevention
  ● Family is able to demonstrate appropriate risk reduction techniques.
  ● Risk of secondary impairments is reduced.
♦ Impact on health, wellness, and fitness
  ● Physical status is improved.
♦ Impact on societal resources
  ● Available resources are maximally utilized.
  ● Documentation occurs throughout patient man-

agement and across settings and follows APTA's *Guidelines for Physical Therapy Documentation.*[62]

♦ Patient/client satisfaction
  • Admission data and discharge planning are completed.
  • Care is coordinated with family and other professionals.
  • Discharge needs are determined.
  • Family has identified surrogate decision maker.
  • Family will be able to identify relevant community resources to meet her discharge needs.
  • Family will verbalize an awareness of the diagnosis, prognosis, interventions, and anticipated goals and expected outcomes.
  • Family's understanding of anticipated goals and expected outcomes is increased.
  • Interdisciplinary collaboration occurs through patient care rounds and patient/family meetings.
  • Referrals are made to other professionals or resources whenever necessary and appropriate.

REEXAMINATION

Reexamination is performed throughout the episode of care.

DISCHARGE

Mrs. Boggs died after 9 days in ICU. Physical therapy was discontinued after a total of nine visits.

Case Study #2: Persistent Vegetative State

Brian Greer is a 16-year-old male who was involved 11 months ago in a head-on collision with a car while riding a dirt bike without a helmet that resulted in a traumatic brain injury, which rendered him quadriplegic and unresponsive. Almost 1 year after his accident, he is being admitted to a long-term care facility.

PHYSICAL THERAPIST EXAMINATION

HISTORY

♦ General demographics: Brian is a 16-year-old right-handed, single black male. He is an only child who was adopted at the age of 2 years old.

♦ Social history: Prior to this injury Brian was a student

who enjoyed being with his friends. He is an only child and has been living with his parents, Elsa (age 40 years) and John (age 42 years). They adopted Brian when he was 2 years of age.

♦ Employment/work: Brian had completed the ninth grade in junior high school prior to the accident, and he was an average student receiving mostly B grades and a few C grades.

♦ Living environment: He had been living with his parents in a second floor walk-up apartment in the city.

♦ General health status
  • General health perception: His health was excellent prior to this injury.
  • Physical function: Normal for his age prior to the injury.
  • Psychological function: Prior to his injury, his parents reported that he had some minor behavioral problems that were concerned primarily with difficulty listening to people in authority.
  • Role function: High school student, son, supportive friend.
  • Social function: Brian had enjoyed being with his friends, riding his dirt bike, playing paint ball, and participating in recreational basketball.

♦ Social/health habits: He had been smoking cigarettes since he was 15 years of age. His parents indicated that Brian did not use alcohol, and alcohol was not a factor in the accident.

♦ Family history: His mother and father are both in good health and involved with Brian's care, but they are in need of a great deal of emotional support.

♦ Medical/surgical history: His history was unremarkable prior to injury. Post injury, Brian's medical history has been as follows:
  • Immediately after the accident he was admitted to an acute medical facility with a diagnosis of tetraplegia and was unresponsive. During the 2.5 months he was in that facility, he had tracheostomy and gastrostomy tubes inserted and required a VP shunt for hydrocephalus.
  • Upon discharge from the acute facility, Brian was then admitted to a rehabilitation hospital for a total of 5 months. He still was unresponsive with a diagnosis of tetraplegia and required insertion of a baclofen pump 8 months post injury due to severe spasticity. He did not make any progress with his therapy in the acute rehabilitation facility. Brian also exhibited increased seizure activity that was classified as focal and secondarily generalized, which required multiple changes in medications. Five months after admission to the rehab hospital, Brian spiked a fever with copious amounts of secretions, and he was transferred back to the acute care hospital.

- His second acute medical care admission lasted 3 weeks. Brian's work-up revealed extensive left-sided pneumonia with a pleural effusion. His sputum culture was positive for *Pseudomonas*. He required a chest tube insertion to drain a left pleural effusion. He was treated with Zosyn and gentamicin for the pneumonia with *Pseudomonas* infection. He also required ventilatory support on and off to maintain his oxygen saturation. Because of his lack of progress in the rehabilitation facility and his inability to return home, he has been admitted to a long-term care facility.

◆ Functional status and activity level: Brian was independent in all functional activities, including ADL and IADL, prior to the head injury. He is currently dependent in all functional mobility skills.

◆ Medications
  - Zosyn 3.375 gm q 6 hr.
  - Gentamicin 7 mg/kg IV q 24 hr.
  - Protonix 40 mg daily.
  - Colace 100 mg bid, Depakene 500 mg q 6 hr, metoprolol 15 mg q 8 hr, Dulcolax suppository q am.
  - Artificial tears prn.
  - Baclofen pump.
  - He has no known allergies.

◆ Other clinical tests: EEG was performed and indicated moderate diffuse slowing that is consistent with a diffuse encephalopathy.

SYSTEMS REVIEW

Note: From the time of admission to long-term care [11 months post injury]).

◆ Cardiovascular/pulmonary
  - BP: 120/72 mmHg
  - Edema: WNL, and Brian is wearing LE compression garments
  - HR: 82 bpm
  - RR: 16 bpm, tracheostomy tube is in place

◆ Integumentary
  - Presence of scar formation
    - Healed scars on his scalp
    - Midline plugged tracheostomy
    - Percutaneous endoscopic gastrotomy tube present in the left abdomen
  - Skin color: WNL
  - Skin integrity
    - Sutures along left hemithorax
    - Stage II decubitus ulcers on elbow and sacrum

◆ Musculoskeletal
  - Gross range of motion: Limitations in all four extremities

- Gross strength: Spasticity in all four extremities
- Gross symmetry: Some asymmetry in postural alignment noted secondary to imbalance of motor control and spasticity
- Height: 6'1" (1.85 m)
- Weight: 156 lbs (70.8 kg)

◆ Neuromuscular
  - Balance: Absent
  - Locomotion, transfers, and transitions: Dependent

◆ Communication, affect, cognition, language, and learning style
  - Communication, affect, and cognition: He responds only to noxious stimuli
  - Learning style: Unknown, but his family indicates that he was a visual learner

TESTS AND MEASURES

◆ Aerobic capacity and endurance
  - Unknown at this time
  - While in the rehabilitation facility he had reached a total of 4 to 6 hours out of bed tolerance in a tilt-in-space wheelchair

◆ Arousal, attention, and cognition
  - Brian follows regular sleep/wake cycles
  - He is not aware of self or environment
  - Glasgow Coma Scale[48]: 6/15 with eye opening=2, verbal response=1, and his best motor response=3

◆ Assistive and adaptive devices
  - Brian is in an electric hospital bed with an air mattress for pressure relief
  - The staff uses a mechanical device for transferring him on and off his wheelchair

◆ Circulation
  - Temperature: 100.0°F rectally
  - Pedal pulse: Intact bilaterally

◆ Cranial and peripheral nerve integrity
  - Unable to formally assess all cranial nerves
  - Minimal testing reveals pupils are dilated and nonreactive indicating involvement of cranial nerve III
  - His gag reflex is absent and an inability to swallow indicates involvement of cranial nerves IX and X

◆ Environmental, home, and work barriers: Brian is unaware of and does not interact in any way with the environment even when family members visit

◆ Integumentary integrity: Brian has Stage II decubitus ulcers on his sacrum and left elbow

◆ Motor function: Absent

◆ Muscle performance: Unable to test

◆ Neuromotor development and sensory integration: Brian has inadequate head and trunk support for any upright supportive sitting

- Orthotic, protective, and supportive devices
  - Brian came from the acute rehabilitation facility with bilateral ankle splints to maintain dorsiflexion, a left elbow splint, and bilateral resting hand splints
  - He is wearing LE compression garments
- Pain
  - Brian's responses are only reflexive
  - He does not exhibit any purposeful movement or response to any painful stimuli
- Posture: Poor head control and slight trunk shortening on the left when sitting in wheelchair resulting in a slight tilt
- Range of motion
  - PROM
    - LEs WNL except for the following
      - Right dorsiflexion=-25 degrees
      - Left dorsiflexion=-20 degrees
      - Right knee flexion=60 degrees
      - Left knee flexion=70 degrees
    - UEs WFL except for the following
      - Left elbow extension=-25 degrees
      - Bilateral wrist extension=0 degrees
      - Bilateral finger extension with passively open hand: Approximately 50% on right and 75% on left
- Reflex integrity
  - Modified Ashworth Scale
    - Spasticity in UEs with grade of 3/5 and is flexor dominate
    - Spasticity in LEs with grade of 2/5 and is extensor dominate
  - Deep tendon reflexes: Decreased throughout
  - Positive Babinski: Silent
- Self-care and home management
  - Patient is dependent in all functional mobility skills
  - Nursing staff uses a mechanical lift for transfers
- Ventilation and respiration/gas exchange
  - Brian is presently off the ventilator
  - He requires suction via the tracheostomy
  - He continues to be on 28% to 30% O_2 via mask
  - Few basal rhonchi on left side

EVALUATION

Brian Greer sustained a head injury 11 months ago when he was hit by a car in a head-on collision while he was on a dirt bike with no helmet. After his acute hospitalization Brian was admitted to an acute rehab facility, but despite daily therapy he continued to be unresponsive. During Brian's rehabilitation he developed pneumonia and was sent back to the acute care facility. Once medically stable, he

was admitted to a long-term care facility with a diagnosis of pneumonia and PVS. Examination revealed absence of any motor or cognitive recovery with secondary impairments including a decline in PROM, out of bed tolerance, and impaired skin integrity. He is unable to clear his airway and requires constant monitoring and intervention by nursing staff. His mother and father are extremely involved, are concerned with their son's lack of progress, and are anxious to see something being done to care for him. Brian should benefit from physical therapy for positioning in bed and wheelchair, for increasing his out of bed tolerance, and for training of nursing staff and family for flexibility exercises and sensory stimulation to improve his level of arousal and awareness.

DIAGNOSIS

Brian Greer is a 16-year old with a diagnosis of tetraplegia and is unresponsive in a PVS. He has impaired: aerobic capacity/endurance; arousal, attention, and cognition; cranial and peripheral nerve integrity; integumentary integrity; motor function; neuromotor development and sensory integration; posture; range of motion; reflex integrity; and ventilation and respiration/gas exchange. He is functionally unable to perform self-care actions, tasks, and activities. He is in need of devices and equipment. These findings are consistent with placement in Pattern I: Impaired Arousal, Range of Motion, and Motor Control Associated With Coma, Near Coma, or Vegetative State and Cardiovascular/Pulmonary Pattern C: Impaired Ventilation, Respiration/Gas Exchange, and Aerobic Capacity/Endurance Associated With Airway Clearance Dysfunction in the APTA's *Guide to Physical Therapist Practice*.[62] The identified impairments, functional limitations, and device and equipment needs will be addressed in determining the prognosis and the plan of care.

PROGNOSIS AND PLAN OF CARE

Over the course of the visits, the following mutually established outcomes have been determined:
- Arousal and attention are improved
- Bilateral dorsiflexion and knee flexion are increased to facilitate positioning in the wheelchair
- Capabilities of the family and nursing staff are improved to provide sensory stimulation, stretching, and positioning programs
- Left elbow extension PROM is increased to minimize skin breakdown
- Respiratory endurance is improved
- Skin condition and integumentary integrity are improved

To achieve these outcomes, the appropriate interventions for this patient are determined. These will include: coordination, communication, and documentation; patient/client-related instruction; therapeutic exercise; prescription, application, and, as appropriate, fabrication of devices and equipment; and airway clearance techniques.

It is anticipated that Brian will need 20 visits over the next 6 to 8 months to establish programs for his family and caregivers and to enable timely reexaminations to monitor the patient's progress with these programs.

INTERVENTIONS

RATIONALE FOR SELECTED INTERVENTIONS

According to the literature, recovery from PVS is most likely to occur during the first year post injury.[63-65] This was the time that Brian received extensive physical therapy in the acute rehabilitation facility, but unfortunately he remained unresponsive. Modest recovery has been reported in a few cases of PVS after 1 year post injury[63,66-68] and for some patients and families this may be significant. A modest recovery may allow Brian to achieve a one- or two-person lift, allowing him to return home without the need for expensive medical equipment or care. This provides the family a glimpse of hope, making a decrease in frequency and/or withdrawal of physical therapy services difficult. Parents will frequently attribute the lack of progress by their child to the withdrawal or reduction of physical therapy services.[69]

Parents often feel that more physical therapy will help their child to "wake up." What is important for the families to understand is that even though aggressive daily physical therapy is not indicated at this stage, there is still a need for ongoing assessment and monitoring.[51,65] Wilson and colleagues[70] surveyed and assessed the care of patients with a diagnosis of PVS or minimally responsive disorder. His results showed that if preventable complications, such as infection, pressure sores, contractures, and poor nutrition, went untreated it limited the patient's potential to improve cognition and quality of life. In long-term care, Brian's rehabilitation will be daily initially to allow for fabrication of necessary splints or to adjust existing splints and to establish programs related to:

- Wheelchair and bed positioning
- Stretching
- Postural drainage
- Multisensory stimulation

Once Brian's services are established and training with family and nursing reveals demonstrated competence with the established program, the physical therapist will continue to see Brian for reexamination, at least one time per month, to monitor and make revisions as indicated to his programs.

Therapeutic Exercise

PROM and prolonged muscle stretching (including application of splints/orthosis and serial casts, bed positioning, wheelchair seating, and standing on tilt tables or standing frames) are common techniques used by physical therapists with patients who are at this low level of functional mobility to improve ROM and reduce spasticity.[71] In a systematic review, Leong[72] looked at the effects of passive stretching for children in vegetative and minimally conscious states. He found that in most studies some improvements were seen using one or a combination of the stretching techniques. The duration of hold and frequency of manual stretch required to make an improvement could not be determined because the levels of evidence for many of the studies were weak, and in some instances only one study was found. Because of the low level of evidence, some findings in the systematic review were based on subject samples that included adults with CVA and TBI and children with CP, so caution should be taken in extrapolating the information for children with PVS. Generally, findings indicated that serial casting and manual passive stretching might be effective in increasing ROM. The parameters for ROM were identified as holding for 20 to 60 seconds per repetition, five repetitions, two to three times per week. Ashford[73] demonstrated that the management of contractures for patients with PVS requires an interdisciplinary approach (physical therapy, nursing, and family) and that PROM exercises alone were not enough. Joint ROM in this patient population was only increased when specific positioning and some pharmacological intervention supplemented it.

Although recovery from a prolonged coma has been reported,[63,66-68] it is rare for someone who has been in a PVS for 11 months and has shown little to no improvement. In the early stages, a multisensory stimulation program is frequently used as a strategy to assist recovery from a coma or PVS.[49,74,75] A systematic review of the literature looked at sensory stimulation in the treatment of individuals with PVS or coma.[59] Specific treatment techniques varied among studies, but they most commonly included vigorous stimulation of the five senses (visual, auditory, olfactory, gustatory, and tactile) and movement. The frequency of treatment ranged from one to two times per day with a duration of 20 to 60 minutes. While this has been shown to be effective in shortening the duration of a coma or PVS,[49,74] it is unclear if changes could be made in late stages of recovery (ie, after 11 months post injury). It was also found that implementation of a sensory stimulation program can be effective in reducing the stress level of family members.[49] This treatment approach has uncertain therapeutic benefits for Brian. However, implementation of such a program, because of its limited detrimental effects, has value as part of a family program.

COORDINATION, COMMUNICATION, AND DOCUMENTATION

Coordination, communication, and documentation with the multidisciplinary team and family members will be ongoing. Communication will occur with nursing staff in each of the following areas: wheelchair and bed positioning protocol including application of positioning devices; proper donning and wearing times for orthotics, including monitoring of skin breakdown; multisensory stimulation program; PROM exercises; pulmonary postural drainage techniques; and transfer training using a mechanical lift.

Monthly reexaminations by the physical therapist will occur to evaluate the effectiveness of the program and modify interventions as needed. Coordination and communication with other team members will occur for each of the monthly reexaminations. Patient care rounds will coordinate needed program changes.

A bed and wheelchair positioning and postural drainage schedule will also be established collaborating with nursing in order to prevent skin breakdown and improve airway clearance.

Referral will be suggested to Brian's mother and father for emotional support. All elements of the patient's management will be documented following APTA and facility guidelines.[62]

Note: Brian's new school district will be notified once he is situated in his long-term care facility. A request will be made to the local educational agency for an educational evaluation to determine educational eligibility, needs, programs, and services that could be provided until he is 21 years of age.

PATIENT/CLIENT-RELATED INSTRUCTION

Brian's family will be given detailed instructions in how to implement each of the following areas of care: multisensory stimulation program including visual, auditory, olfactory, gustatory, and tactile stimulation; wheelchair and bed positioning protocol, including application of positioning devices; PROM exercises; transfer training using a mechanical lift; proper donning and wearing times for his orthotic devices; and monitoring of skin breakdown.

THERAPEUTIC EXERCISE

♦ Flexibility exercises
  • Manual stretching by nursing staff and family members to all joints according to the following parameters
    ▪ 20- to 60-second hold per repetition
    ▪ Five repetitions
    ▪ Two to three times per week
  • Application of splints or fabrication of bivalve cast for prolonged ROM stretch for both ankles and left elbow

  • Bed and wheelchair positioning protocols to maintain joint mobility and prevent skin breakdown
♦ Sensory stimulation
  • Multisensory stimulation program to include the following
    ▪ Stimulation of the five senses including visual, auditory, olfactory, gustatory, and tactile
    ▪ Kinesthetic movement, including changes in position and ROM exercises to all extremities
    ▪ Placing meaningful items in his room (eg, family pictures, trophies, and sports memorabilia)
  • Instruct family to take Brian around the hospital or outside when in the wheelchair

PRESCRIPTION, APPLICATION, AND, AS APPROPRIATE, FABRICATION OF DEVICES AND EQUIPMENT

♦ Application or fabrication of splints/orthoses and serial casts to increase and/or maintain joint mobility
♦ Application of specialized mattress (ie, air, gel) to improve skin integrity
♦ Provision of tilt-in-space wheelchair seating system to improve skin integrity
♦ Tilt table or standing frame to improve ROM and reduce spasticity

AIRWAY CLEARANCE TECHNIQUES

♦ Positioning to maximize ventilation and perfusion
♦ Instruction of nursing staff in pulmonary postural drainage techniques

ANTICIPATED GOALS AND EXPECTED OUTCOMES

♦ Impact on pathology/pathophysiology
  • Tissue perfusion and oxygenation are enhanced.
♦ Impact on impairments
  • Integumentary integrity is improved, and the Stage II decubitus ulcers are reduced to Stage I.
  • ROM is improved.
♦ Impact on functional limitations
  • Transfers from bed to/from wheelchair are achieved by the family with a mechanical lift.
♦ Risk reduction/prevention
  • Risks for skin damage due to loss of movement are fully understood.
  • Safe techniques are demonstrated by nursing staff and family when assisting patient in care and transition activities.
♦ Impact on societal resources
  • Available resources are maximally utilized.

- Documentation occurs throughout patient management in all settings and follows APTA's *Guidelines for Physical Therapy Documentation*.[62]
- Utilization of physical therapy services is optimized.

♦ Patient/client satisfaction

- Care is coordinated with family and other professionals.
- Family understanding of expected outcomes is increased.
- Family will verbalize an awareness of the diagnosis, prognosis, interventions, and expected outcomes.
- Interdisciplinary collaboration occurs through patient care rounds and family meetings.
- Referrals are made to other professionals or resources whenever necessary and appropriate.

REEXAMINATION

Reexamination is performed throughout the entire episode of care. Reexamination will then be performed monthly.

DISCHARGE

Brian had 18 physical therapy visits over 7 months. The patient will be monitored by the interdisciplinary team to determine if any recovery, even a modest one, could result in a discharge to home with family services.

REFERENCES

1. Lundy-Ekman L. *Neuroscience: Fundamentals for Rehabilitation.* 2nd ed. Philadelphia, PA: WB Saunders; 2002.

2. Kandel ER, Schwartz JH, Jessel TM. *Principles of Neural Science.* 4th ed. New York, NY: McGraw Hill Medical; 2000.

3. Purves D, Augustine GJ, Fitzpatrick D, et al. *Neuroscience.* 3rd ed. Sunderland, MA: Sinauer Associates; 2004.

4. Bernat JL. Chronic disorders of consciousness. *Lancet.* 2006;367:1181-1192.

5. Hickey JV. *The Clinical Practice of Neuromedical and Neurosurgical Nursing.* 5th ed. Philadelphia, PA: Lippincott Williams & Wilkins; 2002.

6. Nolan S. Traumatic brain injury: a review. *Critical Care Nursing Quarterly.* 2005;28(2):188-194.

7. McLeod A. Intra- and extracranial causes of alteration in level of consciousness. *British Journal of Nursing.* 2004;13(7):354-361.

8. Brain Injury Association of America Inc. Available at: http://www.biausa.org. Accessed August 20, 2007.

9. Giacino J, Zasler N. Outcome after severe traumatic brain injury: coma, the vegetative state, and the minimally responsive state. *J Head Trauma Rehabil.* 1995;10:40-56.

10. Giacino JT, Ashwal S, Childs N, et al. The minimally conscious state: definition and diagnostic criteria. *Neurology.* 2002;58:349-353.

11. Multi-Society Task Force on PVS. Medical aspects of the persis-tent vegetative state (first part). *N Engl J Med.* 1994;330:1499-1508.

12. National Institute of Neurological Disorders and Stroke (NINDS). Coma Information Page: Available at: http://www.ninds.nih.gov/health_and_medical/disorders/coma_doc.htm. Accessed August 20, 2007.

13. Howard RS, Miller DH. The persistive vegetative state. *BMJ.* 1995;310:341-342.

14. American Academy of Pediatrics Task Force on Brain Death in Children. Report of a special task force: guidelines for the determination of brain death in children. *Pediatrics.* 1987;80:298-300.

15. Bear MF, Connors BW, Paradiso MA. *Neuroscience: Exploring the Brain.* 2nd ed. Philadelphia, PA: Lippincott Williams & Wilkins; 2001.

16. National Institute of Neurological Disorders and Stroke (NINDS). Available at: http://www.nlm.nih.gov/medlineplus/seizures.html. Accessed September 29, 2007.

17. Engle J. ILAE classification of epilepsy syndromes. *Epilepsy Research.* 2006;70(Suppl):S5-S10.

18. Kingsley RE. *Concise Text of Neuroscience.* 2nd ed. New York, NY: Lippincott Williams & Wilkins; 2000.

19. Schachter SC. Adapted from Willmore LJ. Head trauma and the development of post-traumatic epilepsy. In: Ettinger AB, Devinsky O, eds. *Managing Epilepsy and Co-existing Disorders.* Boston, MA: Butterworth-Heinemann; 2002:229-238. Revised April 2004. Available at: http://professionals.epilepsy.com/wi/print_section.php?section=head_trauma. Accessed September 29, 2007.

20. Willmore LJ. Acute traumatic brain injury and seizures. Available at: http://professionals.epilepsy.com/page/head_trauma.html. Accessed September 29, 2007.

21. Medline Plus Drug Information. Available at: http://www.nlm.nih.gov/medlineplus/druginfo/medmaster/a684001.html. Accessed September 28, 2007.

22. Multi-Society Task Force on PVS. Medical aspects of the persistent vegetative state (second part). *N Engl J Med.* 1994;330(22):1572-1579.

23. Schiff ND, Ribary U, Moreno DR, et al. Residual cerebral activity and behavioral fragments can remain in the persistive vegetative state. *Brain.* 2002;125:1210-1234.

24. Greenwood R. Head injury for neurologists. *J Neurol Neurosurg Psychiatry.* 2002;73:i8-i16.

25. Arras JD, Steinbock B. *Ethical Issues in Modern Medicine.* 4th ed. Mountain View, CA: Mayfield Publishers; 1995.

26. Cameron MH, Monroe LG. *Physical Rehabilitation: Evidenced Based Examination, Evaluation and Intervention.* St. Louis, MO: Saunders; 2007.

27. Wijdicks EFM. The diagnosis of brain death. *N Engl J Med.* 2001;344:1215-1221.

28. Jennett B. *The Vegetative State: Medical Facts, Ethical and Legal Dilemmas.* London, England: Cambridge University Press; 2002.

29. Andrews K. Medical decision making in the vegetative state: withdrawal of nutrition and hydration. *NeuroRehabilitation.* 2004;19:299-304.

30. Borthwick CJ, Crossley R. Permanent vegetative state: usefulness and limits of a prognostic definition. *NeuroRehabilitation.* 2004;19:381-389.

31. Strauss D, Shavelle RM, DeVivo MJ, et al. Letter to the editor:

life expectancy after traumatic brain injury. *NeuroRehabilitation.* 2004;19:257-258.

32. *Merck Manual of Medical Information Professional Edition.* 18th ed. Stupor and Coma. The Merck Manuals Online Medical Library for Health Professionals. Last full review/revision November 2005. Available at: http://www.merck.com/mmpe/print/sec16/ch212/ch212a.html.

33. MayoClinic.com. Coma. Available at: http://www.mayoclinic.com/health/coma/DS00724/DSECTION=8. Accessed October 2, 2007.

34. Ashwal S. Pediatric vegetative state: epidemiological and clinical issues. *NeuroRehabilitation.* 2004;19:349-360.

35. Purtillo R. *Ethical Dimensions in the Health Professions.* 4th ed. Philadelphia, PA: Elsevier Saunders; 2005.

36. Sugarman J. *Ethics in Primary Care.* New York, NY: McGraw-Hill; 2000.

37. Jenson AR, Siegler M, Winslade WJ. *Clinical Ethics.* 5th ed. New York, NY: McGraw-Hill; 2002.

38. Guidelines for the determination of death: report of the medical consultants on the diagnosis of death to the President's Commission for the Study of Ethical Problems in Medicine and Biomedical and Behavioral Research. *JAMA.* 1981;246:2184-2186.

39. Johnson GS. While you are waiting. About brain injury: objectives of neurosurgery: 2006. Available at: http://www.waiting.com/neurosurgery.html. Accessed September 25, 2007.

40. Jennett B, Teasdale G. *Management of Head Injuries.* Philadelphia, PA: FA Davis; 1981.

41. Centre for Neuro Skills (CNS). Pharmacology guide. Available at: http://www.neuroskills.com/. Accessed September 28, 2007.

42. RXList: The Internet drug index. Available at: http://www.rxlist.com/script/main/hp.asp. Accessed September 30, 2007.

43. WebMD Medical Reference in Collaboration with The Cleveland Clinic. Epilepsy: medications to treat seizures. Available at: http://www.webmd.com/epilepsy/medications-treat-seizures. Accessed September 28, 2007.

44. Wikipedia, the free encyclopedia. Artificial tears. Available at: http://en.wikipedia.org/wiki/Artificial_tear. Accessed October 3, 2007.

45. MedlinePlus Medical Encyclopedia. Available at: http://www.nlm.nih.gov/medlineplus/ency/article/001423.htm. Accessed April 29, 2008.

46. Montés-Micó R, Cáliz A, Alió J. Changes in ocular aberrations after instillation of artificial tears in dry-eye patients. *J Cataract Refract Surg.* 2004;30(8):1649-1652.

47. Ostwald SK, Wasserman J, Davis S. Medications, comorbidities, and medical complications in stroke survivors: the CAReS Study. *Rehabilitation Nursing.* 2006;31:10-14.

48. Teasdale G, Jennett B. Assessment of coma and impaired consciousness. *Lancet.* 1974;ii:81-83.

49. Mitchell S, Bradley V, Welch JL, Britton PG. Coma arousal procedure: a therapeutic intervention in the treatment of head injury. *Brain Inj.* 1990;4(3):273-279.

50. Robinson LR, Micklesen PJ. Somatosensory evoked potentials in coma prognosis. *Phys Med Rehabil Clin N Am.* 2004;15:43-61.

51. Giacino J, Whyte J. The vegetative and minimally conscious states: current knowledge and remaining questions. *J Head Trauma Rehabil.* 2005;20:30-50.

52. National Institute of Neurological Disorders and Stroke (NINDS). Coma and persistent vegetative state information page. Available at: http://www.ninds.nih.gov/health_and_medical/disorders/coma_doc.htm.

53. Casarett D, Fishman JM, MacMoran HJ, et al. Epidemiology and prognosis of coma in daytime television dramas. *BMJ.* 2005;331:1537-1539.

54. Wijdicks EFM, Wijdicks CA. The portrayal of coma in contemporary motion pictures. *Neurology.* 2006;66:1300-1303.

55. *Merck Manual of Medical Information Home Edition.* 2nd ed. Legal and Ethical Issues: Decision Making (Surrogate). The Merck Manuals Online Medical Library Home Edition for Patients and Caregivers. Last full review/revision February 2003. Available at: http://www.merck.com/mmhe/print/sec01/ch009/ch009f.html.

56. Donatelli LA, Geocadin RG, Williams MA. Ethical issues in critical care and cardiac arrest: clinical research, brain death, and organ donation. *Semin Neurol.* 2006;26:452-459.

57. American Academy of Neurology. *Practice Parameters: Determining Brain Death in Adults (Summary Statement). Report of the Quality Standards Subcommittee of the American Academy of Neurology.* Available at: http://www.aan.com/professionals/practice/pdfs/pdf_1995_thru_1998/1995.45.1015.pdf.

58. Fischer C, Luaute J, Adeleine P, Morlet D. Predictive value of sensory and cognitive evoked potentials for awakening from coma. *Neurology.* 2004;63:669-673.

59. Lombardi F, Taricco M, DeTanti A, Liberati A. Sensory stimulation of brain-injured individuals in coma or vegetative state; results of a Cochrane systematic review. *Clin Rehabil.* 2002;16:464-472.

60. Gruner ML, Terhaag D. Multimodal early onset stimulation (MEOS) in rehabilitation after brain injury. *Brain Inj.* 2000;14(6):585-594.

61. Moffat M, Biggs Harris K, eds. *Integumentary Essentials: Applying the Preferred Practice Patterns.*SM Thorofare, NJ: SLACK Incorporated; 2006.

62. American Physical Therapy Association. Guide to physical therapist practice. 2nd ed. *Phys Ther.* 2001;81:9-744.

63. Kriel RL, Krach LE, Jones-Saete C. Outcome of children with prolonged unconsciousness and vegetative states. *Pediatr Neurol.* 1993;9:362-368.

64. Lipppert-Gruner M, Wedekind C, Klug N. Outcome of prolonged coma following severe traumatic brain injury. *Brain Inj.* 2003;17(1):49-54.

65. Giacino JT, Kalmar K. The vegetative and minimally conscious states: a comparison of clinical features and functional outcomes. *J Head Trauma Rehabil.* 1997;12(4):36-51.

66. Andrews K. Recovery of patients after four months or more in the persistent vegetative state. *BMJ.* 1993;306:1597-1600.

67. Avesani R, Gambini MG, Albertini G. The vegetative state: a report of two cases with a long-term follow-up. *Brain Inj.* 2006;20(3):333-338.

68. McMillan MT, Herbert CM, Further recovery in a potential treatment withdrawal case 10 years after brain injury. *Brain Inj.* 2004;18(9):935-940.

69. Jacobs HE, Muir CA, Cline JD. Family reactions to persistent vegetative state. *J Head Trauma Rehabil.* 1986;1:55-62.

70. Wilson FC, Harpur J, Watwson T, Marow JL. Vegetative state and minimally responsive patients—recovery survey,

long-term case outcomes and service recommendations. *NeuroRehabilitation.* 2002;17:231-236.

71. Leong B. The vegetative and minimally conscious states in children: spasticity, muscle contracture and issues for physiotherapy treatment. *Brain Inj.* 2002;16(3):217-230.

72. Leong B. Critical review of passive muscle stretch: implications for the treatment of children in vegetative and minimally conscious states. *Brain Inj.* 2002;16(2):169-183.

73. Ashford S. Management of a patient diagnosed as PVS. *Physiother Res Int.* 2000;5(3):202-206.

74. Kater KM. Response of head-injured patients to sensory stimulation. *West J Nurs Res.* 1989;11(1):20-33.

75. Gill-Thwaites H, Munday R. The sensory modality assessment and rehabilitation technique (SMART); a valid and reliable assessment for vegetative state and minimally conscious state patients. *Brain Inj.* 2004;18(12):1255-1269.

Abbreviations

6MWT=6-Minute Walk Test

AAROM=active assistive range of motion
ACE=angiotensin-converting enzyme
Ach=acetylcholine
ACL=anterior cruciate ligament
AD=autonomic dysreflexia
ADD=attention deficit disorder
ADHD=attention deficit hyperactivity disorder
ADL=activities of daily living
AFO=ankle-foot orthosis
AFP=alpha-fetoprotein
AHA=American Heart Association
AIDP=acute inflammatory demyelinating polyneuropathy
AMAN=acute motor axonal neuropathy
AMPA=α-amino-3-hydroxy-5-methyl-4-isoxazolepropionic acid
AMSAN=acute motor and sensory axonal neuropathy
APTA=American Physical Therapy Association
AROM=active range of motion
ASIA=American Spinal Injury Association
AVM=arteriovenous malformation

BAPS=Biomechanical Ankle Platform System
BBS=Berg Balance Score
BFO=balanced forearm orthosis
bid=twice a day
BOTMP=Bruininks-Oseretsky Test of Motor Proficiency
BP=blood pressure
BPPV=benign paroxysmal positional vertigo
BSID-II=Bayley Test of Infant Development II
BWS=body weight supported
BWSTT=body weight supported treadmill training

CAT=computerized axial tomography
CDC=Centers for Disease Control and Prevention
CIMT=constraint-induced movement therapy
CIPN=chemotherapy-induced peripheral neuropathy
CMC=carpometacarpal
CMS=Centers for Medicare and Medicaid Services
CN=cranial nerve
CNS=central nervous system
COMT=catecholamine-o-methyltranferase
CO-OP=Cognitive Orientation to Daily Occupational Performance

CP=cerebral palsy
CPG=central pattern generator
CPGs=clinical practice guidelines
CPP=cerebral perfusion pressure
CRPS=complex regional pain syndrome
CSF=cerebrospinal fluid
CT=computed tomography
CTS=carpal tunnel syndrome
CTSIB=Clinical Test of Sensory Interaction on Balance
CVA=cerebrovascular accident

DCD=developmental coordination disorder
DEXA=dual-energy x-ray absorptiometry
DGO=driven gait orthosis
DHI=Dizziness Handicap Inventory
DJD=degenerative joint disease
DS=Down syndrome
DSM-IV=*Diagnostic and Statistical Manual of Mental Disorders, Fourth Edition*
DVT=deep vein thrombosis

ECG=electrocardiography
EDSS=Expanded Disability Status Scale
EEG=electroencephalogram
EMG=electromyography
ENG=electronystagmography
ENog=electroneuronography
EOM=extraocular movements
EPSP=excitatory postsynaptic potential

FDA=Food and Drug Administration
FES=functional electrical stimulation
FSI=Functional Status Index
FSS=Functional Status Scale

GABA=gamma aminobutyric acid
GBS=Guillian-Barré syndrome
GMFCS=Gross Motor Function Classification System
GMFM=Gross Motor Function Measure

HO=heterotopic ossification
HR=heart rate
HSV=herpes simplex virus
HTN=hypertension

IADL=instrumental activities of daily living
ICP=intracranial pressure
ICU=intensive care unit
IDEA=Individuals with Disability Education Act
IEP=individual education plan
IFSP=Individual Family Service Plan
IPSP=inhibitory postsynaptic potential
IS=intercostal space
IVIg=intravenous immunoglobulin

KAFO=knee-ankle-foot orthosis

LE=lower extremity
LLE=left lower extremity
LUE=left upper extremity

MCP=metacarpophalangeal
MDI=multi-dose inhaler
MHR=maximum heart rate
MMSE=Mini Mental Status Exam
MMT=manual muscle testing
MRA=magnetic resonance angiography
MRI=magnetic resonance imaging
MRS=magnetic resonance spectroscopy
MRS=minimally responsive state
MS=multiple sclerosis
MST=maximal stimulation test
MTP=metatarsophalangeal
MVA=motor vehicle accident

NCV=nerve conduction velocity
NDT=neurodevelopmental treatment
NET=nerve excitability test
NICU=neonatal intensive care unit
NPS=numeric pain rating scale
NSAIDs=nonsteroidal anti-inflammatory drugs
NSCISC=National Spinal Cord Injury Statistical Center
NTD=neural tube defect

OH=orthostatic hypotension
ORIF=open reduction internal fixation

PANAS=Positive and Negative Affective Scale
PD=Parkinson's disease
PDMS=Peabody Developmental Motor Scales
PE=plasma exchange
PEDI=Pediatric Evaluation of Disability Inventory
PET scan=positron emission tomography scan
PICC=peripherally inserted central catheter
PNF=proprioceptive neuromuscular facilitation
PNS=peripheral nervous system
PPMS=primary progressive multiple sclerosis
PRE=progressive resistive exercise
PRMS=progressive-relapsing multiple sclerosis
prn=as needed

PROM=passive range of motion
PVL=periventricular leukomalacia
PVS=persistent vegetative state

q=every
qd=every day
qid=four times a day

RGO=reciprocal gait orthosis
RLE=right lower extremity
ROM=range of motion
RPE=rate of perceived exertion
RR=respiratory rate
RRMS=relapsing-remitting multiple sclerosis
RSD=reflex sympathetic dystrophy
RUE=right upper extremity

SCI=spinal cord injury
SDS=simple descriptive scale
SF-36=36-Item Short Form Health Survey
SNAP=sensory nerve action potential
SPECT=single photon emission computed tomography
SPMS=secondary progressive multiple sclerosis
SPMSQ=Short Portable Mental Status Questionnaire
SSRIs=selective serotonin reuptake inhibitors
SSS=Symptoms Severity Scale
sub=subcutaneously

TBI=traumatic brain injury
TCAs=tricylclic antidepressants
TEE=transesophageal echocardiography
TENS=transcutaneous electrical nerve stimulation
THR=target heart rate
TIA=transient ischemic attacks
tid=three times a day
TKR=total knee replacement
TLSO=thoraco-lumbo-sacral orthosis
tPA=tissue plasminogen activator
TSIF=Test of Sensory Function in Infants

UE=upper extremity
UPDRS=Unified Parkinson's Disease Rating Scale
USPHS=US Public Health Service
UTI=urinary tract infection

VAS=visual analog scale
VO$_2$=oxygen consumption
VOR=vestibular-ocular reflex
VP=ventricular-peritoneal
VSR=vestibulo-spinal reflex

WASI=Wechsler Abbreviated Scale of Intelligence
w/c=wheelchair
WFL=within functional limits
WNL=within normal limits

Brand Name Drugs and Products

The brand name drugs and products mentioned in this book are listed below, along with their manufacturer information.

DRUGS

Abbokinase (ImaRx Therapeutics, Tucson, Ariz)

Accutane (Roche Pharmaceuticals, Nutley, NJ)

Activase (Genetech Inc, South San Francisco, Calif)

Adalat (Bayer HealthCare Pharmaceuticals, Morristown, NJ)

Adderall (Shire, Wayne, Pa)

Adriamycin (Pharmacia, Kalamazoo, Mich)

Advair MDI Diskus (GlaxoSmithKline, Philadelphia, Pa)

Advil (Wyeth Pharmaceuticals, Philadelphia, Pa)

Aldactone (Pfizer, New York, NY)

Afrin (Schering-Plough, Kenilworth, NJ)

Ambien (Sanofi Aventis, Bridgewater, NJ)

Anergan 50 (Forest Laboratories, New York, NY)

Antivert (Pfizer, New York, NY)

Apokyn (Vernalis, Morristown, NJ)

Arestin (OraPharma Inc, Warminster, Pa)

Astramorph (Abraxis BioScience, Schaumburg, Ill)

Atamet (Elan, New York, NY)

Ativan (Biovail Pharmaceuticals Inc, Bridgewater, NJ)

Atrovent (Boehringer Ingelheim, Ridgefield, Conn)

Avonex (Biogen Idec, Cambridge, Mass)

Azilect (Teva Pharmaceuticals, North Wales, Pa)

Benadryl (Pfizer, New York, NY)

Benzacot (Truxton, Bellmawr, NJ)

Betaseron (Bayer HealthCare Pharmaceuticals, Morristown, NJ)

Bonine (Insight Pharmaceuticals, Langhorne, Pa)

Botox (Allergan Inc, Irvine, Calif)

BuSpar (Bristol-Myers Squibb, New York, NY)

Calan (Pfizer, New York, NY)

Capozide (Bristol-Myers Squibb, New York, NY)

Carbatrol (Shire, Wayne, Pa)

Cardizem (Biovail Pharmaceuticals Inc, Bridgewater, NJ)

Celebrex (Pfizer, New York, NY)

Clorpres (Mylan Inc, Canonsburg, Pa)

Colace (Purdue, Stamford, Conn)

Compazine (GlaxoSmithKline, Philadelphia, Pa)

Concerta (Alza, Mountain View, Calif)

Copaxone (Teva Pharmaceuticals, North Wales, Pa)

Coumadin (Bristol-Myers Squibb, New York, NY)

Cylert (Abbott, Abbott Park, Ill)

Cytomel (King Pharmaceuticals, Bristol, Tenn)

Cytoxan (Bristol-Myers Squibb, New York, NY)

Dantrium (Proctor and Gamble, Cincinnati, Ohio)

Darvocet (Xanodyne Pharmaceuticals, Newport, Ky)

Darvon (Xanodyne Pharmaceuticals, Newport, Ky)

Demerol (Sanofi Aventis, Bridgewater, NJ)

Depakene (Abbott, Abbott Park, Ill)

Depakote (Abbott, Abbott Park, Ill)

Detrol (Pfizer, New York, NY)

Dexedrine (GlaxoSmithKline, Philadelphia, Pa)

Diazepam Intensol (Boehringer Ingelheim, Ridgefield, Conn)

Didronel (Proctor and Gamble, Cincinnati, Ohio)

Dilacor (Watson Pharmaceuticals, Corona, Calif)

Dilantin (Pfizer, New York, NY)

Dilaudid (Abbott, Abbott Park, Ill)

Ditropan (Alza, Mountain View, Calif)

Diuril (Salix Pharmaceuticals, Morrisville, NC)

Doxinate (Sigma Laboratories, Mumbai, Maharashtra, India)

Dramamine (McNeil Consumer, Fort Washington, Pa)

Dulcolax (Boehringer Ingelheim, Ridgefield, Conn)

Duramorph (Baxter Healthcare Corp, Deerfield, Ill)

Dysport (Ipsen Ltd, Slough, Berkshire, United Kingdom)

Eldepryl (Somerset Pharmaceuticals, Tampa, Fla)

Eltroxin (GlaxoSmithKline, Philadelphia, Pa)

Felbatol (Medpointe Pharmaceuticals, Somerset, NJ)

Flomax (Boehringer Ingelheim, Ridgefield, Conn)

Fragmin (Pfizer, New York, NY)

Gabitril (Cephalon, Frazer, Pa)

Garamycin (Schering-Plough, Kenilworth, NJ)

Haldol (Ortho-McNeil, Raritan, NJ)

HydroDIURIL (Merck, Whitehouse Station, NJ)

Hydrostat IR (Shire, Wayne, Pa)

Imuran (Prometheus Laboratories, San Diego, Calif)

Inapsine (Akorn Inc, Buffalo Grove, Ill)

Inderal (Wyeth Pharmaceuticals, Philadelphia, Pa)

Infumorph (Baxter Healthcare Corp, Deerfield, Ill)

InnoPran XL (GlaxoSmithKline, Philadelphia, Pa)

Keppra (UCB Pharma Inc, Smyrna, Ga)

Klonopin (Roche Pharmaceuticals, Nutley, NJ)

Lamictal (GlaxoSmithKline, Philadelphia, Pa)

Lasix (Sanofi Aventis, Bridgewater, NJ)

Leustatin (Ortho Biotech, Bridgewater, NJ)

Levaquin (Ortho-McNeil, Raritan, NJ)

Levo-T (Alara Pharmaceutical Corp, Caguas, Puerto Rico)

Levotec (Technilab, Pine Brook, NJ)

Levothroid (Forest Laboratories, New York, NY)

Levoxyl (King Pharmaceuticals, Bristol, Tenn)

Lexapro (Forest Laboratories, New York, NY)

Lioresal (Medtronic, Minneapolis, Minn)

Lipitor (Pfizer, New York, NY)

Lopressor (Novartis, Cambridge, Mass)

Lotensin (Novartis, Cambridge, Mass)

Lovenox (Sanofi Aventis, Bridgewater, NJ)

Marezine (Martin Himmel, Lake Worth, Fla)

Melleril (Novartis, Cambridge, Mass)

Meni-D (Seatrace Pharmaceuticals, Rainbow City, Ala)

Metadate CD (UCB Pharma Inc, Smyrna, Ga)

Mevacor (Merck, Whitehouse Station, NJ)

Midamor (Merck, Whitehouse Station, NJ)

Miralax (Schering-Plough, Kenilworth, NJ)

Mirapex (Boehringer Ingelheim, Ridgefield, Conn)

Motrin (McNeil Consumer, Fort Washington, Pa)

Mycostatin (Bristol-Myers Squibb, New York, NY)

Myobloc (Solstice Neurosciences Inc, Malvern, Pa)

Mysoline (Valeant Pharmaceuticals International, Aliso Viejo, Calif)

Navane (Pfizer, New York, NY)

Neurontin (Pfizer, New York, NY)

Norvasc (Pfizer, New York, NY)

Novantrone (Serono, Rockland, Mass)

Nystatin (Altana Inc, Melville, NY)

OxyContin (Purdue, Stamford, Conn)

Parcopa (Schwarz Pharma, Milwaukee, Wisc)

Parlodel (Novartis, Cambridge, Mass)

Pepcid (Johnson & Johnson, New Brunswick, NJ)

Percocet (Endo Pharmaceuticals, Chadds Ford, Pa)

Percogesic (Medtech, Jackson, Wyo)

Permax (Valeant Pharmaceuticals International, Aliso Viejo, Calif)

Prinivil (Merck, Whitehouse Station, NJ)

Proamatine (Shire, Wayne, Pa)

Pro-Banthine (Shire, Wayne, Pa)

Procardia (Pfizer, New York, NY)

Protonix (Wyeth Pharmaceuticals, Philadelphia, Pa)

Proventil-HFA (Schering-Plough, Kenilworth, NJ)

Provigil (Cephalon, Frazer, Pa)

Prozac (Eli Lilly & Co, Indianapolis, Ind)

Rebif (Serono, Rockland, Mass)

Reglan (Schwarz Pharma, Milwaukee, Wisc)

Requip (GlaxoSmithKline, Philadelphia, Pa)

Retavase (Centocor Inc, Horsham, Pa)

Ritalin (Novartis, Cambridge, Mass)

Roxanol (Xanodyne Pharmaceuticals, Newport, Ky)

Ru-Vert-M (Solvay Pharmaceuticals, Marietta, Ga)

Senokot (Purdue, Stamford, Conn)

Serevent MDI Diskus (GlaxoSmithKline, Philadelphia, Pa)

Seroquel (AstraZeneca, Wilmington, Del)

Sinemet (Bristol-Myers Squibb, New York, NY)

Stalevo (Orion, Espoo, Finland)

Strattera (Eli Lilly & Co, Indianapolis, Ind)

Streptase (Aventis Behring, King of Prussia, Pa)

Sudafed (McNeil Consumer, Fort Washington, Pa)

Symmetrel (Endo Pharmaceuticals, Chadds Ford, Pa)

Synthroid (Abbott, Abbott Park, Ill)

Tegretol (Novartis, Cambridge, Mass)

Tenoretic (AstraZeneca, Wilmington, Del)

Tenormin (AstraZeneca, Wilmington, Del)

Thalitone (Monarch Pharmaceuticals, Bristol, Tenn)

Thorazine (GlaxoSmithKline, Philadelphia, Pa)

Ticon (Roberts/Hauck Pharmaceutical Corp, Eatontown, NJ)

Tigan (King Pharmaceuticals, Bristol, Tenn)

Topamax (Ortho-McNeil, Raritan, NJ)

Toprol XL (AstraZeneca, Wilmington, Del)

Transderm scop (Novartis, Cambridge, Mass)

Tranxene (Ovation Pharmaceuticals, Lincolnshire, Ill)

Trileptal (Novartis, Cambridge, Mass)

Tylenol (McNeil Consumer, Fort Washington, Pa)

Tysabri (Elan, New York, NY)

Ultracet (Janssen Pharmaceuticals, Titusville, NJ)

Valium (Roche Pharmaceuticals, Nutley, NJ)

Valrelease (Roche, Basel, Switzerland)

Vaseretic (Biovail Pharmaceuticals Inc, Bridgewater, NJ)

Ventolin HFA (GlaxoSmithKline, Philadelphia, Pa)

Verelan (Elan, New York, NY)

Vistaril (Pfizer, New York, NY)

Vistazine 50 (Keene Pharmaceuticals, Keene, Tex)

Xanax (Pfizer, New York, NY)

Zanaflex (Acorda Therapeutics, Hawthorne, NY)

Zantac (GlaxoSmithKline, Philadelphia, Pa)

Zarontin (Pfizer, New York, NY)

Zelapar (Valeant Pharmaceuticals International, Aliso Viejo, Calif)

Zetran (Roberts/Hauck Pharmaceutical Corp, Eatontown, NJ)

Zocor (Merck, Whitehouse Station, NJ)

Zofran (GlaxoSmithKline, Philadelphia, Pa)

Zosyn (Wyeth Pharmaceuticals, Philadelphia, Pa)

PRODUCTS

Acapella (DHD Healthcare, Wampsville, NY)

Airdyne (Schwinn/Nautilus, Vancouver, Wash)

Biomechanical Ankle Platform System ([BAPS] CAMP, Jackson, Miss)

Disk Criminator (Complete Medical Supplies, Valley Cottage, NY)

ERGYS Rehabilitation Systems (Therapeutic Alliances Inc, Fairborn, Ohio)

Parastep (Sigmedics Inc, Fairborn, Ohio)

Twister (Hasbro, Pawtucket, RI)

Index

acetaminophen, for neurogenic pain, 253
action potential conduction, 116
acute inflammatory demyelinating polyneuropathy (AIDP), 224–225
acute motor axonal neuropathy (AMAN), 224–225
acyclovir, for facial nerve Bell's paralysis, 177
ADL/IADL training
    for Guillain-Barré syndrome, 234
    for Parkinson's disease, 129
    for stroke-central vestibular dysfunction, 106
    for thoracic spinal cord injury, 274
aerobic/endurance conditioning
    for balance loss, 10
    for cerebral palsy, 57
    for cervical spinal cord injury, 261
    for chemotherapy-induced peripheral neuropathy, 240
    for developmental coordination disorder, 35
    for Down syndrome, 28–29
    for Guillain-Barré syndrome, 232
    for Meniere's disease, 202
    for multiple sclerosis, 155–156
    for Parkinson's disease, 128
    for stroke, 82–83, 86–87
    for stroke-central vestibular dysfunction, 105
    for thoracic spinal cord injury, 273
    for traumatic brain injury, 97
aging
    in balance loss and falling, 4
    vestibular dysfunction and, 173
airway clearance techniques
    for cervical spinal cord injury, 260, 263
    for Guillain-Barré syndrome, 231, 234
    for left medial temporal lobe infarct patient, 294
    for persistent vegetative state, 299
    for thoracic spinal cord injury, 272, 275
akinetic mutism, 286
Alberta Infant Motor Scale, 24
albuterol sulfate, 253
alcoholic neuropathy, 224
amantadine, 121
ambulation
    in Down syndrome, 27
    in Meniere's disease, 200
American Spinal Injury Association
    impairment classification scale, 251
    Key Sensory Levels Tested, 250
amitriptyline, 253
amphetamine, 23–24
anaencephalopy, 19
analgesics, causing dizziness, 5
angiotensin-converting enzyme (ACE) inhibitors, 77
ankle-foot orthoses (AFOs)
    for cerebral palsy, 56
    for multiple sclerosis, 157
    for stroke, 89

    for traumatic brain injury, 100
ankle joint, 2
ankle strategy, 3
anti-anxiety drugs
    for impaired consciousness, 289
    for multiple sclerosis, 122
anticholinergics
    for multiple sclerosis, 122
    for Parkinson's disease, 121
    for vestibular dysfunction, 178
anticoagulants
    for hemorrhagic stroke, 76
    for spinal cord injury, 252
anticonvulsants
    for cerebral palsy, 50
    for Down syndrome, 23
    for hemorrhagic stroke, 76
    for impaired consciousness, 289–290
antidepressants
    for multiple sclerosis, 122
    for spinal cord injury, 252–253
anti-emetics, 178
antifatigue agents, 122–123
antifungals, 76
antihistamines
    for hemorrhagic stroke, 76–77
    for vestibular dysfunction, 178–179
antihypertensive drugs
    for carpal tunnel syndrome, 177
    for hemorrhagic stroke, 77
    in impaired consciousness, 290
    for spinal cord injury, 253
anti-inflammatory drugs, 177
antispasticity drugs, 122
antitremor drugs, 122
antivertigo agents, 123
antivirals, 177
Arnold-Chiari malformations, 59
Arnold-Chiari Type II syndrome, 50
arousal
    CNS regions responsible for, 283–285
    impairments of, 285–300
artificial tears
    for facial nerve Bell's paralysis, 177
    in impaired consciousness, 290
assistive/adaptive devices
    for Bell's palsy, 192–193
    for cerebral palsy, 56, 58
    for cervical spinal cord injury, 259–260, 263
    in cervical spinal cord injury, 256–257
    for chemotherapy-induced peripheral neuropathy, 240
    for Guillain-Barré syndrome, 231, 234
    for left medial temporal lobe infarct patient, 294
    for multiple sclerosis, 151, 157

WAIT

...There's More!

SLACK Incorporated's Health Care Books and Journals offers a wide selection of products in the field of Physical Therapy. We are dedicated to providing important works that educate, inform and improve the knowledge of our customers. Don't miss out on our other informative titles that will enhance your collection.

Essentials in Physical Therapy Series

The *Essentials in Physical Therapy* series answers the call to what today's physical therapy students and clinicians are looking for when integrating the *Guide to Physical Therapist Practice* into clinical care.

Essentials in Physical Therapy is led by Series Editor Dr. Marilyn Moffat, who brings together physical therapy's leading professionals to produce the most anticipated series of books in the physical therapy market to cover the four main systems:
- ◆ Musculoskeletal
- ◆ Cardiovascular/Pulmonary
- ◆ Neuromuscular
- ◆ Integumentary

Written in a similar, user-friendly format, each book inside the *Essentials in Physical Therapy* series not only brings together the conceptual frameworks of the *Guide* language, but also parallels the patterns of the *Guide*.

In each case, where appropriate, a brief review of the pertinent anatomy, physiology, pathophysiology, imaging, and pharmacology is provided. Each pattern then details diversified case studies coinciding with the *Guide* format. The physical therapist examination, including history, systems review, and specific tests and measures for each case, as well as evaluation, diagnosis, prognosis, plan of care, and evidence-based interventions are also addressed.

Series Editor: Marilyn Moffat, PT, DPT, PhD, FAPTA, CSCS, *New York University, New York, NY*

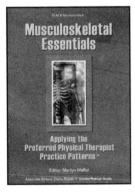
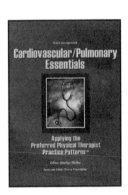
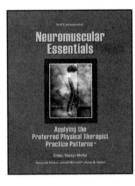
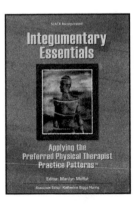

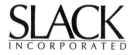